Handbook of Research on Distributed Medical Informatics and E-Health

Athina A. Lazakidou
University of Peloponnese, Greece

Konstantinos M. Siassiakos
University of Piraeus, Greece

Medical Information Science REFERENCE

MEDICAL INFORMATION SCIENCE REFERENCE
Hershey · New York

Director of Editorial Content:	Kristin Klinger
Senior Managing Editor:	Jennifer Neidig
Managing Editor:	Jamie Snavely
Assistant Managing Editor:	Carole Coulson
Typesetter:	Chris Hrobak
Cover Design:	Lisa Tosheff
Printed at:	Yurchak Printing Inc.

Published in the United States of America by
Information Science Reference (an imprint of IGI Global)
701 E. Chocolate Avenue, Suite 200
Hershey PA 17033
Tel: 717-533-8845
Fax: 717-533-8661
E-mail: cust@igi-global.com
Web site: http://www.igi-global.com

and in the United Kingdom by
Information Science Reference (an imprint of IGI Global)
3 Henrietta Street
Covent Garden
London WC2E 8LU
Tel: 44 20 7240 0856
Fax: 44 20 7379 0609
Web site: http://www.eurospanbookstore.com

Library of Congress Cataloging-in-Publication Data

Handbook of research on distributed medical informatics and e-health / Athina A. Lazakidou and Konstantinos M. Siassiakos, editors.

p. ; cm.

Includes bibliographical references and index.

Summary: "This book provides a compendium of terms, definitions and explanations of concepts, processes and acronyms related to different areas, issues and trends in Distributed Medical Informatics, E-Health and M-Health"--Provided by publisher.

ISBN 978-1-60566-002-8 (h/c)

1. Medical telematics--Handbooks, manuals, etc. I. Lazakidou, Athina A., 1975- II. Siassiakos, Konstantinos M.

[DNLM: 1. Telemedicine--methods. 2. Medical Informatics Applications. W 83.1 H236 2009]

R119.95.H36 2009

610.285--dc22

2008014431

British Cataloguing in Publication Data
A Cataloguing in Publication record for this book is available from the British Library.

Editorial Advisory Board

List of Contributors

Table of Contents

Section V
Mobile Health Applications and New Home Care Telecare Systems

Chapter XX
Agile Patient Care with Distributed M-Health Applications 282
Rafael Capilla, Universidad Rey Juan Carlos, Spain
Alfonso del Río, Universidad Rey Juan Carlos, Spain
Miguel Ángel Valero, Universidad Politécnica de Madrid, Spain
José Antonio Sánchez, Universidad Politécnica de Madrid, Spain

Chapter XXI
Mobile Health Applications and New Home Care Telecare Systems: Critical Engineering Issues... 305
Žilbert Tafa, University of Montenegro, Montenegro

Section VI
Distributed Problem-Solving Environments and Medical Imaging

Chapter XXII
A New System for the Integration of Medical Imaging Processing Algorithms
into a Web Environment 325
José Antonio Seoane Fernández, Artificial Neural Networks and Adaptative Systems Group & University of Corunna, Spain
Juan Luis Pérez Ordóñez, Center of Medical Informatics and Radiological Diagnosis & University of Corunna, Spain
Noha Veiguela Blanco, Artificial Neural Networks and Adaptative Systems Group & University of Corunna, Spain
Francisco Javier Novóa de Manuel, Center of Medical Informatics and Radiological Diagnosis & University of Corunna, Spain
Julián Dorado de la Calle, University of A Coruña, Spain

Chapter XXIII
PACS Based on Open-Source Software Components 338
Daniel Welfer, Instituto de Informatica — Universidade Federal do Rio Grande do Sul, Brazil
Jacob Scharcanski, Instituto de Informatica — Universidade Federal do Rio Grande do Sul, Brazil

Section VII
Medical Decision Support Systems

Chapter XXIV
Case Based Reasoning for Customizing Treatment Processes 351
Carolin Kaiser, University of Erlangen-Nuremberg, Germany

Section VIII
Virtual Environments in Healthcare

Chapter XXV
A Holistic Perspective of Security in Health Related Virtual Communities 367
I. Apostolakis, National School of Public Health, Greece
A. Chryssanthou , Greek Data Protection Agency, Greece
I. Varlamis, University of Peloponnese, Greece

Chapter XXVI
Virtual Learning Environments in Health 382
Stamatia Ilioudi, University of Piraeus, Greece
Christina Ilioudi, University of Piraeus, Greece
Konstantinos Siassiakos, University of Piraeus, Greece

Chapter XXVII
Multimedia Distance Learning Solutions for Surgery 390
Jelena Vucetic, Alpha Mission, Inc., USA

Chapter XXVIII
Collaborative Virtual Environments and Multimedia Communication Technologies in Healthcare 399
Maria Andréia F. Rodrigues, Universidade de Fortaleza, Brazil
Raimir Holanda Filho, Universidade de Fortaleza, Brazi

Chapter XXIX
Transforming a Pediatrics Lecture Series to Online Instruction 410
Tiffany A. Koszalka, Syracuse University, USA
Bradley Olson, SUNY Upstate Medical University, USA

Chapter XXX
Quality and Reliability Aspects in Telehealth Systems 425
Anastasia Kastania, Athens University of Economics and Business, Greece
Stelios Zimeras, University of the Aegean, Greece

Section IX
Data Evaluation, Validation, and Quality Aspects

Chapter XXXI
Quality of Health Information on the Internet 443
Kleopatra Alamantariotou, City University London, UK

Chapter XXXII
A Practical Approach to Computerized System Validation 456
Kashif Hussain, University of Valenciennes et Hainaut de Cambrésis, France
Shazia Yasin Mughal, University of Valenciennes et Hainaut de Cambrésis, France
Sylvie Leleu-Merviel, University of Valenciennes et Hainaut de Cambrésis, France

Chapter XXXIII
Organization and Evaluation of Experimental Measurements of Ergophysiological Data with the Method of SF12V2 470
Bill Ag Drougas, HATRLab & Higher Technological Institute of Epirus, Greece
Maria Sevdali, Higher Technological Institute of Kalamata, Greece

Chapter XXXIV
Ubiquitous Risk Analysis of Physiological Data 478
Daniele Apiletti, Politecnico di Torino, Italy
Elena Baralis, Politecnico di Torino, Italy
Giulia Bruno, Politecnico di Torino, Italy
Tania Cerquitelli, Politecnico di Torino, Italy

Section X
Ethical, Legal, and Other Issues in E-Health

Chapter XXXV
Chaotization of Human Systems by Technical Electromagnetic Fields 493
Manfred Doepp, Holistic DiagCenter, Germany

Chapter XXXVI
Demographic Differences in Telehealth Policy Outcomes 500
Mary Schmeida, The Cleveland Clinic, USA
Ramona McNeal, University of Northern Iowa, USA

Compilation of References 509

About the Contributors 550

Index 566

Detailed Table of Contents

This chapter reports the authors' experiences regarding security of the electronic medical record (EMR). Although the EMR objectives are to support shared care and healthcare professionals' workflow, there are some barriers that prevent its successful use. These barriers comprise not only costs, regarding resources and time, but also patient / health professional relations, ICT (information and communication technologies) education as well as security issues. It is very difficult to evaluate EMR systems; however some studies already made show problems regarding usability and proper healthcare workflow modeling. Legislation to guide the protection of health information systems is also very difficult to implement in practice. This chapter shows that access control, as a part of an EMR, can be a key to minimize some of its barriers, if the means to design, develop and evaluate access control are closer to users' needs and workflow complexity.

This chapter outlines the history of medical classifications in a general cultural context. Classification is a general phenomenon in science and has an outstanding role in the biomedical sciences. Its general principles started to be developed in ancient times, while domain classifications, particularly medical classifications have been constructed from about the 16th-17th century. We demonstrate with several examples that all classifications reflect an underlying theory. The development of the notion of disease during the 17th-19th century essentially influenced disease classifications. Development of classifications currently used in computerized information systems started before the computer era, but computational aspects reshape essentially the whole picture. A new generation of classifications is expected in biomedicine that depends less on human classification effort but uses the power of automated classifiers and reasoners.

This chapter provides a brief overview of the most relevant electronic healthcare record standards by examining the level of interoperability and functionality they provide in terms of context, structure, access services, multimedia support, and security. Such evaluations will provide healthcare decision-makers and system integrators with a clear perspective regarding the capabilities and limitations of each standard.

This chapter examines an integrative model of e-health use that connects social disparities at the population level with individual characteristics related to the amount and type of online health information usage, thus providing an account of the ways in which societal disparities play out in individual e-health usage patterns. Based on an overview of the literature on e-health disparities, the authors suggest that social-level disparities are manifested in the form of individual-level differences in health information orientation and health information efficacy, which in turn influence the amount and type of online health use. Exploring the underlying social structures that enable individual-level access, motivation, and ability to utilize the Internet for health and how these structures interact with individual motivation and ability advances our understanding of the Internet, the digital divide, and health disparities.

The authors of this chapter describe a distributed e-healthcare system that uses the Service Oriented Architecture as a basis for designing, implementing, deploying, invoking and managing healthcare services. The e-healthcare system that they have developed provides support for patients, physicians, nurses, pharmacists and other healthcare professionals, as well as for medical monitoring devices, such as blood pressure monitors. The system transmits e-prescriptions from physicians to pharmacists over the Internet. It offers multi-media input and output, including text, images and speech, to provide a human-friendly interface, with the computers and networks hidden from the user.

In this chapter, Mucic provides a brief review of the wide range of telepsychiatry applications. In addition, he offers a completely new and innovative approach regarding assessment and/or treatment of asylum seekers, refugees and migrants in Europe. Experiences from both a Danish telepsychiatry survey

in better organizing and exploiting the bioinformatics resources available online. The authors hope that a concise perspective of the field and a list of selected resources may help interested people quickly understand the main principles of knowledge representation in biomedicine and its high relevance for modern biomedical research and e-health.

The registration of corresponding patient volumes is often a pre-requisite for medical imaging tasks. Accurate alignment, however, usually results in high computational complexity and can hence take a considerable amount of time. This is particularly true with 3-D volume data which adds another dimension to the registration process. One possibility of keeping registration times feasible is to distribute computation among several processors so that it may be accomplished in parallel. This chapter provides a short survey of parallel registration approaches which have been proposed together with some recent research adopting blackboard architecture for distributed high performance image and volume registration purposes.

Within this chapter, the author summarizes literature about online commerce for health products and describes some of the most popular products and the methodology for guiding consumers to quality products. This chapter also presents and analyzes the characteristics and criteria of one particular internet health company and its Web site. Suggestions for encouraging the effectiveness of electronic health commerce are provided and the future of buying and selling products online is investigated.

This chapter introduces and reviews the concept of distributed knowledge management within the Healthcare environment and between healthcare and other partner organizations. As management should not be mistaken for control, distributed should not be identified with multi-centered. Trade-offs between managerial centralism and social contextuality should be allowed. Although the core issues in knowledge management are not technological, tools that can support the central versus social dualism of knowledge management are critical to the effective and appropriate use of generated knowledge. Information tools can significantly affect the user experience and local social wiliness to participation and enhance the managerial trends that make use of knowledge networks and shared logistics. They include service-oriented architectures (SOA), artificial intelligence networks (AIN), multiple agent systems (MAS) and the contextual tools of Web 2.0. All of those tools feed their functionality on the semantic detail, the granularity and the trust levels enjoyed by their information sources.

Section IV
Wireless Telemedicine and Communications Technologies in Healthcare

This chapter describes business and technological challenges and solutions for a successful emergency telemedicine venture called MediComm. Its objective is to provide a new generation of integrated information and communication systems, targeting medical and emergency care organizations. This system enables multi-directional transfer of information (including voice, data, fax, video) between the organization's central information system and its mobile fleet of ambulance vehicles. MediComm enables emergency care personnel to take a patient's vital measurements and personal information in an ambulance on the way to the hospital, send the information to the hospital, and receive from the hospital directions for the patient's treatment during transportation. When the patient arrives into the hospital, his/her information will be already updated in the information system, and the medical personnel will be ready to provide the necessary care immediately. Thus, time will be saved, which for many patients is of critical importance. The treatment of patients will be more effective and simplified, which will result in substantially lower cost of medical care.

This chapter introduces reconfigurable design techniques for lightweight medical systems. The research presented in this chapter demonstrates how the wise use of reconfiguration in small embedded systems is an approach that is beneficial in heterogeneous medical systems. By shrewdly designing embedded systems, one can make efficient use of limited resources through efficient and effective reconfiguration schemes that balance the tradeoffs between power consumption, memory consumption, and interoperability in heterogeneous environments. Furthermore, several reconfigurable architectures and algorithms presented in this chapter will assist researchers in designing efficient embedded systems that can be reconfigured after deployment, which is an essential feature in embedded medical systems.

Evolutions in the field of telecommunications technologies have significantly contributed to the advancement and development of the field of medicine, and they have also brought forth the need for their utilization in the healthcare sector. Thus, the implementation, operational deployment of services, and promising market for telemedicine and e-health has clearly become an important issue. Recognizing this trend, the authors of this chapter attempt to familiarize the readers with the impact that high broadband wireless networks have upon telemedicine services and with the way they facilitate the secure transmission of vital information stemming from bandwidth demanding applications in real time. After providing the readers with an overview of telemedical services and commenting on how they can offer added value to existing healthcare services, they provide an analysis of the wireless infrastructure that has facilitated telemedical services over the years, and point out the significant role that the third generation telecommunications systems can play in the field.

This chapter introduces the usage of telemedicine consultations in daily clinical practice. The author describes the process of teleconsultation along with sample schemes of systems, parties of this process and its roles. Also, the main steps of clinical teleconsultation (determination of necessity for teleconsultation, preparation of medical information, observance of ethics and law conditions, and preparation of conclusion) are shown. The efficiency of teleconsultation is also investigated and, within this discussion, the author proposes a new method for efficiency estimation. Understanding the process of teleconsultation will make it more accessible and easy-to-use for medical practitioners.

Ubiquitous healthcare has become possible with rapid advances in information and communication technologies. Ubiquitous healthcare will bring about an increased accessibility to healthcare providers, more efficient tasks and processes, and a higher quality of healthcare services. Radio frequency identification (RFID) is a key technology of ubiquitous healthcare and enables a fully automated solution for information delivery, thus reducing the potential for human error. This chapter provides an overview of ubiquitous healthcare and RFID applications. In this chapter, the background of ubiquitous computing and RFID technologies, current RFID applications in hospitals, and the future trends and privacy implications of RFID in hospitals are discussed.

Section V
Mobile Health Applications and New Home Care Telecare Systems

This chapter presents an architecture for the integration of various algorithms for digital image processing (DIP) into Web-based information systems. The proposed environment provides the development of tools for intensive image processing and their integration into information systems by means of JAVA applets. The functionality of the system is shown through a set of tools for biomedical application. The main feature of this architecture is that it allows the application of various types of image processing, with different computational costs, through a Web browser and in a transparent and user-friendly way.

This chapter discusses the concept of open-source picture archiving and communication systems (i.e. PACS), which are low cost, and easy to re-configure and customize for specific users' needs. Open-source PACS are based on relatively low cost computational resources and are built by integrating open-source software components that implement basic services of PACS. These services, as well as how to integrate them, are described in this chapter. As an example, a PACS based on open-source software components for angiographic studies is discussed. Using the open-source approach, the authors expect to help diffusing the PACS technology by reducing its development and maintenance costs by using easily available components (e.g. desktop PCs).

Recent advances in medicine, telemedicine, computer technologies, information systems, Web applications, robotics and telecommunications have enabled new solutions for training and continued education in various medical disciplines. This chapter presents the most recent developments and future trends in distance learning for surgeons, focusing on the following goals: (a) Building a comprehensive, worldwide, virtual knowledge base for various disciplines of surgery and telesurgery; (b) Building a virtual knowledge base for rare medical cases, conditions and recommended procedures; (c) Interactive multimedia simulators for hands-on training in all surgical disciplines; (d) Building a worldwide surgical community, which will accelerate the accumulation and sharing of the latest surgical breakthroughs and technological advances. Above all, the most important goal is to improve patient health and convenience, and reduce risks of mortality and complications.

The authors of this chapter show how recent computing technologies such as collaborative virtual environments, high speed networks and mobile devices can be used for training and learning in healthcare providing an environment with security and quality of service. Though a number of studies have been conducted in these research areas, the development of integrated care has proven to be a difficult task. Therefore, we aim also to discuss the promising directions of the current work and growing importance on these subjects. This includes comparative analysis of the most relevant computer systems and applications developed so far that integrate modern computing technologies and health care.

A major issue facing medical education training programs across the USA is the recent advent of universal mandatory duty hour limitations and the time pressure it places on formal face-to-face educational sessions. In response to these mandates, many medical education programs are exploring the use of online instruction. This chapter describes the instructional development process followed to transform a classroom-based pediatrics residency lecture series into an on-demand, video-enhanced, online instructional environment. An overview of the learning principles and instructional sciences that guided the design process is provided. The phases of the designed solution are then described in the context of enhancing the lecture series as it was transformed into online instruction. Implementation logistics are described followed by an overview of the benefits, barriers, and initial project outcomes. Plans for future enhancements and research projects are also discussed.

In this chapter, the authors investigate telehealth quality and reliability assurance. Various models and standards can be applied to assess software quality and reliability in telehealth platforms. Models that assess the quality of the system and the quality of care are presented and approaches based on user satisfaction and expectations. The underlying structural model is based on a modified SERVQUAL approach that consists of five dimensions, which have been consistently ranked by customers to be most important for service quality across all industries. The model can thus be used for evaluation of healthcare services and for planning improvements on services. All these aspects for telehealth systems design are discussed to formulate epistemic criteria for evaluation purposes.

Of the over 100 million Web sites in existence, there are an estimated 100,000 offering health related information. As the amount of health information increases, the public finds it increasingly difficult to decide what to accept and what to reject. The challenge for consumers is to find high quality, relevant information as quickly as possible. The purpose of this chapter is to provide a brief overview of the different perspectives on information quality and to review the main criteria for assessing the quality of health information on the internet. Pointers are provided to enable both clinicians and patients find high quality information sources.

This chapter provides a practical approach to computerized system validation (CSV). Any computer system can be validated utilizing the techniques described. These activities address the organization commitment to implement the underlying system in order to improve, ensure and maintain the quality standards. The CSV is described as a reference and an orientation guide to understand the related quality processes. The activities presented should be useful for initiating and conducting the principal tasks of validation. This chapter reflects a quick guide and addresses one of the "non-technical" aspects of CSV methodology. A clear approach is presented that defines the CSV activities and provides an efficient means of validation to new and existing systems, applications, and environments within the organization.

Ergophysiology, a division of physiology, helps us understand movement in the human body and assists us in creating models and methodologies to understand the mechanisms responsible for movement. Various internal or external conditions impact human movement and if we recognize these problems, we will be able to create scientific methodologies to work to improve the lives of affected individuals. Within this chapter, the authors use the statistical method SF12V2 to organize and select personal information from different individuals and to recognize different problems that affect their daily lives. Using ergophysiological research methodologies, SF12V2 allows researchers to organize the selected data regarding health and kinetics ability level from various individuals.

Current advances in sensing devices and wireless technologies provide an opportunity for improving care quality and reducing medical costs. This chapter presents the architecture of a mobile healthcare system and provides an overview of mobile health applications. Furthermore, it proposes a framework for patient monitoring that performs real-time stream analysis of data collected by non-invasive body sensors. It evaluates a patient's health conditions by analyzing different physiological signals to identify anomalies and activate alarms in risk situations. A risk function for identifying the instantaneous risk of each physiological parameter has been defined. The performance of the proposed system has been evaluated on public physiological data and promising experimental results are presented. By understanding the challenges and the current solutions of informatics appliances described in this chapter, new research areas can be further investigated to improve mobile healthcare services and design innovative medical applications.

Within this chapter the author describes the observation, within his energy diagnostic department, of an increasing number of cases with irrational stimulus-reaction-patterns and with a chaotic regulation state of the autonomous systems. The 'switching phenomenon' was offered as an immediate answer, however, a new cause for this phenomenon also arose— electrosmog exposure. Three criteria were used

Preface

Improvements in healthcare delivery in recent years are rooted in the continued industry-wide investment in information technology and the expanding role of medical informatics. Endeavors to combine medical science and technology have resulted in a growing knowledge base of techniques and applications for healthcare delivery and information management in support of patient care, research and education. Emerging mobile and ubiquitous computing technologies in concert with recent developments in medicine, physiotherapy and psychology have the potential to provide people, especially the elderly and those suffering from chronic diseases, with great opportunities to improve their quality of life and increase independence in daily living. In effect, more and more healthcare will be provided outside of traditional clinical settings in the patient's home and in a proactive, rather than reactive, manner. The main goal of this new publication is to provide innovative and creative ideas for improving communication environments in health and to explore all new technologies in medical informatics and health care delivery systems.

The *Handbook of Research on Distributed Medical Informatics and E-Health* provides a compendium of terms, definitions and explanations of concepts, processes and acronyms. Additionally, this volume features short papers authored by leading experts offering an in-depth description of key terms and concepts related to different areas, issues and trends in various areas of distributed medical informatics, e-health and m-health.

The topics of this handbook cover useful areas of general knowledge including information and communication technologies related to health, new developments in distributed applications and interoperable systems, applications and services, wireless telemedicine and communications technologies in healthcare, mobile health applications and new home care telecare systems, wireless lans and data communications for health care networks, virtual learning environments in health (for patient education, medical students or healthcare professionals), hospital information systems & e-health cards, standardization aspects in e-health related communications, socio/ethical & economic advantages of the new m-health applications, ethical issues in e-health and m-health, evaluation of e-health communication systems, security issues of telemedicine, distributed health telematics applications, space telemedicine and satellite applications and other distributed medical applications.

This handbook is an excellent source of comprehensive knowledge and literature on the topic of distributed health and biomedical informatics.

All of us who worked on the book hope that readers will find it useful.

Athina A. Lazakidou, PhD
Editor

Acknowledgment

The editors express their deep gratitude to the chapter authors whose original contributions served as the foundation for this important handbook.

The editors also would like to acknowledge and express their appreciation to all members of the editorial board who generously allocated their time and expertise to reviewing the manuscripts which was a significant contribution to the overall quality of the publication. Special thanks to Dr. Andriani Daskalaki, Max Planck Institute of Molecular Genetics, Germany, Dr. Sotirios Bisdas, Johann Wolfgang Goethe University, Germany, Dr. Iordanis Evangelou, National Institutes of Health, USA, Dr. Anastasia Kastania, Athens University of Economics & Business, Greece, Dr. Konstantinos Konstantinidis, General Hospital Salzburg, Austria, and Dr. Melpomeni Lazakidou, Institute of Occupational Medicine, Salzburg, Austria.

Kristin Roth, Kristin Klinger and Julia Mosemann, acquisitions/development editors, provided editorial assistance and guidance during the development phase, and Jan Travers, managing director, provided guidance and support over the year since the project began.

Special thanks to IGI Global. Without you, we could not have completed this undertaking.

This book is respectfully dedicated to the newborn baby Marios, who was born during the production of this handbook.

Athina A. Lazakidou, PhD and Konstantinos M. Siassiakos, PhD
Editors

Athina Lazakidou *is lecturer in Health Informatics at the University of Peloponnese at the Department of Nursing in Sparta, Greece. From September 2002 she worked at the University of Piraeus, Greece as a teaching assistant, and at the Hellenic Army Academy & Hellenic Naval Academy, Greece as a visiting lecturer in informatics. Prior to that, she worked also as a visiting lecturer at the Department of Computer Science at the University of Cyprus (2000-2002). She did her undergraduate studies at the Athens University of Economics and Business (Greece) and received her BSc in computer science in 1996. In 2000, she received her PhD. in medical informatics from the Department of Medical Informatics, University Hospital Benjamin Franklin at the Free University of Berlin, Germany. She is also an internationally known expert in the field of computer applications in healthcare and biomedicine, with seven books and numerous papers to her credit. She was also editor of the "Handbook of Research on Informatics in Healthcare and Biomedicine", which is one of the best authoritative reference sources for information on the newest trends and breakthroughs in computer applications applied to healthcare and biomedicine. Her research interests include health informatics, e-Learning in medicine, software engineering, graphical user interfaces, (bio)medical databases, clinical decision support systems, hospital and clinical information systems, electronic medical record systems, distributed medical systems, telemedicine, and other applications in health care.*

Section I
Medical Data and Health Information Systems

Chapter I
Medical Informatics:
Thirty Six Peer-Reviewed Shades

Sanjay P. Sood
C-DAC School of Advanced Computing, Mauritius

Sandhya Keeroo
C-DAC School of Advanced Computing, Mauritius

Victor W.A. Mbarika
Southern University, USA & A&M College, USA

Nupur Prakash
Guru Gobind Singh Indraprastha University, India

Ankur Seth
Adobe Systems, India

ABSTRACT

It is claimed that seeds of 'medical informatics' were sown in 1960s.From this time until the 1990s experts have described the discipline as emerging. This perennial state of advancement can be dedicated to the pioneers of medical informatics who constantly realign its frontiers as the need changes for the rapid developments in the techniques pertaining to organization, processing, management and use of information. During this evolution, researchers and practitioners have made notable attempts to define medical informatics. As a result, today we have a noteworthy collection of peer-reviewed definitions of medical informatics. These definitions not only enlighten us with different perspectives and applications of medical informatics but they also provide a measure of the proliferation of this domain's content. Many of these definitions of medical informatics are unique and explanatory in their respective inferences and contexts. Hence, collectively they can form a larger picture of medical informatics. Lack of clarity about a domain can prove to be counterproductive for new entrants and may also deflect their energies into relatively unrewarding directions. In order to throw light on various perspectives of 'medical informatics' and to understand the evolving meaning of the domain, we carried out a systematic review of formal definitions of medical informatics. An analysis was also performed by mapping 36 peer-reviewed definitions with MeSH (Medical Subject Headings) descriptors relevant to medical informatics. We believe that this research would serve as a handy and an informative resource and may also catalyze further research.

INTRODUCTION

It may be impossible to overlook the influencing role that computers have had on almost all the domains of life – ranging from education through commerce to amusement. This influence is even more pronounced in safety and security critical domains like aerospace and banking. Medicine being a safety as well as a security critical domain is no exception. The booming diffusion of information technology and the emphasis on evidence-based medicine, force the health sector to be an information-intensive industry which desperately hankers for information-driven decisions. Of late, computers and communications technologies have become integral components of medicine and have secured commanding positions in information management in medicine. The is evident from a diverse set applications of computers in medicine, be it hospital information management, patient records, clinical examinations and decision support systems, measurement of physiological parameters, diagnosis, treatment, public health or education computers are omnipresent (Shortliffe, Perreault, Wiederhold & Fagan, 1990; Musen, 2002) and today computers are acting as common thread in the healthcare delivery chain by linking wards to their departments, departments to their hospitals and hospitals to their administrators and branches. In tune with the evolution of information and communications, newer and innovative applications have been joining this technological bandwagon within medicine. Medical informatics is a composite domain that surrounds management of information in medicine. It was perhaps bound to emerge as a discipline primarily because medicine had started to exploit the demanding and extraordinary capabilities of computers to better meet its complex information needs. Currently, medical informatics is a mature discipline and is continually evolving (Patel & Kaufman, 1998). We feel as the discipline matures, there is a need to consolidate past outcomes primarily to educate future practitioners and researchers.

In this era of systems engineering medical informatics is stretching its boundaries and conquering newer boundaries. Today, practitioners of medical informatics include technologists, engineers, clinicians, service providers, regulatory agencies, academicians, professional bodies etc. and their applications of medical informatics are disruptive. For example some of these practitioners have mutually exclusive applications where as others have overlapping applications. This brings with it, to the domain, a wealth of knowledge and promise of further evolution. Because of the many areas of discordance between systems we now have a spectrum of definitions of informatics, yet this in a way reaffirms the dynamism and the continuing evolution of the domain but still there are considerable idiosyncrasies in medical informatics that hamper communication (Patel & Kaufman, 1998) and in certain instances researchers have expressed their concern over the clarity about the very identity of medical informatics (Nagendran, Moores, Spooner & Triscott, 2000; Maojo, Iakovidis, Martin-Sanchez, Crespo & Kulikowski, 2001; Musen, 2002). Interestingly for many clinicians, medical informatics is poorly understood and remains only vaguely equated with computers (Karlinsky, 1999).

During its evolution, numerous attempts have been made to define the field and in many cases these attempts have topped-up existing definitions with some additional details. Since there is no universally accepted definition for medical informatics, the field is evolving in its very own language of communication and in some form is striving for a common ground. Keeping in mind the scope of the domain, it would be meaningful to have a consolidation of existing definition which encompasses, if not all, at least the major components that make up medical informatics. In this paper we have attempted to throw light on various aspects highlighted by researchers and practitioners. This review presents the list of peer-reviewed definitions followed by a qualitative analysis and discussions on the data gathered. This research tries to confirm that the meaning of medical informatics varies with the context in which the term has been used. It is expected that the outcome of the research shall propagate the domain of medical informatics further and the application of this knowledge shall eventually facilitate better quality of life for the populace on our planet.

BACKGROUND

Historically the use of the terminology 'medical informatics' dates back to the second half of the 1970s. The term was influenced from the French expression *informatique médicale*. Till then, other names such as medical computer science, medical information science, computers in medicine, health informatics, and more specialized terms such as nursing informatics, dental informatics, and so on were being used [7] and some of them are still being used. Medical informatics is a field of "applied informatics" whereby its introduction presents itself as being a promise of secure information sharing and communication technologies to upgrade the health sector of the foreseeable future. In the era of 21st century - one of the fast developing and evolving pillars in the health sector, medical informatics is pushing us to live in an "informed society". The nature of medical informatics has been a classical debate now (Masys, Brennan, Ozbolt, Corn & Shortliffe, 2000; Shortliffe & Garber, 2002), without transiting through those debatable topics we would restrict our research to the scope of analyzing definitions only.

Medical informatics is considered to be located at the intersection of information technology and different disciplines of medicine and health care. In the duo-terms of "medicine" and "informatics" the first term indicates the area of research, the second one its methodology (Bemmel & Musen et al., 2002).

Literature published in peer-reviewed journals, Web Sites and various professional and knowledge bodies, was gathered through an extensive systematic search. Definitions from the peer-reviewed literature were extracted and analysed.

Not much has been previously carried out or published on 'standardization of medical informatics' and to the best of our knowledge this research is the first of its kind. Besides facilitating better understanding of medical informatics this research is expected to further its adoption. It is also believed that a better understanding of the meaning of medical informatics could improve communication among the many professionals and organizations and may also encourage them to use and apply the concepts covered by this term. The findings of this research are also expected to contribute towards the alignment of thoughts and achievement of interoperability for the highest possible level of health of an individual, a nation and the world at large.

METHODS

This research is based on a systematic review of the peer-reviewed literature. The criteria laid down for definitions qualifying for the analyses requires that a source be peer-reviewed or comparable in terms of authenticity and correctness, be available in English, and contain text that defines or attempts to define medical informatics in explicit terms.

Search was conducted on the following electronic databases: Pubmed Central, British Medical Journal, Journal of the American Medical Association (JAMA), Journal of the American Medical Informatics Association (JAMIA), Telemedicine and eHealth Journal, Journal of Telemedicine and Telecare. Peer-reviewed publications, papers, reports and case studies on medical informatics were referred from these databases. The search query string "Medical Informatics" OR "Medical-Informatics" OR "Med Informatics" OR "Med-Informatics" were used to search each database. In order to broaden our search we also queried Google search engine with strings like "what is Medical Informatics" and "what is Medical-Informatics". The search was further improved by using the term "definition of" "Med Informatics" and "Med-Informatics" in the Google search engine. These searches were conducted between April 2006 and October 2006. Abstracts of publications in bibliographic databases were also visited and relevant reports, articles, references and Web sites were extracted. The outcome of this review is presented in Table 1. This Table lists definitions of medical informatics in chronological order, duplicate definitions were identified and eliminated. A definition was classified as a unique definition only if the definition highlighted a unique aspect of medical informatics.

Upon completion of all relevant data, a meticulous analysis was performed, the definitions and results were compared to ensure consistency and reliability. This systematic approach was of additional help to look up for patterns, matching words, emerging themes, novel ideas and frequently used words. Different themes found in the definitions of medical informatics were also identified. Details of these are presented in following sections.

RESULTS

Systematic Review

Our searches generated a total of 14,503 results were generated, 1200 abstracts were scanned and roughly 300 publications, reports, proceedings and documents were searched for definitions. The eventual outcome was 36 unique definitions of the term Medical Informatics. These 36 were retrieved from 32 publications, reports etc. definitions have been presented in a chronological order in Table 1. The definitions of medical informatics presented in Table 1 represent a period of 26 years (1977 – 2003) of evolution of the domain.

Qualitative Analysis

The definitions varied in length. The shortest definition comprised of 12 words (Huang & Alessi, 1998) and the longest definition spanned 72 words (Haux, 1996). These 36 definitions included 3 universal themes namely: medicine/medical/biomedicine; health/health care and technology. There were 11 less general themes which comprised : communication; information technology/communication(s) technology; computer technology/computer science; data; information; information science; knowledge; education; research; science and management). These themes were selected on the basis of medical subject headings (MeSH). It should be noted that are some of these 14 themes (like management) may not be MeSH terms but they do get indirectly covered by MeSH. To understand the basic theme of the definition we classified these 14 themes under four headings namely: medicine,

Table 1. Definitions of medical informatics presented in chronological order

No	Year	Author/Source/Organisation	Definition
i.	1977	Levy, A.H. (1977)	Medical informatics is about dealing with the problems associated with information, its acquisition, analysis, and dissemination in health care delivery processes.
ii.	1977	Collen, M.F. (1977)	Medical informatics is the application of computer technology to all fields of medicine – medical care, medical teaching, and medical research.
iii.	1980	Lincoln, T.L. and Korpman, R.A. (1980)	Medical Informatics is the hybrid child of medicine and those logical sciences that are suggested by computer technology.
iv.	1984	Bemmel, J.H.V. (1984)	Medical informatics comprises the theoretical and practical aspects of information processing and communication, based on knowledge and experience derived from processes in medical and health care.
v.	1984	Shortliffe, E.H. (1984)	Medical informatics is a basic science discipline in medicine, although one that has evolved distinct characteristics that have tended to separate it from other traditional academic and research medical specialities. He suggests that medical informatics holds both realized and potential importance for the science and practice of medicine.
vi.	1986	Collen, M.F. (1986)	Medical informatics is a new knowledge domain of computer and information science, engineering and technology in all fields of health and medicine, including research, education and practice.
vii.	1986	Steering Committee on evaluation of medical info. science in medical education, (1986)	Medical informatics combines medical science with several technologies and disciplines in the information and computer sciences and provides methodologies by which these can contribute to better use of the medical knowledge base and ultimately to better medical care.
viii.	1986	Myers, J.D. (1986)	Medical informatics is a developing body of knowledge and set of techniques concerning the organization and management of information in support of medical research, education, and patient care.
ix.	1987	Lindberg, D.A.B. (1987)	a) Medical informatics attempts to provide the theoretical and scientific basis for the application of computer and automated information systems to biomedicine and health affairs.
x.	1987	Lindberg, D.A.B. (1987)	b) Medical informatics studies biomedical information, data, and knowledge - their storage, retrieval, and optimal use for problem-solving and decision-making
xi.	1987	Lindberg, D.A.B. and Schoolman, H.M. (1987)	Medical informatics attempts to provide the theoretic and scientific basis for the use of automated information systems in biomedicine.
xii.	1987	Greenes, R.A. and Siegel, E.R. (1987)	Medical informatics is the field concerned with the cognitive, information processing, and information management tasks of medical and health care, and biomedical research, and with the application of information sciences and technology to those tasks.
xiii.	1988	Shortliffe, E.H. (1988)	Medical informatics draws on, and contributes to, multiple disciplines in the health sciences and information sciences.
xiv.	1990	Blois, M.S. and Shortliffe, E.H. (1990)	Medical informatics is the rapidly developing scientific field that deals with the storage, retrieval, and optimal use of biomedical information, data, and knowledge for problem solving and decision making.
xv.	1990	Greenes, R.A. and Shortliffe, E.H. (1990)	Medical informatics is the field that concerns itself with the cognitive, information processing, and communication tasks of medical practice, education, and research, including the information science and the technology to support these tasks.
xvi.	1993	Seelos, H.J. (1993)	Medical informatics is the science of information processing and the creation of information processing systems in medicine and health care delivery. Its methodological approach is based on the area specific applicability of a multidisciplinary theory of engineering and managing computerized information systems related to its empirical object.
xvii.	1994	Stead, W.W. (1994)	a) Medical informatics is an interdisciplinary field that builds upon a foundation of knowledge developed in the health sciences, biometry, computer science, decision science, engineering, library science, management science, and policy science.

continued on following page

Table 1. continued

xviii.	1994	Stead, W.W. (1994)	b) Medical informatics involves the integrated use of several approaches and techniques from these sciences to solve problems relevant to health research, health education, or health care delivery.
xix.	1994	Collen, M.F. (1994)	Medical informatics is the application of computers, communications and information technology and systems to all fields of medicine - medical care, medical education and medical research.
xx.	1995	Warner, H.R. (1995)	Medical informatics is the study, invention, implementation of structures and algorithms to improve communication, understanding, and management of medical information.
xxi.	1995	Shortliffe, E.H. (1995)	a) Medical informatics examines the effective and efficient use of medical data, information, and knowledge, with computers and communications networks providing a natural technical base for much of what the field involves.
xxii.	1995	Shortliffe, E.H. (1995)	b) Medical informatics deals with the storage and retrieval of biomedical information for the purpose of problem solving and decision making. Under this general theme comes branches such as medical imaging, computer aided surgery, electronic medical records, etc. What all these fields share is the utilisation of computing and communication technologies to produce better health care.
xxiii.	1996	Haux, R. (1996)	Medical informatics is a scientific medical discipline, similar to surgery, internal medicine, epidemiology, or microbiology; and that medical informatics has a strong relationship with the health sciences concerning its field of application, and to informatics concerning its methods and tools. It is a cross-sectional discipline, with relevance for virtually all other specialties of medicine and the health sciences. This is the reason for its impact on research and education in these specialties.
xxiv.	1996	Hasman, A., Haux, R. and Albert, A. (1996)	Medical informatics is defined as the scientific discipline concerned with the systematic processing of data, information and knowledge in medicine and health care.
xxv.	1996	Heinemann, T.D.B. (1996)	Medical informatics is the discipline relating to the management of information and the use of computer systems in health care.
xxvi.	1998	Coiera, E. (1998)	Medical informatics is the rational study of the way we think about patients, and the way that treatments are defined, selected and evolved. It is the study of how medical knowledge is created, shaped, shared and applied.
xxvii.	1998	Morris, T.A. and McCain, K.W. (1998)	Medical informatics is an emergent interdisciplinary field described as drawing upon and contributing to both the health sciences and information sciences.
xxviii.	1998	Huang, M.P. and Alessi, N.E. (1998)	Medical informatics is the study of the use of information in medicine.
xxix.	1998	Patel, V.L. and Kaufman, D.R. (1998)	Medical informatics is an emerging discipline characterized by rapid development and exciting new initiatives that promise to have a significant impact on the practice of medicine.
xxx.	1999	MeSH term, (1999)	Medical informatics is the field of information science concerned with the analysis, use and dissemination of medical data and information through the application of computers to various aspects of health care and medicine.
xxxi.	2000	Shortliffe, E.H. and Perreault, L.E. (eds.) (2000)	a) Medical informatics is the scientific field that deals with biomedical information, data and knowledge—their storage, retrieval and optimal use for problems solving and decision making. In addition to dealing with the biomedical information, data and knowledge. Medical Informatics also includes automated systems for diagnosis, therapy and communicating of medical data.
xxxii.	2000	Shortliffe, E.H. and Perreault, L.E. (eds.) (2000)	b) Medical Informatics is a field that touches on all basic and applied fields in biomedical science and is closely tied to modern information technologies, notably in the areas of computing and communication (medical computer science).
xxxiii.	2000	Kareem, S.A., Baba, A. and Wahid, M.I.A. (2000)	Medical informatics is concerned with the application of computers in the medical and biological sciences and has been considered a field of research in its own right for more than twenty years.

continued on following page

Table 1. continued

xxxiv.	2001	Shortliffe, E.H., Perreault, L.E., Wiederhold, G. and Fagan, L.M. (eds.) (2001)	Informatics is the science that studies the use and processing of data, information, and knowledge, and medical informatics as informatics applied to medicine, health care, and public health.
xxxv.	2002	Wyatt, J.C. and Liu, J.L.Y. (2002)	Medical informatics is the study and application of methods to improve the management of patient data, clinical knowledge, population data, and other information relevant to patient care and community health.
xxxvi.	2003	Beolchi, L.(Ed). (2003)	Medical informatics is the combination of computer science, information science and the health sciences (medicine) designed to assist in the management and processing of data to support the delivery of health care.

Table 2. Classification of themes

	Medicine	Technology	Academics	Miscellaneous
1.	Medicine (Medical) / Biomedicine			
2.	Health / Health care			
3.		Technology		
4.		Communication		
5.		Information technology / communication/ s technology		
6.		Computer technology / Computer science		
7.		Data		
8.		Information		
9.		Information Science		
10.			Knowledge	
11.			Education	
12.			Medical research / biomedical research	
13.				Science
14.				Management

technology, academics and miscellaneous. The classification of the themes has been depicted in Table 2.

Medical informatics has been defined in various ways whereby 27 definitions (Levy, 1977; MEDINFO-80; Lincoln & Korpman, 1980; Shortliffe, 1984; Collen, 1986; Myers; 1986; Greenes & Siegel, 1987; Blois, & Shortliffe, 1990; Greenes, Shortliffe, 1990; Seelos, 1993; Stead, 1994; Collen, 1994; Warner, 1995; Haux, 1996; Hasman, Haux & Albert, 1996; Heinemann, 1996; Coiera, 1998; Morris & McCain, 1998; Huang & Alessi, 1998; MeSH term; Shortliffe & Perreault, 2000; Kareem, Baba, & Wahid, 2000; Shortliffe, Perreault, Wiederhold, & Fagan, 2001; Wyatt & Liu, 2002) start with the word 'is' immediately after the word medical informatics, and others make use of verbs like 'comprises (Bemmel, 1984), combines (Steering Committee for Symposium on Medical Informatics, 1986), studies (Lindberg, (1987), at-

Table 3. Analysis of definitions

No	Year	Author/Source/Organisation	Themes (MeSH Terms)													
			1	2	3	4	5	6	7	8	9	10	11	12	13	14
I.	1977	Levy, A.H. (1977)		x						x						
II.	1977	Collen, M.F. (1977)	x					x						x		
III.	1980	Lincoln, T.L. and Korpman, R.A. (1980)	x					x							x	
IV.	1984	Bemmel, J.H.V. (1984)	x	x		x				x		x				
V.	1984	Shortliffe, E.H. (1984)	x											x	x	
VI.	1986	Collen, M.F. (1986)	x	x	x			x			x	x	x	x		
VII.	1986	Steering Committee on evaluation of medical info. science in medical education, (1986)	x		x			x			x	x			x	
VIII.	1986	Myers, J.D. (1986)	x							x		x	x	x		x
IX.	1987	Lindberg, D.A.B. (1987)	x	x											x	
X.	1987	Lindberg, D.A.B. (1987)	x						x	x		x				
XI.	1987	Lindberg, D.A.B. and Schoolman, H.M. (1987)	x							x					x	
XII.	1987	Greenes, R.A. and Siegel, E.R. (1987)	x	x			x			x	x			x		x
XIII.	1988	Shortliffe, E.H. (1988)		x							x				x	
XIV.	1990	Blois, M.S. and Shortliffe, E.H. (1990)	x						x	x		x			x	
XV.	1990	Greenes, R.A. and Shortliffe, E.H. (1990)	x		x	x				x	x		x	x		
XVI.	1993	Seelos, H.J. (1993)	x	x						x					x	
XVII.	1994	Stead, W.W. (1994)		x				x				x			x	x
XVIII.	1994	Stead, W.W. (1994)		x									x	x	x	
XIX.	1994	Collen, M.F. (1994)	x				x						x	x		
XX.	1995	Warner, H.R. (1995)	x			x				x						x
XXI.	1995	Shortliffe, E.H. (1995)	x			x			x	x		x				
XXII.	1995	Shortliffe, E.H. (1995)	x	x			x			x						
XXIII.	1996	Haux, R. (1996)	x	x									x	x	x	
XXIV.	1996	Hasman, A., Haux, R. and Albert, A. (1996)	x	x					x	x		x			x	
XXV.	1996	Heinemann, T.D.B. (1996)		x						x						x
XXVI.	1998	Coiera, E. (1998)	x									x				
XXVII.	1998	Morris, T.A. and McCain, K.W. (1998)		x							x				x	
XXVIII.	1998	**Huang, M.P. and Alessi, N.E.** (1998)	x							x						
XXIX.	1998	Patel, V.L. and Kaufman, D.R. (1998)	x													
XXX.	1999	MeSH term, (1999)	x	x					x	x	x					

continued on following page

Table 3. continued

XXXI.	2000	Shortliffe, E.H. and Perreault, L.E. (eds.) (2000)	x						x	x		x			x	
XXXII.	2000	Shortliffe, E.H. and Perreault, L.E. (eds.) (2000)	x			x	x	x							x	
XXXIII.	2000	**Kareem, S.A., Baba, A. and Wahid, M.I.A.** (2000)	x											x	x	
XXXIV.	2001	Shortliffe, E.H., Perreault, L.E., Wiederhold, G. and Fagan, L.M. (eds.) (2001)	x	x					x	x		x			x	
XXXV.	2002	**Wyatt, J.C. and Liu, J.L.Y.** (2002)		x					x	x		x				x
XXXVI.	2003	Beolchi, L.(Ed). (2003)	x	x				x	x		x				x	x

tempts to provide (Lindberg & Schoolman, 1986; Lindberg, (1987), draws on (Shortliffe, 1988), involves (Stead, 1994), examines (Shortliffe, 1995) and deals with (Shortliffe, 1995).

Table 3 presents the analysis of all the 36 definitions of medical informatics as mapped against 14 themes (MeSH terms) listed in Table 2.

Medical Perspective

Out of these 36 definitions, 13 include the word 'medicine' (MEDINFO-80; Lincoln & Korpman, 1980; Shortliffe, 1984; Collen, 1986; Seelos, 1993; Collen, 1994; Haux, 1996; Hasman, Haux & Albert, 1996; Patel & Kaufman, 1998; Huang & Alessi, 1998; MeSH; Shortliffe, Perreault, Wiederhold, & Fagan, 2001; Beolchi, 2003) and 2 (Lindberg & Schoolman, 1986; Lindberg, 1987) have referred to biomedicine.

In general, the word 'medicine' has been used from 'medical' perspective in 15 definitions (MEDINFO-80; Bemmel, 1984; Shortliffe, 1984; (Steering Committee for Symposium on Medical Informatics, 1986) ; Myers, 1986, Greenes & Siegel, 1987; Greenes, Shortliffe, 1990; Collen, 1994; Warner, 1995; Shortliffe, 1995; Haux, 1996;Haux, 1996; Coiera, 1998; MeSH term; Shortliffe & Perreault, 2000; Kareem, Baba, & Wahid, 2000; of which 5 were referred as medical care (MEDINFO-80; Bemmel, 1984; Steering Committee for Symposium on Medical Informatics, 1986; Greenes & Siegel, 1987; Collen, 1994), 4 as medical research (MEDINFO-80; Myers, 1986; Greenes, Shortliffe, 1990; Collen, 1994), 3 as medical education (Myers, 1986; Greenes, Shortliffe, 1990; Collen, 1994), 3 as medical knowledge; Steering Committee for Symposium on Medical Informatics, 1986); Shortliffe, 1995; Coiera, 1998), 3 as medical data (Shortliffe, 1995; MeSH term; Shortliffe & Perreault, 2000), 3 as medical information (Warner, 1995; Shortliffe, 1995; MeSH term), 1 as medical teaching (MEDINFO-80), 1 as medical practice (Greenes, Shortliffe, 1990), 1 as electronic medical records (Shortliffe, 1995), 2 as medical science (Steering Committee for Symposium on Medical Informatics, 1986); Kareem, Baba, & Wahid, 2000), 1 as medical specialties (Shortliffe, 1984), 1 as medical discipline (Haux, 1996), 1 as medical imaging (Shortliffe, 1995) and 1 as medical computer science (Shortliffe & Perreault, 2000).

The term 'medical' has further been associated to the term 'biomedical' as biomedical information (Lindberg, 1987; Blois, & Shortliffe, 1990; Shortliffe, 1995; Shortliffe & Perreault, 2000), biomedical data (Lindberg, 1987; Blois, & Shortliffe, 1990; Shortliffe & Perreault, 2000;Kareem, Baba, & Wahid, 2000), biomedical knowledge

(Lindberg, 1987; Blois, & Shortliffe, 1990; Shortliffe & Perreault, 2000), biomedical research (Greenes & Siegel, 1987) and biomedical science (Shortliffe & Perreault, 2000).

Eleven out of the 36 definitions refer to health care (Levy, 1977; Bemmel, 1984; Greenes & Siegel, 1987; Seelos, 1993; Stead, 1994; Shortliffe, 1995; Hasman, Haux & Albert, 1996; Heinemann, 1996; MeSH term; Shortliffe, Perreault, Wiederhold, & Fagan, 2001; Beolchi, 2003). The term 'health care' has been used in relation to health care delivery (Levy, 1977; Seelos, 1993; Stead, 1994), and deliver health care (Beolchi, 2003); which suggests that health care may refer more to health care processes and systems rather than to the health of people. Furthermore the term 'health' was reflected in 9 definitions (Collen, 1986; Lindberg, 1987; Shortliffe, 1988; Stead, 1994; Haux, 1996; Morris & McCain, 1998; Shortliffe, Perreault, Wiederhold, & Fagan, 2001; Wyatt & Liu, 2002; Beolchi, 2003) out of which 5 were referred as health sciences (Shortliffe, 1988; Stead, 1994; Haux, 1996; Morris & McCain, 1998; Beolchi, 2003), 1 as health research (Stead, 1994), 1 as health education (Stead, 1994) 1 as health affairs (Lindberg, 1987), 1 as public health (Shortliffe, Perreault, Wiederhold, & Fagan, 2001) and 1 as community health (Wyatt & Liu, 2002).

Technological Perspective

Out of 36 definitions, 9 included the term 'technology' (MEDINFO-80; Lincoln & Korpman, 1980; Collen, 1986; Steering Committee for Symposium on Medical Informatics, 1986; Greenes & Siegel, 1987; Greenes, Shortliffe, 1990; Collen, 1994; Shortliffe, 1995; Shortliffe & Perreault, 2000). The word communication has been explicitly mentioned 5 times (Bemmel, 1984; Greenes, Shortliffe, 1990; Warner, 1995; Shortliffe, 1995; Shortliffe & Perreault, 2000). The use of the word technology has further been enhanced in the strings 'information technology', 'communication/s technology', 'computer technology' and 'computer science'. The string information technology has been used in 3 definitions (Greenes & Siegel, 1987; Collen, 1994; Shortliffe & Perreault, 2000); communication/s technology shows up in 2 definitions (Collen, 1994; Shortliffe, 1995); computer technology has been used twice (MEDINFO-80; Lincoln & Korpman, 1980) ; while the words computer science have been used 5 times (Collen, 1986; (Steering Committee for Symposium on Medical Informatics, 1986) ; Stead, 1994; Shortliffe & Perreault, 2000; Beolchi, 2003). In all the definitions, technology has been used as a noun.

To add another dimension to medical informatics, concept of information science has appeared 8 times (Collen, 1986; Steering Committee for Symposium on Medical Informatics, 1986; Greenes & Siegel, 1987; Shortliffe, 1988; Greenes, Shortliffe, 1990; Morris & McCain, 1998; MeSH term; Beolchi, 2003).

Academic Perspective

Few researchers have associated medical informatics with activities such as education, research and management. Education (Collen, 1986; Myers, 1986; Greenes, Shortliffe, 1990; Stead, 1994; Collen, 1994; Haux, 1996) has been associated with medicine as medical education in 3 instances (Myers, 1986; Greenes, Shortliffe, 1990; Collen, 1994) and with health as health education (Stead, 1994). Research has been reflected 10 times (MEDINFO-80; Shortliffe, 1984; Collen, 1986; Myers, 1986; Greenes & Siegel, 1987; Greenes, Shortliffe, 1990; Stead, 1994; Collen, 1994; Haux, 1996; Kareem, Baba, & Wahid, 2000); out of which 4 depict medical research (MEDINFO-80; Myers, 1986; Greenes, Shortliffe, 1990; Collen, 1994), 1 refers to biomedical research (Greenes & Siegel, 1987) and 1 refers to health research (Stead, 1994).

Miscellaneous Perspectives

Medical informatics has also been defined by referring to the term management which appeared in 7 definitions (Myers, 1986; Greenes & Siegel, 1987; Stead, 1994; Warner, 1995; Heinemann, 1996; Wyatt & Liu, 2002; Beolchi, 2003) out of which 5 refer to the management of information or information management (Myers, 1986; Greenes & Siegel, 1987; Warner, 1995; Heinemann, 1996; Wyatt & Liu, 2002), 2 refer to management of data (Wyatt & Liu, 2002; Beolchi, 2003), 1 refers to management of clinical knowledge (Wyatt & Liu, 2002) and another one refers to management science (Stead, 1994).

Others referred to medical informatics in more general nouns (eg. data, information and knowledge,). Data as a noun has been used 9 times (Lindberg, 1987; Blois, & Shortliffe, 1990; Shortliffe, 1995; Hasman, Haux & Albert, 1996; MeSH term; Shortliffe & Perreault, 2000; Shortliffe, Perreault, Wiederhold, & Fagan, 2001; Wyatt & Liu, 2002; Beolchi, 2003) it also has been used twice as medical data (Shortliffe, 1995; MeSH term), thrice as biomedical data (Lindberg, 1987; Blois, & Shortliffe, 1990; Shortliffe & Perreault, 2000), once as patient data (Wyatt & Liu, 2002) and once more as population data (Wyatt & Liu, 2002). 17 definitions have come up with the term information (Levy, 1977, Bemmel, 1984; Myers, 1986; Lindberg, 1987; Greenes & Siegel, 1987; Blois, & Shortliffe, 1990; Greenes, Shortliffe, 1990; Seelos, 1993; Warner, 1995; Shortliffe, 1995; Hasman, Haux & Albert, 1996; Heinemann, 1996; Huang & Alessi, 1998; 37; Shortliffe & Perreault, 2000; Shortliffe, Perreault, Wiederhold, & Fagan, 2001;Wyatt & Liu, 2002), out of which 3 defined information as information processing (Bemmel, 1984; Greenes & Siegel, 1987; Greenes & Shortliffe, 1990), information processing systems (Seelos, 1993), medical information (Warner, 1995; Shortliffe, 1995; MeSH term), biomedical information (Lindberg, 1987; Blois, & Shortliffe, 1990; Shortliffe, 1995; Shortliffe & Perreault, 2000), information systems (Lindberg & Schoolman, 1986; Lindberg, 1987; Greenes & Siegel, 1987), information management (Greenes & Siegel, 1987) and management of information (Myers, 1986; Heinemann, 1996; Wyatt & Liu, 2002).

13 of the definitions include the term 'knowledge' (Bemmel, 1984; Collen, 1986; Steering Committee for Symposium on Medical Informatics, 1986; Myers, 1986; Lindberg, 1987; Blois, & Shortliffe, 1990; Stead, 1994; Shortliffe, 1995; Hasman, Haux & Albert, 1996; Coiera, 1998; Shortliffe & Perreault, 2000; Shortliffe, Perreault, Wiederhold, & Fagan, 2001; Wyatt & Liu, 2002) it has been used in relation to medical knowledge (18; Shortliffe, 1995; Coiera, 1998), biomedical knowledge (Lindberg, 1987; Blois, & Shortliffe, 1990; Shortliffe & Perreault, 2000) and clinical knowledge (Wyatt & Liu, 2002).

Science and information science further described medical informatics in explicit terms. The term science appears 12 times (Lincoln & Korpman, 1980; (Shortliffe, 1984; Steering Committee for Symposium on Medical Informatics, 1986; Shortliffe, 1988; Seelos, 1993; Stead, 1994; Haux, 1996; Morris & McCain, 1998; Shortliffe & Perreault, 2000; Kareem, Baba, & Wahid, 2000; Shortliffe, Perreault, Wiederhold, & Fagan, 2001; Beolchi, 2003) and has been used in relation to health sciences (Shortliffe, 1988; Stead, 1994; Haux, 1996; Morris & McCain, 1998; Beolchi, 2003), medical science (Steering Committee for Symposium on Medical Informatics, 1986; Kareem, Baba, & Wahid, 2000), biomedical science (Kareem, Baba, & Wahid, 2000), logical sciences (Lincoln & Korpman, 1980), basic science (Shortliffe, 1984), decision science (Stead, 1994), library science (Stead, 1994), management science (Stead, 1994), policy science (Stead, 1994), biological science (Kareem, Baba, & Wahid, 2000); certain definitions also pertained to scientific basis (Lindberg, 1987; Lindberg & Schoolman, 1986), scientific field (Blois, & Shortliffe, 1990; Shortliffe & Perreault, 2000) and scientific discipline (Haux, 1996; Hasman, Haux & Albert, 1996).

While most of the definitions concentrated on information, about one quarter of them focused on information retrieval too. These definitions lay much emphasis in the medical sector and its role in academics like research, education, including science.

Although this research does not measure the impact of various definitions, but based on our experience, most commonly used definitions are those from authors like Shortliffe E.H. (Shortliffe, 1984; Shortliffe, 1988; Blois, & Shortliffe, 1990; Greenes, Shortliffe, 1990; Shortliffe, 1995; Shortliffe & Perreault, 2000; Shortliffe, Perreault, Wiederhold, & Fagan, 2001) and M.F. Collen (MEDINFO-80; Collen, 1986; Collen, 1994). Upon analysing the nature of these definitions, a fact that surfaces is these seven definitions touch all the four (or at least 3) perspectives of medical informatics and can be classified as explicit definitions. Besides these, two more definitions (Collen, 1986; Greenes, Shortliffe, 1990; Wyatt & Liu, 2002;) can be considered as comprehensive definitions as these definitions also cover all the four perspectives of medical informatics.

DISCUSSION

Medical informatics includes discrete concepts such as medicine, technology, academics, science/s and management. Various perspectives are reflected in these definitions with varying degrees of concentration. In these definitions, 'health care' very explicitly refers to health care as a process, rather than to health as a state of being free from illness. Similarly, the term 'medicine' does not refer to drugs, rather it reflects medical care. The definitions show that technology, communication technology and computers are only a means to help better communications in the field of medical sector rather than a tool of computerization. Thus, computer technology is more used in medicine as the means to help achieve interoperability amongst various systems within the medical field. The themes that have dominated the definitions are medicine, technology (information technology and information science), and science.

Finding 1: these definitions are indicative of the fact that medical informatics is more about education, research, science, decision support and management and not merely computerisation.

An in-depth understanding of medical informatics depicts a positive sign. Most of the definitions referred to problem solving (Lindberg, 1987; Blois, & Shortliffe, 1990; Stead, 1994;

Shortliffe, 1995) and decision making (Lindberg, 1987; Blois, & Shortliffe, 1990; Shortliffe, 1995) as well as terms like 'improve' (Warner, 1995); Wyatt & Liu, 2002), improve communication, understanding, and management of medical information (Warner, 1995), improve the management of patient data, clinical knowledge, population data (Wyatt & Liu, 2002); effective and efficient use (Shortliffe, 1995); better use of the medical knowledge base (Steering Committee for Symposium on Medical Informatics, 1986), better medical care (Steering Committee for Symposium on Medical Informatics, 1986) and better health care (Shortliffe, 1995). None of these 36 definitions referred to any cautious, harmful, disadvantageous effects or warnings to humanity.

Finding 2 : Medical informatics is seen as a domain that may not have adverse effects.

Barring 4 definitions (Levy, 1977; Patel & Kaufman, 1998; Huang & Alessi, 1998; MeSH term) out of 36 rest all definitions touch at least three of the four perspectives. In all 8 definitions ((Steering Committee for Symposium on Medical Informatics, 1986; Myers, 1986; Greenes & Siegel, 1987; Blois, & Shortliffe, 1990; Hasman, Haux & Albert, 1996; Shortliffe & Perreault, 2000; Shortliffe, Perreault, Wiederhold, & Fagan, 2001;Wyatt & Liu, 2002) touch all four perspectives of medical informatics. Interestingly, three out of these eight definitions (Blois, & Shortliffe, 1990; Shortliffe & Perreault, 2000; Shortliffe, Perreault, Wiederhold, & Fagan, 2001) have E.H. Shortliffe as one of the authors.

Finding 3: Medical informatics is a domain that can be explicitly defined if the explanation highlights at least 3 perspectives (namely Medical, Technological (informatics), Academics).

Besides these definitions, the overwhelming number of hits which resulted in so many informal definitions of medical informatics on the Internet reveals that medical informatics is indeed an important concept and a consensus over the definition needs be reached. This is so because various authors, sources and organisations perceive medical informatics in their own way even more so as no consensus has been reached on its universal meaning. Most of these informal definitions were correct but some were quite vague which tend to give a limited explanation especially to non-IT literate people. A unanimous definition would enhance the aspect of interoperability and communication among organisations and other entities.

CONCLUSION

Being such a widely used topic by so many organizations, medical informatics is indeed an issue of great concern. A systematic approach used to carry out the search and collection of definitions, shows the degree to which these versions of medical informatics varied. Very subtly the research conveys that there is a strong need for a universally acceptable definition. It is hoped the effort put forward shall be helpful in furthering medical informatics in order to have a better view of the concept and shall eventually lead to a better quality of life for mankind.

The research has prompted us to come up with an analytically crafted definition of medial informatics. On the basis of what we have learned from this research our version of medical informatics is as follows:

"Medical informatics is knowledge domain of computers and information science that originates from the intersection of medicine and information technology in all fields of health and medicine. It deals with medical information management tasks like storage, cognition, information processing, retrieval, optimal use of biomedical information, data and knowledge to further research, to improve accuracy, timeliness and reliability of medical problem solving and decision-making processes. This is achieved by application of computers and associated technologies"

Furthermore, key concepts, sub-domains and applications of medical informatics include (Bemmel & Musen et al. 2002):

- Information Systems
- Electronic Health Record
- Electronic Patient Record
- Data Acquisition Systems
- Data Communication Systems
- Data Processing Systems
- Inference Support Systems
- TeleHealth including Telemedicine, Tele-Education, etc.
- Picture Archival & Communication System
- Biomedical Instrumentation
- Public Health Informatics
- Nursing Informatics
- Virtual Reality Applications in Medicine
- Medical Knowledge & Decision Support

We would like to consider this definition to be an initial step towards the consolidation and investigation of the definitions and their perspectives. It can be classified as a vital step the more so, as it shows the way in which different researchers and practitioners treat medical informatics. This compilation of existing definitions can be a useful resource to facilitate communication, discussion, and stimulate further research that may be aimed at answering queries such as, What do people expect from medical informatics? Does the medical sector make provision for its promotion? Do health care providers want medical informatics? How does medical informatics change the relationship, understanding and interaction within the medical sector? Time, patience, and further in-depth research within the field would provide at least provisional answers to these questions, and to the overwhelming number of questions still unasked.

REFERENCES

Bemmel, J.H.V. (1984). *The structure of medical informatics - Medical Informatics. (9)*, p. 175.

Bemmel, J.V. and Musen, M.A. (eds.). *Handbook of medical informatics*, Springer.

Beolchi, L.(Ed). (2003). *Medical informatics in : Telemedicine glossary 5th edition, working document*, p. 748.

Blois, M.S. and Shortliffe, E.H. (1990). The computer meets medicine: Emergence of a discipline in Medical Informatics. *Computer Applications in Health Care, 20.*

Coiera, E. (1998). Guide to medical informatics, the internet and telemedicine. *Chapman and Hall Medical 2nd Edition*, ISBN 0 412 75710 9 (book review. BMJ. 316, 158).

Collen, M.F. (1986). Origins of medical informatics. *West J Med. (145)6*, 778–785.

Collen, M.F. (1994), The origins of informatics. *Journal of the American Medical Informatics Association, (1)2* 91-107.

Greenes, R.A. and Siegel, E.R. (1987). Characterization of an emerging field, In: approaches to defining the literature and disciplinary boundaries of medical informatics. *Symp Comp Appl Med Care*, 411–415.

Greenes, R.A. and Shortliffe, E.H. (1990). Medical Informatics, In: An emerging academic discipline and institutional priority. *Journal of the American Medical Association, (263) 8*, 1114-1120.

Hasman, A., Haux, R. and Albert, A. (1996). *A systematic view on medical informatics, (51)* 3,131-139.

Haux, R. (1996). Medical informatics. In, once more towards systematization. *Methods Inf Med., (35)*3, 189-92 (abstract).

Heinemann, T.D.B. (1996). Medicine and books. In: *Medical Informatics. BMJ* (313), 1270.

Huang, M.P. and Alessi, N.E. (1998), An informatics curriculum for psychiatry. *Academic Psychiatry (22)*, 77-91.

Kareem, S.A., Baba, A. and Wahid, M.I.A. (2000). Research in medical informatics. *Health Informatics Journal, (6)*2, 110-115.

Karlinsky, H. (1999). Feature : *medical informatics, information technology, and psychiatry, bulletin canadian psychiatric association.*

Levy, A.H. (1977). *Is informatics a basic medical science?* Proceedings of MEDINFO, 979.

Lincoln, T.L. and Korpman, R.A. (1980). *Computers, health care, and medical information science. Science, (210)*4467, 257–63.

Lindberg, D.A.B. and Schoolman, H.M. (1986). The National Library of Medicine and Medical Informatics. *West J Med., (145)*6, pp786–790.

Lindberg, D.A.B. (1987). *NLM long range plan.* Report of the Board of Regents, 1987, p.31.

Maojo, V., Iakovidis, I., Martin-Sanchez, F., Crespo, J. and Kulikowski, C. (2001). Medical informatics and bioinformatics :European efforts to facilitate synergy. *Journal of Biomedical Informatics, (34)*, 423–427.

Masys, D.R., Brennan, P.F., Ozbolt, J.G., Corn, M., and Shortliffe, E.H. (2000). Are medical informatics and nursing informatics distinct disciplines? The 1999 ACMI debate. *Journal of the American Medical Informatics Association, (7)*3, 304-312.

MEDINFO, *Preliminary announcement for the Third World Conference on Medical Informatics*, MEDINFO 80, 1977. Retrieved from http://www.amia.org/history/what.html

MeSH (medical subject headings) definition of medical informatics as defined in NLM's. Retrieved 10th January, 2007 from http://www.nlm.nih.gov/tsd/acquisitions/cdm/subjects58.html

Morris, T.A. and McCain, K.W. (1998). *The Structure of Medical Informatics Journal Literature. J Am Med Inform Assoc, (5)*5, 448–466.

Musen, M.A. (2002). Medical informatics: searching for underlying components. *Methods Inf Med., (41)1*, 12-19.

Myers, J.D. (1986). Medical education in the information age, Proceedings of the Symposium on Medical Informatics. p. 3.

Nagendran, S., Moores, D., Spooner, R. and Triscott, J. (2000). Is telemedicine a subset of medical informatics? *Journal of Telemedicine and Telecare, (6)*2, pp51-52.

Patel, V.L. and Kaufman, D.R. (1998). Medical informatics and the science of cognition. *Journal of the American Medical Informatics Association, 5(6)*, 489-492.

Seelos, H.J. (1993). The empirical object of medical informatics. J Med Syst., vol.17, 2, 87-96.

Shortliffe, E.H. (1984). The science of biomedical computing, In: Pages JC, Levy AH, Gremy F, Anderson J (eds.), *Meeting the Challenge: Informatics and Medical Education*. Amsterdam, The Netherlands: North-Holland, 1-10.

Shortliffe, E.H. (1988). The state of the art in medical information sciences. In: Kuhn RL (Ed) *Frontiers of Medical Information Sciences*. New York: Praeger, pp 11–18.

Shortliffe, E.H., Perreault, L.E., Wiederhold, G. and Fagan, L.M. (1990). *Medical Informatics: computer applications in health care*, MA: Addison-Wesley.

Shortliffe, E.H. (1995). *Medical informatics meets medical education. JAMA (273)*, 1061-1065.

Shortliffe, E.H. and Perreault, L.E. (eds.) (2000). *Medical informatics: computer applications in health care and biomedicine*. New York: Springer-Verlag.

Shortliffe, E.H., Perreault, L.E., Wiederhold, G. and Fagan, L.M. (eds.) (2001). *Medical Informatics: Computer Applications in Health Care and Bio*medicine, 2nd Edition, New York: Springer-Verlag.

Shortliffe, E.H. and Garber, A.M. (2002). Training synergies between medical informatics and health services research, successes and challenges. *Journal of the American Medical Informatics Association, vol. 9*, 133-139.

Steering Committee on the evaluation of medical information science in medical education. (1986). In *Proceedings of the symposium on medical informatics* (pp. 2-3). Washington, DC: Association of American Medical Colleges.

Stead, W.W. (1994). JAMIA – Why? *J Am Med Informatics Assoc., Vol. 1*, 75-76.

Warner, H.R. (1995). Medical informatics: A real discipline? *J Am Med Informatics Assoc., vol. 2, 4*, 207-214.

Wyatt, J.C. and Liu, J.L.Y. (2002). Basic concepts in medical informatics. *Journal of Epidemiology and Community Health, vol. 56*, 808-812.

KEY TERMS

Computer: Is a machine for manipulating data according to a list of instructions.

Decision Support Systems: Are a class of computer-based information systems including knowledge based systems that support decision making activities.

Health Care (Healthcare): Is the prevention, treatment, and management of illness and the preservation of mental and physical well-being through the services offered by the medical, nursing, and allied health professions.

Information: Is the result of processing, manipulating and organizing data in a way that adds to the knowledge of the receiver. In other words, it is the context in which data is taken.

Information Science: Is an interdisciplinary science primarily concerned with the collection, classification, manipulation, storage, retrieval and dissemination of information. Information science studies the application and usage of knowledge in organizations, and the interaction between people, organizations and information systems. It is often (mistakenly) considered a branch of computer science. It is actually a broad, interdisciplinary field, incorporating not only aspects of computer science, but also library science, cognitive, and social sciences.

Information Systems: Is the discipline concerned with the development, use, application and influence of information technologies. An information system, following a definition of Langefors, is a technologically implemented medium for recording, storing, and disseminating linguistic expressions, as well as for drawing conclusions from such expressions.

Information Technology: Is "the study, design, development, implementation, support or management of computer-based information systems, particularly software applications and computer hardware."

Knowledge: Is (i) facts, information, and skills acquired by a person through experience or education; the theoretical or practical understanding of a subject, (ii) what is known in a particular field or in total; facts and information or (iii) awareness or familiarity gained by experience of a fact or situation. Philosophical debates in general start with Plato's formulation of knowledge as "justified true belief" .

Methodology: Is (i) the analysis of the principles of methods, rules, and postulates employed by a discipline" or (ii) the development of methods, to be applied within a discipline or (iii)a particular procedure or set of procedures.

Science: Refers to any systematic methodology which attempts to collect accurate information about reality and to model this in a way which can be used to make reliable, concrete and quantitative predictions about future events and observations. In a more restricted sense, science refers to a system of acquiring knowledge based on the scientific method, as well as to the organized body of knowledge gained through such research.

Chapter II
Medical Privacy and the Internet

D. John Doyle
Cleveland Clinic Foundation, USA

ABSTRACT

E-health technology has started to become commonplace in the clinical world, with practitioners setting up their own Web sites to disseminate educational information to patients, with physicians and nurses working as team members to access clinical information about a patient using an electronic patient chart, and with patients even conducting their own research to make informed decisions about clinical options.However, these potential benefits must be tempered from the perspective of medical privacy. Ever since the Hippocratic Oath of antiquity, protecting the privacy of patients has been an important precept of medical ethics. With technological developments, however, health information has come into use by many organizations and individuals that may be unsensitized to medical privacy concerns. This report is concerned with these issues.

INTRODUCTION

Whatsoever things I see or hear concerning the life of men, in my attendance on the sick or even apart therefrom, which ought not be noised abroad, I will keep silence thereon, counting such things to be as sacred secrets. (Oath of Hippocrates, 4th Century, B.C.E)

E-health technology based on the Internet has much to offer to the clinical world: integrated and easily-accessible electronic medical records, educational resources for clinicians, patient education Web sites, e-mail communication between patients and care givers, and a great deal more. The abundance of such capabilities and resources, it has been argued, has had a salutatory effect on patient empowerment, at least in the case of individuals on the endowed side of the "digital divide" (Pitts V, 2004; Sadan B, 2002; Akerkar SM & Bichile LS, 2004).

Such technologies can potentially benefit clinical care and patient education in a number of ways. Patients just given diagnoses of conditions such as diabetes mellitus or migraine headaches can be referred by their physicians or by health agencies to reliable sites to further learn how to manage their conditions and review the latest treatment developments. Patients can also conduct their own research to make a more informed decision about clinical options. Practitioners sometimes set up their own Web sites to disseminate educational information to patients, as well as to provide more mundane information such as office hours. Clinical Web sites can play a fundamental role in patient education and can be cheaper, more convenient, and more readily updated than the paper brochures that are ordinarily used to provide health care information, practitioner credentials, and advertising.

E-health technologies can also allow physicians working as team members, perhaps in geographically disparate locations, to access clinical information about a patient by using an electronic patient chart similar to the current paper record. By using this model, for instance, a doctor could annotate a digitized radiograph as to a possible fracture site and then send the radiograph file to a radiologist at home, with a request for a quick verbal reply by telephone. This would allow for quick second-opinion consults without requiring the doctor to leave his or her home. Laboratory reports could also automatically be sent to physicians carrying e-mail capable pagers to ensure that they are immediately notified of important test results.

However, these numerous potential benefits must also be viewed from the perspective of medical privacy. Just as privacy issues of a more general nature (such as a person's demographic information, shopping habits, travel interests, etc.) are a matter of concern with the Internet (Crichard M, 2003; Oliver H, 2002; Pincus LB & Johns R, 1997), so is the privacy of medical information. Ever since the Hippocratic Oath of antiquity, protecting the privacy of patients has been an important precept of medical ethics. However, with technological developments, health information has come into use by many organizations and individuals that may be less sensitive to medical privacy concerns. These include employers, insurers, police agencies, government administrators, vendors of health products, attorneys and others.

A CLINICAL ANECDOTE

Now that Internet access has become more commonly available, some patients are using this technology to assist in their medical care. The following personal anecdote (Doyle DJ, 1996) illustrates this point. A middle-aged man noted that for several years food would get caught in what he believed to be a pouch in his esophagus. Although usually not problematic, he noted with increasing frequency that filling of the pouch would sometimes lead to vomiting in socially embarrassing circumstances. Not having a family doctor, he sought information on his condition via friends, relatives, and the "Merck Manual", a well-respected medical reference available in both paper and electronic format. Suspicious that the description of "Zenker's diverticulum" given there matched his condition, he then did a search over the Internet (using the Lycos search engine), and came upon a reference to Zenker's diverticulum in an online article written by the author (Doyle DJ, 2007). As a result, the patient searched the Internet for my address and telephone number and later contacted me by telephone seeking clinical advice. As this patient was not in a locale where I had a medical license, this information was provided informally, outlining what investigations might be done and providing the patient with the names of some clinicians known to be experienced in esophageal conditions.

This story illustrates some of the novel ways in which patients may sometimes acquire clinical information. As the Internet and e-health continue to increase in popularity, patients will increasingly search for information about their condition and may even compare different forms of medical treatment. Blogs, discussion groups, and organization Web sites (e.g., the American Cancer Society) allow those suffering from severe medical conditions to receive medical information and emotional support for themselves, their families, and friends from those affected by the same medical condition. But the situation also raises issues related to medical privacy and confidentiality. These issues are the subject of this paper.

CATEGORIES OF INDIVIDUALS USING THE INTERNET FOR MEDICAL / E-HEALTH PURPOSES

Individuals using the Internet for medical / e-health purposes tend to fall into five categories: (1) patients and their families looking for easily understood, nontechnical health information, (2) patients wishing to make their personal health information electronically available to authorized individuals via the Internet, (3) healthcare providers looking for clinical information for their practice (such as might be part of a practitioner's "Continuing Medical Education"), (4) healthcare providers looking to provide easily understood clinical information directed at their patients, and (5) healthcare educators looking for high-quality resources that can be recommended to their students, be they patients or care givers. In all five settings potential privacy issues arise that have important policy implications.

For patients and their families looking for health information, one special advantage of using the Internet is the ease of participating in discussion forums concerning a wide range of clinical topics. This makes for useful exchanges of information and ideas, and explains the popularity of on-line services such as Yahoo! Groups (e.g., groups.yahoo.com and groups.google.com). Medically-related discussion groups can provide patients with a relatively easy way of seeking and receiving information about a specific medical condition from those familiar with the condition from personal perspectives. Such discussion groups offer the capacity for significant gains in distributing medical information, but at the same time have potential for serious drawbacks. One part of the problem is that most information offered in medical discussion groups is anecdotal and distributed by lay people who, while they may be very knowledgeable about a particular individual's condition, may lack the knowledge and resources to provide accurate and comprehensive information of a more general or more technical nature. Also, individuals suffering from chronic or terminal diseases have sometimes had their hopes raised by the prospect of a "miracle" cure, only to find that such cures are actually quack remedies. Finally, and particularly pertinent to the current discussion, when personal information such as one's e-mail address is posted at such sites, obvious privacy issues arise. For instance, a marketer of a quack remedy for AIDS (or even a legitimate charitable organization) might attempt to get e-mail addresses of visitors to an AIDS discussion forum, either directly from the postings, or indirectly from the site administrator.

Patients can also use the Internet to locate area physicians (e.g., through the American Medical Association Web site), check their credentials, and to access disciplinary reports, malpractice judgments, and arbitration awards on a particular physician. Such data are often provided in the United States through state licensing authorities. One US Web site (www.docboard.org), maintained by Administrators in Medicine (AIM), has links to state regulatory bodies, including some osteopath and podiatry licensing bodies. Local magazines in many major American cities (e.g., *Minneapolis St. Paul Magazine, Boston Magazine*) have published their surveys of best area doctors, often grouped by specialty. In Canada, the Web sites of licensing organizations often provide lists of member doctors, including those who are accepting new patients.

THE PERSONAL CLINICAL WEB PAGE

Access to emergency medical information (allergies, summaries of past hospital admissions, old electrocardiogram records, etc.) is often required when travelers are admitted to a hospital far from home. The need for such information is likely to be especially strong when a patient is unconscious at the time of entry into hospital, such as might occur following a head injury or stroke. To a substantial degree this problem has been addressed by the MedicAlert System (www.medicalert.org), which provides a very limited amount of clinical information as an inscription on a bracelet (or other device), with a phone number to call where further information can be obtained. However, Web pages have now become a common way to organize this information on the Internet. Some of these Web pages are private and require password access. This same approach might be used to provide patient information to clinicians, almost all who have access to the Internet. A brief explanation of the concept, which I originally proposed in 1995 (Doyle DJ, 1995), follows.

Essentially, the concept is that clinicians would be able to use Internet browser software to access an (unpublished) Web page whose address (URL) is given on a patient's bracelet. When prompted, the clinician would be required to enter a password, which would be provided on the patient's bracelet (and possibly at another secure place). This password arrangement would prevent unauthorized access to the Web page should someone happen to stumble upon the patient's unpublished Web page address. Once the clinician had accessed the patient's Web page, he or she would be presented with relevant clinical information placed there, including text information such as lists of medications and even hospital discharge summaries, as well as graphical images such as electrocardiograms or radiographs.

Such an arrangement would offer several potential advantages. Less human intervention would be needed to access the patient's information, as opposed to the need for an individual to answer the telephone, provide verbal information, and fax documents to the clinician. The proposed method also eliminates the need for a fax machine and is available on a 24-hour basis, essential in emergency situations. Finally, data encryption would ensure that the information would remain private, helping to ensure security beyond the use of a password.

While this concept was originally proposed a decade ago by the author (Doyle DJ, 1995), to my knowledge such a service remains commercially unavailable in the USA. While it may be that privacy concerns may be at least partly responsible for this fact, it is also likely that the potentially high costs that would necessarily be incurred in adeptly summarizing a patient's medical record and converting it to Web format would also be an important impediment, especially if such a service were not covered by medical insurance.

The above notwithstanding, the Australian site, YourHealthRecord.com (which redirects to http://www.mynetrecord.com) allows patients to maintain their own online record system, with information such as current health, past health, medications, allergies etc. made available online. Since this site is hosted in Australia, users in other nations must be sure to not to make false assumptions, based on local law, about the privacy and confidentiality of any information they enter. Similar concerns may exist at www.yourdiagnosis.com, a companion site to YourHealthRecord.com that is also hosted in Australia.

INTERNET MEDICAL DISCUSSION GROUPS

Although numerous discussion groups exist on the Internet on topics from astronomy to zoology, the development of professional discussion groups on medical topics is a more recent development. Simply stated, an Internet Medical Discussion Group (IMDG) is a network of users with Internet access sharing a common interest in some medical field. For example, IMDGs for AIDS, cancer treatment, chronic fatigue syndrome, dentistry, epilepsy, forensic medicine, medical physics, nursing and occupational medicine are all available. These discussion groups offer participants the opportunity to meet colleagues from all over the world, share clinical experiences, obtain advice, and learn new perspectives on a variety of clinical topics. Because participants tend to be distributed internationally, fresh perspectives on clinical issues are often offered.

Participation in an IMDG usually begins by posting a note to the group's participants - in essence, sending an electronic letter to all group members. To save the writer the need to keep a mailing list for all members, the letter (in actuality, an e-mail message) is sent to a list server or list processor that takes care of message distribution. Once distributed, the letter is available to all IMDG members for reading and commentary. Because responding to a message is very straightforward (merely a few keystrokes), lively helpful discussions often follow. Members can usually also reply privately, rather than to the whole group, where appropriate. The sequence of messages following an originating message is known as a thread.

Postings made to IMDGs are usually not edited or moderated, and may include accidental postings intended for other recipients, as well as postings of limited information value or postings with grammatical or factual errors. Often, postings result in further commentary from others, clarifying an issue or perhaps presenting an alternative perspective to the discussion. Still, there is usually no systematic means by which postings are scrutinized to determine suitability for the list recipients.

Before the advent of the IMDG, one could only resort to telephone communication with known experts and literature searches to find out some specialized clinical information. The IMDG serves as yet another source of topical and current information. The author has personally used an IMDG known as the Anesthesiology Discussion Group on several occasions to obtain and provide information difficult to get by other means. In one instance, after an anesthetic for liver transplantation that required the administration of 142 units of blood, I described the case to the discussion group, initiating a lengthy discussion that provided clinical hints to all who do liver transplantation anesthesia. In another case, I asked about the clinical use of pentastarch for cardiac surgery and was put in touch with clinicians experienced with use of the product. In yet another instance, in preparation for a planned animal experiment, I wrote privately to a veterinary anesthetist who frequently contributes to the list to inquire about using propofol for canine anesthesia.

Naturally, in all such instances special care must be taken to ensure that privacy of medical information is maintained, especially when clinicians communicate with one another to discuss or debate various management options in complex cases. In addition, besides the privacy tradition established by Hippocrates *(What I may see or hear in the course of the treatment ... I will keep to myself, holding such things shameful to be spoken about)*, clinicians may be bound by specific national regulatory requirements (*vide infra*).

INTERNET-BASED PATIENT PORTALS

Some clinics have implemented Internet-based patient portals for communication between patients and health-care workers (Liederman EM & Morefield CS, 2003). Such portals allow patients to send messages directly to their physicians in a secure manner in order to request advice, obtain appointments, get prescription refills, and obtain referrals. In addition, such portals may offer information such as clinic hours, as well as advice for dealing with commonly encountered clinical problems such as headaches, diarrhea, etc.

In a study by Lin et al. (Lin CT, Wittevrongel L, Moore L, Beaty BL, & Ross SE, 2005) the authors conducted a randomized controlled trial involving 606 patients to study the impact of a patient portal "on patients' satisfaction with access to their clinic and clinical care" and "the content and volume of email messages and telephone calls from patients to their clinic". The "portal" users were able to "send secure messages directly to their physicians and to request appointments, prescription refills, and referrals" while the control patients received standard care. The authors found that the portal users "demonstrated increased satisfaction with communication and overall care" and that they "particularly valued the portal's convenience, reduced communication barriers, and direct physician responses".

Although use of such portals remains somewhat limited, initial experiences have been positive, both from the perspective patients and of care-givers. Still, some health-care workers remain reluctant to communicate online with patients, citing concerns of an increased workload, perils to patient privacy and increased medico-legal concerns.

CLINICAL USE OF E-MAIL

One particularly important medical-technical issue concerns the use of e-mail in healthcare environments, where matters of privacy, security and confidentiality in relation to medical information exist. In response to these concerns, the American Medical Informatics Association (http://www.amia.org) has published guidelines for e-mail communication and for administrative and medico-legal aspects of the use of e-mail (Kane B & Sands DZ, 1998). These guidelines include: (1) not using e-mail for urgent matters (where telephone contact is preferred), (2) informing patients about who actually handles received e-mail messages (a job often handled by receptionists), (3) establishing the types of transactions permitted using e-mail, and (4) instructing patients to note the type of transaction in the subject line of the message to allow filtering. The association also provides guidelines on instructing patients on when to escalate to phone calls or to go to the hospital, on not forwarding patient-identifiable information to a third party without prior patient permission, on carefully checking all "To" fields prior to sending e-mail messages, and on matters of e-mail encryption and backup.

Since the use of e-mail and the Web by patients would be expected to be among the most popular means of electronically communicating with clinicians, it is of interest to consider the experiences and attitudes of patients in this regard. Hassol et al. (Hassol A et al., 2004) sought to "evaluate patients' values and perceptions regarding Web-based communication with their primary care providers in the context of access to their electronic health care record". This was done via an online survey sent to 4,282 patients using an electronic health record system known as "MyChart", where data was collected on user satisfaction, ease of use, communication preferences, and other matters. The authors found that "only a minority of users were concerned about the confidentiality of their information" and that "patients preferred e-mail communication for some interactions (e.g., requesting prescription renewals, obtaining general medical information), whereas they preferred in-person communication for others (e.g., getting treatment instructions)".

In February 2005, the Canadian Medical Association (CMA) created a policy entitled *Physician Guidelines for Online Communication with Patients* which is available at http://policybase.cma.ca/dbtw-wpd/PolicyPDF/PD05-03.pdf. This document is rich in practical advice, such as the following advice about providing advice to individuals who are not part of a physician's medical practice:

> **Non-patients:** Physicians should take care to avoid appearing to provide medical advice to non-patients and inadvertently establishing a patient–physician relationship through the exchange of information. Devices such as notices on open Web sites describing who the information on the site is for, the use of closed (password protected) Web sites and a standard automated response to non-patients can be used to this end.

Another interesting piece of advice in this document concerns "virtual patients":

> **Virtual patients:** Currently, a variety of guidelines appear to discourage or forbid a purely online or virtual patient–physician relationship. Emphasis is generally placed on the importance of face-to-face, in-person encounters and the use of electronic communications only as a means of follow-up, clarification, monitoring, etc., within the context of an existing relationship. However, through telehealth technology, clinicians have been developing practice protocols that are allowing them to provide care at a distance. This is an emerging field and as the sophistication of technology and the users of it increases, the current reluctance may well be revisited. This may be especially so in cases where physical access to a physician is severely limited or non-existent (for example, in remote or emergency settings) and the benefits of a virtual relationship are demonstrably better than no access at all.

In addition, the CMA has also developed a "privacy tool" which allows clinicians to create a personalized patient confidentiality policy for their practice. This tool is available at http://www.cma.ca/index.cfm/ci_id/40833/la_id/1.htm (registration required).

TELEMEDICINE AND THE INTERNET

The use of the Internet as an aid to clinical care has been especially valuable for the practice of telemedicine, where patients are often located at great distances from care givers (White P, 2004; Hyler SE & Gangure DP, 2004). This is especially in the realm of radiology, where x-ray, CT-scan and MRI images may be sent as ordinary e-mail attachments to clinical consultants.

However, the popularization of telemedicine has introduced a number of special issues in the realm of medical licensing and jurisdiction. In the USA, several states have recently adopted legislation that addresses licensing requirements for interstate practice. In some cases these statutes have required out-of-state physicians to obtain a license to provide medical services to patients located in the state that are being treated using electronic communications and have placed restrictions on the nature of physician-to-physician consultations, such as second opinions on the interpretation of biopsies and tests or imaging interpretations for x-ray or ultrasound studies.

For instance, in Texas the practice of medicine act was modified in 1995 to include the following provision: "A person who is physically located in another jurisdiction but who, through the use of any medium, including an electronic medium, performs an act that is part of a patient care service initiated in this state, including the taking of an x-ray examination or the preparation of pathological material for examination, and that would affect the diagnosis or treatment of the patient, is engaged in the practice of medicine in this state for the purposes of this Act. (2007). This means that individuals who practice telemedicine on Texans must have a Texas medical license. Similar issues also exist in Europe and elsewhere.

Such issues raise many medico-legal issues. If state lines are crossed through telemedicine, which physician is liable in the event of substandard care: the consulting physician or the referring physician? And which state licensing board should bring the suit? It may be that in cases of malpractice, the patient has the option to bring a malpractice suit against the physician using telemedicine in three states: the physician's state, the patient's state, or any state with which the physician has established sufficient telemedicine business links.

A related matter concerns difficulties raised by the possible need to obtain special consent from telemedicine patients. This concern may be of special importance in the practice of tele-psychiatry (Gritzalis S, 2004). While some of the processes that take place during a telemedical visit consultation will be unique, it is likely that the legal principles that apply to the conventional, face-to-face, doctor-patient relationship are equally as valid in the context of the practice of telemedicine.

In a loosely related matter, Nelson (Nelson SB, 2006) provides a cautionary tale about American hospitals and clinics that may wish to subcontract medical records work to individuals and institutions outside the USA, where the legal and regulatory environment can be very different:

A recent incident at a California hospital illustrates this problem. The hospital contracted with a Florida company to transcribe dictation. The Florida company subcontracted to a Texas company that further subcontracted to a woman in Pakistan, who became frustrated by slow payment for her work. The woman tried to blackmail the hospital by threatening exposure of patient records if she was not paid immediately. Data paths and control can be difficult to follow in an era of international out-sourcing.

SEXUAL HEALTH AND THE INTERNET

It is sometimes claimed that sex and health matters are the two most popular subjects for Internet browsing. If it is true, then the use of the Internet as an aid to the marketing of Viagra® (sildenafil) and other pharmaceutical products to treat erectile dysfunction must surely be an concern. Not only is there literally thousands of sites offering information on Viagra®, Levitra® and Cialis® (with many sites offering information of dubious value), but the drugs themselves can be sometimes be bought on the Internet without a prior prescription (see for instance, http://kwikmed.com/).

The medico-legal issues in this practice are obvious. For instance, in many cases the patient does not receive a traditional physical exam by a physician, but rather completes a detailed online questionnaire and communicates with a physician using secure online communication. In fact, specifically in response to these concerns, the American Medical Association has issued a warning about this practice, pointing out that drug information at these sites is often written in medical terminology that the lay person cannot understand, and noting that the patients are provided neither with a proper physical nor a follow-up visit to determine whether the drug worked or exhibited side-effects (Baldwin G, 1999).

It appears that the manufacturers of Viagra, Levitra and Cialis have not ignored the use of the Internet to boost sales. For instance, at the official Levitra site (www.levitra.com) visitors can learn about their free trial program, how to get a prescription filled online, and answers to common questions. For individuals who are shy with their doctor, the site also offers a number of suggestions and opening scripts to help address the topic of erectile dysfunction *("My erections just aren't as hard and lasting as they used to be. What can LEVITRA do to improve my erectile function?")*. A past version of the site even allowed users to send free electronic greeting cards bearing the

Levitra logo. Finally, a section for health care professionals is also provided.

While this site is uncommonly well-designed and informative (possibly a consequence of regulatory matters), users who want to participate in special offers must enter personal information (name, address, date of birth, e-mail address, racial group, health status, sexual matters etc.) that raises obvious privacy issues.

So commercially valuable is the Internet traffic related to erectile dysfunction that even the misspellings of erectile dysfunction related Web sites have been taken for marketing purposes (examples: cialsi.com, viagar.com, levitar.com and countless others).

UNPROVEN TREATMENTS

The Internet has been especially useful to individuals wishing to promote unproven clinical treatments. An Internet search using the term "alternative medicine" will produce hundreds upon hundreds of hits covering chiropractic, homeopathy, iridology, reflexology and many other controversial therapies. Many of these sites offer useless or even dangerous products for sale. Many sites also have a legal disclaimer such as the following (from http://www.aviva.ca):

The products, information, services and other content provided on and through this site, including without limitation any products, information, services and other content provided on any Linked Site, are provided for informational purposes only to facilitate discussions with a healthcare professional regarding treatment. The information on this Web site is often provided in summary or aggregate form, and may not be construed as medical advice or instruction. All information and product descriptions on this website are provided for educational purposes only. No action should be taken solely on the content of this website, regardless of perceived scientific merit. Users should consult their health care professionals on any matter related to their health.

Presumably, the authors feel that this warning is sufficient to ward off any legal trouble should any misinformation provided lead to harm.

Associated with the concern of patient safety in this setting is that of the privacy of any communications between an individual and those offering such treatments. While some well-established Web sites like www.alternativemedicine.com have privacy policies, many (perhaps most) such sites do not. A natural concern is that patients seeking information or therapies at such sites have confidential information shared with other vendors as a means of developing more sales leads.

PRIVACY OF CARE GIVERS

One interesting related privacy issue concerns the privacy of care givers. A number of US states now put malpractice data on the Internet. For instance, the State of Virginia makes practitioner information available at http://www.vahealthprovider.com, while the Federation of State Medical Boards of the United States offers a national fee-based service at http://www.docinfo.org. The Health Grade site at http://www.healthgrades.com provides data on disciplinary actions against doctors taken for medical incompetence, sexual misconduct, criminal convictions, ethical lapses and other offenses. Other sites such as http://www.medicalmalpractice.com and www.sue-a-doctor.com are offered as resources to individuals who are unsatisfied with the medical care they have received. Such sites raise obvious concerns to some individuals. Although some care givers embrace such developments in theory, many are worried about the use of malpractice information as an indicator of competence or quality. Cynics argue that the medico-legal systems in Canada and the USA are so haphazard that good doctors are just as likely to be sued as those who may be practicing below the standard of care. Others contend that the public may misinterpret malpractice history data and punish capable doctors who happen to treat a large number of high-risk patients. Finally, concerns may be raised as to the accuracy of the information provided and the means available for care givers to correct inaccuracies that might arise in the public record.

THE QUEST FOR SOLUTIONS

In response to privacy and confidentiality concerns, governments and regulatory agencies around the world are taking a serious look at protecting medical data from unauthorized scrutiny. Consequently, as the uses and users of sensitive medical information have multiplied, so have proposed and implemented regulatory and technical protections. In some countries, increased accountability is now being required of organizations that collect, market, or distribute medical and related information. In the USA the recent implementation of the Health Insurance Portability and Accountability Act (HIPPA) (Rovner JA, 2004; Gunn PP et al., 2004) has had a major impact on how medical information is handled. Patients in many countries now have the right to see who has examined their health records and to correct inaccurate or incomplete data, similar to how consumers in many countries can review and correct their credit and financial records. In particular, HIPAA provides a lengthy list of information items that are considered to be privileged and require special handling. These are listed in Table 1.

In addition to regulatory guidelines, a variety of potential technological solutions exist that can be adapted to help maintain the privacy of medical information. For instance, data encryption and secure data transmission methods can prevent the interception of personal information by anyone, including even law enforcement and intelligence

Table 1. Information classified as protected health information by the Health Insurance Portability and Accountability Act of 1996 (HIPAA).

• Name
• Geographic subdivisions smaller than a state
• Dates, including date of birth, admission, discharge, death
• Telephone number
• Fax number
• E-mail address
• Social Security number
• Medical record number
• Health-plan beneficiary number
• Account number
• Certificate/license number
• Vehicle identification, including license plate
• Device identifiers and serial numbers
• Web site addresses, uniform resource locators (URLs)
• Internet Protocol (IP) addresses
• Biometric identifiers, including voice and finger prints
• Full-face photos and comparable images
• Any other unique identifying number or characteristic

From Nelson SB. Privacy and medical information on the Internet. Respir Care. 2006;51:183-7 and based on Standards for privacy of individually identifiable health information. US Department of Health and Human Services, Office of Civil Rights. 45 CFR §164.514(b)(2)(i) December 28, 2000. Amended April 17, 2003. (Available online at http://www.hhs.gov/ocr/combinedregtext.pdf)

agencies (at least if done with adequate knowledge and care) (Gritzalis S, 2004).

With information interception addressed, the next questions to be answered are what kinds of medically related information should be collected and what use of this information is acceptable? For example, the use of "cookies" in Web browsers may allow one to track a person's use of a particular Web site. Should such information be sold to third parties, there is potential for the violation of one's privacy. For instance, information about an individual's repeated visits to sites for AIDS (acquired immune deficiency syndrome) information, herpes information, drug addiction resources etc., could potentially be sold to insurance companies or others by unscrupulous site owners. Consider also a marketer of a quack remedy for AIDS who gets e-mail addresses of visitors to an AIDS Web site from a dishonest site owner in an effort to generate sales (or seek contributions in the case of a charitable organization).

The complexities of using the Internet to support clinical care raises many issues which will only be resolved as legislation is passed and as common law rulings accumulate. If a patient is harmed or injured by a physician's (or even their own) misinterpretation of information posted on the Web, who is responsible? What about the case where the information posted is incorrect? If e-mail is "intercepted" containing confidential patient information, what are the liability issues? Legal liability issues also figure prominently in any discussion of inaccurate and potentially harmful medical information. Jurisdiction becomes relevant, given the international nature of the Web. Questions arise as to who is responsible if unverified and ultimately harmful information is distributed via a discussion group. Is the person volunteering that information liable, or is it always *caveat emptor*? What onus is there on individuals who use this content? What responsibility, if any, do Web site and UseNet administrators bear? In cases of international communication, in whose legal jurisdiction would liability proceedings take place? Should liability claims apply only to peer-reviewed or organization certified sites? These questions must ultimately be addressed so the legal and medical communities can best utilize the enormous potential the Internet offers. Until these issues are adequately addressed, many physicians and patients will avoid or restrict their use of the Internet for medical purposes.

CONCLUSION

As emphasized earlier, Internet technology has the potential to offer much to the clinical world. But these many benefits must also be viewed from the perspective of medical privacy. Fortunately, technological solutions already exist that can be readily adapted to maintain patient privacy.

Figure 1.

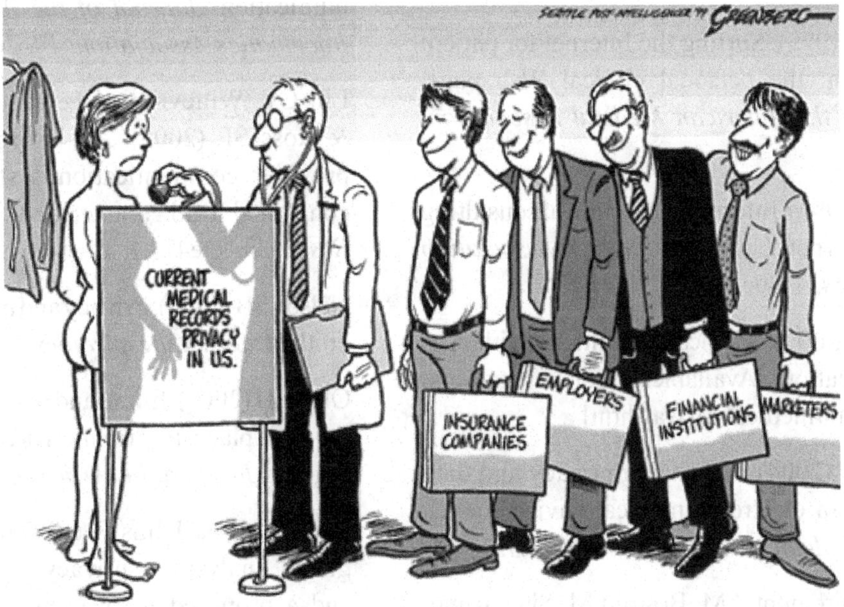

From http://www.reuben.org/greenberg/.Toons/.Toons,%20social/qqxsgMedical%20privacy.gif. Reproduced with permission.

For instance, data encryption and secure data transmission technologies can help prevent the interception of personal information by anyone other than authorized individuals. Coupled with this are supporting government regulations (such as the US Health Insurance Portability and Accountability Act) that have been passed in recent years. Correctly implemented, such developments will help guarantee medical privacy on the Internet.

REFERENCES

Akerkar SM & Bichile LS (2004). Health information on the internet: patient empowerment or patient deceit? *Indian Journal of Medical Sciences, 58,* 326.

Baldwin G (1999). AMA warns doctors on dangers of Web pill pushing. amednews.com *The Newspaper for America's Physicians.* Retrieved from www.ama-assn.org/amednews/1999/pick_99/biza0719.htm

Crichard M (2003). Privacy and electronic communications. *Computer Law and Security Report, 19,* 299-303.

Doyle DJ (1995). Surfing the Internet for patient information: the personal clinical Web page. *Journal of the American Medical Association, 274,* 1586.

Doyle DJ (1996). Informational clinical consulting via the Internet. *Canadian Medical Association Journal, 154,* 1180.

Doyle DJ (2007). Medical Conditions with Airway Implications. Available: http://anestit.unipa.it/anestit/gta/medical-airway.html

Gritzalis S (2004). Enhancing privacy and data protection in electronic medical environments. *Journal of Medical Systems, 28,* 535-547.

Gunn PP, Fremont AM, Bottrell M, Shugarman LR, Galegher J, & Bikson T (2004). The Health Insurance Portability and Accountability Act Privacy Rule: a practical guide for researchers. *Medical Care, 42,* 321-327.

Hassol A, Walker JM, Kidder D, Rokita K, Young D, Pierdon S et al. (2004). Patient experiences and attitudes about access to a patient electronic health care record and linked web messaging. *Journal of the American Medical Informatics Association, 11,* 505-513.

Hyler SE & Gangure DP (2004). Legal and ethical challenges in telepsychiatry. *Journal of Psychiatric Practice, 10,* 272-276.

Kane B & Sands DZ (1998). Guidelines for the clinical use of electronic mail with patients. The AMIA Internet working group, task force on guidelines for the use of clinic-patient electronic mail. *Journal of the American Medical Informatics Association, 5,* 104-111.

Legislation affecting telemedicine licensure (1995-1997) (2007). *Council on Licensure, Enforcement and Regulation.* Retrieved from www.clearhq.org/teletable2.htm

Liederman EM & Morefield CS (2003). Web messaging: a new tool for patient-physician communication. *Journal of the American Medical Informatics Association, 10,* 260-270.

Lin CT, Wittevrongel L, Moore L, Beaty BL, & Ross SE (2005). An Internet-based patient-provider communication system: randomized controlled trail. *Journal of Medical Internet Research, 7,* e47.

Nelson SB (2006). Privacy and medial information on the Internet. *Respiratory Care, 51,* 183-187.

Oliver H (2002). Email and internet monitoring in the workplace: Information privacy and contracting-out. *Industrial Law Journal, 31,* 321-352.

Pincus LB & Johns R (1997). Private Parts: A global analysis of privacy protection schemes and a proposed innovation for their comparative evaluation. *Journal of Business Ethics, 16,* 1237-1260.

Pitts V (2004). Illness and Internet empowerment: writing and reading breast cancer in cyberspace. *Health (London), 8,* 33-59.

Rovner JA (2004). Making sense of HIPAA Privacy: solutions for complex compliance dilemmas. *Journal of Health Law, 37,* 399-427.

Sadan B (2002). Patient empowerment and the asymmetry of knowledge. *Studies in Health Technology and Informatics, 90,* 514-518.

White P (2004). Privacy and security issues in teleradiology. *Seminars in Ultrasound, CT, and MR, 25,* 391-395.

KEY TERMS

Blog: A blog ("Web log") is a journal, often of a personal nature, published on the web, and usually updated periodically using a "blogging" software package.

Cookie: A small text file that some Web sites place on a user's computer, containing information such as one's user ID, user preferences, shopping cart information, etc so that preferences can remembered on future visits to the Web site.

E-Mail: Electronic mail composed on a computer system and transmitted over a network. Messages sent may include attached files.

IP Address: A number that uniquely identifies each sender or receiver of information on the Internet.

Linked Site: A web site or other resource that is easily accessed via hyperlink using a Web browser.

Search Engine: A software program that searches documents (usually Internet documents) for specified words or phrases and provides a list of the documents where the specified words or phrases were found.

Telehealth: An all-encompassing term describing the use of telecommunications, information technology, and health education to improve health care.

Telemedicine: The use of telecommunications technology such as video conferencing for clinical diagnosis and treatment, especially where the clinician and patient are physically far apart.

URL: An acronym for "Uniform Resource Locator" or address of a resource on the Internet.

Chapter III
Security of Electronic Medical Records

Ana Ferreira
University of Kent, UK & University of Porto, Portugal

Ricardo Cruz-Correia
CINTESIS, Portugal & University of Porto, Portugal

Luís Antunes
LIACC, University of Porto, Portugal

David Chadwick
University of Kent, UK

ABSTRACT

This chapter reports the authors' experiences regarding security of the electronic medical record (EMR). Although the EMR objectives are to support shared care and healthcare professionals' workflow, there are some barriers that prevent its successful use. These barriers comprise not only costs, regarding resources and time, but also patient / health professional relations, ICT (information and communication technologies) education as well as security issues. It is very difficult to evaluate EMR systems; however some studies already made show problems regarding usability and proper healthcare workflow modeling. Legislation to guide the protection of health information systems is also very difficult to implement in practice. This chapter shows that access control, as a part of an EMR, can be a key to minimize some of its barriers, if the means to design, develop and evaluate access control are closer to users' needs and workflow complexity.

INTRODUCTION

Healthcare is information and knowledge driven. Good healthcare depends on taking decisions at the right time and place, according to the right patient data and applicable knowledge (Friedman C and Wyatt J, 2006). Communication is of most relevance in today's healthcare settings, as health related activities, such as delivery of care, research and management, depend on information sharing and teamwork (Coiera, 2003).

Providing high-quality health care services is an information-dependent process. Indeed, the practice of medicine has been described as being dominated by how well information is processed or reprocessed, retrieved, and communicated (Barnett, 1990). An estimated 35 to 39 percent of total hospital operating costs has been associated with patient and professional communication activities (Richart, 1970). Physicians spend over a quarter (Commission, 1995, Mamlin and Baker, 1973) and nurses half (Korpman and Lincoln, 1998) of their time writing up patients' charts.

Patient records exist to memorize and communicate the data regarding a particular individual and to help deliver care to him or her. Records are not only an information system but also a communication system, to enable communication between different health professionals and between the past and present (Dick and Steen, 1997, Nygren et al., 1998). Patient records, the patient and published evidence are the three sources needed for the practice of evidence-based medicine (Friedman C and Wyatt J, 2006).

After decades of development of information systems, designed primarily for physicians and other healthcare managers and professionals, there is an increasing interest in reaching consumers and patients directly through computers and telecommunication systems (Chuva Mt et al., 2006). Consumer health informatics is designed to empower consumers by putting health information into their hands, including information on their own health, such as diagnoses, lab results, personal risk factors and prescribed drugs. All this information requires strong security means.

Information security is usually defined by three main characteristics (Cen/Tc251), (Harris S, 2003): confidentiality – the prevention of unauthorized disclosure of the information; integrity – the prevention of unauthorized modification of the information; availability – the prevention of unauthorized withholding of the information. Confidentiality is often used interchangeably with privacy but they are not exactly the same. Privacy is the right of an individual to not have their private information exposed (and this is usually enforceable by law), whilst confidentiality is limiting access to information to authorised individuals only.

The complexity of building secure information systems relates mainly to three fundamental and competing factors: the complexity of the security technology itself; the difficulty of classifying the information that is to be protected; and the use of the technology by humans (usually the most problematic factor (Schneier B, 2004)). Other important but secondary competing factors are: protecting information from unauthorised access whilst needing to be able to access it for audit or law enforcement purposes; and making it easy for an authorised user to gain access to the information but complex for an unauthorised user to do the same.

LEGISLATION

The Health Insurance Portability and Accountability Act (HIPAA) of 1996 (USA Congress, 1996) is the American legislation that provides for the security and privacy as well as health insurance for American workers and their families. Title I of HIPAA protects health insurance coverage for workers and their families when they change or lose their jobs. Title II of HIPAA, the Administrative Simplification (AS) provisions, requires the establishment of national standards for electronic health care transactions and national identifiers for providers, health insurance plans, and employers. The AS provisions also address the security and privacy of health data. The standards are meant to improve the efficiency and effectiveness of the nation's health care system by encouraging the widespread use of electronic data interchange in the US health care system. Despite all this defined legislation, and no matter the status of IT or financial resources, compliance with HIPAA and functional implementation of EMR systems requires a change in the culture of an organization (Knitz M, 2005).

The European experience on the same matters is described in a 1997 recommendation (Ministers Committee, 1997) from the European Community that established to all its members a set of principles and recommendations regarding the protection of medical data. From these we highlight the following security recommendations:

9.2: In order to ensure in particular the confidentiality, integrity and accuracy of processed data, as well as the protection of patients, appropriate measures should be taken:

- **e:** with a view to selective **access to data** and the security of the medical data, to ensure that the processing as a general rule is so designed as to enable the separation of: identifiers and data relating to the identity of persons; administrative data; medical data; social data; genetic data

In 2004 the European Community (Ministers Committee, 2004) made some more recommendations on the impact of information technologies on health care – the patient and Internet.

As an example, in October 1998 Portugal adopted all these recommendations (law 67/98 —Personal Data Protection, and later law 12/2005 on Personal Genetic Health Information). It is, however, interesting to present the summary of two studies made in Portugal on this subject. The first one was made by the Portuguese National Data Protection Commission (CNPD) in 2004, and is a report on the health information processing status of most Portuguese Hospitals; the second is a study made by some medical students at Hospital de São João, Porto, regarding the opinions of medical doctors about access control, further described in the Access Control Section within this chapter (Pinho C et al., 2006).

Regarding the CNPD report we highlight the following conclusions: (note that this study was made in 2004 and since then some anomalies are bound to have been corrected):

- The CNPD was not notified, as is mandatory by law, in 50% of the cases where health information is processed.
- Patients where not informed when their data was used for research purposes.
- In 35% of the applications, there was not a logical separation between health information and administrative data.
- Regarding passwords, 172 applications had it whilst 12 did not. The most commonly used password is the users' name.
- In 136 applications only 2 followed the conservation time enforced by the CNPD.
- Regarding the health information that was kept in paper, confidentiality was not a concern. Requests and information travel through the hospital without any kind of protection.

Furthermore, the European Union's data protection directive (in effect since October 1998) requires all member countries to enact legislation enabling patients to have access to their medical records (Eysenbach, 2000). This Recommendation (Ministers Committee, 1997) also defines that patients should be able to access their clinical information whenever they request and have means to control who can see and change that information. However, this is still not common practice mostly because of logistic and also cultural issues. The general idea is that healthcare professionals think that patient's access to their medical records may negatively affect their relationship with the patients. Patients themselves do not know if they want to see their medical record and if they do, will it be helpful and will they understand it anyway.

There are however some studies that show that patients' access to their medical records brings more benefits than not, and so the authors believe this is prone to become more common in the years to come (Ferreira A et al., 2007a).

EMR INTEGRATION AND SECURITY

The introduction of the EMR within healthcare organizations depends on integrating heterogeneous information that is usually scattered over different locations (Waegemann C, 2003, Cruz-Correia R et al., 2005). This is why the EMR is becoming an essential source of information and an important support tool for the healthcare professional. There is also an increasing need to access healthcare information at remote locations (Institute, 2005). This and the distributed nature of the information stress the need for security requirements to be taken seriously (Bakker A, 2004). In healthcare organisations that require intra and inter-organizational interactions, authorisation and access control mechanisms cannot only be organized at a user level, but need also to be defined at other levels that can reflect those dynamic interactions. To do this, a series of structured and formal policies, models and roles must be defined (Blobel, 2004).

Although standardization and data exchangeability are topics that receive global attention, many of the healthcare applications are highly dedicated and specific to the environment in which they are used. Their functions range from pure administrative and billing to the creation of research databases, decision support, picture archiving, and image analysis.

Experience has shown that physicians are horizontal users of information technology (Greenes and Shortliffe, 1990). Rather than becoming power users of a narrowly defined software package, they tend to seek broad functionality across a wide variety of systems and resources. Thus, routine use of computers, and of EMR, will be most easily achieved if the computing environment offers a critical mass of functionality that makes the system both smoothly integrated and useful for essentially every patient encounter. Also, many computer applications today use information from several data sources.

With the introduction of networked systems within our healthcare organizations, there are new opportunities to integrate a wide variety of resources through single clinical workstations. In such an environment, diverse clinical, financial, and administrative databases need to be accessed and integrated, typically by using both networks to tie them together and a variety of standards for sharing data among them. Thus the clinical data repository has developed as an increasingly common idea.

Patient data quality in computer-based patient records has been found to be rather low in several health information systems (Hogan and Wagner, 1997, Hammond et al., 2003, Hohnloser et al., 1994). Furthermore, the assessment of the correctness of collected patient data is a difficult process even when we are familiar with the system in which it was collected (Berner and Moss, 2005). Therefore, one of the main challenges of health information systems or networks is to be able to gather the different parts of the medical record of a patient without any risk to mix them with those of another patient (Quantin et al., 2004, Arellano and Weber, 1998). Erroneous patient identification has also an impact on hospital charging, as subsidiary partners refuse to pay for misidentified medical procedures.

In May 2003, the Department of Biostatistics and Medical Informatics implemented a virtual electronic patient record (Cruz-Correia et al.,

2005) for the Hospital S. João (HSJ), a university hospital with over 1350 beds. The system integrates clinical data from 10 legacy hospital departments information systems (HDIS) and the diagnosis related groups (DRG) and hospital administrative databases (HAD), aiming to deliver the maximum information possible to health professionals. Over 800 medical doctors use the system on a daily basis and the HSJ-VEPR retrieves an average of 3000 new reports each day (in PDF or HTML formats).

To detect and prevent possible problems in the HSJ-VEPR, Nagios (Koffler and Galstad, 2002) version 2 (a system and network monitoring application) was installed and configured (Cruz-Correia et al., 2006). Sometimes a HDIS sends an abnormal number per day (either too big or to small) of reports to HSJ-VEPR. This normally reflects some kind of HDIS problem. It was decided to develop a dynamic system that learns from the number of reports received previously in the same weekday and implement it as a Nagios plug-in. To define an initial knowledge base, a table was created where each record included the number of reports of a particular HDIS in a particular week day (Table 1). The system calculates percentile 2.5 and 97.5 to be used as lower and higher margins of the normality interval.

The comparison of current and previous IS behavior allows the detection of irregularities. In this case the knowledge used to trigger alerts is build from past experience. We feel that as the time goes, we will have more records and consequently the percentiles for normality the range can be changed from [2.5, 97.5] to [1, 99] increasing even more the method specificity.

Table 1. Percentiles 2.5 and 97.5 of reports sent in 2005 by a particular HDIS

Percentile	Mon.	Tue.	Wed.	Thu.	Fri.	Sat.	Sun.
2.5	82	100	148	121	99	45	40
97.5	561	595	560	674	668	300	364

One of the main challenges of health information systems integration is to gather parts of the medical record without jeopardizing patient data quality. The HSJ-VEPR indexes all information to a unique hospital patient number. Identification problems occur when the hospital patient number or the hospital encounter number that are being sent by the HDIS are wrong (Cruz-Correia R et al., 2006). These errors could lead to associating the report to a different patient.

The idea of detecting identification errors is based on checking the name and date of birth sent by the HDIS against the hospital administrative database (HAD). The main difficulty arises from small changes in patient names, which would originate false identification errors (e.g.: "Jessica Maria Smith Murphy" <=> "Jessica Maria S. Murphy").

The patient data quality algorithm is triggered with the arrival of a new clinical report from a particular HDIS, and is divided in three phases: 1st detect errors in hospital patient number, 2nd detect errors in hospital encounter numbers and 3rd store report in HSJ-VEPR .

When errors occur, a report is generated and sent to the HDIS administrators. This report includes a description of the error along with all information sent by HDIS and retrieved from HAD. By doing so, the origin of the error can be traced and corrected.

This module has been deployed in July 2005, and is being configured for each HDIS. Currently it scans an average of 65.000 reports per month (2.100 per day). In the first 6 months 423 patient identification errors were found within 391.258 reports checked.

The detection of these errors has triggered both their correction on each HDIS as well as a change on department workflow which resulted in less identification errors. Two errors where also found on HAD, caused by inappropriate re-utilization of a unique hospital patient number.

Cross-checking between integrated distributed systems may be used to guarantee global patient data quality and integrity. As proper checking methods are put in place, the number of inconsistencies in integrated systems tends to decrease as people awareness of these silent problems increases.

As stated in (Institute, 2005) the main factor that is driving the need for EMR systems to be implemented is the need to improve clinical processes or workflow efficiency. Also, as stated in (Lehoux P, 2006), information technologies are used in healthcare to record, transmit and provide access to administrative and clinical information, so this should imply that access to and use of information respects confidentiality and brings efficiency and quality to healthcare. For now, the reality is that EMRs still do not integrate easily among healthcare professionals' daily workflow (Miller R. H and Sim I, 2004) in order to be efficiently used.

One obstacle mentioned by healthcare professionals for the use and integration of EMR within healthcare is patient privacy (Knitz M, 2005). As stated above, in order to protect patients' privacy it is essential to at least provide for information confidentiality. When asked, healthcare professionals say they think EMR have problems in terms of security due to its ease of distribution and wider online access (Miller R. H et al., 2004).

There are also other barriers that impede the effective integration of EMR within the healthcare practice. These barriers can be grouped in: time/cost, relational and educational (Sprague L, 2004, Miller R. H and Sim I, 2004). Apart from the cost of EMR integration and the time healthcare professionals spend using the system in order to access and insert information there are other issues that relate more with human processes and their daily tasks. These are the relational and educational barriers explained below.

The relational barrier includes the perceptions that the physician and the patient have about the use of the EMR and how their relationship may be affected by it. As an example, when the physician uses the computer during a consultation, the patient may be uncomfortable with the lack of attention given to him and have doubts about the information being written.

The educational barrier comprises the lack of proficiency and difficulties that healthcare professionals have in interacting with the EMR in order to perform their daily tasks (Becker and Sewell, 2004). Because healthcare professionals do not participate in the design and development of working tools (in this case the EMR), they usually have to redesign their practice workflow and processes, which is very challenging and consumes more time and costs (Miller R. H and Sim I, 2004). In order to facilitate their daily workflow, since they access and use the EMR, the users must be involved in its design and development as they were within the case study described above in the HSJ (Ferreira A et al., 2005).

Although there is usually an initial plan describing the rules to access an EMR, devised by engineers, promoters and implementers, its access in practice is often different from what was envisaged and decided at first (Kling R, 1991, Lehoux P et al., 1999). Users may have to reorganize their tasks and routines to accommodate the system; or they may even circumvent the rules that have been established for accessing the system (Lehoux P et al., 1999, Akrich M, 1994) because they were too cumbersome or time-consuming or both (e.g. by sliding in a personal ID card and keying in a password).

An EMR should focus on helping and facilitating users to follow their daily processes without much effort and time. It should improve the working life of the health care professionals and bring benefits to them and their patients, rather than imposing costs on them, in terms of time and effort, with no perceivable benefits to either them or their patients. Therefore new security models and technologies to be implemented should focus on human processes and needs rather than on theoretical studies.

INFORMATION SYSTEMS EVALUATION

Many of the problems presented previously could be avoided if proper systems' evaluation could be provided and means to redesign and improve the system were easy to apply. This evaluation should be done, ideally, before, during and after information system's development and installation. How do we know if a system is really working and performing the way it is supposed to? How can we know how to improve and better adapt that system either because the circumstances or the objectives changed? The answer is, of course: evaluation.

The developing and good design of usable technology is very important as these can make users more productive and comfortable when using the system. Once more, the emphasis is usually on technology and not on users when systems are developed. Developers do not usually understand users, their tasks, workflow and environment. A system interface is the bridge between both the world of technology and the world of the user, the means by which the user interact with the system (Hackos Joann and Redish Janice, 1998). What can be more important than making sure people use the system in their natural physical, social and cultural environment?

For example in (Brostoff et al., 2005) usability and design methods were used to evaluate a specific software tool. Questionnaires were also applied to achieve a more generic feeling for the tool. According to their results, this evaluation and interface redesign improved its efficiency, making the tool easier to use and understand.

Another example is briefly described in (Hackos Joann and Redish Janice, 1998) where programmers designing a medical records' system completely changed their initial software interface after they visited the site. They discovered that the workflow among departments and individuals proceeded in a different manner to what they had imagined. They watched people performing their tasks and interviewed medical records' staff about the nature of their work. The message then is to design from reality and not from assumptions. In conclusion, evaluation methods must focus on users' behaviour as well as attitudes and opinions.

However, healthcare information systems' evaluation is not trivial (Friedman C and Wyatt J, 2006). Medical informatics is a combination of domains that makes any evaluation very complex and never definitive. There is not a specific method for all cases and one of the most important things to take into account is to choose the right method at the right moment in time. The following section presents a review about IS evaluation.

The authors performed a brief review about evaluation methods used for information systems (IS), most of them in healthcare. This review

Table 2. Results for the review on IS evaluation

Objectives	Total
Presents methods to evaluate information systems	13
Evaluate evaluation methods	10
Improve technologies or applications	
Information System's Evaluation	4
Methods of evaluation	
Others	6
Usability	4
Questionnaires/interviews	4
Literature review	3
Not mentioned	3
Cognitive science	2
Quantitative/qualitative	2
Soft-systems	2
Heuristics	2
Ergonomic methods and tools	1
Problems encountered	
No proper evaluation methods	12
Applications are difficult to use	6
Complex workflow analysis and decisions	5
Costs and insufficient policies	2
Insufficient infrastructure	1

comprised 27 articles about this subject from 1999 till 2006, 3 of which are websites. Some of the articles described new evaluation methods, others the results and application of some methods and yet others the evaluation of the methods themselves.

The main results of this review are presented in Table 2.

In a similar proportion, the reviewed articles either try to introduce new methods of evaluation or the result of analyzing some existing evaluation methods. There is a split worry in order to find the most adequate evaluation methods as well as trying to check what the main problems are with the existing ones.

The most common used methods to evaluate IS, besides proprietary ones, are usability methods, questionnaires or interviews.

The most frequent problems encountered within the articles reviewed regarding evaluation methods are that these are usually not right for the evaluation that needs to be performed. Also, regarding the IS that were evaluated, the results show that the problems of the evaluated applications are not, as was probably expected, the costs that these applications incur. Results of evaluation show that applications are often difficult to use and that workflow and decisions that those applications are supposed to help are usually too complex and cannot be implemented.

There are many issues regarding IS evaluation and this is becoming very challenging as still no adequate methods can be used in a generic fashion. The problems encountered are recurrent. They deal with the fact that IS are not developed according to users' needs, workflow tasks and complexity. This justifies why it is so difficult to choose or develop the right evaluation methods for IS. There seems to be a problem from conception and not on the evaluation side. This makes it hard to decide which methods to choose and apply, and first of all, what is needed to evaluate in first place.

If it is so hard to do this within the IS, it is harder to do this within parts of the IS as is for example security, and more specifically access control.

ACCESS CONTROL

In order to securely access information within a system three steps are usually required: identification (where a user says who he is, e.g. with a login username); authentication (where a user proves his identification given in the first step, e.g. with a password or a PIN number); and authorisation (where access rights are given to the user).

Access control is conceptually part of the authorisation process that checks if a user can access the resources he requested.

The design of access control systems is very complex and should start with the definition of structured and formal access control policies as well as access control models (Blobel, 2004). An access control policy must describe the rules that need to be enforced in order to provide the information security requirements of the organization. Afterwards, an appropriate access control model must be chosen in order to model the rules defined within the policy. Examples of common access control models are: role-based access control (RBAC) that associates rights to groups of users according to their roles within the organization; identity based access control (IBAC) that associates rights to specific users depending on their needs; and mandatory access control (MAC) that defines mandatory rules for all the users of the system. A model can also be hybrid and include more than one model in order to tackle the more heterogeneous needs of an organization. Only after the access control model is chosen can the right technology and both authentication and access control mechanisms be selected and implemented. Authentication mechanisms provide for the identification and authentication of a user to the system - the first

2 steps above - (e.g. login/password; fingerprint) while access control mechanisms protect against unauthorized use of the requested resources (e.g. access control lists, security labels) (ISO, 1989). Both mechanisms should perform in a correct and consistent way according to the access control policy and model defined.

The means of providing access control has become more challenging as policies and user needs become more complex. These need to be studied carefully within the healthcare environment so that access control can be correctly developed and applied without hindering the system's use.

We are including all three steps to access an IS within the scope of the review presented in this section since the first two steps are necessary precursors to the third. Furthermore many implementations combine the three steps together into one access control decision, by having the implicit access control policy that everyone who is successfully authenticated can have access to the resource. This is the coarsest granularity of access control policy, in which everyone has the same access rights. Thus the authentication mechanism becomes a combined authentication and authorisation mechanism.

This review comprised full articles from the last 10 years (1996 until mid 2006) whose content covered access control policies, models and authentication mechanisms (that incorporated an implicit access control function) in general and applied to the healthcare environment (Ferreira A et al., 2007b). Searches were made in medical databases such as Medline (that included the BMJ-British Medical Journal) as well as IEEE Xplore and ACM.

As can be seen in Table 3, from the 17 articles that mentioned the definition and use of an access control policy only in 1 case was it implemented, and this was a prototype system. From the 59 articles that mentioned access control models, 52 concentrated on the study of an access control model and in only 8 cases were these studies implemented, mostly as prototypes with only 1 of these being implemented in a real scenario

The most commonly used access control model was RBAC, being covered in 38 articles out of 52. The most commonly studied and prototyped authentication mechanism was digital signatures with public key certificates (9 out of 15). During the last ten years the 3 countries with more publications in this particular area are the USA with 40, UK with 8 and Germany with 7.

With the healthcare articles, 59 were deemed to be appropriate and were included in the review. From a total of 27 articles that refer to the system's

Table 3. Number of papers reviewed covering access control policies, models and mechanisms between 1996 and 2006.

	1996-99	2000-03	2004-06	Total
Access control policy				
Study/Analysis		4	12	**16**
Implementation			1	**1**
Access control model				
Study/Analysis	4	11	37	**52**
Implementation		2	6	**8**
Authentication mechanisms with an implicit access control function				
Study/Analysis		5	10	**15**
Implementation		1	2	**3**

Table 4. Number of papers reviewed covering access control policies, models and mechanisms in healthcare between 1996 and 2006.

	1996-99	2000-03	2004-06	Total
Access Control Policy				
Study/Analysis	2	8	12	**22**
Implementation		3	1	4
Access Control Model				
Study/Analysis	6	10	8	**24**
Implementation	1	6	1	**8**
Authentication Mechanisms with an implicit access control function				
Study/Analysis	6	10	8	**24**
Implementation	1	6	1	**8**

Table 5. Healthcare institutions, information systems and user groups.

	1996-99	2000-03	2004-06	Total
Healthcare Institution				
Hospital	3	10	7	**20**
Hospital Department		2		**2**
Primary Care		1	1	**2**
Private Care		1	3	**4**
Other		2	5	**7**
Total	3	16	16	**35**
Healthcare Information System				
EPR/EMR/CPR	5	14	15	**34**
Prescription		2	1	**3**
Consultation			1	**1**
Total	5	16	17	**38**
Portal/Internet Access				
Healthcare professionals		1	1	**2**
Patients		1		**1**
Total		2	1	**3**
User groups				
Medical doctors		2	2	**4**
Nurses		3	2	**5**
Patients		1	4	**5**
Others (HPs,GPs,IT,Pharmacists)	2	13	9	**24**
Total	**2**	**19**	**17**	**38**

implementation, 25 were built as prototypes whilst 2 were built in a real life scenario.

From the 34 published articles that mention access control policies, Table 6 shows that 22 refer to the study and analysis of those policies, whilst only 4 of them actually implemented policy based systems as prototypes. In 14 out of these 34 papers, the policies were institutionally or legislatively defined, whilst in only 4 of those 34 articles is it mentioned that end-user can set policies. But none of these 4 policies were actually implemented, not even as prototypes. Further, none of the 34 articles that mention access control policies included the end-users of the system as part of the group that designed and developed those policies.

Finally, 7 articles refer to the need for an override policy definition i.e. an access control system which allows the user to override the current policy in times of emergency, and gain access to patient confidential information that they would not otherwise be able to see (Ferreira A et al., 2006). As for access control models, from the 40 articles that refer the use of access control models, 24 of these mention its study and analysis whilst in 8 articles the models were implemented as prototypes only.

The most commonly used access control model was RBAC (22 from 40) whilst the most tested authentication mechanism was digital signatures with public key certificates (29 from 41).

Focusing now on the EMR and its users, Table 5 shows the type of information systems that were implemented and in which healthcare institutional setting they were implemented. It also presents the most common types of user groups for those systems.

Most of the information systems are EMR (34 from 38 articles) and were implemented within hospitals (20 from 35 articles). The end users of the system are mostly healthcare professionals (HPs), general practitioners (GPs), IT and pharmacists. Only in 5 articles is it mentioned that patients might have access to their healthcare information but none of these systems were being used in a real environment. During the last ten years the 3 countries with more publications in this particular area were the USA with 15, UK with 10 and Greece with 7.

Table 6. Problems regarding EMR integration encountered in the revised articles

Problem type	Number of occurrences
Disruption to workflow & performance	7
Educational Barriers	5
Management problems	4
Cultural barriers	2
Security concerns	1
Relational Barriers	1
Increase in time for patient session	1

Table 6 shows the usability problems that were encountered as described in the published articles. Not surprisingly, most of them relate mainly with the disruption of workflow and performance when the EMR is used as well as with educational problems.

As an example, in order to find out more about end users' opinion on access control to EMR, this study (Pinho C et al., 2006) applied a survey to medical doctors within a university hospital. Most respondents agree that access control levels must exist for EMR and that not all doctors must have total access to all patient records. They indicate that more sensitive information (e.g. HIV) must only be accessed by doctors that treat those patients.

A great number of doctors also revealed that patients should not have total access to their own medical records (Figure 1). This must be further analysed as patients should have the right to access all their medical information, if they require. It is surprising that most doctors think they can access all the information about a patient they are treating and, at the same time, feel the patients themselves cannot have the same right regarding their own information.

Figure 1. Doctors' response regarding full access to patients' records

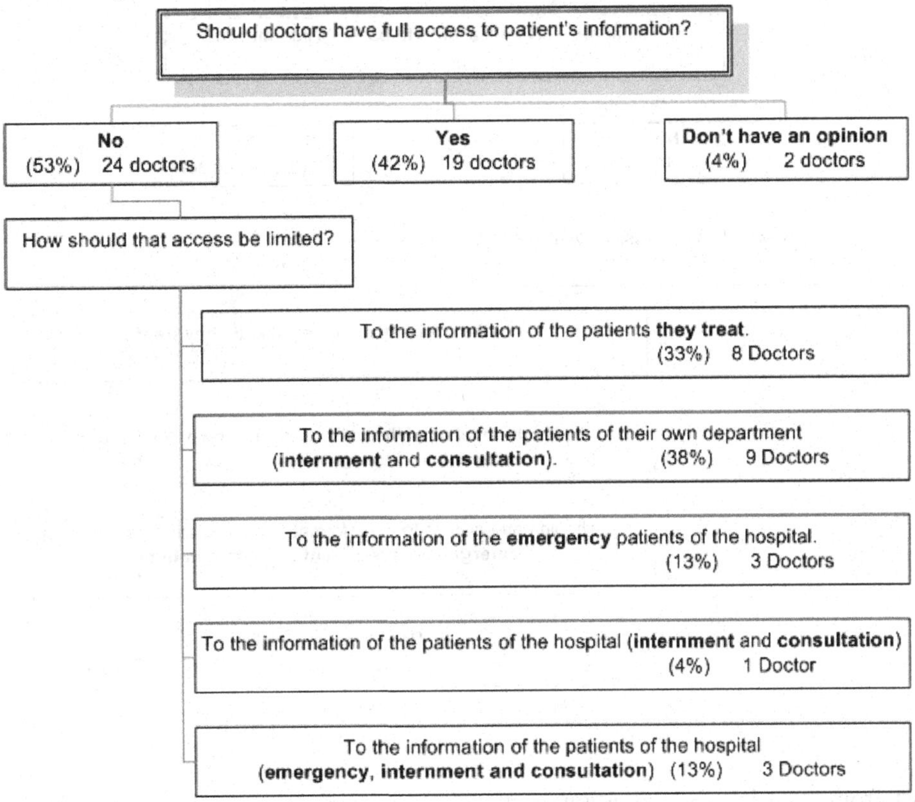

Further, most doctors thought that nurses should not access all patient information (Figure 2). But how different would these results be if the same questionnaire was applied to the nurses or other category of healthcare professionals?

As a reflection of this specific study, the authors' experience within this field by having contact with both healthcare and IT professionals in various lectures and workshops shows that healthcare professionals have great difficulty in defining the best policies to control the access to IS.

Although there is legislation and healthcare professionals know the way they perform their daily tasks, it is quite hard for them to define accurately, the correct access rights to an IS. Nevertheless, healthcare professionals feel that their participation is essential in order to adapt access control policies to their needs.

They further agree that access control needs to be defined by a multidisciplinary team, including themselves, and reach a consensus to the best of their ability. Only this way can access control and the right usage of EMR be achieved.

DISCUSSION

EMR are essential to today's shared care and although security is very difficult to achieve it is regarded as having a fundamental role to play.

An EMR should focus on facilitating users to follow their daily processes without much effort and time. These processes must be taken into account when new security models and technologies are implemented. Further, automatic verification of data quality must be provided and used to trigger alerts of malfunctions and inconsistencies, ensuring data integrity and better health care.

Figure 2. Doctor responses regarding nurses' full access to patients' records

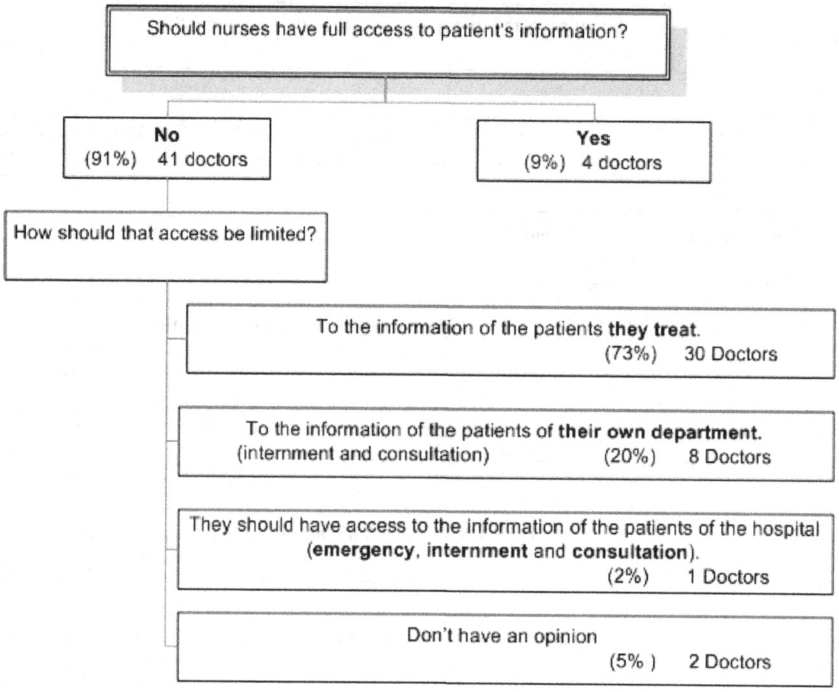

Apart from security, IS evaluation is an essential requirement to build proper and efficient IS. However, this is very challenging as still no adequate methods can be used in a generic fashion. Some evaluations that are made encounter problems that deal mainly with the fact that IS are not developed according to users' needs, workflow tasks and complexity. This justifies why it is so difficult to choose or develop the right evaluation methods for IS. There seems to be a problem from conception and not on the evaluation side. This makes it hard to decide which methods to choose and apply, and first of all, what is needed to evaluate.

Regarding access control, although there is legislation and healthcare professionals know the way they perform their daily tasks, it is quite hard for them to define accurately, the correct access rights to an IS. From legislation to practice, the development of access control (as well as other healthcare IS such as EMR) has several problems. Nevertheless, healthcare professionals feel that their participation is essential in order to adapt access control policies to their needs. They further agree that access control needs to be defined by a multidisciplinary team, including themselves, and reach a consensus to the best of their ability.

CONCLUSION

It is a fact that the end users of a product seldom participate in its design and definition although everybody agrees that this would probably save a lot of costs and time. In healthcare, these problems go further and interfere with the appropriate use of the EMR, its security and furthermore, with the provision of proper patient healthcare.

The authors believe that if healthcare professionals and patients support and participate in the access control systems' design and development process, more specifically the access control policy definition that defines and links security from legislation to practice, then some of the problems regarding EMR integration and use that were described within this chapter could be minimized.

REFERENCES

Akrich M. (1994). Comment sortir de la dichotomie technique/société : Presentation des diverses sociologies de la technique. De la préhistoire aux missiles balistiques : De líntelligence sociale des techniques. *La Découverte Latour & Lemonnier*, 105-131.

Arellano, M. G.,Weber, G. I.. (1998). Issues in identification and linkage of patient records across an integrated delivery system. *J Healthc Inf Manag, (12)*, 43-52.

Bakker A. (2004). Access to EHR and access control at a moment in the past: a discussion of the need and an exploration of the consequences. *Int J Med Inform, (73)*, 267-70.

Barnett, O. (1990). Computers in medicine. *JAMA, (263)*, 2631-2633.

Becker, M. Y.,Sewell, P. (2004). Cassandra: flexible trust management, applied to electronic health records.

Berner, E.,Moss, J. (2005). Informatics Challenges for the Impending Patient Information Explosion. *J Am Med Inform Assoc,* 12, 614-7.

Blobel, B. (2004). Authorisation and access control for electronic health record systems. *Int J Med Inform,* 73, 251-7.

Brostoff, S., Sasse, M. A., Chadwick, D., Cunningham, J., Mbanaso, U.,Otenko, S. (2005). "R-What?" Development of a role-based access control (RBAC) policy-writing tool for e-scientists. *Software - Practice and Experience, (38)*, 835-856.

CEN/TC251 (1999). ENV 12251: Health Informatics - Secure user identification for health care management and security of authentication by passwords. *European Standards in Health Informatics.* CEN.

Chuva MT, Fernandes MT, Correia C, Barbosa L, Silva MJ, Gomes MJ, Moreira MM, Gomes MM, Vinhas MS, Dias M, Moreira M,Ferreira A. (2006). Attitudes and opinions of patients and healthcare professionals about the use of coomputers in primary care – systematic review. *IX Jornadas Científicas dos Estudantes de Medicina. Faculdade de Medicina da Universidade do Porto.*

Coiera, E. (2003). *Guide to health informatics*, Arnold.

Commission, A. (1995). For your information: a study of information management and systems in the acute hospital.

Cruz-Correia R, Vieira-Marques P, Costa P, Ferreira A, Oliveira-Palhares E, Araújo F,Costa-Pereira A. (2005). Integration of Hospital data using Agent Technologies – a case study. *AICommunications special issue of ECAI, (18)*, 191-200.

Cruz-Correia R, Vieira-Marques P, Ferreira A, Oliveira-Palhares E, Costa P,Costa-Pereira A. (2006). Monitoring the integration of hospital information systems: how it may ensure and improve the quality of data. *Stud Health Technol Inform (121)*, 176-182.

Cruz-Correia, R., Vieira-Marques, P., Costa, P., Ferreira, A., Oliveira-Palhares, E., Araujo, F.,Costa-Pereira, A. (2005). Integration of hospital data using agent technologies - a case study. *AI Communications, (18)*, 191-200.

Cruz-Correia, R., Vieira-Marques, P., Ferreira, A., Oliveira-Palhares, E., Costa, P.,Costa-Pereira, A., 2006. Monitoring the integration of hospital information systems: how it may ensure and improve the quality of data. *Stud Health Technol Inform, (121)*, 176-182.

Dick, R.,Steen, E., 1997. *The Computer-based patient record: An essential technology for healthCare.*

Eysenbach, G. (2000). *Consumer health informatics. BMJ, (320)*, 1713-16.

Ferreira A, Correia A, Silva A, Corte A, Pinto A, Saavedra A, Pereira A, Pereira AF, Cruz-Correia R,Antunes L. (2007a). Why facilitate patient access to medical records. *Studies in Health Technology and Informatics, (127)*, 77-90.

Ferreira A, Cruz-Correia R, Antunes L,Chadwick D W. (2007b). Access Control: how can it improve patients' healthcare? *Studies in Health Technology and Informatics, (127)*, 65-76.

Ferreira A, Cruz-Correia R, Antunes L, Farinha P, Oliveira-Palhares E, Chadwick D. W,Costa-Pereira A. (2006). How to Break Access Control in a Controlled Manner. *CBMS2006.* Salt Lake City, USA.

Ferreira A, Cruz-Correia R, Antunes L, Oliveira-Palhares E, Farinha P,Costa-Pereira A. (2005). How to start modelling access control in a healthcare organization. *10th International Symposium for Health Information Management Research.* Greece.

Friedman C,Wyatt J. (2006). *Evaluation methods in biomedical informatics*, Springer.

Greenes, R.,Shortliffe, E. (1990). Medical Informatics: an emerging academic discipline and institutional priority. *JAMIA, (263)*, 1114-20.

Hackos JoAnn,Redish Janice. (1998). *User and task analysis for interface design* Wiley.

Hammond, K., Helbig, S., Benson, C.,BM, B.-S. (2003). Are electronic medical records trustworthy? Observations on copying, pasting and duplication. *AMIA Annual Symposium.*

Harris S, 2003. *CISSP All-in-one exam guide.* McGraw-Hill Osborne Media.

Hogan, W.,Wagner, M. (1997). Accuracy of data in computer-based patient records. *J Am Med Inform Assoc, (4)*, 342-355.

Hohnloser, J., Fischer, M., Konig, A.,Emmerich, B. (1994). Data quality in computerized patient records. Analysis of a haematology biopsy report database. *Int J Clin Monit Comput, (11)*, 233-40.

Institute, M. R., 2005. 7th annual survey of electronic health record trends and usage for 2005, Medical records institute. (2005). *Medical records institute, medical records institute.*

Kling R, 1991. Computerization and social transformations. Science, technology and human values. *Science, Technology and Human Values, (16)*, 342-267.

Knitz M. (2005). *HIPPA compliance and electronic medical records: are both possible?* . Bowie State University: Maryland, Europe.

Koffler, D.,Galstad, E. (2002). *Nagios 1.x documentation.*

Korpman, R.,Lincoln, T. (1998). The computer-stored medical record: For whom ? *J Am Med Inform Assoc, (259)*, 3454-3456.

Lehoux P, 2006. *The Problem of Health Technology: Policy Implications for Modern Health Care*, Routledge.

Lehoux P, Sicotte C,Denis J. (1999). Assessment of a computerized medical record system: disclosing its scripts of use. *Evaluation and Program Planning, (22)*, 439-453.

Mamlin, J.,Baker, D., 1973. Combined time-motion and work sampling study in a general medicine clinic. *Medical Care, (11)*, 449-456.

Miller R. H, Hillman J. M,Given R. S, 2004. Physician use of IT: results from the Deloitte Research Survey. *J Healthc Inf Manag, (18)*, 72-80.

Miller R. H,Sim I, 2004. Physicians' use of electronic medical records: barriers and solutions. *Health Aff (Millwood), (23)*, 116-26.

Ministers Committee (1997). Recommendation No. R (97) 5 of the Committee of Ministers to Member States on the Protection of Medical Data. IN Europe, C. o. (Ed.).

Ministers Committee (2004). Recommendation Rec(2004)17 of the Committee of Ministers to member states on the impact of information technologies on health care – the patient and Internet IN Europe, C. o. (Ed.).

Nygren, E., Wyatt, J. C.,Wright, P. (1998). Helping clinicians to find data and avoid delays. *Lancet, (352)*, 1462-6.

Pinho C, Sá C, Mendes E, Santos E, Silva F, Sousa F, Gomes F, Abreu F, Mota F, Aguiar F, Faria F, Macedo F,Martins S. (2006). Electronic patient records - who should access what? Doctors' view. *Biostatistics and Medical Informatics Department - Faculty of Medicine of Porto.*

Quantin, C., Binquet, C., Bourquard, K., Pattisina, R., Gouyon-Cornet, B., Ferdynus, C., Gouyon, J. B.,Allaert, F. A., 2004. A peculiar aspect of patients' safety: the discriminating power of identifiers for record linkage. *Stud Health Technol Inform, (103)*, 400-6.

Richart, R., 1970. Evaluation of a medical data system. *Computers and Biomedical Research, (3)*, 415-425.

Schneier B, 2004. *Secrets and Lies: digital security in a networked world*, Wiley.

Sprague L, 2004. Electronic health records: How close? How far to go? *NHPF Issue Brief*, 1-17.

USA Congress, 1996. HIPAA - Health Insurance Portability and Accountability Act IN Government, U. (Ed.), Public Law (pp. 104-191) 104th Congress.

Waegemann C, 2003. EHR vs. CPR vs. EMR. *Healthcare Informatics online*.

KEY TERMS

Access Control: Set of security features that control how users and systems communicate and interact with other systems and resources. They protect systems and resources from unauthorized access and can be a component that participates in defining the level of authorisation after an authentication is successful. Access control is extremely important because is one of the 1st lines of defence used to fight against unauthorized access to systems and network resources. *Shon Harris, CISSP. All in one CISSP Certification. MCGrawHill, Osbourne, 2003.*

EMR: Electronic medical record (EMR) is a medical record in digital format. A Medical record is a systematic documentation of a patient's medical history and care. The term 'Medical record' is used both for the physical folder for each individual patient and for the body of information which comprises the total of each patient's health history. Although medical records are traditionally compiled and stored by health care providers, personal health records maintained by individual patients have become more popular in recent years.

Information Security: Is the process of protecting data from unauthorized access, use, disclosure, destruction, modification, or disruption. This means protecting the confidentiality, integrity and availability of data regardless of the form the data may take: electronic, print, or other forms.

IS: An information system (IS) is a system, automated or manual, that comprises people, machines, and/or methods organized to collect, process, transmit and disseminate data that represent user information.

Medical Informatics: The rapidly developing scientific field that deals with biomedical information, data, and knowledge - their storage, retrieval, and optimal use for problem solving and decision making. The emergence of this new discipline has been attributed to "advances in computing and communications technology, to an increasing awareness that the knowledge base of medicine is essentially unmanageable by traditional paper-based methods, and to a growing conviction that the process of informed decision making is as important to modern biomedicine as is the collection of facts on which clinical decisions or research plans are made." *Edward Shortliffe, M.D., Ph.D. What is medical informatics? Stanford University, 1995.*

Section II
Standardization and Classification Systems in Medicine

Chapter IV
The Cultural History of Medical Classifications

György Surján
National Institute for Strategic Health Research, Hungary

ABSTRACT

This chapter outlines the history of medical classifications in a general cultural context. Classification is a general phenomenon in science and has an outstanding role in the biomedical sciences. Its general principles started to be developed in ancient times, while domain classifications, particularly medical classifications have been constructed from about the 16th-17th century. We demonstrate with several examples that all classifications reflect an underlying theory. The development of the notion of disease during the 17th-19th century essentially influenced disease classifications. Development of classifications currently used in computerised information systems started before the computer era, but computational aspects reshape essentially the whole picture. A new generation of classifications is expected in biomedicine that depends less on human classification effort but uses the power of automated classifiers and reasoners.

INTRODUCTION

This chapter outlines the history of medical classifications in a general cultural context. While classification and medical terminology is a hot topic of current biomedical informatics, our aim is to show, that nearly all problems we face currently originates from the past. The modern computer era however offers more efficient techniques although the principles of these techniques have been developed through many centuries.

Classification is an essential issue in all scientific activity. Its importance is emphasised by R.A Crowson in his book titled *Classification and biology* (Crowson R. A., 1970). He argues, that it is often thought that the essence of science is to count or measure things. But before we could do so we have to select *what* we want to count or measure (and what not). And this distinction presupposes a *classification*. Indeed, all scientific activity requires a clear scope definition: a distinction between relevant and irrelevant phenomena. This distinction – either made consciously or unconsciously – is at least a dichotomous classification. But this is usually not the last step – even if the aim is not to classify the phenomena of the given domain. This is particularly true in life sciences. If someone – let say – wants to study the alimentary habits of frogs (either in a qualitative or quantitative way), it is necessary to classify the things in the world as frogs and non frogs. But the habit of one particular frog at a particular time is probably not a real scientific issue: science is more about the general rules than about particular phenomena. So we study the habits of a number of frogs. Then we realise that there are many different kinds of frogs, each kind probably having different habits: many different species, but also young and old, male and female ones etc. And now we are in the middle of the sea of the problem of classification:

Which distinctions are relevant and which are not for an actual problem?
Which distinctions are relevant in general?
Which categories are real, which are arbitrary?
Are we able to classify all phenomena correctly – are the categories well defined?

This is no more the problem of a scope definition: we have to define classes *within* the scope of our research in order to properly interpret our observations. This is very characteristic to all life sciences, mostly due to the amazing variability of life. Medicine is no exception. Medical classification is not a solved problem, and perhaps never will be totally solved. Beyond the fact, that the rapid development of medicine reshapes classifications from time to time, it points to several philosophical, linguistic and logical problems. Philosophically it is related to the questions about the basic nature and structure of existence, the ontological nature of medical entities etc. The linguistic aspect deals with the naming conventions and the language used to describe medical phenomena, while the logical aspect is related to the problem of reasoning over medical facts.

The goal of this chapter is to show that all problems around medical classification and terminology have historical roots. This history can be seen in a wider and a narrower context. A narrower context would focus on biomedical and health problems, while a wider context includes the development of the theory of classification in general.

While we prefer the wider context, we do not want to provide an exhaustive description of the whole history of classifications and all cultural problems around it. Through selected examples we just want to show, that nearly all the problems we are facing now, already emerged in the past, and that the lessons learnt from this history can help to avoid traps in present and future development. This approach determines the structure of this chapter: first we want to describe the development of a general theory of classifications, pointing to the mentioned philosophical, linguistic and logical aspects. Then we will show how specific domain classifications emerged, particularly in life sciences. The third part of the chapter will go through the history of classifications in the medical domain while the fourth deals with current trends and achievements.

DEVELOPMENT OF A GENERAL THEORY OF CLASSIFICATIONS

The Beginnings

We believe that classification (i.e. identification of discrete entities of the world and grouping them into categories) is an inherent property of human intelligence. In that sense the history of classifications is as long as the history of mankind. Later on, this inherent and often subconscious intellectual activity became subject of scientific investigation. The known history of this conscious investigation, the *theory of classifications,* started in ancient Greek philosophy. After the initial steps of Plato, Aristotle carried out foundational work by drawing up the principles of categorisation that are still more or less valid. Before his substantial work there was a lack of language necessary to describe the theory of classifications. The fifth book of Aristotle's Metaphysics (a series of his studies collected by his students) provides a vocabulary of fundamental notions, like *principle, substance, quality and quantity, necessary and accidental properties, unity, identity, part and whole,* etc. Many of the words e.g. *category (κατεγωρια)* used today to describe classifications were coined by Aristotle. Perhaps his most influential work was the invention of the conceptual hierarchy that is the structure that stems from the arrangement of existing things into species and genera (i.e. specific and generic classes). This structure serves as the basis of the definitions of entities by specification of a "*genus proximum*" and a "*differentia specifica*". It was recognised rather early that a superior category might have many different, partially overlapping subdivisions. To avoid confusion it is important to find proper 'differentiae' (properties that divide generic categories into non-overlapping subcategories). These differentiating criteria were called *fundamentum divisionis* (basis of division).

The main goal of ancient philosophers was to make clear how the true nature of certain things can be defined and to find ways to understand the nature of being. None of the known ancient classifications gave an exhaustive, fully comprehensive representation of its domain, since there was no need for any practical use of classifications. The detailed classifications (e.g. the classification of animals developed by Aristotle) served as a testbed of the theory (Ogle, 2001).

In the 3rd century A.D. the Neo-Platonist philosopher, Porphyry wrote an introduction to Aristotle's Categories. This work is known today as *Isagoge* from the Greek word "Εισαγωγε" that means introduction. This work was discussed and rewritten in Latin by several early medieval thinkers, e.g. Boetius and Peter of Spain. The text is available in English translation by George McDonald Ross (Ross, n.d.) The Isagoge explains the basic notions of Aristotelian classification theory, such as individuals, species and genera. An illustration of this is known through Peter the Spain as "Tree of Porphyry". Its logical structure is shown in (Figure 1).

This early 'conceptual graph' provides a strictly dichotomous tree structure. Each category has exactly two "differentiae" that lead

Figure 1 The Tree of Porphyry

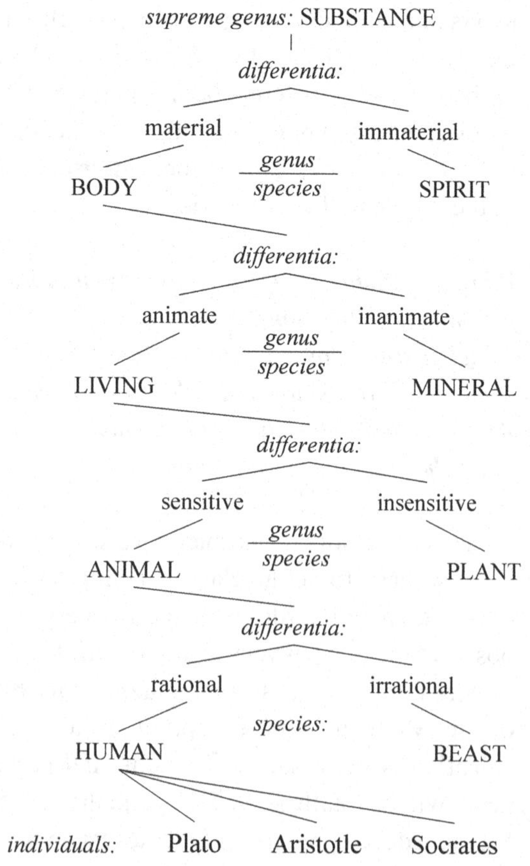

to two subcategories. The "differentiae" are attribute-pairs based on presence or lack of some property (e.g. rational – irrational, or material – immaterial, etc). Another important feature of the graph is that there is one single highest genus (i.e. the topmost category; the *Substance*). There are several layers of subordinate genera and the lowest category, called species: *Human* and *Beast*, have no further subcategories. Only individuals may belong to species. Except the topmost and the lowest categories all intermediate categories are genera of their subcategories and species of their super-categories:

What has been said will become clearer if we consider just one category. Substance is in itself a genus, and under it there is body; under body, animated body; under animated body, animal; under animal, rational animal; under rational animal, the human being; and under the human being, Socrates, Plato, and all particular human beings. Of these, substance is so general that it can only be a genus, and the human being is so specific that it can only be a species; whereas body is a species of substance, and the genus of animated body. But animated body is also a species of body, and the genus of animal; and again animal is a species of animated body, and the genus of rational animal; and rational animal is a species of animal, and the genus of human being; and the human being is a species of rational animal, but it is not the genus of any sub-division of humanity, so it is only a species; and anything which is immediately predicated of the individual it governs will be only a species, and not a genus. So, just as substance is the most general genus, being the highest, with nothing else above it; so the human being is only a species, and the lowest, or (as we said) the most specific species, since it is a species under which there is no lower species or anything which can be divided into species, but only individuals (such as Socrates, Plato, or this white thing)... (Ross, n.d.)

These distinctions between types are often used even in modern medical and non-medial classifications. The lowest level categories that have no subcategories just direct instances are called today 'concrete class', while all categories above this that have but indirect instances are called 'abstract classes', while the modern name of the supreme genus is 'top level category'.

The strict dichotomy (i.e. each class must have exactly two direct subclasses with one and only one differentiating criterion) was a Platonic idea; As D. Ross points out Aristotle argued against this strict dichotomy in the 'De partibus animalium' (Ross, 1977).

The Ars Magna

The middle ages were strongly influenced by ancient Greek philosophers. Great thinkers of the scholastic period tried to synthesize this philosophical tradition with Christianity, but it was not a straightforward discipline. Perhaps the strangest, somewhat odd but obviously exciting example was the "Ars Magna" written by Ramón Lull (1235-1315). Lull (or Raymond Lully or Raymundus Lullus) lived in a religiously heterogeneous (Jewish, Islamic and Christian) environment, and wondered why the obvious truth of his own religion (Christianity) was not convincing enough for others. He thought that this must be due to the weakness of language, so he tried to invent a system that is able to represent all truth and reason in an obvious, convincing and language independent way.

To achieve this goal, he tried to build up a structure of the ultimate general knowledge, onto which all other more specific sciences are built. Highly influenced by Aristotle, he sought the most general principles, to which all particular principles belong as parts of a whole. To structure this general knowledge, Lullus selected nine letters (from 'B' to 'K'), arranged them onto two disks, labelled with letters '**A**' and '**T**'. Each letter assigns one absolute, one relative principle, one

Table 1. The Lullian alphabet

	General Principles Disk 'A'	Relative Principles Disk 'T'	Questions	Subjects	Virtues	Vices
B	Goodness	Difference	Whether	God	Justice	Avarice
C	Greatness	Concordance	What	Angels	Prudence	Gluttony
D	Duration	Contrariety	Of what	Heaven	Fortitude	Lust
E	Power	Begin	Why	Man	Temperance	Conceit
F	Wisdom	Middle	How much	Imagination	Faith	Acidy
G	Will	End	What quality	Senses	Hope	Envy
H	Virtue	Major	When	Vegetation	Charity	Wrath
J	Truth	Equal	Where	Elements	Patience	Lies
K	Glory	Minor	How, with what	Instruments	Compassion	Inconstancy

question, one subject, one virtue and one vice as is shown in Table 1

The nine letters on disk **'A'** refer to the nine absolute principles, the disk indicates them in both in noun and adjective form (goodness and good, wisdom and wise etc.), and all the nine letters are linked by connecting lines to all the others, forming a fully connected graph (See Figure 2).

The lines connecting each letter to all other letters refer to statements like Goodness is durable, Power is great, Greatness is powerful etc. The letters on the second disk are arranged in a different way, they form three triangles. This disk T depicts the relative principles, as is shown in Figure 3

Each relative principle has different sorts. E.g. difference may exist between sensual and sensual, between sensual and intellectual, and between two intellectual things. These sorts are also indicated on disk T.

Then Lullus creates a table containing all bi-grams (combinations of two letters) without

Figure 2. Figure The absolute principles

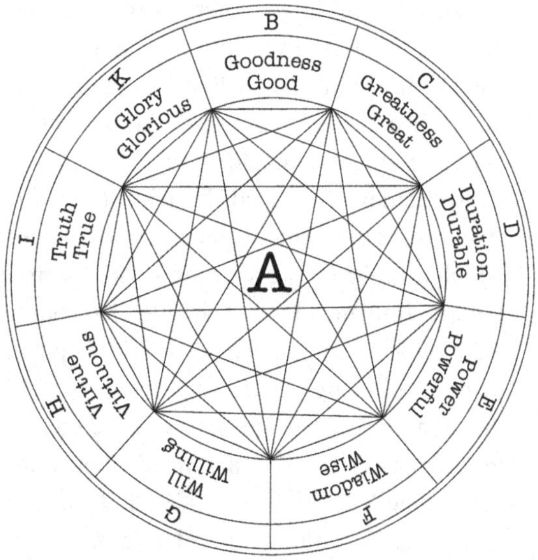

Figure 3. The relative principles

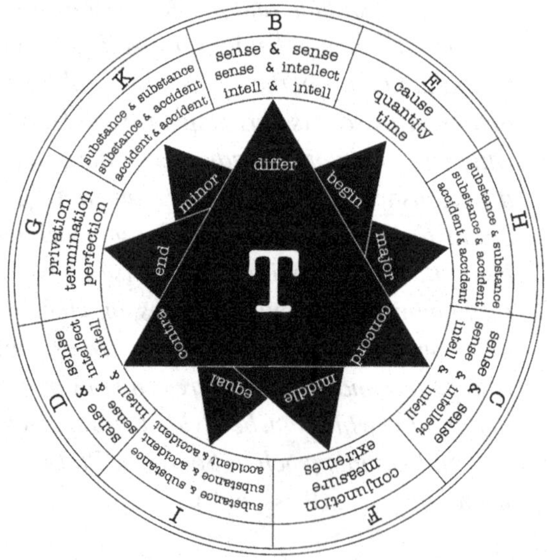

Figure 4 The bi-grams

BC	CD	DE	EF	FG	GH	HI	IK
BD	CE	DF	EG	FH	GI	HK	
BE	CF	DG	EH	FI	GK		
BF	CG	DH	EI	FK			
BG	CH	DI	EK				
BH	CI	DK					
BI	CK						
BK							

repetition, irrespectively to the order or the letters (Figure 4).

The whole 6th part of the Ars Magna deals with that. The letters may refer either to general or relative principles, but to questions, subjects, virtues and vices as well. For instance BF means 36 different statements and one or two questions about each statement (*'whether it is'* and *'how much'*). Let we see some examples:

Statements:

Goodness is Knowable; Wisdom is Good; Wisdom is Different; Difference is Good; Faith is good; Faith has knowledge; God is wise; God is good; God is different; Avarice has knowledge; Avarice is evil;

Questions:

Is goodness knowable? How knowable is goodness? How much knowledge does justice have? Is faith good? How wise is God? Is avarice evil?

Lullus slightly modifies the meanings of the letters depending on the subject of the statements or questions, or in case of vices he changes sometimes the propositions to their opposite without any explanation. So God is wise, faith and avarice has knowledge, God and faith are good, but avarice is evil (why not good?). Lullus apparently admired the "combinatorial explosion" (the high number of possible derived meanings of just two letters taken from a set of nine), but he fails to achieve the real goal: to create a tool to discriminate false and true statements. He must sometimes violate his own rules to avoid combinations that are controversial with his belief.

Further on he creates a third disk that consists of three coaxial wheels; each of them contains the nine letters. By rotating the three wheels independently, it is possible to generate all possible tri-grams (729 variations). Lullus extends each trigram using an additional letter 't'. The letters, preceding this 't', refer to the disk A, the following letters refer to disk T. So a trigram, e.g. 'bcd' can be interpreted in different ways: 'bcdt', 'bctd', 'btcd' and 'tbcd'. Lullus provides a table that lists all these possibilities. Still, the meaning of these 'codes' are not unambiguous, since the letters may refer to the disks, but also to the questions, subjects, virtues and vices, according the 'alphabet'. Lullus perhaps intentionally allows this 'flexibility'.

...each science has principles different from those of other sciences, the human intellect requires and seeks one general science with its own general principles in which the principles of all other sciences are contained as particulars of a universal that regulates the principles of other sciences so that the intellect can repose in those sciences by really understanding them and banishing all erroneous opinions. This science helps to establish the principles of all other sciences by clarifying their particular principles in the light of the general principles of this art, to which all particular principles belong as parts of a whole. (Dambergs, 2003)

This is something like what we call in our days 'top level ontology. In spite of all peculiarities, the ideas of Lullus influenced many thinkers not only in his own age but through many centuries. He had followers and also serious opponents and perhaps parodists as well. Even today many people admire his work. John Sowa mentions him as the inventor of first device for automated reasoning (Sowa, 2000). His work is converted to a software application that allows studying his ideas (Abbott & Dambergs, 2003).

From our aspect, the following features of this work are important:

Lullus used letters to signify concepts – in the same way as we use codes nowadays. However he used the same letter for several different entities, so his codes were not unique.

He created a combinatorial system that is able to generate a number of complex entities (or statements) very similar to our combinatorial coding systems.

He tried to formally discriminate true and false statements, or formally approve what he thought to be true. This is what we now do with reasoners that are able to make inferences on formally described statements.

In a later work, the "Arbor Scientiae" (The Tree of Science or the Tree of Knowledge) Lullus drew up a categorial structure of all sciences and disciplines of his age. This treelike structure was based on the nine principles described in the Ars Magna. The structure is not a true tree structure in the geometric sense, but a lattice, since some of the branches or sub-trees cross over. (Eco, 1993) This is the problem of poly-hierarchy that also present in recent medical classifications. (The definition of poly-hierarchy is that it occurs whenever an entity has more than one super-ordinate entities that are hierarchically not related to each other).

The efforts of Lull reappeared three centuries later in the work of Leibnitz, who himself studied Ars Magna thoroughly.

The Real Character

Further important developments can be observed in the work of Bishop John Wilkins (1614-1672): *An Essay towards a Real Character and a Philosophical Language*, published in London 1668 (Wilkins, 1668).

The 'real character' is a writing system, in which all elements (each single character) have direct meaning (i.e. syntax and semantics have an unambiguous one to one relation). Wilkins was concerned not only about the variety of languages, but also about the alternations of the language over time (e.g. he compared many English versions of the Lord's Prayer as something that should be stable but it is not). After investigating the history of languages and language variations, Wilkins turns to study the history of letters, supposing that all alphabets originate from Hebrew. He states that there are less variations and differences in letters than in languages, because letters much younger. Anyway, the variety of letters he thought to be an appendix to the curse of Babel. Then he mentions examples in which letters – just for brevity – are used to signify words instead of sounds. (Sort of shorthand writing) Then he continues:

Besides these, there have been some other proposals and attempts about a real universal character that should not signify words, but things and notions, and consequently might be legible by any nation in their own tongues. (Wilkins, 1668)

This was the aim why he created his own system. To achieve this goal he thought it necessary to start from a generally accepted systematisation of the world, at least those things that are general, elementary entities. Once there is an unambiguous system of symbols that refer to these elementary things, the combination of the characters will allow representing all other entities. So the second part of his work has this title: '*Conteining a regular enumeration and description of all those things and notions to which names are to be assigned*'. This second part is a system of categories, that follows Aristotelian principles of categorizations and somewhat resembles the Tree of Porphyry. It starts from 40 top level categories, called genera arranged into a tree structure. These genera are subdivided into "differences" and further into "species" (The word 'difference' refers to 'differentia specifica' but often refers to the subcategory defined by the differentiating criterion, as it is the case here).

In total he had 2030 species. Wilkins tried to fix the number of "differences" for a genus to six (i.e. one category can have at most six subcategories), but he admits that this is sometimes not possible (especially in case of living beings), because they *"are of too great variety to be comprehended in so narrow a compass."* The species under each "difference" are arranged into pairs *"just for better helping memory"* The proposed hierarchy is much more complex than a simple three level tree: the top level categories are themselves arranged into a tree and many of the species also have subdivisions. Wilkins apparently tried to enforce an artificial structure on the system but recognised that reality often does not obey this.

The third part of his work is titled *'Concerning natural grammar'*. In this part Wilkins tries to set up a general grammar that is independent from each particular language but preserves all features that he thought to be common in all languages. This grammar gives a combinatorial nature to his system, and allows describing many more things than the 2030 entities covered by his categorial structure. This 'grammar' conveys something that we currently call *relations*. E.g. this allows him to describe butcher as flesh +merchant, carpenter as wood + manufacture and mathematician as quantities + artist.

The fourth part of his work deals with the writing system. Wilkins propose actually two alphabets; the first is solely for writing, that contains unpronounceable symbols, the second is created for speaking, and contains Latin and Greek letters and diphthongs. It arranges consonants and vowels in such a way that it helps pronunciation. All of the characters are significant: either they signify a category or a grammatical construct. In the fourth chapter of this part Wilkins gives two examples of the usage of his language: he "translates" the Lord's Prayer and the Credo into this language, explaining the translations word by word.

As an appendix, Wilkins included an alphabetical dictionary of approximately 15000 English words, that are either indexed to his "philosophical tables" (i.e. the system of his categories or grammatical entities), *"or explained by such Words as are in those tables"*. Homonyms are indexed to different places according to the different meanings, as the following extract shows:

Abolish.
[a. Nothing] T.I.1.O.
[Annihilate] AS.I.1.O.
[Destroy] AS.I.4.O.Abate

The letter 'a.' stands for 'active' that is the given meaning is a verb (makes something nothing).

By this dictionary Wilkins tries to demonstrate, that his "philosophical language" is really able to express everything that is expressible in English.

Beyond the important improvement (compared to Lull) that the codes of Wilkins are unique, he also discovered that codes can express the hierarchy of a system of categories. This strategy of code value assignments is used today in e.g. ICD codes, the Read Clinical Classification (version 2) and versions 2 and 3 of SNOMED. This code value assignment has an obvious computational benefit (it is easy to decide if one entity is subsumed by another) but enforces a strict tree structure. Wilkins also drew up classification trees, trying to follow the principles of the Tree of Porphyry, but he could not help violating both the dichotomous principle and the tree structure: the same things appear several times even in the same table (in the same sub-tree). Once the principle of dichotomy is given up, the number of subdivisions of a single category might increase, but the strategy of assigning a single English letter to a subdivision leads to a restriction of the number of subclasses of a category, since in this way it is not possible to represent more than 26 subcategories at a given node, since the English alphabet has no more letters.

The principle of mutually unique codes has another drawback: any misspelling or typing error leads immediately to misunderstanding. (Eco, 1993) Natural coding systems, e.g. genetic code and natural language, are usually redundant and hence there is some degree of fault tolerance. (The use of check digits was not invented at that time of course, and would be of little help without using computers).

The system set up by Wilkins was quite large: navigation in the space of 2030 entities in a paper based representation is difficult. And still – as he realised – this system was far from complete. In our modern time we also have to realise, that maintenance problems increase rapidly with the size of classifications, and completeness seems to be never achievable in building medical classifications.

When to Think Will Mean to Calculate

In the 17th century, two extraordinary scientists, Gottfried Wilhelm Leibnitz (1646 - 1716) and Isaac Newton independently invented the infinitesimal calculus (differential and integral calculus). Both of them were polyhistors, working not only in various fields of mathematics but also in several scientific disciplines like philosophy, linguistics, physics and theology. A century before Charles Babbage, the 'father of computers', Leibniz developed a mechanical calculator that was able to multiply and divide. He was heavily influenced by the thoughts of Lullus, and was seeking for a better mathematical foundation of his ideas. A dream of Leibnitz was to eliminate all uncertainty from mathematical proofs, so that true and false statements could be distinguished in a formal way, simply by calculations. "To think will mean to calculate" he claimed. In order to achieve this, he proposed to decompose the whole knowledge into elementary entities and assign prime numbers to them. In other words, he used numeric codes, contrary to the alphabetic codes of Lullus and Wilkins. Complex entities can be coded by multiplication of the codes of their components. Following the idea of Sowa (Sowa, 2000) with some minor modification, let us take the Tree of Porphyry as an example and assign 1 to *Substance* and the subsequent prime numbers to the differentiae. We get the Table 2 in this way.

Table 2. Prime numbers representing differentiae (after Sowa)

SUBSTANCE	1
Material	2
Immaterial	3
Animate	5
Inanimate	7
Sensitive	11
Insensitive	13
Rational	17
Irrational	19

Then HUMAN as a rational, sensitive, animate, material SUBSTANCE gets the code 2x5x11x17= 1870, while LIVING, as animate material SUBSTANCE is 2x5=10, and PLANT as insensitive LIVING is 10x13=130. The benefit of this representation is that the truth of such statements, like "*HUMAN is a LIVING being*" can be investigated by division of the corresponding code numbers. Since 1870 is divisible by 10, the statement is true. To investigate the statement "*HUMAN is a PLANT*" we have to divide 1870 by 110; the result is not a natural number, so the statement is false. This representation has the obvious benefit that it makes certain types of syllogism calculable. But, as Sowa claims, still many logical operations, such as implication and negation, can not be calculated in this way. Leibnitz had further concerns about his own invention. While Wilkins thought that due to the high number of entities, setting up a categorical system is a huge work that requires co-operation of many scientists, Leibnitz realised that not only the number of entities that have to be assigned is infinite, but any smallest piece of world is infinitely complex (Eco, 1993).

Therefore he felt that the entirety of prime numbers is insufficient to represent the world. This view is not surprising for somebody who invented the infinitesimal calculus. Modern studies of human thinking do not confirm his concern unanimously. E.g. Sowa argues that all representations in our mind – even the representations of continuums are discrete (Sowa, 1984). If he is right, it is possible to map all concepts to natural numbers or prime numbers – at least theoretically.

The idea of Leibnitz about the formalisation of thinking came back in 19-20th century mathematics in the form of formal languages, and especially in the work of Gödel, who showed the inherent limitations of the dream of Leibnitz.

"Concept Writing": Towards Formal Languages

One of the most interesting aspects of the *Ars Magna* is that three components: the classification itself, the system of codes to denote categories, and the rules of the used "language" (i.e. the logic and reasoning) were present and developed simultaneously. After Leibnitz, these aspects became separated from each other. The first important steps towards formal languages were made by Gottlob Frege (1848-1925) with his *Begriffsschrift* (concept-writing); but this was only about the syntactic rules that enable the representation of the logical structure of any statement, and not about how the symbols denote concepts nor about how to categorise of the concepts. The Begriffschrift contains the following four primitives only:

├ *p* assert *p*
┬ *p* not *p*
┬ p
└ *q* if *p* than *q*
x
P(*x*) for every *x* P(*x*)

These graphical symbols proposed by Frege are not in use today because of the difficulty to map them to spoken natural language. For instance the following symbol (See Figure 5) stands for the simple statement that some men are tall, but must be read as

Figure 5 Frege's concept writing

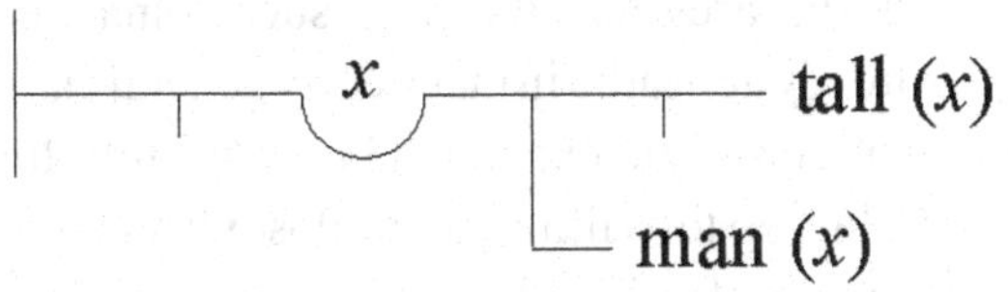

"It is not true that if x is a man then x is not tall."{S1}

In the recently used syntax of predicate calculus it is:

$\exists x(\mathrm{tall}(x) \wedge \mathrm{man}(x))$
that is to be read as:
"There exist x, where x is tall and x is man." {S2}

Note, that {S1} and {S2} are semantic equivalents.

The syntax evolved through the works of Peirce, Peano, Russell and others. We do not follow here this story in detail, but will return to formal languages when we discuss modern biomedical classifications. We also do not follow the philosophical chain of developing top level categories (the so called top level ontologies) that aim to provide a general framework, under which all classifications can be arranged in a consistent way. A summary of this story is given by Sowa (2000). Instead we turn to domain classifications.

Domain Classifications

Domain classifications do not aim to represent the whole world or the universe of human knowledge, which was an obvious aim e.g. of both Lullus and Wilkins. Rather, domain classifications – as the term itself indicates – focus on a single, well described domain, e.g. plants, chemicals, minerals, diseases etc. Of course, such domain entities already appeared in many early general classifications, mostly as examples. From Aristotle through Lullus up to Wilkins, all philosophers built some domain classifications; biology, later medicine was a favourite test-bed for them. When early philosophers tried their hands on domain classifications, this was done mainly to test whether their theory – on which the classification was built – suited the entities of the given domain.

A real domain classification however is not only a restriction of the scope; at the same time such a classification aims to be comprehensive. They are designed for some practical use within the given domain, and to achieve this all entities of a domain should be classifiable, even if arbitrary collective categories ("not elsewhere classified") are used. In other words, the difference between top level (general) and domain classifications is not just the difference of their scope, but also the difference in purpose: general classifications aim at the proper understanding of reality, domain classifications aim at some practical use, often for some statistical *data collection*. This last point is especially significant for medical classifications. Domain classifications have been developed in a number of different fields. There are classifications both for natural and artificial things; e.g. minerals, clouds, poetry, folk music and transport vehicles. Now let us review some examples from biology, since historically they are the closest relatives of medical classifications.

Carl von Linné

Perhaps the first pure domain classification that satisfied the criteria mentioned above of which parts are even used today, was the system developed by Carl von Linné (1707-1778) known also as Carolus Linnaeus. He studied medicine at various European universities and was fond of plants. At that time botany was an integral part of medical curricula because of the wide use of medicinal plants. Linnaeus graduated and practised medicine, but his scientific work concentrated on the classification of living organisms, mostly of plants. Linnaeus is often referred to as the father of taxonomy. He arranged plants into a *system* of hierarchically arranged categories (taxa) following Aristotelian principles. Contrary to Porphyry, Linnaeus restricted the term 'species' to the lowest level categories and 'genus' to the first level above 'species'. (As we mentioned, for Porphyry all intermediate levels are genera of their subcategories and species for their super-ordinate categories) The levels above genus were called Orders, Classes and Kingdom by Linné. While contemporary biology still uses this structure, the number of levels has been extended, by introducing Phyla, Superclasses, Superorders, Infraorders, Families, Superfamilies and Tribes.

It was also the idea of Linné, that species should be named according to their place in the classification. This system of names he proposed is called the *binominal nomenclature* as the names consist of two parts: the first name denotes the genus and the second is used for distinguishing the given species from others within the same genus. This fits with the Aristotelian principle of defining things by the '*genus proximum*' and the '*differentia specifica*'. Linnaeus did not use any *codes* for his classification, but the proposed names refer to the place of the named thing in the hierarchy of the classes – similarly to many recent medical coding systems, where code values reflect the place of the category in the hierarchy.

From Aristotle up to Linnaeus the systematisation of living organisms was based on the so called *scala naturae,* (the natural scale), a continuous chain of organisms, with humans on the top and the simplest living organism at the bottom. The ranking of this list of species was based on their complexity, and the different species were not arranged into classes. So this hierarchy was an *exclusive hierarchy* of categories, like military ranks. A higher ranked category does not subsume the lower ones. In other words: the *scala naturae* was not a chain of generalisation-specialisation. It was something like a disease classification in which diseases were arranged into a ranked list according to their seriousness.

Contrary to that, the Linnaean system (published in several editions of his *Sytema naturae*) was an *inclusive (subsumption) hierarchy* that had two important features that followed Porphyry's principles: (1) The structure he proposed was a strict tree structure. (2) He tried to find a "diagnostic criterion" that is a sufficient and necessary condition for the membership of each taxon (category). The hierarchical tree structure he proposed had some weak points: it failed to represent hybrid species that inherit essential properties of two independent species. This is the poly-hierarchy problem that frequently occurs in many classifications and often disturbs developers of classifications even today. Before the age of computers it was a source of technical difficulty, since a poly-hierarchy is hard to represent on paper; nowadays it is a modelling challenge.

Another weakness of the Linnaean taxonomy is that it can not explain the phenomenon that features characteristic of a genus ("diagnostic criteria") sometimes are missing from certain species (or subordinate genera) of that genus. E.g. fleas are pterygote insects with no wings, whales are mammalians with no hair etc. (Panchen 1992). This is what biologists call *polythetic taxa.*

The essence of the Linnaean "revolution" was the move from a ranked scale to an inclusive hierarchy. The basis of this step was a scientific theory saying that biological species show not only different levels of complexity but show common essential properties and these properties constitute a reasonable basis for classification.

Developmental Theory and the Classification of Species

In 1859 the publication of the "Origin of species" by Charles Darwin (1809-1882) resulted in an immediate outbreak of a revolution in biology, not only in the sense of rapid development but also in the sense of a heavy fight between supporters and opponents of the theory. While Darwin was a diligent observer who himself collected many facts supporting his theory, most– if not all – of his statements were already stated by different researchers. In the introduction of his work, he lists 34 researchers that contributed to his theory. His ultimate merit was the careful selection not only of the facts but also of the contemporary scientific works that could be arranged as mosaic pieces into a whole and consistent picture.

Darwin's theory served as a new principle of the whole biological classification.

The natural diagnostic criterion of a taxon became: having an ancestor in common. But this is not necessarily a visible, intrinsic property: it hardly can be established just by investigating visible features of existing living organisms, but requires knowledge about the phylogenesis. (Nowadays the sequencing of the DNA can essentially contribute to this research, but Darwin could not even dream of it.) Phylogenetic inheritance is different from the inheritance of object properties along ontological hierarchies: descendants of a species may loose essential properties (necessary conditions) of their ancestor (see the problem of polythetic taxa of Linnaeus); different descendants may loose different essential properties, but still belong to the same taxon due to having common phylogenetic roots. Contemporary classification of species in biology is still based on Darwinian principles; just it is more and more based on the analysis of DNA sequences today. However in many cases biologists are increasingly concerned about the definition of species. The classical definition says that individuals of the same species are able to interbreed producing reproductive descendants. This definition hardly can be defended in case of micro-organisms, like bacteria. On the other hand there are some examples of interbreeding individuals from different species that are able to produce reproductive descendants

From our perspective three important lessons have to be learned from the history of the biological classification of species.

1. As was shown, developments in biology reshaped the biological classifications. All biological classifications reflected the contemporary theory of life.
2. An important step in the development of biological classification was the introduction of an inclusive hierarchy instead of an exclusive rank of species.
3. The pattern of classification itself – a mere geometrical structure - reflects a basic philosophical view of the world. There are two basic patterns of inclusive hierarchies: logical division and clustering

Logical division (e.g. the Tree of Porphyry) starts from some unity: that is a generic top level category, the "summum genus". Then this unity is gradually divided into smaller and smaller subcategories according to strict rules of sufficient and necessary attributes that are inherited by all subsumed classes; until finally we arrive to unique individuals or instances.

Clustering moves in the opposite direction. It starts with the observation of individuals and seeks for groups of individuals that share common properties. On that basis it defines classes, and then – still based on common properties – several classes are merged into superclasses, etc until we arrive at a supreme class that covers all observed individuals of the domain of interest.

In principle these two approaches may lead to the very same categorial systems. At first sight one can imagine a third classification pattern. This is the pragmatic classification. E.g. things that require a certain action could be classified into one category, regardless of their properties. This is important for us, since medical classifications are not so much theory-driven, but pragmatically oriented. But if it is true that certain different things really require the *same* action, then there must be a theory that explains why this is the case. And this theory will show what is common in those apparently heterogeneous or dissimilar things. Exactly in the same way that the theory of evolution explains what is common in dissimilar species belonging to the same taxon.

Development of Medical Domain Classifications

Ancient Time

Undoubtedly early physicians tried to *categorise* diseases. But no trace of a real ancient medical domain classification was found in the literature. None of the known works of Hippocrates – the most famous ancient physician who lived about two centuries before Aristotle – concentrates on classification. Neither his ancient followers like Galen worked heavily on disease classification.

The known history of medical domain classifications begins in the 17th century with the classification of diseases. Other medical domain classifications (procedures, drugs, medical devices, etiologic agents, social factors, etc.) were not developed until the 20th century.

John Graunt and the London Bills of Mortality

During the early 1600-s around the great plague epidemic in London, it was decided to collect systematically data of all death cases. Some periodic data collection was started in 1592, but it became continuous about ten years later. The obvious reason was early detection of a plague epidemic outbreak. It was quite a challenging enterprise at that time, since there were not enough medically trained personnel. Moreover there were no practical or theoretical foundations or any guidelines how to do such things. Practically the work was done by so-called searchers, usually women, nominated at each parish. They had to examine all corpses to decide what the person died of. They had no predefined list of diseases; neither were they medically educated. No wonder that some of the recorded causes were really odd. The records they made were collected by each parish and published in print weekly as the London Bills of Mortality for more than a century (Greenberg, 1997).

John Graunt, (1620-1674), later often referred to as the father of demography, analysed the data published in the Bills. His study entitled Natural and Political Observations (made upon) the Bills of Mortality was first published in 1662. In this work he presented a number of substantial observations based on the analysis of the figures of the Bills. E.g. he tried to estimate the proportion of live-born children dying before the age of six. At that time the Bills of Mortality did not record the age at death of the person. He defined a set of causes that he supposed never occur after the age of six and another set of causes that he supposed to occur under six in half of the cases. With these postulates he was able to calculate the approximate proportion of young children who died. Whether or not such an approach can be justified, the idea, that such data can tell more about a population than what is directly expressed by the numbers – is obviously interesting. This is an early example of the reuse of information: data collected for one specific purpose was used for another. Later investigations revealed that Graunt's estimates were quite good. (World Health Organisation, n.d.) He also observed that the number of deaths due to other reasons than plague also increased during periods of a plague epidemic. This was surprising and conflicted with what everyone would expect. Graunt concluded that death due to plague was significantly underreported. Other sources confirm that families of persons died of plague often bribed searchers to report death due to something else to avoid being locked up in their house. By analysing the numbers Graunt was able to estimate that the number of death due to plague was 25% higher than reported. Then he concludes that the true number of plague deaths could not be defined without reporting all diseases. "*A true Accompt* (=account) *of the Plague cannot be kept, without the Accompt of other Diseases*" and also that "*The ignorance of the Searchers* [is] *no impediment to the keeping of sufficient, and useful Accompts.*" A facsimile of the original edition can be found on the web (Stephan, 1996).

These early experiences highlight two important aspects of disease classifications that are relevant even today – needless to say in a very different form.

One aspect is the lack of knowledgeable personnel. In that time it concerned the lack of medical knowledge and the low number of trained physicians; today the problem is that in many countries there is a shortage of professionals that are knowledgeable in the theory of classification and medicine (at least in nosology) as well. *Nosology* comes from the Greek word νοσος (nosos = disease). It means a branch of medicine that deals with the classification of diseases.

The other interesting problem was that *financial incentives* distorted the data: searchers were paid for not making records of plague. Even today there is a huge literature of the distorting effect of financing incentives, especially with case mix based systems. See (Hsia, Kurshat, Fagan, Tebbut & Kusserow, 1988), (Hsia, Ahern, Ritchie, Moscoe, & Kurshat, 1992) and many others.

We can also learn from Graunt, that under certain conditions, data are reusable, and also that important and reliable observations about a population are possible even if the data are seriously distorted at the individual level.

The London Bills of Mortality practically lacked any theoretical, scientific foundation. Today it is difficult to judge how effective this system was in preventing plague epidemics. We just have to stress that classification in medicine is not a purely academic exercise. The question is not merely how to describe or categorise the reality. Classifications in medicine are tools used for interventions that improve the health of the population.

Development of the Notion of Disease in the 18th century

The naïve, layman approach to disease suggests that diseases are entities that can be named. But this was not always thought to be obvious during centuries. Consider that we do not necessarily name situations when our car or computer brakes down. Similarly it is not self evident that various conditions that are considered as illness of our body should have names. During the history of medicine various theories emerged that did not consider diseases as defined or definable entities. The so called 'Galenism' explained all diseases as a disturbance of the balance of the four humours (blood, bile, phlegm, and choler) and the four qualities: heat, cold, wet and dry (corresponding to the four elements: fire, air, water, earth). According to this theory, diseases are not distinct, identifiable "things" but rather some degree of a process that does not display well defined forms. E.g. fever was thought to be a consequence of excess of hot fluids. Just as extreme weather conditions, floods, drought periods, storms usually do not have specific type-names, similarly disease-types in this view do not require names. Miasma theory explained diseases as consequences of some imbalance of the air and these conditions again hardly could be classified into named entities. Such views were strong amongst academically trained physicians through medieval and early modern centuries. A more evidence based theory developed slowly.

In the second half of the 17th century the famous English physician Thomas Sydenham was seriously concerned about the inefficiency of contemporary medicine. He stated that instead of wasting time with studying the basic sciences of medicine (at this time anatomy, physics, chemistry and botany) physicians ought to spend most of their time at the bedside, and make direct observations about the nature of diseases. He suggested that diseases '*were to be reduced to certain and determinate kinds with the same exactness as we see it done by botanic writers in their treatises of plants*' Sydenham considered diseases as entities having definite properties, in alignment with the naïve approach. As he continues:

Nature, in the production of disease, is uniform and consistent; so much so, that for the same disease in different persons the symptoms are for the most part the same; and the self-same phenomena that you would observe in the sickness of a Socrates you would observe in the sickness of a simpleton. (Fischer-Homberger, 1970)

But his view was not unanimously acknowledged by the scientific community at that time. The whole period was characterised by the co-existence of contradictory theories. Besides Galenism, another important theory was contagionism. As early as in 1546 Girolamo Fracastoro published his theory of epidemic diseases that he thought to be caused by small particles that could be transferred from one patient to another. Beyond that, he supposed that these 'spores' are specific to the given type of epidemic disease; hence plague can cause only plague, small pox only small pox etc. But the debate on Galenism, contagionism, miasma theory and some other theories (like iatromechanism, that considered the human body as a mechanical machine) continued for centuries, and even at the time of the plague epidemic in Marseille in 1720 many did not believe that plague was contagious (Delacy, 1999).

Nearly one century after Sydenham, in the midst of the 1700s, – among others – three highly respected physicians tried to follow Sydenham's recommendation to create taxonomies of diseases in the same or similar way as botanist did with plants.

1. François Bossier de Lacroix, alias Sauvages (1706-1777) first published anonymously his *Nouvelles Classes de Maladies* in 1731, and about 30 years later a more elaborated version entitled *Nosologica Methodica* (1763). Its

full title was *Nosologia Methodica Sistens Morborum Classes, Genera et Species, juxta Sydenhami mentem et Botanicorum ordinem.* In this work he grouped 2400 diseases into 315 genera, 44 orders, and 10 classes (Lesh, 1990).

2. Carol von Linné (1707-1778), who had good contact with Sauvages, also published a classification called *Genera Morborum* (1759, 1763) that was strongly founded on Sauvages' work. Linné listed more or less the same diseases, but classified them differently into 325 genera and 11 classes.
3. Some year later in Scotland, William Cullen published his *Synopsis Nosologicae Methodicae* (1769). This was an integrative work of the several previous taxonomies (including Sauvages and Linnaeus) and Cullen's own classification. The latter entitled *Genera Morborum Praecipua Definita.* This work was published several times in Latin, and in English and in a number of European languages, the last time as late as in 1823. We show with the example of Linné's *Genera Morborum,* how such 'botanical classifications of diseases' were constructed.

An edition of the *Genera Morborum* from Italy is available electronically (Linneaus, 1776). In this edition he classified 325 diseases into a three level hierarchical structure that has eleven supreme categories. All the diseases are assigned serial numbers. These code numbers form a continuous series that does not reflect the hierarchy. Each classified condition has a short symptomatic description (informal definition). These descriptions are often cross-referenced: a description of one condition uses another one. E.g. Cholera is defined as a combination of vomiting, diarrhoea and colic. These cross-references are made explicitly by indicating the numbers of referenced entities.

50.Colica
Intestini dolor umbilicalis cum torminibus
....
183. Vomitus
Rejectio ingestorum convusliva
...
186. Cholera
vomitus .183. cum diarrhoea .187. colica .50.
187 Diarrhoea
dejectio faecum liquidarum frequens

So the *Genera Morborum* can be seen as a hierarchical mono-axial cross-referenced coding system of the diseases. It is not a mere tabular list of the diseases known at that time, because all the conditions are defined by symptomatic criteria — this latter feature is something that we even miss in today's form of the ICD! The *Genera Morborum* was merely a scientific enterprise. We are not aware of any public health usage of it. This also seems to be true for the Sauvages' *Nosologia Methodica.* Their purpose of classification was to improve efficiency of medical treatment by better understanding the nature of diseases:

It was not only hoped that a working therapy would evolve from a systematic nosology of diseases; it was also hoped that such a nosology would facilitate communication between doctors and thus be of didactic use. (Fischer-Homberger, 1970)

The latter point became more important. As she continues:

The significance of the communicatory value of nosology is, for instance, clearly stressed by Vincenzo Chiarugi (1759-1820), the nosologist of psychiatry. In the introduction to the systematic part of his work he wrote that considering the prevailing uncertainty and confusion in matters of terminology, it seemed necessary to establish a set of terms with which everyone would associate the same meanings. And Johann Peter Frank (1745-1821), although considering nosological systems as such to be worthless from a scientific point of view, nevertheless conceded that 'they make medical language accessible to the most diverse nations from pole to pole'.

We have to note, that this was the time when the language of science slowly turned from Latin to national languages. Anyway the goal to make medical texts intelligible regardless from nationality and mother tongue is something what we can read in many recent works on the interoperability of health information systems.

None of these three classifications were maintained further in the following 19th century, which was the century of pathology. Autopsies became more and more common, the dissection of corpses was performed not to study the normal anatomy – since this was already well known at the time – but to study the pathological alterations causing death. Medical observations were not anymore restricted to the surface of the body. This was the time, when Semmelweis made his influential observations about the death of women due to puerperal sepsis that was caused by the fact that physicians and medical students performed autopsies and treated patients without disinfection. Disinfection hand washing improved the development of surgery and this achievement in turn revealed many observations on internal changes of the body under living conditions. Instead of observing external symptoms it became possible to observe the internal pathological alterations that explain the external symptoms and characterise the various diseases. Botanic type classifications that were based on observable superficial properties of diseases were no more the interest of physicians. In the light of pathology it became clear, that many of the 'diseases' listed in the 18th century classifications were only symptoms that could be caused by a number of diseases, often rather different ones. At the same time, the medical profession started to specialise, and classification of diseases slowly became an enterprise of public health physicians instead of clinicians. Public health – at that time – was mostly concerned with mortality statistics.

So far we have seen two different and more or less independent threads in the history of disease classifications:

The early mortality statistics required a classification of causes of death. This practical goal was apparently different from the goal of those philosophers who founded the principles of the theory of classifications. It was not about understanding the nature of the existence or the metaphysical status of entities, but to provide a basis for statistical analysis in order to study and improve public health. In that sense, medical (diagnostic) classifications are different from other domain classifications: they are used to *provide evidence of need for intervention.*

The other thread seems to be a continuation of the work of philosophers; it was a scientific enterprise even in lack of a suitable theory of diseases that could be used as a foundation of the classification. The *Genera Morborum* and the *Systema Naturae* are very similar in the sense that both are based on observable properties that in lack of a proper theory did not lead to a rigorous and consistent classification. Linné's botanic classification is still respected today, while all similar botanic enterprises of that time and all its contemporary disease classifications have been forgotten. The reason of this perhaps is that Linné was lucky enough to find and select observable properties for plants that later became explained by phylogenetic facts, so many of his taxa are still valid, while other botanic classifications were not so lucky. And nobody was lucky enough to find categories of diseases that could remain defendable in the light of the inventions of the next century.

The two threads gradually converged in the history of ICD, the International Classification of Diseases, but even up to now did not result in a fully satisfactory solution.

The Roots of ICD from the 19th Century

From the 19th century on statistics – including health statistics – became more and more official: institutions and organisations were established in various European countries and in the States to collect and publish statistical demographic and health data. One of these institutes was the General Register Office of England and Wales founded in 1837. The head of this office – the Registrar General – was obliged to present a report to "both houses of Parliament by Command of Her Majesty" on births, deaths and marriages. The first report that covered the second half of the year 1837 was published in 1839. (Farr, 1839). This report contained several appendices, one of them was written by William Farr (1807-1883) the first health statistician of the Register Office. This appendix was a letter to the Registrar General, containing many valuable observations on the mortality data presented in the report. From our point of view the most important observation is that Farr realized that the usefulness of mortality statistics strongly depends on an appropriate nosology. He gave a short summary of nosology from Sauvages to Cullen and up to his contemporary nosologists. He demonstrated that there are a number of different nosologies sometimes differing from each other essentially only in the number of classes, but sometimes differing in the principal "fundamentum divisionis". Most often, the main differentiating criterion is the localization of disease, but sometimes it is the severity of disease, the underlying pathological process or even the typical age of onset of the disease. Farr criticised all these classifications and proposals from the point of view of mortality statistics, and pointed out that the Cullen classification that was then in general use in public services became outdated because of the substantial development of pathological anatomy since the time of Cullen. Then he introduced the notion of 'statistical nosology' (i.e. a nosology that suits the requirement of population studies and mortality statistics). His principal "fundamentum divisionis" was the 'mode in which diseases affect the population'. In that sense he discriminates three basic classes of maladies: (1) contagious diseases either endemic that prevail in particular localities, or epidemic that spread over countries and (2) sporadic that arise in an isolated manner and originate internally from the body and (3) violent causes of death

Figure 6. Farr's categories

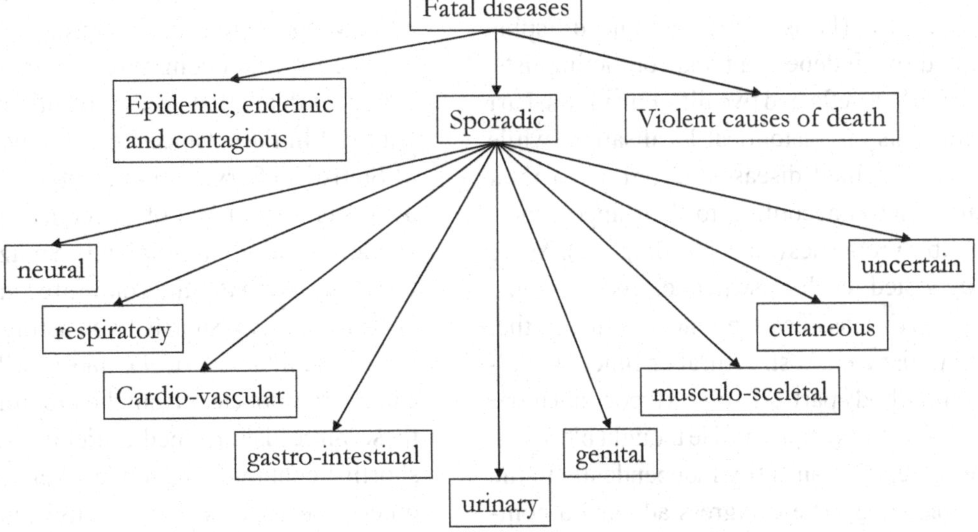

caused by external agents: injuries or poisoning. (The term 'sporadic' means that the cases appear independently from each other; sporadic diseases are usually but not necessarily rare.) Figure 6 illustrates the proposed structure (using somewhat modernised terminology)

The Structure of "*Statistical Nosology*" Proposed by W. Farr

As Figure 6 shows, he classified sporadic diseases according to their anatomical localisation.

Farr paid attention not only to the structure of classification but also to the terms used to identify the categories. He did not use numbers or any sort of codes to designate a class.

Another concern of Farr was that primary disease causing death often was mistaken for its complications. The problem of selecting one and only one principal cause of death – which is medically not always sensible – will be discussed later when we will describe the coding rules of ICD.

In the 19th century health statistics became an international issue. This fact also emphasized the importance of a standard nomenclature. The first International Statistical Congress (Brussels) in 1853, decided to request Farr and Marc d'Espine to prepare an internationally applicable, uniform classification of causes of death. Even at that time standardisation was a difficult enterprise: at the next Congress (Paris 1855) Farr and d'Espine presented two independent and conflicting lists. These two lists reflected two different views. Farr put emphasis on anatomical localisation, while d'Espine classified diseases according to their "nature" that is according to their appearance, observable properties (gout, bleeding, etc). As we already stated, each classification reflects some theory. Farr's classification reflects a theory that says that disease is a structural or functional alteration of a body part. d'Espine's theory put more emphasis on the symptoms. He thought bleeding, for instance, to be an entity independently to the site of bleeding. The Congress adopted a compromise of the two proposals. I do believe that this compromise had serious consequences for the structure of ICD that is present even today: still there is no clear "fundamentum divisionis" in ICD, the uppermost division (into chapters) is still a mixture of anatomical, etiological and pathological division. In the later revisions of ICD, Farr's approach became dominant. But Farr himself was not quite consistent: his basic categorisation consisted of five groups: epidemic, general (systemic), local, developmental diseases and consequences of violence. (Note that this proposal of Farr was somewhat different from what he described in his first letter to the Registrar General.). Only the third group was really classified according to anatomical manifestation. This classification was adopted and updated several times by the International Statistical Congress, but never became unanimously accepted.

The International Statistical Congress was later succeeded by the International Statistical Institute. This organization established a committee in 1891, led by Jacques Bertillon (1851-1922), charged with the task of preparing a classification of causes of death. We have to emphasize the importance of the fact that from this point on the construction of the classification was not a work of one single expert: the elaboration of the classification was done by a committee, which necessarily represented different views, philosophies and interests, and always led to some compromise.

The Bertillon committee composed a list of causes of death that predominantly reflected the list used in Paris (since Bertillon was the Chief of Statistical Services in the city of Paris), but it also was a synthesis of different national classifications used in England, Switzerland and Germany. Actually the committee created three classifications: a shortlist consisting of 44 entities, a medium list of 99, and a full list of 161 causes. It is not clear from the literature, whether these three lists formed a hierarchy, where the shortlist contained the top level entities, and the others consisted of their subdivisions. It is also possible, that the shorter lists simply disregarded the less important causes or collected them into some "other" garbage categories. In any case this system reflected the fact, that different questions (different problems in health care) require different levels of granularity. The Bertillon Classification of Causes of Death was accepted by the meeting of the International Statistical Institute in Chicago in 1893. Up to his death in 1922 Bertillon was involved in several revisions of the system that became more and more accepted and widely used in many countries. The need for revision from time to time was obviously motivated by the growing number of improvements in medicine. On the other hand, stability of a statistical classification is crucial in order to obtain comparable data over time (backward compatibility). Following the proposal of the American Public Health Association, the International Statistical Institute decided on decennial revisions.

After the death of Bertillon, the Health Organisation of the League of Nations – the ancestor of the WHO of the UN – had taken more and more interest in classification, (not only in mortality but more and more in morbidity). The work was therefore continued by a so called "Mixed Committee" consisting of representatives both of the Health Organisation and the International Statistical Institute. For a relatively long period classification of causes of death and disease classifications (mostly for hospital statistics) had been developed more or less separately. In 1856, in his sixteenth Annual Letter to the Registrar General, Farr himself proposed to extend his system to diseases that are not fatal but causes public health problems. At the first and second International Conference for the Revision of the Bertillon Classification (1900, 1909) a parallel list for morbidity statistics had been adopted. Non-fatal diseases were represented as subdivisions of certain categories of causes of death. But these early experiment did not result in an internationally accepted, satisfactory morbidity classification. Therefore a number of national classifications emerged, until finally, the World Health Organisation (WHO), founded after the Second World War created the first proposal of the *International Classification of Diseases, Injuries, and Causes of Death*, as the sixth revision of the Bertillon classification. The accepted classification was supplemented with an alphabetic list of disease names and a manual that described the *coding rules.* Even in very common and simple cases more then one code may apply to describe different aspects of that case. Therefore it is necessary to define certain rules that explain how to select the single statistically appropriate "principal diagnosis" code for each case.

One may wonder why one and only one principal diagnosis is allowed for a case, since one person might suffer from several lethal diseases and there are no evident rules to find out which of them actually caused death. The traditional way of thinking in mortality statistics was apparently the following: There is a total number of deaths in a given population in a given period of time. This number can be broken down according to different attributes like age, gender and cause of death. Of course, we expect that the number of male and female death cases should be equal to the total number of death cases. Similarly the sum of the death cases due to all causes is expected to be equal to the total number of death cases. To extend the list of causes with combinations of diseases could be a theoretically possible solution, but a list containing all possible combinations would be too long and unmanageable in paper based systems. This is a good example of the serious difference between clinical and public health views. Today when we more and more often speak about reuse of clinical information, we have to be aware that in many cases there is no easy and straightforward way from clinical records to public health information.

Through the following revisions, ICD became a more and more comprehensive system, while some of the features of the original structure were still preserved. In spite of all the constructional problems the coding system became more and more widely used, not only for the original purposes, but for many others, ranging from clinical data management through resource allocation, financing, reimbursement to health policy decision making.

This expansion of uses generated a need for a much more detailed representation than necessary for health statistics both at an international or national level. Since a fine grained system would not be suitable for statistical purposes, the ninth revision introduced an additional hierarchical level: all statistically relevant entities are represented by a three digit code while finer distinctions can be made as subdivisions, using the fourth (or for some categories even an optional fifth) digit. The former (7th and 8th) versions used basically three digit codes, and only a part of the three digit items were subdivided using a 4th digit character. The so called *dagger asterisk* notation is also an invention of the 9th edition. This notation is used to cross reference items from different chapters representing the anatomical and pathological categorisation of the same disease. This enables to describe conditions by combined codes, but still keeping the rule that only one principal cause of death (or one principal disease in case of morbidity statistics) is allowed. This issue goes back to the dispute between Farr and d'Espine about the organisation principle. Unfortunately this dagger-asterisk system did not lead to a consistent combinatorial solution. Daggers are used to mark codes that describe etiology or pathology aspect, while asterisks are used to mark codes that describe the localisation of the disease. But these marks are applied only in a limited number of the cases where ICD allows combining codes. Even in such cases the allowed combinations are strictly defined. E.g. the first chapter of ICD describes infectious diseases. This chapter contains a whole section for tuberculosis from codes A15.0 to A19.9. The entities listed here contain some information about the localisation of the disease and also about the diagnostic method. For instance A15.1 means 'Tuberculosis of lung confirmed by [bacteriological] culture only'. Some of the codes in this section are marked with a dagger. E.g. A17.0 means 'Tuberculous meningitis' and it is allowed to combine with G01 that stands for 'Meningitis in bacterial diseases classified elsewhere'. Note that in case of A17.0 the specification of the diagnostic method is missing. A17.0 is not allowed to combine with anything else then G01, but this combination says nothing more than A17.0 alone. On the other side, G01 (that is marked with asterisk) is allowed to be used in combination with a number of codes. Some of them are reasonable combinations (e.g. A69.2 + G01 means Lyme meningitis while A69.2 means Lyme disease only without specification of the localisation), but some are not (A39.0 + G01 means meningococcal meningitis, but A38.0 alone means the same). So instead of offering a freedom for the users to select codes that describe the infective agent (and the diagnostic method if necessary) and combine it with codes describing the localisation, the allowed combinations are 'printed in the stone' in advance, and carry very few or no information. (These examples are taken from the currently used 10th version, but the problem in the 9th version was the same).

Around the development of the 9th version it was recognised that important aspects of diseases are not reflected in ICD at all. To overcome this shortcoming, additional classifications (e.g. for functions and disabilities, for morphology of tumours, for medical procedures) were proposed.

The current version of ICD is the tenth revision that preserves the above mentioned hierarchy and realises that health statistics may go further than mortality and morbidity: sometimes there are conditions where a person may require some health service without having an illness. These conditions are also included in ICD-10. (e.g. Pregnancy or being in contact with a patient having infective disease).

The development of ICD is described in a document published by WHO (World Health Organisation, n.d.).

Current Issues in Medical Classifications

Computers Step In

Computers reshape our life nearly in all aspects. This is particularly true for medical classifications. A number of constraints arose in the past from the limitation of paper based information management. Enforcing tree structures to avoid multiple inheritance and the need of a single principal cause of death are just examples. But the traditions inherited from the past are strong, and changes come slowly. We are not at the end of this story. Until now, the use of computers reformed medical classifications in the following ways:

a. Classifications increased in number, and extended in scope. From the midst of the 20th century more and more medical domains (procedures, laboratory concepts, social conditions, medical devices, drugs etc.) were classified. Wikipedia currently lists more than 20 medical classifications under the title 'medical classifications'. And this is obviously not an exhaustive list. (We provide a brief of internet resources related to current medical classifications in the appendix.) These classifications often overlap because there is no universally accepted, universally suitable coding system in the medical domain. This is partially a consequence of the lack of a general theory of medicine. However, contemporary classifications are not theory-driven but practically oriented: various classifications have been developed to serve various practical needs.
b. The use of classifications became manifold. While early classifications were used nearly exclusively to create statistical tables (perhaps additionally for educational purposes) in the modern health care systems coded data are often re-used for a number of purposes, e.g. for financing, quality assurance, policy making, medical decision support, document and information retrieval etc.
d. Classifications increased in size. Computers made them more easily manageable, so much larger classifications could emerge. This also means that the granularity of coding systems became more and more fine-grained: nomenclatures emerged. Before the age of computers, very detailed coding systems were useless due to their inconvenience of use.
e. Large combinatorial systems emerged. While a vision of a combinatorial coding system already appeared in the work of Lullus, before the age of computers such systems could not spread and develop because of their inconvenient use in paper based systems.
The idea of a two-axial combinatorial system was raised first at a symposium at the New York Academy of Medicine in 1929 (Chute, 2000). The resulting classification was called standardized nomenclature of diseases, SND for short. The two axes were the topology (i.e. the anatomical localisation of the disease) and the aetiology (in reality it contained pathological and patho-physiological entities) describing the nature of the alteration. Pretty soon, in 1933, the system was extended with operations, resulting in the standardized nomenclature of diseases and operations (SNDO). In this system diseases can be described as combinations of the codes of the appropriate anatomical site and pathological entity. Since the Operation axis contained only generic categories (like 'removal' or 'incision') actual operations could be coded also by combinations of the code of the anatomical site and the generic operation. The first medical use of a combinatorial system was followed by a number of multi-axial coding systems, since compositionality offered higher flexibility and expressivity than mono-axial

systems can ever achieve. New inventions, e.g. newly invented operations can be coded immediately without any modification of the coding system. (Since maintenance of classifications require consensus building in a large community, modifications of medical classifications are rather slow and often seriously behind the rapidly developing medical science).

In the sixties, when computers appeared on the horizon, American pathologists developed the system further according to their needs, creating SNOP, the systematized nomenclature of pathology, that later developed further and extended beyond the need of pathology as SNOMED, Systematized Nomenclature of Medicine. Subsequent versions have been published in 1979, 1982 and 1994. The history of the development of the three versions highlights the pros and cons of multi-axial approach.

When humans create classifications manually, multiple inheritance always causes problems. For the human mind it is much easier to deal with pure tree structures. Unfortunately reality usually does not obey this wish. The multi-axial approach has the promise to get rid of multiple inheritance. The author has published a paper demonstrating that multiple inheritance can always be eliminated by introducing new dimensions (Surján & Balkányi, 1996). It is very clear in the case of ICD for instance, that a disease can be classified according to the affected body part (anatomy), according to the nature of pathological alteration (pathology), and also according to the cause of the disease (aetiology). This is the cause of polyhierarchy e.g. in case of pneumonia, which is a lung disease, and an inflammation as well. A multi-axial approach can make this situation very clear: represent the lung as a respiratory tract organ, and – in a separate axis – inflammation as a given pathological condition, and pneumonia as a combination of these entities.

On the other hand, multi-axial systems have serious limitations. There is a lack of a grammar that could provide clear semantics to the combinations. E.g., the juxtaposition of codes of 'incision' and 'trachea' together does not necessarily *mean* 'tracheotomy'. At least theoretically it could mean 'incision *of* trachea' but 'incision *by* trachea' or even 'trachea *of* incision'. Of course human knowledge prevents us from such comic misinterpretations, but computers lack the required common sense and medical knowledge. They need an explicit specification of the semantics. As soon as the location of the disease differs from the location of the intervention, what commonly occurs in medical practice, some syntactic rules are required to make clear how to connect pathology and intervention codes to locations. If a given semantic interpretation adheres to an axis, e.g. 'location' means that something exists in the given location. Then there is the problem that one axis can represent one semantic role only. In reality however a certain thing that has a given ontological nature, may play different roles. E.g. in the second version of SNOMED there was an axis for aetiology. This included chemical substances among others, since they can play an etiological role in case of poisoning. Being a 'chemical substance' is the ontological property while being a poisoning agent is a role in a disease. One chemical substance that causes poisoning in one case can be a medicine as well as a component of some drug in other situations. In the 3rd version of SNOMED the Etiology axis has been split up into three dimensions, namely physical agents, chemicals, and living organs. This was a shift from the actual role to the ontological nature of the entities. But at the same time the notion of 'unknown aetiology' disappeared, since there was not an axis any more where such a notion could be placed.

f. Recognition of the above mentioned limitations lead to steps towards a formal representation and formal definitions of the categories, in order to benefit from the potential of reasoners (programs that enables computer to reason automatically).

All these changes originate from the essential change in paradigm of using such systems. Before the age of computers, the goal always was to create tabulations for statistical, financial or any other purposes. But the new paradigm, as Rector emphasises, is to use codes in 'patient centred' software systems (Rector, 1999). As pointed out by Slee and others, earlier classifications were designed for grouping cases to create some *output* from diagnostic information; while the new coding systems aim at using them for *input* information into electronic health records. (Slee, Slee & Schmidt, 2005).

During the past several decades the talk moved from 'classification' to 'terminology' then to 'concept or knowledge representation' and finally to 'ontology'. These were the favourite terms at various scientific events. In spite of this shift of wording, the problem remained the same: how to make medical descriptions semantically computable? Using codes instead of names to identify classes means that we map our semantic units to natural numbers (whether we use numeric or alphanumeric codes they are countable and hence can be mapped to natural numbers). This allows computers to manipulate the information independently from the ambiguity of language. This is an important prerequisite of semantic computing, that makes it possible to use categories of classifications as variables in any formal language. (Formal languages consist of a defined, usually strongly limited number of symbols, a set of syntactic rules, and an unlimited number of free variables). Once it is achieved, it opens the way towards a formal description of the *meaning* of the categories. The first robust system of formally defined medical entities was the GALEN core model, produced by a project funded by the European Union. (Rector, Nowlan & Glowinski, 1993). Actually GALEN does not use codes, the categories are identified by human readable strings, but the content of a category does not depend on these strings but on their formal definition. GALEN brought three new inventions:

- To represent a new entity it is not necessary to seek its proper place in the whole classification, it is 'enough' to define the entity according to the strict formal rules of GALEN.
- The formal definitions enable the use of automated reasoners to classify all entities, eliminating human errors.
- Users can compose new entities according to their need while the formalism ensures that the new entities will have a clear semantics intelligible for everybody acquainted with the system.

Co-Existence of Classifications – The Problem of Mapping

In the previous section we saw that there are many concurrent, partially overlapping medical classifications, often used in parallel. The reason for this – as we mentioned – is that different classifications serve different tasks. All classifications are abstractions (i.e. details thought to be irrelevant for the given task are rejected). But certain details can be relevant for one task while irrelevant for another. In principle, a very fine-grained representation could carry all information that could be relevant for all conceivable purposes. Then it would be possible to extract the relevant information as required in a given situation. But there is no hope in the close future to develop such single totally satisfying 'omnipotent' classification. So we have to learn how to live with the variety of classifications.

One often mentioned way to solve this problem is the 'mapping' of various classifications to each other. But it is easy to see, that if two classifications are really different (i.e. they consist of different entities) such a mapping can not be done without distortion of the information. Let us illustrate this problem with a sheet of paper that is divided into squares on one side and into triangles on the other. (Look at the illustration on Figure 7) Squares are coded by numbers and triangles by letters. A given point of this sheet can be 'classified': instead of describing its precise co-ordinates we can say that it falls let say, in the square '4' or triangle 'g'. It is very clear, that a mapping from squares to triangles or vice versa is not possible without some distortion: once we do not know the co-ordinates of a point but only the code of the corresponding triangle, we can not tell precisely in which square the point falls. Of course we can create a conversion table using the maximal overlap. E.g. most of the triangle 'e' overlaps square '3'. In some lucky and exceptional cases, the whole triangle overlaps a square, like triangle 'a'. In such exceptional situations mapping is possible in one direction. A mapping of all entities in one direction is possible without distortion only if one system consists merely of subdivisions of the other.

In 1986 the National Library of Medicine (NLM) of the USA started the Unified Medical Language System (UMLS) project. The project strongly built on the experiences with MESH (Medical Subject Headings), a thesaurus used for document retrieval in MEDLINE, the scientific literature database of NLM. (Lindberg, Humphreys, & McCray, 1993).

The background of the project was the recognition that the use of MESH is limited by the fact that the language of users often differs from the language used in the requested documents (McCray, Aronson, Browne, Rindflesch, Razi & Srinivasan, 1993) and also from the terms of MESH. Searchers are more willing to use their own search term than map their terms to MESH entries. To overcome this barrier it was decided to integrate all relevant thesauri, classifications and terminological systems into UMLS. This forms the first so called knowledge source of UMLS, the Metathesaurus. This is a huge repository of concepts, their preferred names and synonyms, and relations among the concepts. Unfortunately, many of the relations (e.g. 'broader than' or 'oth-

Figure 7. The problem of mapping

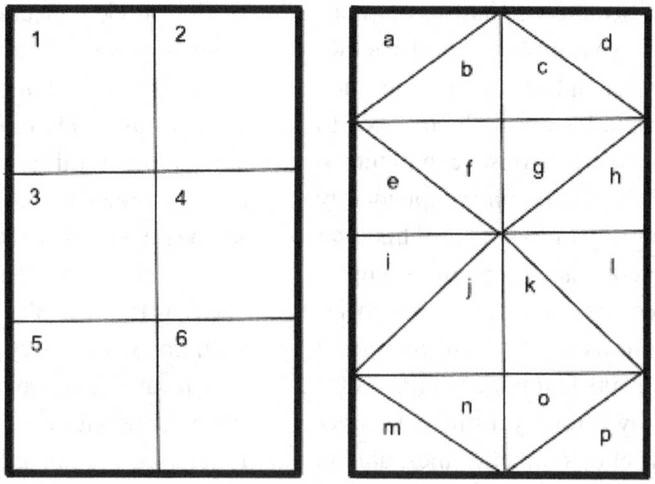

erwise related') have no clear semantics. The second knowledge source of UMLS, called Semantic Network, was created to arrange concepts collected form various sources into an integrated space of broad semantic types. Originally, the third knowledge source, the Information Source Map, was created to provide information about the sources that are integrated into UMLS. It was hoped that the UMLS enterprise can help to map categories from one classification to another. Partly due to the lack of explicit semantics (and the consequent inconsistencies) but partly because of the inherent theoretical limitations, this could not be fully achieved. Bodenrider et al. report a 50-65% success rate in mapping (Bodenreider, Nelson, Hole & Chang, 1998).

Of course this does not mean that the whole UMLS project failed. To the contrary, the system was growing through many years, and grows continuously till now. Hundreds of publications report applications of UMLS in various fields from nursing informatics to natural language processing etc. ...

End of the Story? The Medical Viewpoint

We argued, that all domain classifications reflect an underlying theory of the given domain. From this point of view one may wonder how a disease classification can exist at all, since a scientifically sound general theory of diseases is something that is missing even in modern medicine. A partial answer is that while there is no such a general and defendable theory of diseases, still from the very beginning physicians had some theory, however vague, by which they hoped to explain the causes of diseases. We do not state that in lack of a proper theory classifications cannot exists, but very likely they are not well structured and consistent. Indeed all disease classifications show some inconsistency and arbitrariness. But the other part of the answer is that classifications not only reflect a theory but often are used to improve the theory. If somebody tries to classify entities of an obscure domain this can help in identifying the weak points in the corresponding theory; and often indicates the topics that require further research.

Fischer-Homberger argues that medicine found its theoretical basis in pathology around the 19th century and the importance of nosology decreased from this time on (Fischer-Homberger, 1970) She refers to Sydenham, who first proposed that classification of diseases should follow the way of classification in botany, and at the same time he was sceptical about the usefulness of basic medical sciences, e.g. anatomy. At the time of Sydenham basic sciences could not really help the practical work of physicians. So Sydenham suggested going to the bedside instead of studying anatomy, botanics, and chemistry. Fisher-Homberger points out that the development of pathological anatomy in the 19th century reshaped this picture; in pathological anatomy a science had been found on which medicine could base itself. The sceptical attitude of Sydenham and his followers became unjustified, since from that time on the cause of many diseases had been discovered. According to Fisher-Homberger, this achievement made nosology obsolete and unnecessary. She mentions psychiatry and dermatology as two exceptions, as medical fields where causes of many diseases are still unknown.

This view suggests that nosology is nothing else than a surrogate for sound knowledge. The early nosologists had to follow an empiricist way: their classifications were based on the observable properties of the diseases, pretty in the same way that Linnaeus followed in classification of plants. But recognition of causes of diseases does not mean the end of nosology, like the Darwinian theory of the origin of species did not lead to the end of biological classification. The development in the 19th century medicine led to the end of the symptomatic disease classifications only.

We do not believe that medical classifications will be useless and become obsolete. On the contrary, we expect better classifications in the future. The emergence of ontologies (here in the sense of formal representations of entities and their relations) opens the way to get rid of many consistency errors that necessarily occur when either individual experts or committees construct classifications without appropriate theoretical foundations. The goal is not to find the right classes and super-classes any more. The goal is to find the primitives, and to formally define all other entities based on the primitives. This is a challenging new way, that has of course certain limitations (whether a formal system is theoretically and practically decidable is always a question), but obviously new experiences will be obtained. Formal ontologies can be considered as realisations of the dream of Leibnitz ('to think will mean to count') in the sense that they make logical reasoning computable.

Development of Code Value Assignment

Early classifications sometimes used numbers to identify the entities, sometimes not. The consistent use of these identifiers *instead of* the names of the entities is a relatively late invention. The obvious aim of using codes is to get rid of language dependency and ambiguity of names. Early health statisticians, like Farr, recognised that inconsistent use of disease names often leads to statistical errors. Even today it is often thought, that synonyms and homonyms are the major obstacles for comparing data and for the interoperability of heterogeneous information systems. While this is only one – and perhaps not the most serious – aspect of the problem, use of codes in computerised data processing has well known obvious benefits.

Whenever (either numeric or alphanumeric) codes are to be assigned to the categories of a classification, the question emerges, how this assignment has to be done. Linnaeus used a simple sequential numbering in the *Genera Morborum*. But once a categorial system is organised, it seems to be reasonable to use code values that express the structure of the system (hierarchy, combinations). Such a tendency is present in many current medical coding systems, like ICD and SNOMED version 3 for instance. This code value assignment strategy has obvious benefit both for human users and computers. It makes it easy to move up and down in the hierarchy, and to decide whether a hierarchical relation holds or not between two entities, etc.

However this assignment strategy often leads to irrational constraints: it makes it difficult to represent poly-hierarchies; and causes a restriction on the number of possible subclasses because of the limited number of available characters. To get rid of this limitation Read codes version 2 uses both numbers and letters and discriminates upper and lowercase letters to be able to represent up to 62 subclasses for each entity. (Note that Read codes – like the Real Character of Wilkins – are organised in a way that each single character has actual meaning).

More complex coding systems developed recently are not intended for manual use. Once human usage is not the goal, this "expressive" code assignment strategy can be replaced by other solutions. For computers all strings are meaningless but string searching can be done very fast. So to find a super-ordinate class can be done easily

Table 3 Representation of two forms of pneumonia in SNOMED and ICD

Entity	ICD code	SNOMED CT concept ID
Bacterial pneumonia	J15	53084003
Pneumonia caused by staphylococcus	J15.2	22754005

not only by manipulating the code (e.g. removing some rightmost characters) but also by looking up in a table that describes the hierarchical relationships. Let us show this with the example how ICD and SNOMED CT represent bacterial and staphylococcal pneumonia (Table 3).

From the ICD codes it is easy to infer from J15.2 that it is a subordinate category of J15, simply by removing the two last characters ('.2') from the code of staphylococcal pneumonia. Such a simple formal inference is not possible with SNOMED identifiers. In case of SNOMED a relational table or some other data source should be used to list all subsumption hierarchies. But computers can process such sources in a fast and effective way, so there is no absolute need for expressing the hierarchy formally by code values. Using a separate data source instead of expressive codes to describe the hierarchy has the following benefits:

- It is easy to represent poly-hierarchies.
- There is no limitation on the number of subdivisions for a single category.
- It gives freedom to modify the structure of the system without changing the codes.

For instance, Barry Marshall and Robin Warren (Nobel Laureates in physiology in 2005) discovered the fact, that gastric ulcer is caused by Helicobacter pylori. Earlier it was thought to be a usually psychosomatic disease. Consequently gastric ulcer should be moved from its current place to gastro-intestinal infections. Or when the HIV virus was identified as the etiological agent of AIDS (Acquired Immune Deficiency Syndrome), this condition had to be moved from immunological disorders to viral infections. In case of expressive codes such situations result in the change of code values due to the change of our knowledge but without change of the meaning. If the hierarchy is represented in separate tables, it is enough to correct the corresponding rows while the meaning of the codes remains the same.

But even this does not mean that random code assignment is the best choice. The problem of code value assignment can be well demonstrated by the example of ASCII codes that are used to represent letters in computers. ASCII codes are arranged in alphabetic order: the ASCII code of A is 65, B is 66, C is 67 etc. The code of a lowercase letters is equal to the code of corresponding upper case letter + 32. This arrangement has the following benefits:

- It is makes it easy to order strings (e.g. names) in alphabetic order, since it follows the order of corresponding code numbers.
- It makes it easy to convert strings from upper case to lower case and vice versa.
- Since $32=2^5$ in case of binary digital representation the rightmost five digits are equal for all upper and lowercase letters (e.g. the binary code for 'A' is 0100 0001, for 'a' is 0110 0001). That makes case insensitive processing easy.

All these things work properly with the English alphabet. As soon as other languages, like French, German, or Hungarian have to be dealt with, an extension of the original ASCII code table should be used and the above mentioned systematic arrangement disappears. In the Hungarian alphabet for instance 'A' is followed by 'Á'. In the so called 852 code page the corresponding codes for 'Á' and 'á' are 181 and 160. So, if there is a need to arrange strings according to the Hungarian alphabet an auxiliary table should be used that describes the order of letters. The same happens when additional tables describe the hierarchy (i.e. a partial order) of classes in case of some current medical classifications.

The history of the development of code value assignment shows two things:

1. If code values convey some additional information beyond the direct meaning of an entity, there is a risk that in case of change of

our knowledge some code values should be changed without changing of the meaning. Therefore use of 'mute' codes that merely identify an entity without conveying additional information is recommended, at least in case of generally used systems.

2. Certain value assignment strategies can support effective computing, but this depends on the given task. In local applications this can be a useful technique.

Lessons From the History

'*Historia est magistra vitae*' (history is the teacher of life) says an ancient Latin sentence. Understanding that certain problems persisted over centuries may help us to redefine our research targets to avoid everlasting disputes that lead nowhere.

Nearly all the problems we face nowadays in the fields of medical terminology, classification, coding systems and knowledge representation already emerged in the past. What we are looking for – currently and throughout the centuries – is a tool that enables us to represent the world, at least the medically relevant phenomena in an unambiguous, comparable, relevant, and – since computers emerged – processible way. The representational techniques used currently and in the past fail to satisfy the entirety of these requirements. I try here to summarise the reasons of failure:

The problem of size: none of the medical classifications and terminological systems created so far was complete. Building large terminologies and classifications is a time and resource consuming enterprise. The necessary consensus building also requires a lot of time, while medicine is changing rapidly.

The problem of representation: before large scale classifications could achieve an acceptable level of comprehensiveness the used representation became obsolete. The first classifications were represented in plain paper based tables, later converted to simple database table structures. Then relational databases, conceptual graph formalisms, various knowledge representations (description logic (DL) and first order logic (FOL) languages) emerged. Recently the development of web technology seems to be a driving force for standard implementations of these languages; OWL (Web Ontology Language) is the most common example. Not only the representation but medicine itself develops fast: new terms and categories emerge; old ones become obsolete at a speed that is hard to follow.

Structural problem: all approaches in the field provided a structure to arrange the entities. But none of the proposed structures seems reasonable and convincing to everyone. All structures appear to be somewhat arbitrary and accidental. When someone looks at such a structure it is always questionable why this and not another structure was used. The worst case is when the structure represents a compromise of different aspects, resulting in a hotchpotch of '*fundamenta divisionis*'.

The poly-hierarchy problem: as we mentioned, the human mind apparently strives to see tree structures in all hierarchies, while reality is more complex and seems to form lattices instead of trees: nearly always there are several options to find a basis of divisions. Before the age of computers it was simply too hard to represent poly-hierarchies. Computers can easily cope with them. But perhaps human thinking still adheres too much to paper based representations, or human thinking is genuinely bound to tree hierarchies, and we intuitively refuse more complex structures. In principle it is easy to say, that at least at one level of divisions we must not mix more than one discriminating criterion. But apparently the consistent application of this simple rule in a large system often fails. Today in modern ontology engineering it is a modelling challenge whether manual assertion of poly-hierarchy is allowed or not. Usually it is recommended that users should create only a tree structure manually and additional relations should be inferred by automated reasoning.

Use and reuse: it is relatively easy to create a classification that serves one definite goal satisfactorily. We saw historical examples that data collected for one specific purpose *under certain circumstances* and *with certain limitations* can be used for a different purpose. But the general rule is that the better the classification fits one purpose the less chance of its reuse for another.

Conflict between representational power and ease of use: coding systems with a finer granularity allow the representation of more details and to express rich semantic content. But increasing the representational power can only be done at the expense of ease of (human) use, and usually also at the expense of increasing coding and classification errors. The problem of coding errors was studied in a number of publications. A review of them was presented by the author (Surján, 1999). Here I would like to show only the historical aspect of validity: The practical use of disease classifications stems from mortality statistics. Individual errors in mortality classification can not directly harm the individual, since the subject of the classification already died. John Graunt showed already in the 17th century, that it is possible to get correct conclusions from statistical data even if there is a high number of individual errors. When the classification was expanded to morbidity statistics, individual harm was still not possible since the data were not used in the treatment process. But this usage of classifications opened the way towards using codes in individual patient management. The inherited potential of errors then became a source of possible danger to individuals.

The importance of the human factors: The story of the London Bills of Mortality has shown that the reliability of classification data strongly depends on human factors, including the knowledge of the person who classifies the cases, and also the financial incentives. Nowadays many automated or semi-automated coding software are available, promising that human factors can be eliminated in the future. However none of them have general acceptance. None of them are prefect but many of them exceed the performance of human coders. Still the general opinion is that we should trust humans more than computers. We have no space here to discuss the reasons for that. But it is very clear that the classifications will become more and more complex, and humans will not be able to manage them, so coding (or more precisely translating medical text to some formal language) should be left to computers in the future. This is true for medical classifications also. There are hot issues today in this field that require some solution. But we can not be sure that these problems ever can be solved.

Today and Tomorrow

More than thirty years after the publication of Fisher-Homberger's sceptic paper about the end of medical classification (Fischer-Homberger, 1970) we have to see that, in spite of her prediction, the story has not ended. It is true, that clinicians are not strongly interested in large, comprehensive disease classifications. Their attention turns to the details: they classify forms and variations of a disease: types of lymphomas or fractures of a bone etc. I would use the term 'micro-classification' for them, since their scope is rather limited, and they usually consist of a small number of classes. The importance of comprehensive disease classifications shifted from clinical medicine to public health and health information science. And the development did not stop. WHO is preparing the 11th version of ICD (Üstün & al., 2007) and there is a movement to introduce an international standard medical terminology based on SNOMED-CT. Unfortunately neither GALEN nor SNOMED-CT is represented using some standard formal language. Currently the most popular formal language is OWL (the Web Ontology Language) that was designed to be used in World Wide Web technology. There are some experiments to transform GALEN from its original language (GRAIL) to OWL (Héja,

Surján, Lukácsy, Pallinger, Gergely, 2007). Top level ontologies are developed to ensure the consistency and inter-operability of various domain ontologies. Certain domains appear to be crucial for nearly all biomedical domains. Anatomy is a good example. In such domains re-usable, foundational or reference ontologies are developing, that could be built in several applications., The foundational model of anatomy (FMA) is perhaps the best known example (Rosse, C., Mejino, J.L. Jr., 2003). The rapid development of molecular biology (genomics and proteomics) produces a huge number of newly described entities (gene and protein sequences, cell-components, molecular functions etc.) that are arranged into the fast growing gene ontology (GO) for short (Ashburner, et al., 2000) The word 'classification' is used perhaps less frequently for these systems. The current buzzword is 'ontology' instead. This reflects two important considerations:

1. It is not enough to create and order classes; categories require formal definitions.
2. The term 'ontology' comes from philosophy, and expresses a sort of philosophical commitment. This means that categories should not be based on human ideas or simply observable properties, but on the substantial properties of the entities.

These statements outline current trends and movements in the field. In any branch of informatics it is hazardous to try to predict the future. In some years dramatic and totally unexpected changes can happen. And – as we stated above – medical classifications shifted partly to the field of information science. The development of medical science is also speeding up, and it also contributes to the unpredictability of the future of medical classifications. But based on the current trends we can draw a picture, without being sure that this will really happen. According to this picture in the foreseeable future we can not expect one single, robust medical classification, but perhaps we can develop a system of interoperable classifications. My expectation is to get a generally accepted standard top level ontology that ensures the consistency of all other classifications, and a number of standard foundational ontologies that are used as building component of various application specific ontologies used for different practical purposes. This is illustrated in Figure 8

Figure 8. Synergy of ontologies

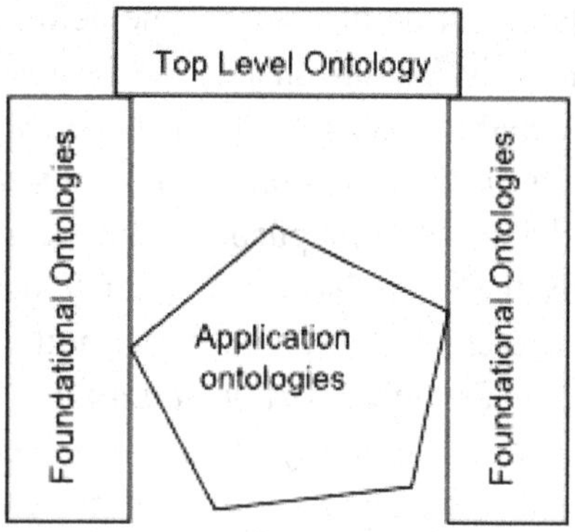

Whatever will happen in the closer or more distant future, it is obvious that we always have to keep in mind, what happened in the past. This was my intention with this chapter.

Acknowledgements

The author has to express his special thanks to Arie Hasman for his valuable comments, and all members of Health Ontology Forum, a working group of the Medico- biological Section of John von Neumann Computer Society, for their contribution to the fertilising atmosphere in which this work could be carried out.

REFERENCES

Abbott, S & Dambergs, Y. (2003). *Raymond Lull's ars magna*. Retrieved December 28, 2006 from http://lullianarts.net/cont.htm

Ashburner, M., Ball, C.A., Blake, J.A., Botstein, D., Butler, H., Cherry, J.M., Davis, A.P., Dolinski,

K., Dwight, S.S., Eppig, J.T., Harris, M.A., Hill, D.P., Issel-Tarver, L., Kasarskis, A., Lewis, S., Matese, J.C., Richardson, J.E., Ringwald, M., Rubin, G.M., Sherlock, G. (2000). Gene ontology: tool for the unification of biology. *The Gene Ontology Consortium. Nature genetics, 25* (1):25-9

Bodenreider, O., Nelson, S.J., Hole, W.T. & Chang, H.F. (1998). Beyond synonymy: exploiting the UMLS semantics in mapping vocabularies (pp. 815-819). *Proceedings AMIA Fall Symposium* American Medical Informatics Association

Chute, C. (2000). Clinical Classification and Terminology -Some History and Current Observations *Journal of the American Medical Informatics Association, 7*(3), 298–303.

Crowson, R. (1970). *Classification and biology* London: Heinemann Educational Books Ltd.

Dambergs, Y. translator. (2003). *Raymond Lull: ars magna* Retrieved December 28, 2006 from http://lullianarts.net/agu/contents.htm

Delacy, M. (1999). Nosology, mortality and disease theory in the eighteenth century *Journal of the History of Medicine, 54*, 261-284.

Eco, U. (1993). *La ricerca della lingua perfetta nella cultura europea* Rome-Bari: Gius Laterza & Figli

Farr, W. (1839). *First Annual report of the Registrar General* London: W. Clowes and Sons

Fischer-Homberger, E. (1970). Eighteenth-century nosology and its survivors *Medical History, 14*(4), 397-403.

Greenberg, SJ. (1997). The "Dreadful Visitation": public health and public awareness in seventeenth-century London. *Bulletin of the Medical Library Association 85(4)*, 391-401.

Héja, G., Surján, G., Lukácsy, G., Pallinger, P., Gergely, M. (2007). GALEN based formal representation of ICD10. *International Journal of Medical Informatics, 76,* 118–123

Hsia, D.C., Ahern, C.A., Ritchie, B.P., Moscoe, L.M. & Kurshat, W.M. (1992). Medicare Reimbursement accuracy Under the Prospective Payment System, 1985-1988 *Journal of the American Medical Association, 268*(7), 896-899.

Hsia, D.C., Kurshat, W.M., Fagan, N.B., Tebbut, J.A. & Kusserow, R.P. (1988). Accuracy of Diagnostic Coding for Medicare Patients under the Prospective Payment System *New England Journal of Medicine 318(6)*, 352-355.

Lesh, J. (1990). Systematics and the geometrical spirit. In Frangsmyr, T., Heilbron, J. L., & Rider, R.E. (eds). *The quantifying spirit in the 18th century.* Berkley: University of California Press. Retrieved June 29, 2007 from http://content.cdlib.org/ark:/13030/ft6d5nb455/?&query=quantifying%20spirit&brand=ucpress

Lindberg, D.A., Humphreys. B.L. & McCray. A.T. (1993). The Unified Medical Language System. *Methods of Information in Medicine, 32*(4), 281-291.

Linneaus, C. (1776). *Genera Morborum* Retrieved June 13, 2006 from http://fermi.imss.fi.it/rd/bd#

McCray, A.T., Aronson, A.R., Browne, A.C., Rindflesch, T.C., Razi, A. & Srinivasan. S. (1993). UMLS knowledge for biomedical language processing. *Bulletin of the Medical Library Assocation, 81*(2), 184-194.

Ogle, W. (2001). transl. *Aristotle: De Partibus Animalium.* Retrieved June 24, 2007 from http://etext.lib.virginia.edu/toc/modeng/public/AriPaan.html

Panchen, A.L. (1992). *Classification Evolution and the Nature of Biology* Cambridge: University Press

Rector, A. (1999). Clinical terminology: why is it so hard? *Methods of Information in Medicine 38*(4–5), 239–252.

Rector, A., Nowlan, W. & Glowinski A. (1993). *Goals for concept representation in the GALEN project.* Proceedings of annual symposium of computer applications in medical care. (pp 414-418). American Medical Informatics Association

Ross, D. (1977). *Aristotle.* London: Methuen & Co Ltd.

Ross, G (n.d.) Porphyry, Introduction to Aristotle's categories Retrieved June 9, 2007 from http://www.philosophy.leeds.ac.uk/GMR/hmp/texts/ancient/porphyry/isagoge.html

Rosse C, Mejino JL Jr. (2003) A reference ontology for biomedical informatics: the Foundational Model of Anatomy. *Journal of Biomedical Informatics 36,* (6):478-500.

Slee, V.N., Slee, D. & Schmidt, H.J. (2005). The tyranny of the diagnosis code. *North Carolina medical journal, 66*(5), 331-337.

Sowa, J (1984). *Conceptual Structures: Information Processing in Mind and Machine.* Reading: Addison Wesley

Sowa, J. (2000). *Knowledge representation – Logical philosophical and computational foundations* Pacific Grove: Brooks/Cole cop.

Stephan, E. (1996). *Observations on the bills of mortality.* Retrieved December 28, 2006 from http://www.ac.wwu.edu/~stephan/Graunt/graunt.html

Surján, G. & Balkányi, L. (1996). Theoretical considerations on medical concept representation. *Medical Informatics (London,) 21*(1), 61-68.

Surján, G. (1999) Questions on validity of International Classification of Diseases-coded diagnoses. *International Journal of Medical Informatics, 54(2),* 77-95.

Üstün, B., Jakob, R., Çelik, C., Lewalle, P., Kostanjsek, N., Renahan, M., Madden, R., Greenberg. M.., Chute, C., Virtanen, M. Hyman, S., Harrison, J., Ayme, S. & Sugano, K. (2007). *Production of ICD-11: The overall revision process* Geneva: World Health Organisation. Retrieved June 21 2007 from http://extranet.who.int/icdrevision/help/docs/ICDRevision.pdf

Wilkins, John (1668). *An essay towards a real character, and philosophical. language* london: brouncker press. Retrieved from: http://reliant.teknowledge.com/Wilkins/

World Health Organisation (n.d.) *History of the development of the ICD* Retrieved June 27, 2006 from http://www.who.int/classifications/icd/en/HistoryOfICD.pdf

KEY TERMS

Categorial Structure: A system, that consist of a number of categories or classes arranged in a hierarchical relation, based on subsupmtion

Class: A class or category is the entirety of individual entities that share some common exclusive property. It differs from set in the sense, that the change of the number of individuals belonging to a class does not change the class itself. E.g. 'human' is a class. Many people may dye or born, but this does not change the class human. While a set of humans e.g. that stay in a room changes as soon as somebody leaves or enters the room.

Coding System: A coding system is a plain list of classes or a categorial structure where all classes assinged by some unique symbol sequence.

Hierarchy: Hierarchy is a structural feature of systems formed from entities among which a transitive, assymmetric and reflexive relation is defined. If the relation is represneted with the > sign, than transitivity means that:

If a>b and b>c then a>c
Assymmetric means that
If a>b is true than b>a is flase
Reflexivity means that for all 'a' it true that a>a.

The assymetric (or directed) relation defines sub- and superordinated entity pairs. The term 'hierarchy' is often used also for system of categories arranged into a hiearchy.

Nomenclature: A system of canonic terms used to described entities of a domain. The term also used for coding systems designed to represent as much entites of a domain as possible. (Contrary to classifications that aim to represent a limited number of abstract categories within the given domain.

Poly-Hierarchy: Is hierarchy where at least one entity has two independent superordinates. Independent means here that there is no hierarchical relation among them.

Subsumption: Is a relation between classes, where all individuals belong to one class, belong to another by necessity. E.g. all humans are mammalians by necessity (i.e. it can not be otherwise) therefore mammalians subsume humans.

APPENDIX

A short inventory of internet resources related to current medical classifications:

ATC/DDD Drug Classification:
http://www.whocc.no/atcddd/
CPT-4 Current Procedural Terminology:
http://www.ama-assn.org/ama/pub/category/3113.html
DSM Diagnostic and Statistical Manual of Mental Disorders:
http://allpsych.com/disorders/dsm.html
HCPCS Health Care Procedure Coding System:
http://www.cms.hhs.gov/MedHCPCSGenInfo/
ICD International Classification of Diseases;
ICD-O-3 International Classification of Diseases for Oncology, Third Edition;
ICD-10-NA Application of the International Classification of Diseases to Neurology;
ICD-10 for Mental and Behavioural Disorders;
ICD-DA Application of the International Classification of Diseases to Dentistry and Stomatology:
http://www.who.int/classifications/icd/en/
ICD-10-PCS American Procedure Codes:
http://www.cms.hhs.gov/ICD9ProviderDiagnosticCodes/08_ICD10.asp
ICECI International Classification of External Causes of Injury:
http://www.who.int/classifications/icd/adaptations/iceci/en/index.html
ICF International Classification of Functioning, Disability and Health:
http://www.who.int/classifications/icf/en/
ICHI International Classification of Health Interventions — under development:
http://www.who.int/classifications/ichi/en/
ICPC-2 International Classification of Primary Care:
http://www.who.int/classifications/icd/adaptations/icpc2/en/index.html
LOINC Logical Observation Identifiers Names and Codes:
http://www.regenstrief.org/medinformatics/loinc/
MedDRA Medical Dictionary for Regulatory Activities;
http://www.meddramsso.com/MSSOWeb/index.htm;
MeSH:
http://www.nlm.nih.gov/mesh
NANDA North American Nursing Diagnosis Association International Taxonomy:
http://www.nanda.org/html/taxonomy.html
Technical Aids for Persons with Disabilities: Classification and Terminology ISO9999:
http://www.who.int/classifications/icf/iso9999/en/
SNOMED;
SNOMED International;
SNOMED Clinical Terms:
http://www.snomed.org/
TNM Classification of Tumour Size, Lymph Node Involvement and Metastasis:
http://www.uicc.org/index.php?id=508

UMLS Unified Medical Language System:
http://umlsinfo.nlm.nih.gov/

Chapter V
Overview and Analysis of Electronic Health Record Standards

Spyros Kitsiou
University of Macedonia Economic and Social Science, Greece

Vicky Manthou
University of Macedonia Economic and Social Science, Greece

Maro Vlachopoulou
University of Macedonia Economic and Social Science, Greece

ABSTRACT

A fundamental requirement for achieving continuity of care is commonly accepted to be the integration and interoperability of different clinical oriented systems towards the realization of a "longitudinal" Electronic Healthcare Record. To enable seamless integration of various kinds of IT applications into a healthcare network, a commonly accepted framework based on international relevant standards has become an urgent need. However, there is much marketplace confusion today in the healthcare domain, due to the variety of overlapping or complementary interoperability standards and initiatives, which have evolved over the years addressing integration of applications at different levels. This chapter provides a brief overview of the most relevant Electronic Healthcare Record standards, by examining the level of interoperability and functionality they provide, in terms of context, structure, access services, multimedia support, and security, to provide healthcare decision-makers and system integrators with a clear perspective regarding the capabilities and limitations of each standard.

INTRODUCTION

In order to manage the safe and effective delivery of complex and knowledge intensive healthcare, clinical practitioners increasingly require timely access to detailed, accurate, and complete patient healthcare records, along with efficient communication methods to share segments of a patient's record within and between care teams (Smith, 1996). Also, as the focus of healthcare delivery, over the years, has shifted progressively from medical centres of excellence to primary care, community settings, and to the patient's personal environment (e.g., home care), patients nowadays require as well access to their own healthcare records to an extend that allows them to play an active role in their health management (Lewis et al., 2005). The development of a longitudinal, patient-centred electronic healthcare record (EHR), which has been a key research field in the health informatics domain for many years, is a much anticipated solution to these issues.

According to Tang and McDonald (2006), "an EHR is a repository of electronically maintained information about an individual's lifetime health status and health care, stored such that it can serve the multiple legitimate users of the record". Iakovidis (1998) also argues that the purpose of an EHR should be toward the support of continuity of care, education and research. On the other hand, an EHR system is defined as a set of interoperable information system components establishing appropriate mechanisms to generate, use, store and retrieve an EHR, while ensuring confidentiality at all times (Blobel, 2002). Ideally, an EHR shall include information such as patient identification, observations, vital signs, physical examinations, treatments, therapy interventions, administered drugs, allergies, diagnostic and laboratory tests, as well as imaging reports.

Yet, much of these fine-grained clinical information on which quality care depends is usually stored in distributed, isolated clinical systems and databases in different kinds of proprietary formats within healthcare organizations. Typical formats may include mixtures of narrative, structured, coded, and multimedia entries, unstructured or structured document-based storage, relational database tables, as well as digitized hardcopies maintained in a document management system. One of the major impediments towards the realization of an EHR is the fact that healthcare organizations, all too frequently, consist of a large number of disparate and heterogeneous information systems, which have been deployed to support specific departmental needs Most of these information systems today are proprietary and have been designed autonomously by different vendors, in order to optimize specific processes within various departmental units. Therefore, each system, required to participate in the co-operative healthcare process and facilitation of an EHR, usually differs in technological and architectural aspects (e.g., user interface, functionality, presentation, terminology, data representation and semantics), preserving the problem of system integration prevalent and of significant complexity (Xu et al., 2000; Lenz and Kuhn, 2002). This has constituted a severe interoperability problem in the healthcare informatics domain, allowing healthcare organizations to be left with islands of heterogeneous systems and technologies that are difficult to integrate. Thus, the requirements to provide clinical professionals of any speciality with an integrated, and relevant to their profession, view of the complete health care history of each patient under their care has so far proved to be a significant challenge. Nevertheless, this need is now widely recognised to be a major obstacle to the safe and effective delivery of healthcare services, by clinical professions, by health service organisations and by governments internationally.

There are many perceived benefits of making EHR systems interoperable. EHRs can contribute to more effective and efficient patient care by facilitating the retrieval, acquirement, organization, processing, communication, and view of patient health record data from different sites (Tang and McDonald 2006). Duplicate data entry and prescribing can be avoided, while real-time transferring of patient data between care sites can be improved, if information is captured, maintained, and communicated securely and consistently, in line with clinical needs. Moreover, EHR systems complimented by clinical decision support tools are capable of reducing errors, improve productivity and decision-making choices, benefit patient care by providing automatic reminders, alerts to possible drug interactions, flag of abnormal values and lists of possible explanations for those abnormalities, along with other possible functions too numerous and constantly evolving to mention (Garg et al., 2005). Nevertheless, meeting these potential requirements and benefits necessitates the interoperability among various clinical oriented information systems that support the seamless communication of health record data, while preserving faithfully the clinical meaning of the individual authored contributions within it.

Generally speaking, interoperability is the ability of different information technology systems and software applications to communicate by exchanging data accurately, effectively, and consistently, and to use the information that has been exchanged. More specifically, according to Brown and Reynolds (2000), the term interoperability is defined as follows:

Interoperability with regard to a specific task is said to exist between two applications when one application can accept data (including data in the form of a service request) from the other and perform the task in an appropriate and satisfactory manner (as judged by the user of the receiving system) without the need for extra operator intervention.

The above definition implies the following

- The ability to communicate data (connectivity).
- The data received by the receiving system is sufficient to perform the task and the meaning attached to each data item is the same as the understood by the creators and users of the sending and receiving systems.
- The task is performed to the satisfaction of the user of the receiving system

Given the continuous evolution of technological innovation and the important need for EHR interoperability, over the years a number of interoperability standards have been developed and continuously refined, in order to improve the compatibility among a variety of healthcare applications and systems. Standards such as the Health Level 7 (HL7) Clinical Document Architecture (CDA), CEN EN 13606 EHRcom, and the OpenEHR initiative, aiming to structure the clinical content of an EHR with the purpose to facilitate the exchange of meaningful clinical data, as well as industry initiatives and de facto standards such as integrating the healthcare enterprise (IHE), and digital imaging communications in medicine (DICOM), have played so far a significant role towards the development of interoperable EHR systems. However, given the plethora of international standards and industry initiatives, and also the fact that different types of integration requirements, all too frequent, can not be satisfied by one standard or integration approach only, selecting the most appropriate solution can be a complex task both for system and service providers (Mykkanen, et al., 2003).

This chapter aims to provide an analysis of the aforementioned prominent EHR standards, in order to provide healthcare decision-makers and system integrators with a clear perspective regarding the capabilities and limitations of each standard by examining the level of interoperability and functionality they provide, in terms of context, structure, access services, multimedia support, and security.

The GEHR/OpenEHR Initiative

Realising the electronic health record has been at the heart of the EU health telematics programmes for the past fifteen years (Iakovidis, 1998). Considerable research has been undertaken, in order to explore the user requirements for adopting EHRs, as well as proposed architecture formalisms to capture healthcare data comprehensively and in a manner which is medico-legally rigorous and preserves the clinical meaning intended by the original author.

One of the most well known Research and Development Projects, funded by the EU Health Telematics research programme in 1991, is the Good European Health Record (GEHR) initiative (Ingram 1995; Griffith et al., 1995). From 1991-1995, the GEHR Project, who's consortium involved 21 participating organisations in seven European countries, and included clinicians from different professions and disciplines, computer scientists in commercial and academic institutions, and major multi-national companies, explored a wide range of clinical requirements for the wide-scale adoption of electronic health records (EHRs), in place of paper records within primary and secondary care and across different specialities. The outcome of this effort was the development and evaluation of different EHR prototypes, which were based on a set of architecture models, exchange formats, specifications of access and integration tools and a standard architecture, all made available and placed in the public domain. This initiative was later continued under the name Good Electronic Health Record with strong participation from Australia. Currently, this initiative is maintained by an international online, non-profit organization, called the OpenEHR Foundation[1], whose aim is to promote and facilitate progress towards the development of high-quality and interoperable EHRs to support the needs of patients and clinicians.

The most noteworthy concept of these initiatives, proposed and defined independently by the Australian GEHR team, is a knowledge-based model, also known as the archetype modelling technique, which facilitates on one hand the specification of a generic clinical record structure, and on the other hand the specific semantic definitions of clinical contents that need to be standardized (Beale, 2002). This model utilizes a dual-level methodology to define the EHR structure. More specifically, the first level is used to define a small, but constant in time, Reference Object Model (ROM) for an EHR, which typically contains only a few generic, non-volatile, concepts/classes (e.g., role, act, entity, participation, observation, etc). In addition, at this level (the level of the ROM), additional methods on how to organize and group clinical information, capture contextual information, query and update the health record, and use of versioning to safely manage clinical information from a medico-legal point of view, are specified (Beale, 2005; Beale and Heard, 2005). Although the ROM has rich capabilities, it is generic enough to store any type of clinical information. Subsequently, in order to overcome the problem of modelling and specifying the concepts and semantic definitions of clinical contents (e.g. blood pressure, lab results, etc.), the proposed methodology utilizes a second level, in which the constraint rules and mechanisms, called archetypes, specialize the generic data structures that have been implemented using the ROM. Figure 1, illustrates a simple example of the dual-methodology concept. A generic class called "Observation_Content" (implemented in the ROM) can be constraint and restricted by an archetype model class called "A_Observation_Content". This later class is further defined and constraint by an instance archetype called "Blood Pressure". The "Blood Pressure" archetype in turn specifies to the Archetype Model and subsequently to the ROM that the first element in the blood pressure group of elements, will have the name "systolic", and its value must be an integer between 40 and 300 mm[Hg], while the second element will have the name "diastolic" with the

Figure 1. Blood pressure instance in the dual-methodology approach

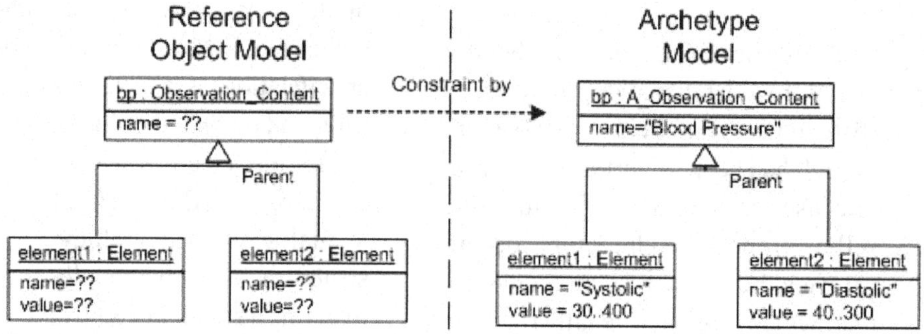

same constraints on its value. Of course it has to be noted that in real clinical practice much richer and complicated models usually exist.

A formal language called Archetype Definition Language (ADL) (Beale and Heard, 2003) has been introduced by the OpenEHR initiative in order to describe for each archetype three basic parts: descriptive data, constraint rules, and ontological definitions. Descriptive data usually contain a unique identifier for the archetype, a machine readable code describing the clinical concepts modelled by the archetype, as well as various metadata such as author, version, and purpose. Also, due to the fact that an archetype may be a specialization of another archetype, the ADL language also states probable specializations. In turn, the constraint rules are the core aspects of each archetype, defining the potential restrictions on the valid structure, cardinality, and content of the EHR component models. In addition, the ontological part defines the controlled vocabulary that can be used in specific places within an instance archetype.

The main advantage of the dual-level methodology and the archetypes approach is that clinical concepts (represented by the archetypes) are modelled externally and separately from the reference information model of the EHR system.

Figure 2. Meta-architecture of the OpenEHR methodology approach (Beale 2002).

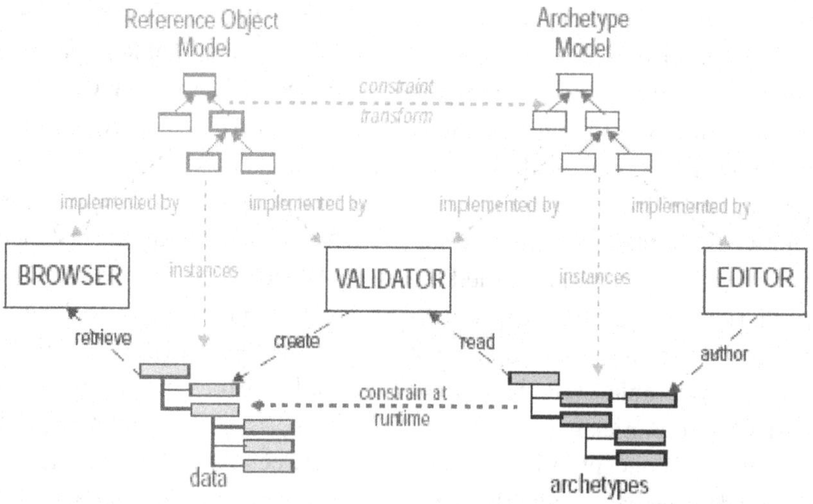

In other words, instead of following the traditional "single-level" development method of a clinical information system, where the domain concepts and semantics which the system has to process are hard-coded directly into its software and database models, the archetype methodology allows domain concepts to be defined separately by domain specialist (e.g., doctors, nurses, clinical bodies, etc.) without worrying about the internal mechanics of the static application software model (the ROM). Derived from this perspective, a basic requirement of an EHR system, illustrated in Figure 2, is to provide three building blocks that are specific to the archetype approach:

- An editor for creating and maintaining the archetypes
- A validator that enforces the constraints are runtime, and
- A browser component who will allow an optimized display of specific archetypes, such as the example archetype illustrated in Figure 1.

Based on the above building blocks, user data entries that need to be stored into an EHR system are guided and validated at runtime against the constraints which are defined in the archetypes for each specific concept. The dual-methodology also allows for the development of "OpenEHR templates". Templates aim to describe the organization and order of models and entries into a record or document (e.g. discharge summaries, antenatal examination, etc.) by using a set (a specified number) of archetypes that can be used for a particular data collection. The OpenEHR foundation maintains libraries of validated templates and archetypes, which can be re-used as a starting point towards the easier and faster development of an EHR system as opposed to a development from scratch approach.

Overall, the framework of the OpenEHR foundation includes a Reference Information Model, the ADL language specification for expressing archetypes, an archetype library, implementation technology specifications such as XML schemas, IDL specifications, and a collection of open source implementations for OpenEHR specifications, all published in the OpenEHR web site (www.openehr.org).

The CEN/TC 251 AND ENV/EN13606 EHRcom

Much of the work and experience of the GEHR project and the OpenEHR foundation, along with other European research and development projects such as the EHCR Support Action (Dixon et al, 2001), and the Synapses project (Grimson et al, 1998), have provided significant input and opportunities for progress on the CEN and ISO standardization organizations.

The CEN/TC 251 (CEN/TC 251), supported by the European Commission DGIII (industry), healthcare organizations, suppliers of ICT-solutions and users, is the technical committee on Health Informatics for the European Committee for Standardization. Its mission is to achieve compatibility and interoperability between independent health information systems and to enable modularity by means of standardization. The TC 251 team comprises of four working groups, which cover: information models, systems of concepts and terminology, security, and technologies for interoperable communications. In particular, the overall scope of the CEN Working Group I (WPI) focuses on standards for the representation of the electronic healthcare record and standards for messages to meet the specific business needs for the communication of healthcare information. In the framework of this working group two work items in the 1990s were intended to be studied and further defines. The first work item, developed as the pre-standard ENV 12265 was the Electronic Healthcare Record Architecture (EHCRA). The ENV 12265 was a foundation standard defining the basic principles upon which electronic healthcare records should be based (CEN ENV 12265). The majority of the requirements for this work item were mainly derived from the GEHR mentioned in the previous section. The second work item, called Electronic Healthcare Record Extended Architecture, published in 1999, was a four-part EHCR successor standard called ENV 13606.

The CEN standard ENV 13606 Electronic Healthcare Record Communication, is predominantly a message-based standard for the exchange of electronic healthcare records. This is mainly due to the fact that the ENV 13606 does not attempt to specify a complete EHR system, but instead, it focuses on the following main parts:

- The Domain Termlist, which provides a set of measures to be used in order to structure the EHR content.
- The Distribution rules, which specify a set of data objects that represent the rules under which certain EHR content may be shared with other systems, and finally.
- The Messaging, which defines a set of request and response messages enabling the partial or entire communication and also the updating of a patient's EHR.

Several EHR demonstrator projects and few suppliers in the UK (Booth et al., 1999; Markwell et al., 1999), Spain, the Netherlands, Denmark (Bredegaard, 2000), and Greece (Deftereos et al., 2001) have selected to use the ENV 13606, however, implementation efforts and experiences were not successful due to the fact that the standard suffered many weaknessess. The single-level modeling approach made the information model extremely complex with lots of optionatiality and levels of abstraction. These weaknesses unfortunately enforced the implementor parties to pursue several adaptations to the ENV 13606, made in an ad hoc approach, defeating therefore the main objective of the standard.

In December 2001, the Health Informatics Technical Committee of the European standards organisation CEN appointed a Task Force, known as EHRcom, to review and revise its 1999 four-part pre-standard ENV 13606 relating to EHR Communications, to produce a definitive European Standard. The mission of the EHRcom Task Force is to produce a rigorous and durable information architecture for representing the EHR, in order to support the interoperability of systems and components that need to interact with EHR services (Kalra, 2006):

- As discrete systems or as middleware components;
- To access, transfer, add or modify health record entries;
- Via electronic messages or distributed objects;
- Preserving the original clinical meaning intended by the author;
- Reflecting the confidentiality of that data as intended by the author and patient.

The revised ENV 13606 (CEN ENV 13606:2000), also called EHRcom, is a five-part standard consisting of the following parts:

- **Part 1—The Reference Model:** A comprehensive, generic EHR model drawing on 14 years of R&D and 2 previous CEN standards. The Reference Model will also be mapped to the HL7 RIM and Clinical Document Architecture (see next section about HL7 and CDA).
- **Part 2—The Archetype Interchange Specification:** An information model and exchange syntax for communicating archetypes; this specification is an adoption of the OpenEHR archetype approach, and will also be compatible with the emerging HL7 Template specification.
- **Part 3—The Reference Archetypes and Term Lists:** Contain a set of vocabularies and term lists to support the Reference Model. It also contains guidelines on how to use the Reference Model classes and attributes, and how to design archetypes.

Part 4—The Security Features: Defines measures to support access control, consent and audit of EHR communications.

- **Part 5—The Exchange Models:** Define messages and service interfaces to enable EHR and archetype communication.

Currently, parts 1 and 4 are officially approved and published as European Standards, while parts 2,3, and 5 are still in work progress and are expected to be approved in 2008. It should also be noted that there is a wide international interest in this CEN work, and the Reference Model (Part 1) has been adopted by the International Organisation for Standardisation (ISO) as a draft standard for consultation and subsequent voting. In general, the CEN Reference Model for EHR communication is a generic model capable of representing the structure and context of part or all of the electronic health record of one subject of care, to support interoperable communications between systems and services that might request or provide EHR data. It is not intended to specify the internal architecture or database design of such systems. Figure 3, shows the logical hierarchy of building blocks which allows EHR content to be mapped.

On the highest level, folders may contain compositions by reference. A composition, ideally corresponds to a clinical document, and usually contains various sections defined by section headers and different entries, which in turn consists of specific elements or in some cases consist of clusters of elements. Each element contains values, and each value is based on a specific data type.

Similarly, with the GEHR/OpenEHR initiative, the most important approach that the EHRcom establishes, as opposed to the 1999 version, is dual-methodology based on archetypes. As described in the previous section, archetypes are used to specify clinical concepts (e.g. blood pressure, heart rate, ECG measurements, etc.) that work as constraint rules to restrict possible values or even relationships of the record components in an EHR composition. An Archetype Definition Language, similar to the one utilized

Figure 3. Main hierarchy of classes of the EHR in the EHRcom (Kalra 2006).

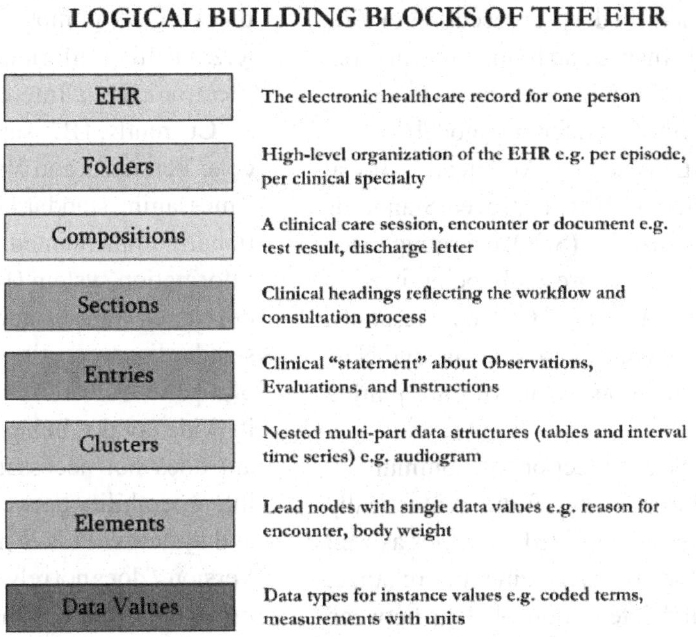
LOGICAL BUILDING BLOCKS OF THE EHR
EHR
The electronic healthcare record for one person
Folders
High-level organization of the EHR e.g. per episode, per clinical specialty
Compositions
A clinical care session, encounter or document e.g. test result, discharge letter
Sections
Clinical headings reflecting the workflow and consultation process
Entries
Clinical "statement" about Observations, Evaluations, and Instructions
Clusters
Nested multi-part data structures (tables and interval time series) e.g. audiogram
Elements
Lead nodes with single data values e.g. reason for encounter, body weight
Data Values
Data types for instance values e.g. coded terms, measurements with units

by the OpenEHR will be defined by the EHRcom. Efforts are also made by the EHRcom group to harmonize the concept of archetypes with other standards, such as that of the HL7 and the Clinical Document Architecture, which is further described in the next section.

Overall, the completion of the EHRcom standard, which have drawn important lessons from the previous ENV 13606 standard as well as the experiences from several R&D projects, is very much anticipated by the European health informatics industry, since it will provide a revolutionary solution to the EHR interoperability issues. However, at this point there is no evidence neither for implementation outcomes or market acceptance, since the standard is not fully completed.

The HL7 and Clinical Document Architecture

Health Level 7 (HL7) is an ad hoc standards group organization that was formed in 1987, as a result of efforts to develop an integrated Hospital Information System by interconnecting function specific systems that deal with several aspects of patient's care in a hospital (e.g., patient admission, transfer or discharge, orders for drugs, procedures or tests and their results, finance and billing information, etc). The number "7" in its name refers to the application layer in the OSI reference model (Tanenbaum, 1988). HL7 is now an American National Standards Institute (ANSI) approved Standards Developing Organization (SDO) operating in the healthcare area. HL7 is presently being used in the United States, Australia, Canada, Germany, the Netherlands, Greece, Israel, Japan, and New Zealand, while additional countries are joining each year[2].

HL7 provides a collection of communication standard formats specifying syntactically and semantically standardized messages as well as interfaces for the electronic interchange, management, and integration of data between computer applications from different vendors within a healthcare network. It does not assume or make any assumption of data storage within applications; neither comprises an architectural framework for health information systems. For this reason, it doesn't tackle any aspects of functional integration between different software components, but only integration at the data level. Moreover, the HL7 standard does not focus on the requirements of a particular department within a healthcare organization. It simply supports various healthcare systems by specifying the precise messaging syntax to be used, including definitions of segments and internal code strings. In general, it can be viewed as a message oriented standard designed to support communication among distributed systems by utilizing a trigger event model that causes the sending system to transmit a standard pre-defined message to the receiving unit with a subsequent response by the receiving unit. For example, when an event occurs, such as the admission of a patient in a healthcare facility, in an HL7 compliant system (e.g., and admission discharge transfer (ADT) system), an HL7 message is prepared by collecting the necessary data (e.g. demographics data) from the underlying application system and it passes them on to a number of other requestor systems (e.g. a Billing Information System), usually as an Electronic Data Interchange message.

Currently, HL7 supports two message protocols, Version 2 and Version 3. The HL7 Version 2 messaging standard is the most widely, internationally implemented standard within a hospital information system (HL7 2.5: 2000). It has been developed and refined over the years to reflect standardised reporting data sets for several aspects of a patient's care in hospital. However, despite its wide uptake, being an HL7 Version 2 compliant does not necessarily guarantees full scale interoperability between healthcare applications and systems. This is mainly due to the fact that Version 2 does not rely on an underlying reference information model. The definitions for many data are rather vague, and there are also multiple optional fields that can be used or excluded from the implementation. Although, these optional fields provide a degree of flexibility, any implementation effort towards the interoperability between healthcare systems requires primarily a detailed bilateral agreement, also known as a "conformant statement". However, this solution is not scalable and requires a great effort of analysis work. In many cases, the use of HL7 Version 2 standard has created the problem of inconsistent implementations due an enormous and unsystematic growth of message segment definitions that have limited the realization of interoperability.

In order to remedy this problem, the HL7 has created a Version 3 standard (HL7 V3). The key feature of Version 3 is an object-oriented model, called the Reference Information Model (RIM) (HL7 RIM). The RIM is a formal information model representing the core classes and attributes, which specify and ensure the validity of content for any Version 3 messages that need to be exchanged between healthcare systems. In general, the RIM defines four major classes of information:

- Entities, (e.g., for persons, organisations, places and devices)
- Roles (e.g. a patient or an employee;
- Participation relationships (e.g. a patient and a clinician relationship), and
- Acts, (e.g. for the recording of appointments, patient encounters, procedures, etc).

In addition, the HL7 organization in Version 3 has introduced the Clinical Document Architecture (CDA), previously known as Patient Record Architecture (PRA), in order to facilitate the exchange of messages between medical information systems. CDA is currently on its second release and was approved as an ANSI standard in May 2005 (HL7 CDA Release 2:2005). The CDA is a document markup standard that defines a generic structure of messages and semantics for the communication and exchange of clinical documents (e.g. discharge summaries, progress notes, etc.), encoded in Extensible Markup Language (XML). By leveraging the use of XML, the CDA makes documents both machine-readable for XML-aware Web browses, so they are easily parsed and processed electronically, and also human-readable so that they can be easily retrieved and used by the people who need them. CDA documents derive their meaning (coded vocabulary) and data types from the HL7 Reference Information Model. More specifically the CDA, based on its letter "A", which stands for Architecture, can be thought of as a set of hierarchically related XML Document Type Definitions (DTDs) or schemas. In the current CDA standard three levels of hierarchy are defined:

- **Level One—Document Header and Body:** The document header, which is derived from the RIM, is consisted of four parts: the document information, encountered data, service actors and service targets (Dolin et al., 2001). It defines the semantics of each entry in the document and conveys the context in which the document was created. Its primary purposes are to make clinical document exchange possible across and within institutions and also facilitate the compilation of an individual patient's clinical documents into an EHR. The Body contains the clinical document context and can comprise either an unstructured text or nested containers such as sections, paragraphs, lists and tables through structured markup.
- **Level Two—Section Level Templates:** In this level the fine-grained observations and instructions within each heading are defined, through a set of RIM Act classes. In level two a set of Templates that can be layered on top of the CDA Level One specification specify or else constraint both the structure and the content of a document, supporting in this way the interoperability since the receiver knows what to expect. A Template may specify a document type (e.g. physical

examination) and further define its sections (e.g. Vital signs, or Cardiovascular examination, etc.), however the specific semantics of each entity are defined in Level Three.

- **Level Three—Entry Level Templates:** This label enables clinical content and semantics to be formally specified to the extend that they can be expressed in an HL7 Version 3 message based on the RIM model. For instance, this level can allow messages to be extracted from a clinical document for a laboratory order or a representation of symptoms findings.

Many national and international implementation projects, as well as commercial products, use the HL7 CDA as a formal format for defining clinical documents, particularly those who have used the HL7 standards for clinical information systems. However, it has to be pointed out that the HL7 clinical document architecture (CDA) is not an EHR standard per say, since it only defines parts of an EHR architecture. Nevertheless, it can form an important component of an EHR, and for this reason, efforts are made to harmonize the release two with the equivalent components of the EN 13606 Reference Model as well as the OpenEHR initiatives.

Digital Imaging and Communications in Medicine

The digital imaging and communications in medicine (DICOM) (DICOM, 2004) is a de facto standard published in 1993 jointly by the American College of Radiology (ACR) and the National Electrical Manufacturers Association (NEMA), building on two previous ACR-NEMA specifications originating from 1985. It addresses the issue of vendor-independent data formats and data transfers for digital medical images, in order to achieve compatibility and to improve workflow efficiency between imaging systems and other clinical information systems within the healthcare environment. Both CEN and ANSI have adopted DICOM by reference in their imaging standards. Nevertheless, given the fact that the DICOM standard was published in 1993, it precedes the development of Web Technologies, such as XML and Web services. Thus, it utilizes a binary encoding, as opposed to the aforementioned standards, with lists of hierarchy for data elements that are identified by numerical tags. In order to remedy this problem, DICOM issued two additional supplementary standards, called Web Access to DICOM Persistent Objects (WADO), and DICOM Structured Reporting (SR).

Web Access to DICOM Persistent Objects (WADO)

Web Access to DICOM Persistent Objects (WADO) standard was published in 2004, as an extension to the initial DICOM standard, and was a collaboration effort among DICOM and ISO (DICOM Supplument 85, 2004; ISO 17432, 2004). Generally speaking, WADO defines a Web-service that can be utilized by web clients who do not speak DICOM, in order to access particular DICOM objects (e.g. radiology images) via HTTP or HTTPS from a Web server. Although, this may sound a straight forward and simple process, it has to be pointed out that DICOM does not support any query mechanisms, and for this purpose every time a client wants to retrieve an object, it has to specify that object by its unique identifiers. In order perform this task the standard provides a method to harmonize the HTTP query syntax with pre-existing DICOM-enabled servers. In addition, there are a number of other options that can be passed on to the web server. The first and most common option, used for teaching purposes and clinical trials, is a request by the client to the server to hide during the transition any fields containing names or other unique identification data from that specific object. Other options include the conversion of the image presentation (e.g. from DICOM to JPEG), the selection of the size transformation for the requested image, the quality, the selection of a specific region of that image, and so on.

The WADO standard provides a good approach to be utilized by EHR web-based system that need to gain access to DICOM objects, and make them available to other systems (e.g. via email) within and between healthcare organizations. A number of commercial implementations of the standard are already available.

DICOM Structured Reporting (DICOM-SR)

Another extension to the initial DICOM standard is the DICOM structuring reports (SR) specification, which was published in 2000 (Hussein, 2004a, 2004b). The SR specification provides primarily a standard information model for the electronic representation of medical image structured reports in DICOM's tag-based format for inclusion within an EHR. Based on this model, the actual content of a structured report is represented by a document tree, which specifies the structure (nesting level), the depth, and in a hierarchical way, the relationships among contents. Every content works as a node and comprises its own information (semantics), which are described based on machine-readable codes. In addition, the standard, just like other standards, specifies a range of different templates (e.g. template for diagnostic imaging report) in order to facilitate improved document structuring and harmonization among implementations. Although, its information model provides a high degree of flexibility to store different kinds of data, ranging from text reports to completely structured documents, it is not sufficiently rich in medico-legal and revision attributes to satisfy the requirements of an EHR. Thus, it is highly unlikely that the standard will be accepted in the near future by commercial implementers away from the imaging field.

ISO/TC 215 Health Informatics and the EHR Architecture (ISO TS 18308)

The ISO Technical Committee 215 (Health Informatics) was formed in 1999 to support the compatibility and interoperability of independent information and communication technology (ICT) systems in healthcare. This scope includes also the development of EHR standards. However, the ISO committee is still somewhat in a phase of trying to define its role, since relatively few work items have been formally approved, although a number of projects have been initiated. Regarding the focus on the development of an EHR architecture the ISO committee has only provided individual building blocks but not yet a complete comprehensive standard that defines the architecture itself. One of these standardization building blocks has been the Web Access to DICOM persistent object, mentioned in the previous section, which was a joint-effort with the DICOM.

In addition, the technical committee 215 published in 2004 another important specification the TS 18308 – Requirements for an electronic health record Architecture (ISO/TS 18308). This specification lists and collates a set of clinical and technical requirements for the implementation of an electronic health record architecture that shall support the use and communication of EHRs across different health sectors, countries, and models of healthcare delivery. However, the TS 18308 provides only requirements and not the actual technical architecture itself. Thus, the primary target groups of this specification document are developers of EHR reference architecture standards such as the CEN EN 13606 and other the OpenEHR. In fact the OpenEHR has harmonized its own requirements for the development of the EHR architecture with the TS 18308. In addition, the TS 18308 is complemented by a technical recommendation draft (ISO/TR 20514), published by the ISO Committee in 2005. This draft describes "a pragmatic classification of electronic health records" and furthermore provides "simple definitions for the main categories of EHR and supporting descriptions of the characteristics of electronic health records and EHR systems." These definitions also support legislative and access control requirements that are applicable to all kinds of EHRs.

Integrating the Healthcare Enterprise (IHE)

Integrating the healthcare environment (IHE)[3] is a recently-formed industry sponsored organization, founded in 1998, in the USA by the Radiological Society of North America and the Healthcare Information and Management Systems Society (HIMSS). Overall, the IHE is seeking to promote interoperability between systems within specialist departments such as radiology, and the conventional hospital systems used to order such investigations and to receive imaging study reports. It is working closely with standards organisations such as CEN and HL7. The IHE initiative does not develop standards, however, it selects and promotes appropriate standards from other organizations for specific cases, while also develops application profiles that work as restrictions for these standards. Among these integration profiles, describe in the next subsections, are the "retrieve information for display (RID)" and the "cross-enterprise document sharing (XDS)". Both address methods on how to access EHRs in various formats (IHE, 2005a).

Retrieve Information for Display (RID)

The RID is best described as a Web service and provides through its WSDL (Web Service Description Language) a simple and rapid read-only access to patient-centric clinical information located outside a user's application. It supports access to existing persistent documents in well-known presentation formats such as HL7 CDA Level One, PDF or JPEG, as well as access to specific key patient-centric information for presentation to clinicians. Overall, the main focus of the RID integration profile is visual presentation and not a complete integration of structured databases. It is the responsibility of the information source to convert the healthcare specific semantics into a suitable presentation format. The display, on the other hand, may process and render this presentation format with only generic healthcare semantics knowledge, but will in general not be able to provide any processing of the healthcare information beyond document display. In addition to the above, the RID integration profile does not address access control or security measures for the transmitted information. Other integration profiles offered by the IHE, such as the enterprise user authentication (EUA) and audit trail and node authentication (ATNA) can be used to facilitate these tasks. The RID profile was initially published in August 2003 and has seen a rather quick market uptake. Several prototype implementations from different vendors have been successfully tested for their interoperability at the IHE cross-vendor testing events, and several commercial products are already available on the market.

Cross-Enterprise Document Sharing (XDS)

Another IHE specification aiming to provide means for EHR document archiving is the cross-enterprise document charing (XDS). XDS is a rather new since the final implementation documentation was released in 2005 (IHE 2005b). It defines registry and repository services, by using an ebXML registry with one or more attached repository systems, and can function as a centralised or distributed warehouse for clinical documents. However, XDS is document centric and "content agnostic" in the sense that any kind of document can be stored in an XDS archive, provided that the metadata for the document, for which XDS has a detailed specification, are available. Figure 1, offers a simple view of the systems (actors) and transactions (interfaces) that are defined by the

Figure 4. Actors and transactions of the IHE XDS integration profile (IHE 2005b)

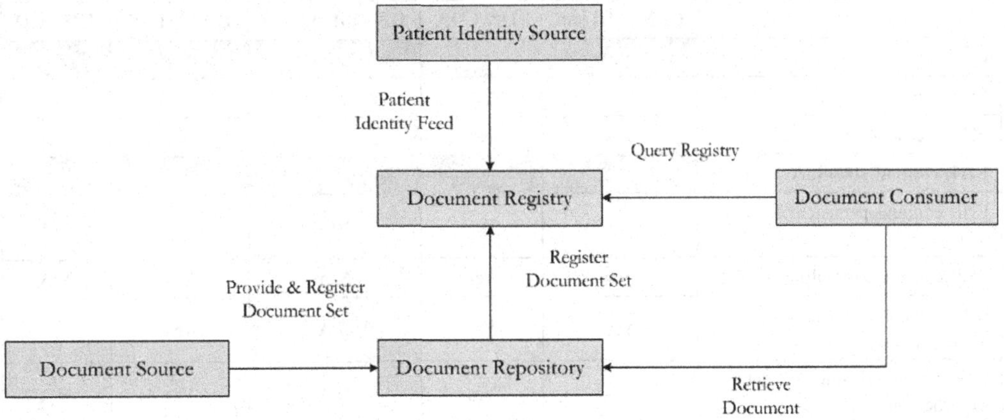

XDS integration profile. A *Document Source* represents a healthcare information system that acts as a point of service where care is provided and clinical information is collected. Subsequently, a document source provides clinical documents (along with metadata) to one or more *Document Repositories* which store the document and then forward the metadata to the central *Document Registry,* in order to register the document. In other words, the document registry does not actually store any document per say, it simply stores the related to the document meta information along with reference regarding the repository from which a document can later be retrieved. A *Document Consumer* is a service application system where care is provided and access to clinical documents is needed. The document consumer queries the central registry for certain documents and receives as a response a list of corresponding to the query documents. Access to the documents and retrieval is then possible through direct access to the document repositories where the documents are stored. The *Patient Identity Source*, finally, is the central system that assigns and manages patient identifiers for one XDS installation.

Based on this simple description it becomes evident that the XDS integration profile mainly provides a storage, indexing and distribution mechanism. However, through specific collaborations between the involved parties, it will be capable of supporting and complementing HL7 CDA documents and EHRcom (13606) equivalent structures, but not a full EHR system.

DISCUSSION

Based on the above overview of the standardization efforts toward the realization of interoperable and compatible EHRs, it becomes evident that the related standards vary widely with regard to their scope and content. Some of them offer a specific content and structured format while others do not. Moreover, some standards define access services, and security features for retrieving and submitting EHR content. For this reason, it is necessary to provide the readers with a simple yet comprehensive guide, presenting all the standards described earlier along with their most important capabilities (Table 1).

Table 1, initially assesses the EHR scope of each standard in terms of content structure and access services. Afterwards, it investigates each standard by utilizing specific EHR aspects (e.g. for content structure, access services, and security features). Features that are not supported by specific standards are characterized with the initials N/A, meaning "Not Applicable". In addition,

Table 1. Overview of features and service of EHR standards (Adapted by Eichelberg et al., 2005)

	CEN EHRcom	HL7 CDA	DICOM WADO	DICOM SR	IHE RID	IHE XDS
EHR Scope						
EHR content structure	Yes	Yes	No	Yes	No	No
EHR access services	Yes	No	Yes	No	Yes	No
EHR content structure						
EHR contains persistent documents	Yes	Yes	N/A	Yes	N/A	N/A
EHR can contain multimedia data	Yes	Yes	N/A	Yes	N/A	N/A
EHR can contain references to multimedia data	Yes	Yes	N/A	Yes		
EHR structured content suitable for processing	Yes	Yes	N/A	Yes	N/A	N/A
EHR supports archetypes /templates	Yes	Yes	N/A	Yes	N/A	N/A
EHR specifies library of archetypes/templates	Yes	Yes	N/A	Yes	N/A	N/A
EHR specifies distribution rules	Yes	No	N/A	No	N/A	N/A
EHR standard covers visualization	No	Yes	N/A	No	N/A	N/A
EHR supports digital signatures on persistent documents	No	No	N/A	Yes	N/A	N/A
EHR access services						
Service for querying EHR content	Yes	N/A	No	Yes	Yes	Yes
Service for retrieving EHR content	Yes	N/A	Yes	Yes	Yes	Yes
Service for submitting EHR content	Yes	N/A	No	Yes	No	Yes
Document-Centric storage/retrieval	No	N/A	Yes	Yes	Yes	Yes
Content format agnostic	No	N/A	No	No	Yes	Yes
EHR security features						
Supports transport level encryption	Yes	N/A	Yes	Yes	Yes	Yes
Protocol allows to transmit user credentials	Yes	N/A	Yes	Yes	Yes	Yes
Protocol enforces access rules	Yes	N/A	No	No	No	Yes

bearing in mind that some EHR standards have overlapping areas, it makes an absolute sence to consider the combination of different aspects of EHR standard functions and services. However, this is a complicated task with many hidden risks, since implementation project needs, scope and targeted areas may vary. Nevertheless, an important initiative that can work as a source for finding a plethora of important information regarding not only the technical specifications and capabilities of each standard, but also the possibility of standard's combination, is the RIDE

Project[4] (Funded by the European Union). RIDE is "a roadmap project for interoperability of eHealth systems leading to recommendations for actions and to preparatory actions at the European level". This roadmap will "prepare the ground for future actions as envisioned in the action plan of the eHealth Communication COM 356, by coordinating various efforts on eHealth interoperability in member states and the associated states".

CONCLUSION

The ever increasing demand for cost containments and provision of quality patient care has led to making healthcare organizations heavily dependent on Information and Communication Technology (ICT). However, the rapid evolution of software applications and healthcare information systems has created an urgent demand for standardization in the healthcare IT market. This demand for standards has also become an urgent need, in order to enable EHR information to be shared between different healthcare facilities. Standards to support EHR communication are at an advanced stage of development, however, further research and implementation work to refine and improve these standards is a must. Overall, standards can support affordable and scalable systems that can be upgraded, as opposed to risky investments in proprietary solutions. Communication standards can allow products from multiple vendors to easily exchange clinical information and contribute to the improved compatibility and interoperability among a variety of applications and systems. Moreover, by utilizing standardized products, healthcare organizations can start with low-entry systems for single departmental solutions and gradually build up larger scale systems up to a comprehensive Electronic Health Record spanning across healthcare enterprises.

REFERENCES

Beale, T. (2002). Archetypes: constraint-based domain models for future-proof information systems. In *OOPSLA 2002 Workshop on Behavioural Semantics*. Retrieved from http://www.deepthought.com.au/it/archetypes/archetypes new.pdf

Beale, T. (2005). The openEHR Integration Information Model. openEHR Reference Model. *The openEHR foundation*.

Beale, T. and Heard, S. (2003). Archetype definitions and principles. *The openEHR foundation*.

Blobel, B. (2002). Evaluation and harmonisation of electronic healthcare record architecture approaches. *Business Briefing: Global Healthcare*, 1-5.

Booth, N., Jain, N.L., and Sugden B. (1999). *The TextBase project—implementation of a base level message supporting electronic patient record transfer in English general practice*. Proceedings of the AMIA Annual Symposium, 691-5.

Bredegaard, K. (2000). National standardisation of electronic health care records in Denmark. *Toward an Electronic Health Record Europe 2000*, 98-102.

Brown, N. and Reynolds, M. (2000). Strategy for production and maintenance of standards for interoperability within and between service departments and other healthcare domains. *Short Strategic Study CEN/TC 251/N00-047, CEN/TC 251 Health Informatics*. Brussels: Belgium.

CEN ENV 12265. (1997). *Medical informatics { electronic healthcare record architecture*. European Prestandard ENV 12265. European Committee for Standardization. Brussels: Belgium.

CEN ENV 13606. (2000). *Medical informatics { electronic healthcare record communication. european prestandard ENV 13606*. European Committee for Standardization. Brussels: Belgium.

CEN/TC 251. *European committee for standardization - technical committee on health informatics.* Retrieved from http://www.centc251.org/.

Deftereos, S., Lambrinoudakis, C., Andriopoulos, P., Farmakis, D., and Aessopos, A. (2001). A java-based electronic healthcare record software for beta-thalassaemia. *Journal of Medical Internet Research, 3*(4), e33.

DICOM Supplement 85 (2004). Web Access to DICOM Persistent Objects (WADO). *Joint DICOM standards committee / ISO TC215 Ad Hoc WG on WADO, final text.* Retrieved from ftp://medical.nema.org/medical/dicom/_nal/sup85 ft.pdf.

DICOM. (2004). Digital imaging and communications in medicine. *NEMA Standards Publication PS 3, National Electrical Manufacturers Association*. Rosslyn: VA, USA.

Dixon R, Grubb PA, Lloyd D, Kalra D. (2001). Consolidated list of requirements. *EHCR Support Action Deliverable 1.4. European Commission DGXIII.* Retrieved from http://www.chime.ucl.ac.uk/HealthI/EHCR-SupA/ del1-4v1_3.PDF.

Dolin RH, Alschuler L, Beebe C., et al. (2001). The HL7 clinical document architecture. *J Am Med Inform Assoc., 8*(6), 552–69.

Eichelberg, M., Aden, T., Riesmeier, J., Dogac, A., and Laleci, G. B. (2005). A survey and analysis of Electronic Healthcare Record standards. *ACM Computing. Surveys, 37*(4), 277-315.

Garg, A.X., Adhikari, N.K.J., McDonald, H., Rosas-Arellano, M.P., Devereaux, P.J., Beyene, J., Sam, J., and Haynes, R.B. (2005). Effects of computerized clinical decision support systems in practitioner performance and patient outcomes: A systematic review. *Journal of the American Medical Association, 293*, 1223–1238.

Griffith S., Kalra D., Lloyd D., and Ingram D. (1995). A portable and communicable architecture for electronic healthcare records: The good European Healthcare Record Project (AIM project 2014). Greenes, R. A. and others, eds. *Medinfo 8*(1995), 223-226.

Grimson, J., Grimson, W., Berry, D., Stephens, G., Felton, E., Kalra, D., Toussaint, P., and Weier, O.W. (1998). A CORBA-based integration of distributed electronic healthcare records using the synapses approach. *IEEE Trans Inf Technol Biomed, 2*(3), 124-38.

HL7 2.5 (2000). HL7. Application protocol for electronic data exchange in healthcare environments, version 2.5. *ANSI Standard.* Ann Arbor: MI, USA.

HL7 CDA Release 2.0 (2005). The HL7 version 3 standard: Clinical data architecture, release 2.0. *ANSI Standard.*

HL7 RIM. HL7. *Reference information model.* Retrieved from http://www.hl7.org/library/data-model/RIM/modelpage non.htm

HL7 V3. HL7. *Version 3 message development framework.* Retrieved http://www.hl7.org/library/mdf99/mdf99.pdf

Hussein, R., Engelmann, U., Schroter, A., and Meinzer, H.P. (2004a). DICOM structured reporting: Part 1. Overview and characteristics. *Radiographics, 24*(3), 891-96.

Hussein, R., Engelmann, U., Schroter, A., and Meinzer, H.P. (2004b.). DICOM structured reporting: Part 2. Problems and challenges in implementation for PACS workstations. *Radiographics, 24*(3), 897-909.

Iakovidis, I. (1998). Towards personal health record: Current situation, obstacles and trends in implementation of electronic healthcare records in Europe. *International Journal of Medical Informatics, 52*(128), 105-117.

IHE. (2005a). *IT infrastructure technical framework revision 2.0.* Retrieved from http://www.ihe.net/Technical Framework/index.cfm.

IHE. (2005b). *Cross-enterprise document sharing for maging (XDS-I)*. IHE Radiology TechnicalFramework, Supplement 2005-2006, Trial Implementation, Integrating the Healthcare Enterprise. Retrieved http://www.ihe.net/Technical Framework/upload/IHE RAD-TF Suppl XDSI TI 2005-08-15.pdf

Ingram D., Griffith S., Maskens A.P., Kalra D., Lloyd D., and Southgate L. (1995). The Good European healthcare record project - the results of a three year project to design a common architecture for healthcare records across Europe AIM project A2014. *Future of Patient Records - Care for Records of Care. May 1995*, 415-419.

ISO 17432. (2004). *Health informatics - messages and communication - Web access to DICOM persistent objects*. International Standard IS 17432, International Organization for Standardization, Geneva, Switzerland.

ISO/TR 20514. (2005). *Health informatics - electronic health record - definition, scope and context*. Technical Report TR 20514. International Organization for Standardization. Geneva: Switzerland.

ISO/TS 18308. (2004). *Health informatics - requirements for an electronic health record architecture*. Technical Specification TS 18308. International Organization for Standardization, Geneva: Switzerland.

Kalra, D. (2006). Electronic health record standards. *IMIA Yearbook of Medical Informatics*, 136-144.

Lenz, R., Kuhn, K. (2002). *Integration of heterogeneous systems in hospitals*. Business briefing: data management and storage technology

Lewis, D., Eysenbach, G., Kukafka, R., Stavri, Z., Jimison, H.B. (2005). *Consumer health informatics informing consumers and improving health care* (Eds.). Health Informatics Series, Springer Science+Business Media, Inc., USA, 2005.

Mykkanen, J., Porrasmaa, J. Rannanheimo, J., and Korpela, M. (2003). A process for specifying integration for multi-tier applications in healthcare. *International Journal of Medical Informatics, 70*, 173-182.

Smith, R. (1996). What clinical information do doctors need? *British Medical Journal, Oct. 313*, 1062-1068.

Tanenbaum A. S. (1988). *Computer networks, 2nd ed*. Englewood Cliffs, N.J: Prentice-Hall, .

Tang, P.C., McDonald, C.J. (2006). Electronic health record systems. In Cimino, J. J. and Shortliffe, E. H. (eds.) *Biomedical Informatics: Computer Applications in Health Care and Biomedicine (Health Informatics)*. Springer-Verlag, New York, Inc.

Xu, Y., Sauquet, D., Zapletal, E., Lemaitre, D., and Degoulet, P. (2000). Integration of medical applications: the mediator service of the SynEx platform. *International Journal of Medical Informatics, 58-59*, 157-166

KEY TERMS

E-Health: It is a relatively recent term for healthcare practice which is supported by electronic processes and communication. The term is inconsistently used: some would argue it is interchangeable with health care informatics and a sub set of Health informatics, while others use it in the narrower sense of healthcare practice using the Internet. The term can encompass a range of services that are at the edge of medicine/healthcare and information technology like electronic health records, telemedicine, evidence-based medicine, virtual healthcare teams etc.

Electronic Health Record: An electronic health record (EHR) refers to an individual patient's medical record in digital format. Electronic health record systems co-ordinate the storage and retrieval of individual records with the aid of computers. EHRs are usually accessed on a computer, often over a network. It may be made up of electronic medical records (EMRs) from many locations and/or sources. A variety of types of healthcare-related information may be stored and accessed in this way.

Health Level Seven (HL7): It is an all-volunteer, not-for-profit organization involved in development of international healthcare standards. HL7 is also used to refer to some of the specific standards created by the organization (i.e. HL7 v2.x, v3.0, HL7 RIM etc.).

Electronic Health Record (EHR) Standards: Standards are documented agreements containing technical specifications or other precise criteria to be used consistently as rules, guidelines, or definitions of characteristics, to ensure that materials, products, processes and services are fit for their purpose. There are three main organizations that create standards related to EHR- HL7, CEN TC 215 and ASTM E31. HL7, operating in the United States, develops the most widely used healthcare-related electronic data exchange standards in North America, while CEN TC 215, operating in 19 European member states, is the preeminent healthcare information technology standards developing organization in Europe.

Interoperability: Interoperability is the ability of information and communication systems and business processes to support data flow and to enable the exchange of information and knowledge. Interoperability must be secured at the technical (norms and standards for linking computer systems and services), semantic (meaning of data) and process levels (defining business aims, modelling business processes and actualizing cooperation between various management units). Interoperability can be achieved by adopting national and international technical norms.

ENDNOTES

1. OpenEHR available at http://www.openehr.org.
2. See http://www.hl7.org for current information on HL7 and its evolution.
3. IHE. Integrating the Healthcare Enterprise. http://www.ihe.net/.
4. For more information you can visit http://www.srdc.metu.edu.tr/webpage/projects/ride/index.php.

Section III

Distributed E-Health Communication Systems and Applications

Chapter VI
The Integrative Model of E-Health Use

Graham D. Bodie
Louisiana State University, USA

Mohan J. Dutta
Purdue University, USA

Ambar Basu
University of South Florida, USA

ABSTRACT

This chapter overviews an integrative model of e-health use that connects social disparities at the population level with individual characteristics related to the amount and type of online health information usage, thus providing an account of the ways in which societal disparities play out in individual e-health usage patterns. Based on an overview of the literature on e-health disparities, we suggest that social-level disparities are manifested in the form of individual-level differences in health information orientation and health information efficacy, which in turn influence the amount and type of online health use. Exploring the underlying social structures that enable individual-level access, motivation, and ability to utilize the Internet for health and how these structures interact with individual motivation and ability advances our understanding of the Internet, the digital divide, and health disparities.

INTRODUCTION

Since its early history in the 1960s, the Internet has grown to contain some 80 million Web sites with a projected 137 million Americans using the Internet as of June 2005 (Fox, 2005a). Obtaining health information is one of the most widespread uses of the Internet. This category increased 59 percent between 2000 and 2003 (Madden & Rainie, 2003), and the most current Pew Internet and American Life Project data (Fox, 2005b) indicates that eight in ten Internet users have gone online to search for health-related information. Other uses of the Internet for health include, but are not limited to, participating in online support groups, consulting with health professionals, purchasing medication, and different levels of involvement in telemedicine and/or telehealth projects (Cline & Haynes, 2001; Dutta-Bergman, 2004c).

In addition to the sheer volume of individuals using the Internet for health purposes, health-focused Internet use patterns have quickly evolved from consumers viewing static information-based pages to engaging in interactive health management initiatives. These developments support the need for scholars to investigate issues related to the Internet and its increasing use for health-related outcomes. In addition, in 2001, approximately 47% of consumers reported having used the health information gathered from sources beyond their doctor in a treatment decision (Cline & Haynes, 2001). This active consumer participation in health-related decision making marks a dramatic shift in the conceptualization of the patient from a passive receiver of health services to an active collaborator or co-participant in health care decision making (Eysenbach & Diepgen, 1999; Marks & Lutgendorf, 1999). Increasingly, researchers are addressing the role of e-health use in the context of medical decision making because its usage ultimately influences the health of the consumer by impacting the quality of the health-care decision, knowledge of and access to healthcare resources, confidence in the decision, the quality of care received, and the quality of health outcomes associated with the health-care decision (Brody, Miller, Lerman, Smith, & Caputo, 1989; Cotten & Gupta, 2004; Pontes & Pontes, 1996).

One of the areas of growing interest in healthcare is the role of the digital divide in the realm of health outcomes, particularly in the context of access to and utilization of health resources (Dutta-Bergman, 2004b). Several lines of work explore the intersections between the research areas of digital divide and health disparities, suggesting that the distribution of health disparities mirror the distribution of communication technologies; furthermore, the distribution of health information seeking and processing skills also tend to map the broader patterns of differences in health (Dutta, Bodie, & Basu, 2008). For instance, studies continually show that when compared to Whites, racial and ethnic minorities are less likely to have access to healthcare and are more likely to be impacted by and die from most major diseases (e.g., cancer, diabetes) (Bassett & Krieger, 1986; Feldman & Fulwood, 1999; Smith & Kington, 1997). This is even more discouraging considering that the majority of chronic diseases are preventable (CDC, 2004). Racial and ethnic differences in health disparity are mirrored by an equally troubling disparity in access to and use of online health information (Talosig-Garcia & Davis, 2005) and other e-health services (Hsu et al., 2005).

The purpose of this chapter is to explore the role of individual and situational differences in the motivation and ability to use the Internet for health purposes and to show how these differences relate to similar differences in health status and well-being, reflecting broader patterns of socio-structural disparities. We examine the Integrative Model of E-Health Use (IMEHU) (Dutta-Bergman, 2006) and extend its theoretical ambit and practical implications by exploring the underlying social structures that enable some individuals access and motivation to utilize the Internet for health and how these structures interact with individual motivation and ability. In the process, we advance our understanding of the intersection between the Internet, the digital divide, and the impact such an interlope has on health disparities. Furthermore, we extend current understanding of the digital divide literature by suggesting that the question of usage goes beyond simple access/inaccess to the realm of patterns of usage and skills needed to use health-based technologies.

The theoretical framework we propose in this chapter connects the social disparities at the population level with the individual level characteristics that are directly related to the amount and type of health information usage on the Internet (Dutta & Bodie, 2008; Dutta et al., 2008). We suggest that social disparities are manifested in the form of individual-level differences in health information orientation and health information efficacy; individual-level differences, in turn, influence the amount and type of online health use. Our chapter will pull together several lines of research and show how the IMEHU can help to advance theory building and to propose useful policy recommendations. So that the model is grounded in relevant research, the concept of the digital divide will be introduced and expanded beyond simple but widespread conceptualizations. Then, we present our theoretical model, elucidate core components of the model, and then discuss ongoing research based on the model. A concluding section suggests areas for future research and offers policy recommendations stemming from the model.

DIGITAL DIVIDE: IMPORTANCE TO E-HEALTH

Digital Divide is the term used to define the gap between people who have and people who do not have access to Internet technology (NTIA, 2000); it is the differences between the technological "haves" and "have nots" (Gunkel, 2003). The digital divide literature is based on the argument that access to and use of the Internet is pivotal to the success of an individual in the information age (NTIA, 2000; Hindman, 2000). In this sense, the Internet is an enabler that catalyzes and contributes to economic, professional, and social success of individuals and communities (NTIA, 1999). Unfortunately, patterns of computer and Internet penetration levels show substantive differences between different racial, ethnic, and socioeconomic groups in the United States (Czerwinski & Abramowitz, 2001; Fogel, Albert, Schnabel, Ditkoff, & Neugut, 2003; Fox, 2005a). Moreover, simply giving people access to the Internet does not seem to remedy deep-seated social disparities. For example, Jackson, et al. (2004) provided low-income families with home-based Internet access. Racial differences in use, with African-Americans reporting less overall use than White participants, were present at the first 3-month follow-up and actually increased at the 6-month survey. Thus, it seems that with the dissemination of computers also comes the responsibility to motivate their use, train users best practice strategies, offer hardware and software that is user friendly, provide low-cost and helpful technical support, and offer help in understanding material and assessing information quality (Dutta et al., 2008).

Given the health and well-being outcomes associated with e-health use, investigating the division between "haves" and "have nots" takes on extra import within this context. However, scholars and other advocates who principally appeal to either social divisions or to individual differences miss part of the overall picture—that structurally reinforced communicative inaccess influences health outcomes through the mediation of individual predispositions, which are simultaneously reinforced by structural-level disparities. Thus, we argue, there is a need to highlight the multi-level and integrative nature of e-health use (Dutta-Bergman, 2006); such a focus incorporates individual motivation and ability to use the Internet for health purposes as well as structural-level issues that are often assumed or not problemetized in current treatments of this phenomenon.

THE INTEGRATIVE MODEL OF E-HEALTH USE

Fundamentally, the IMEHU (Dutta-Bergman, 2006) suggests that macro-level disparities in social structures are manifested in individual-level differences in motivation and ability, thus connecting the broader structures in social systems with the micro-level contexts within which these structures constrain and enable human agency. Individual-level variances in motivation and ability to use the Internet for health purposes, accompanied by within-population differences in technological efficacy reflect the broader structural disparities within the population; these specific technology-based differences, in other words, are reflective of broader structural patterns of differentials in opportunities for learning the skills for utilizing technologies. The individual-level differences in motivation and ability become the conduits through which the structural inequities reinforce themselves and continue to contribute to healthcare disparities.

Within this model, the digital divide is not only represented by direct differentials in access to certain healthcare infrastructures within the larger social system, but they are further reinforced and sustained by disparities in access to and usage of communication infrastructures. Figure one presents the IMEHU based on the literature on media effects (Dutta-Bergman, 2006). According to this model, both motivation and ability are key contributors to online health use. Although motivation and ability are most likely to be accurately represented by a combination of variables, the discussion below will focus on a single proxy for each; these have been the foci of past theorizing and research and thus constitute the best representatives of the two concepts.

Motivation for E-Health: Health Information Orientation

Past theorizing suggests that patterns of technology usage for health are predicated upon the intrinsic interest in the topical area (i.e., health). This is represented in the current model by the construct *health orientation*, or the intrinsic interest in health-related issues. Health-oriented consumers are more likely to seek out Internet-based health resources compared to their less health-oriented counterparts (Dutta-Bergman, 2004a, 2004b, 2004c).

Research on health information orientation suggests variances in the types of channels through which high and low health information oriented individuals learn health content (Dutta-Bergman, 2004d). Specifically, the health information oriented individual is more likely to learn health information from active and information-rich channels as opposed to his or her low health information oriented counterpart.

Health information orientation not only influences quantity of e-heath use, but it also influences the information processing strategies used while engaged with e-health channels. In other words, the motivation to seek out and process health information is also related to information processing strategies adopted by individuals and the cues attended to by highly involved individuals as compared to those individuals who have low levels of involvement in health-related topics (Petty & Cacioppo, 1986a;, 1986b). Specifically, a heightened level of motivation activates individual

Figure 1.

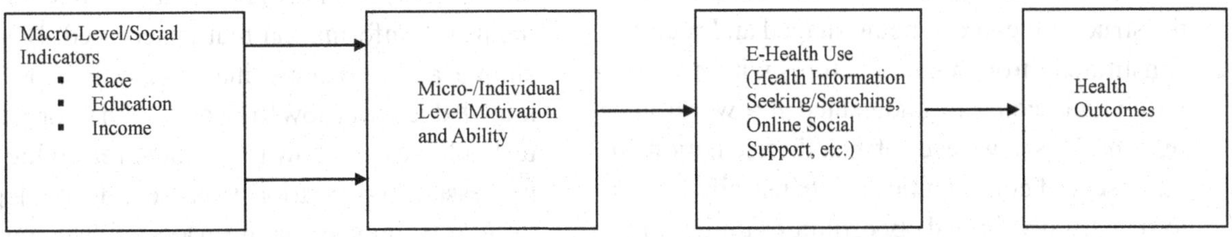

engagement in information processing, decision making, and adoption of behavioral choices based on the consideration of message content. High levels of motivation increase the attention paid by the individual to relevant information and the comprehension of such material. It also increases the active information search for issue-based information. Therefore, a health motivated individual actively participates in health-related issues and actively searches out relevant health information (Dutta-Bergman, 2004b, 2004c; MacInnis, Moorman, & Jaworski, 1991; Moorman & Matulich, 1993; Park & Mittal, 1985).

Existing scholarship documents a strong relationship between traditional socio-economic indicators (race, education, income) and health orientation, pointing out that the motivation in health-related issues is greater among certain segments (White, college-educated, and upper class citizens) of the population as compared to other segments (racial minority, non college-educated, economically challenged). Johnson & Meischke (1991) and Rice (2001) have both noted that people with a lower socioeconomic status (SES) tend to report lower levels of health orientation; they are less motivated to seek out health information than those with greater access to health information resources. Likewise, individuals who have reason to seek out health information or for whom health is highly salient (those who are extrinsically motivated) should be more likely to pay attention to such information. Therefore, variables such as illness diagnosis, state of disease, and caregiving responsibilities of aging parents might influence the motivation to search out health information online as do variables typically studied in research on the digital divide. Thus, individual motivation to seek out and use e-health is embedded within the structural context, being shaped and socially constituted through the structures within which individuals come to understand the world and live in. This low level of health orientation in underserved communities is intrinsically linked to structurally limited opportunities for learning about health information resources and the ways to utilize these resources.

To design, implement, and evaluate preventive health interventions it is imperative to have knowledge about the link between health information orientation and e-health use as well as the interwoven structural disparities elucidated within this framework. Most fundamentally, understanding these important relationships allows a higher level of theoretical sophistication and a recognition of the communication system surrounding high and low health information oriented individuals. More specifically, it allows planners and campaign managers to understand ways in which these systems might be structurally improved in order to meet the information needs of individuals, groups, and communities, and create opportunities for learning that promote interest in health-related issues and support this interest in a sustainable fashion. By investigating the role of motivation in the context of e-health use, the IMEHU provides an explanatory pathway for articulating the process underlying the use of the Internet for health purposes. It also offers a mechanism for understanding the ways in which social disparities influence health outcomes through their impact on information seeking and information processing strategies.

E-Health Ability: Health Information Efficacy

Along with being motivated to seek out health resources on the Internet, an individual's e-health use patterns are influenced by her or his ability to seek out the desired resources. Ability includes (a) having access to health information on the Internet and (b) being able to understand the health information that is accessed. Beyond simple access versus inaccess, this taps into knowledge about how to locate health information technologies and how to go about retrieving and processing information from such technologies once the technology has been located. The concept of efficacy taps into the individual's belief in his or her ability to engage in a particular behavior. The twin concepts of *health information efficacy* and *technological efficacy* capture the perceived ability to seek out health information and use new communication technologies respectively. Greater the efficacy, stronger the likelihood of health information seeking under felt motivation.

Efficacy, like health information orientation, is structurally constituted. The perceived ability to seek out health information is lower among racial minorities as compared to Whites. Similarly, the perceived ability to use communication technologies to meet felt needs is lower among racial minorities compared to Whites (Dutta et al., 2008). These perceptual barriers in using technologies and seeking out health information are very much constituted within the realm of real differentials in access to communication infrastructures (Dutta-Bergman, 2006). Finally, the motivation and efficacy components are interlinked, such that they each shape the other within the structural environment.

The concept of health information efficacy is built on the existing research on self-efficacy which refers to the degree of confidence individuals have in their ability to perform a health behavior and positively predicts the adoption of the preventive behavior (Bandura, 2002). It is the perceived ability to exert personal control, and in this case, captures the extent of confidence individuals feel in their ability to engage with e-health resources. Self-efficacy influences the likelihood of health information seeking and health information processing (Dutta-Bergman, 2006). Health information efficacy varies with the extent to which people feel empowered to make health choices and the extent to which they feel they have access to the basic resources of health that are critical to survival.

Health information efficacy varies with race such that members of ethnic minority groups have been shown to perceive lower levels of efficacy as compared to Whites (Dutta et al., 2008). Such lower levels of efficacy are tied to the material absence of tools and resources in the African American and Latino segments of the population. In addition, the structural absence of critical resources contributes to the perceptions of barriers to engaging with e-health technologies; these barriers are, however, tangible and are connected to the material absence of resources from underserved communities.

Health Outcomes

Ultimately, the IMEHU offers a theoretical framework for understanding population-level health-related disparities by suggesting mediating mechanisms through which health information orientation, health information efficacy and technological efficacy influence e-health use. From a policy standpoint, the model also lays out key foundations for addressing healthcare and communication infrastructures with the goal of reducing the inequities in healthcare. The motivation and perceived capacity to navigate online health resources tends to be lower among the marginalized communities, thus reinforcing existing disparities within the social systems (Dutta-Bergman, 2006). We observe complementary patterns in disparities such that communicative disparities mirror other disparities including healthcare disparities (Dutta-Bergman, 2006). Using health and communication technologies are critical competencies in today's society and are closely tied with a variety of health outcomes (Cline & Haynes, 2001; Dutta-Bergman, 2006); therefore, the extent to which certain segments of the population utilize multiple health resources significantly affects the health outcomes of these segments.

For instance, research suggests that searching for health information on the Internet equips consumers with the ability to engage in preventive behaviors, empowers them in the context of their ability to navigate physician-patient relationships, empowers active healthcare consumer participation in the realm of policies that impede health outcomes, and fosters community platforms for social change by presenting possible communicative spaces for engaging the health active segment of the population (Dutta-Bergman, 2004d). Similarly, research in the area of telemedicine has shown this technology to be capable of reducing cost of healthcare while simultaneously increasing patient care and decreasing rates of morbidity, mortality, and health complications (Currell, Urquhart, Wainwright, & Lewis, 2000; Rendina, Downs, Carasco, Loonsk, & Bose, 1998; "Virtual medical worlds", 2006, April; Wainwright & Wootton, 2003).

Several elements of e-health infrastructure influence the likelihood that any one individual (or group of individuals) will experience such positive outcomes. Two interrelated issues, equity in access and patterns of Internet usage, are explored here. These issues, although discussed under the umbrella of the digital divide, have really yet to be incorporated under any real theoretical framework. Thus, they are briefly presented below in light of the IMEHU.

Access and equity. Digital divide research continually shows significant differences in Internet access along socioeconomic and racial lines (Dutta-Bergman, 2006). Moreover, since these demographic factors are a proxy for barriers such as cost, location, and literacy, (Rice, 2001), when strict access is equivalent, the quality (or equity) of that access is disparate (Dutta et al., 2008). As the IMEHU highlights, the differential demographic distribution of both health information orientation and health information efficacy further suggests differential patterns of access to health information resources on the Web, and differential utilization patterns of such technologies.

Similar to the distribution of communication technologies, access to healthcare resources typically reflects sociodemographic and racial differentials. These patterns of inaccessibility to healthcare services are also replicated on the World Wide Web, such that those with minimal access to healthcare structures also have minimal access to health information infrastructures such as health Web sites, thus demonstrating a complementary pattern of inaccess (Dutta-Bergman, 2006; Dutta et al., 2008).

The differential patterns of healthcare access are a growing area of concern for policy members, practitioners and academics working in the healthcare sector. Increasingly, scholarly articles continue to document the disparities in access to basic healthcare; whereas healthcare is accessible for some population segments, such care and its benefits are typically inaccessible to the marginalized segments of society (Dutta-Bergman, 2004a). Related to the previous discussion about reaching marginalized populations with health campaigns, knowledge gap research documents that public information campaigns, although documenting improvement in overall outcome levels, simultaneously increase the gaps between the "haves" and the "have nots" (Viswanath & Finnegan, 1995). The availability, placement, and use of health information systems on the Internet are likely to contribute to such gaps. Motivation serves an important role as a mediating variable because higher SES groups and Whites are typically more health information oriented as compared to lower SES groups and minority populations (Dutta-Bergman, 2004a; , 2004c; Johnson & Meischke, 1993). As a result, more privileged groups are more likely to seek out health information resources on the Internet, process information from such resources, and adopt healthy behaviors as compared to lower SES groups (Dutta-Bergman, 2004c).

This suggests the need for public and governmental efforts that are specifically targeted at reducing the gaps between the health "haves" and "have nots" in society. One such attempt in bridging the digital divide is the creation of Community Technology Centers (CTCs) that are public access computer facilities located in low income neighborhoods (Breeden, Cisler, Guilfoy, Roberts, & Stone, 1998). By creating sustainable technological resources for health information access and developing initiatives for increasing awareness of and interest in such resources (Freimuth, Stein, & Kean, 1989), such efforts can highlight issues of access and motivation. In addition, the development of sustainable communication skills for seeking out and processing health information should be added to these efforts to increase efficacy.

Patterns of usage. Patterns of usage refers to Internet functions, or, in this context, the ways in which the Internet is used by the health consumer. As documented by more recent inquiries into the digital divide (e.g., Dutta-Bergman, 2006), variation in Internet usage patterns for health purposes should also be considered as an important determinant of health outcomes (Dutta-Bergman, 2004c; Dutta et al., 2008). In fact, recent scholarship on the digital divide questions the simplistic notion of the digital divide being conceptualized in terms of basic access or inaccess, and calls for further exploration of the ways in which various segments of the population use the Internet. In other words, we ought to look beyond ownership of computer and Internet connection to explore the ways in which computer access is put to use.

Published scholarship documents critical disparities within the population in terms of patterns of usage among various consumer segments. As previously reported, the motivation to search for health information is higher among more highly educated consumers compared to consumers with lower levels of education. Individuals with lower levels of education experience a greater number of barriers in using the Internet for health purposes as compared to individuals with higher levels of education. Health information efficacy should, therefore, also be lower among lower SES groups as compared to higher SES groups.

Similarly, racial divides are significantly evident in patterns of health information usage, with African Americans being significantly less health information oriented compared to Caucasians and Asian Americans. The fact that Internet health information seeking disparities mirror the broader patterns of disparities in the population suggests the relevance of investing in capacity building in underserved communities that have low levels of health information orientation and health information efficacy (Dutta-Bergman, 2006).

In addition to investing in infrastructures in such communities, health communicators and policy makers ought to focus on creating educational resources that foster health information orientation and health information efficacy in the communities. Specific programs addressing the barriers faced in the underserved ethnic groups need to be put into place; also efforts need to be targeted toward building efficacy through skills training. For instance, educational programs seeking to provide training in searching, evaluating, and deciphering health information would help address the barriers related to the extent of overload that the underserved groups face. Similarly, design opportunities need to be created for the developers of online health information to respond to the communities that are in most need for health information.

CONCLUSION

There is little doubt that the proliferation of the Internet has opened up and continues to widen possibilities of accessing health information and processing such information to impact health outcomes. However, extant research in e-health suggests that this important medium of health information exchange also significantly contributes to the existing knowledge gaps in society and the resulting structural and health disparities. Internet use and its impact on any individual's and community's health are predicated upon the availability of structural resources like healthcare and means of accessing relevant health information outside a healthcare setting; such differences are mediated through disparities in individual-level factors such as motivation and ability. The integrative model proposed in this chapter suggests a pathway that depicts this mediation. Motivation to use the Internet for health is seen to be typically patterned around an individual's structural context such that people in the high SES bracket tend to be more motivated to use the Internet for seeking out health-related information. At the same time, this orientation is also dependent on an individual's perceived ability to not only have access to the Internet, but also on her or his sense of being able to use the technology to seek out the required information. Thus, motivation has to be complemented with ones perceived ability to use the Internet for the desired effect. And perceived ability is directly related to living structures such as income, education, race, and skills required to navigate the Internet. In all structures in the macro realm — infrastrucutural and communicative — play out and are intertwined with individual-level characteristics like orientation and efficacy.

Empirical validation of the model presented in this chapter and elsewhere is underway. By using secondary data from the National Cancer Institute and structural equation modeling, Bodie, Dutta, Basu, and Anderson (2007) found evidence for the pathway leading from demographics (i.e., race, gender, age, education, income) to health information orientation to health information seeking on the Interent. The pathway from demographics to efficacy did not achieve a conventional level of significance; however, this result is likely due to low levels of reliability in the proxy measure used for efficacy. Other work is underway and should provide added insight into the multi-level nature of the phenomenon under study. This work should also lead to theoretical refinement and a deeper understanding of the ways in which structural level disparities are played out in and reinforced by individual differences in motivation and ability to use e-health resources.

From an applied standpoint then, the IMEHU supports past documentation that simply equipping communities, households and/or individuals with communication technologies is not enough to motivate their use. Certainly, creating access points is an important first step. However, in light of the literature reviewed above, it is merely a first step, one that helps to but does not fully address health disparities; for disparities to be meaningfully addressed, root causes ought to be theorized and reconfigured. This is particularly noticeable within the section on usage patterns.

Ultimately, this chapter suggests that in order to address disparities in technology uses for health, there is a need to attend to existing broader structural and communicative disparities. These structural and communicative disparities work hand in hand to create, sustain, and reinforce health disparities in underserved communities. Key policy formulations need to extend beyond providing underserved communities basic access to health communication technologies to looking at building basic structural capacities. Along with it, such communities should be ensured access to communication platforms and modalities that guide them towards more efficacious ways of navigating available technologies to achieve the desired results in the realm of health and well-being. Emphasis needs to be placed on creating sustainable learning opportunities for using the technologies, and for seeking out and using e-health technologies in underserved communities. To this effect, the model we present serves as an important tool to guide health communication practitioners and policy formulators as it integrates the macro with the micro and presents a composite picture of factors that impact Internet use for an individual's health and well-being.

REFERENCES

Bandura, A. (2002). Social cognitive theory of mass communication. In J. Bryant & D. Zillman (Eds.), *Media effects: Advances in theory and research* (pp. 121-154). Mahwah, NJ: Erlbaum.

Bassett, M. T., & Krieger, N. (1986). Social class and black-white differences in breast cancer survival. *American Journal of Public Health, 76*, 1400-1403.

Bodie, G. D., Dutta, M. J., Basu, A., & Anderson, J. G. (2007, November). *Explaining demographic differences in online health information seeking: An initial test of the integrative model of e-health Use.* Paper presented at the annual convention of the National Communication Association, Chicago, IL.

Breeden, L., Cisler, S., Guilfoy, V., Roberts, M., & Stone, A. (1998). *Computer and communications use in low-income communities: Models for the neighborhood transformation and family development initiative*. Baltimore, MD: Annie E. Casey Foundation. .

Brody, D. S., Miller, S. M., Lerman, C. E., Smith, D. G., & Caputo, G. C. (1989). Patient perception of involvement in medical care: Relationship to illness attitudes and outcomes. *Journal of General Internal Medicine, 4*, 506-511.

Center for Disease Control and Prevention (CDC). (2004). Fact sheet: Racial/Ethnic health disparities. Retrieved April 24, 2006, from http://www.cdc.gov/od/oc/media/pressrel/fs040402.htm

Cline, R., & Haynes, K. (2001). Consumer health information seeking on the Internet: The state of the art. *Health Education Research, 16*, 671-679.

Cotten, S. R., & Gupta, S. S. (2004). Characteristics of online and offline health information seekers and factors that discriminate between them. *Soc Sci Med*, 1795-1806.

Currell, R., Urquhart, C., Wainwright, P., & Lewis, R. (2000). Telemedicine versus face to face patient care: Effects on professional practice and health care outcomes. Retrieved June 4, 2007, from http://www.cochrane.org/reviews/en/ab002098.html

Czerwinski, S. J., & Abramowitz, A. D. (2001). *Telecommunications: Characteristics and choices of internet users*. Retrieved April 8, 2006. from http://www.gao.gov/new.items/d01345.pdf.

Dutta-Bergman, M. J. (2004a). A descriptive narrative of healthy eating: A social marketing approach using psychographics in conjunction with interpersonal, community, mass media and new media activities. *Health Marketing Quarterly, 20*, 81-101.

Dutta-Bergman, M. J. (2004b). Developing a profile of consumer intention to seek out additional health information beyond the doctor: Demographic, communicative, and psychographic factors. *Health Communication, 17*, 1-16.

Dutta-Bergman, M. J. (2004c). Health attitudes, health cognitions, and health behaviors among Internet health information seekers: Population-based survey [Electronic Version]. *Journal of Medical Internet Research*, 6, e15. Retrieved August 22, 2005 from http://www.jmir.org/2004/2/e15.

Dutta-Bergman, M. J. (2006). Media use theory and internet use for health care. In M. Murero & R. Rice (Eds.), *The internet and health care: Theory, research, and practice* (pp. 83-103). Mahwah, NJ: Erlbaum.

Dutta, M. J., & Bodie, G. D. (2008). Web searching for health: Theoretical foundations and connections to health related outcomes. In A. Spink & M. Zimmer (Eds.), *Web searching: Interdisciplinary perspectives.* New York: Peter Lang Publishing.

Dutta, M. J., Bodie, G. D., & Basu, A. (2008). Health disparity and the racial divide among the nation's youth: Internet as an equalizer? In A. Everett (Ed.), *The MacArthur Foundation Series on Digital Media and Learning: Race and Ethnicity*: MIT Press.

Eysenbach, G., & Diepgen, T. L. (1999). Labeling and filtering of medical information on the Internet. *Methods of Information in Medicine, 38*, 80-88.

Feldman, R. H. L., & Fulwood, R. (1999). The three leading causes of death in African Americans: Barriers to reducing excess disparity and to improving health behaviors. *Journal of Health Care for the Poor and Undeserved, 10*, 45-71.

Fogel, J., Albert, S. M., Schnabel, F., Ditkoff, B. A., & Neugut, A. I. (2003). Racial/Ethnic differences and potential psychological benefits in use of the internet by women with breast cancer. *Psycho-Oncology, 12*, 107-117.

Fox, S. (2005a). *Digital divisions.* Washington, DC: Pew Internet & American Life Project.

Fox, S. (2005b). *Health information online: Eight in ten internet users have looked for health information online, with increased interest in diet, fitness, drugs, health insurance, experimental treatments, and particular doctors and hospitals* Washington, DC: Pew Internet & American Life Project.

Freimuth, V. S., Stein, J. A., & Kean, T. J. (1989). *Searching for health information: The Cancer Information Service Model.* Philadelphia: University of Pennsylvania Press.

Gunkel, D. J. (2003). Second thoughts: Toward a critique of the digital divide. *New Media & Society, 5*, 499-522.

Hindman, D. B. (2000). The rural-urban digital divide. *Journalism & Mass Communication Quarterly, 77*, 549-560.

Hsu, J., Huang, J., Kinsman, J., Fireman, B., Miller, R., Selby, J., et al. (2005). Use of e-Health services between 1999 and 2002: a growing digital divide. *Journal of the American Medical Informatics Association, 12*, 164-171.

Jackson, L. A., Barbatsis, G., Biocca, F., Zhao, Y., von Eye, A., & Fitzgerald, H. E. (2004). Home Internet use in low-income families: Frequency, nature, and correlates of early Internet use in the HomeNetToo Project In E. P. Bucy & J. E. Newhagen (Eds.), *Media access: Social and psychological dimensions of new technology use*. Mahwah, New Jersey: Erlbaum.

Johnson, J. D., & Meischke, H. (1991). Cancer information: Women's sources and content preferences. *Journal of Health Care Marketing, 11*, 37-44.

Johnson, J. D., & Meischke, H. (1993). A comprehensive model of cancer-related information seeking applied to magazines. *Human Communication Research, 19*, 343-367.

MacInnis, D. J., Moorman, C., & Jaworski, B. J. (1991). Enhancing and measuring consumers' motivation, opportunity, and ability to process brand information from ads. *Journal of Marketing, October*, 32-53.

Madden, M., & Rainie, L. (2003). *America's online pursuits: The changing picture of who's online and what they do.* Washington D.C.: Pew Internet and American Life Project. Accessed on April 24 from http://www.pewinternet.org/pdfs/PIP_Online_Pursuits_Final.PDF.

Marks, G. R., & Lutgendorf, S. K. (1999). Perceived health competence and personality factors differentially predict health behaviors in older adults. *Journal of Aging and Health, 11*, 221-239.

Moorman, C., & Matulich, E. (1993). A Model of consumers preventive health behaviors: The role of health motivation and health ability. *Journal of Consumer Research, 20*(2), 208-229.

National Telecommunications and Information Administration (NTIA). (1999). *Falling through the net: Defining the digital divide.* Washington, DC: US Department of Commerce.

NTIA. (2000). *Falling through the net: Defining the digital divide.* Washington, DC: US Department of Commerce.

Park, C. W., & Mittal, B. (1985). A theory of involvement in consumer behavior: Problems and issues. In J. N. Seth (Ed.), *Research in Consumer Behavior* (Vol. 1, pp. 201-231). Greenwich, CT: JAI Press.

Petty, R. E., & Cacioppo, J. T. (1986a). *Communication and persuasion: Central and peripheral routes to attitude change*. New York: Springer-Verlag.

Petty, R. E., & Cacioppo, J. T. (1986b). The elaboration likelihood model of persuasion. *Advances in Experimental Psychology, 19*, 123-205.

Pontes, M. C. F., & Pontes, N. M. H. (1996). Variables that influence consumers' inferences about physician ability and physician accountability for adverse health outcomes. *Health Care Management Review, 22*, 7–20.

Rendina, M. C., Downs, S. M., Carasco, N., Loonsk, J., & Bose, C. L. (1998). Effect of telemedicine on health outcomes in 87 infants requiring neonatal intensive care. *Telemedicine Journal, 4*, 345-351.

Rice, R. (2001). The Internet and health communication: A framework of experiences. In R. Rice & J. Katz (Eds.), *The Internet and health communication* (pp. 5-46). Thousand Oaks, CA: Sage.

Smith, J. P., & Kington, R. S. (1997). Race, socioeconomic status, and health in late life. In L. G. Martin & B. J. Soldo (Eds.), *Racial and Ethnic Differences in the Health of Older Americans*. Washington, DC: National Academy Press.

Talosig-Garcia, M., & Davis, S. W. (2005). Information-seeking behavior of minority breast cancer patients: an exploratory study. *Journal of Health Communication, 10*(Supplement 1), 53-64.

Virtual medical worlds. (2006, April). Retrieved June 8, 2007, from http://www.hoise.com/vmw/06/articles/contentsvmw200604.html

Viswanath, K., & Finnegan, J. R. (1995). The knowledge gap hypothesis: Twenty-five years later. In B. R. Burleson (Ed.), *Communication Yearbook 19* (pp. 187-227). Thousand Oaks, CA.: Sage.

Wainwright, C., & Wootton, R. (2003). A Review of Telemedicine and Asthma. *Disease Management & Health Outcomes, 11*, 557-563.

KEY TERMS

Digital Divide: Digital Divide is the term used to define the gap between people who have and people who do not have access to Internet technology; it is the differences between the technological "haves" and "have nots". In recent years this term has been extended to include differentials in Internet usage patterns.

Health Information Orientation: The intrinsic interest in health-related issues.

Health Information Efficacy: The intrinsic consumer belief in his or her ability to search for and process health information. It is the perceived ability of an individual to seek out health information and to do so in a way that is beneficial, given seeking purposes.

Integrative Model of E-Health Use (IMEHU): A theoretical framework based on several information processing, media use, and channel complementarity theories that suggests that macro-level disparities in social structures are manifested in individual-level differences in motivation and ability, thus connecting the broader structures in social systems with the micro-level contexts within which these structures constrain and enable human agency.

Internet Usage Patterns: Internet functions, or the ways in which the Internet is used by the consumer to achieve certain goals.

Marginalization: The process whereby a group of individuals who share physical, cultural, or other characteristics is ostracized from other societal groups which leads to differential and unequal treatment and the population being underserved in one or more ways.

Social/Structural Disparities: The differences between certain segments of the population in terms of access and usage of core benefits such as healthcare and Internet. Such differences include socioeconomic status (education, income), race, gender, and age. When individuals of one demographic have fewer opportunities to engage with structural elements of society there is said to be a social/structural disparity at play.

Chapter VII
A Distributed E-Healthcare System

Firat Kart
University of California, Santa Barbara, USA

Gengxin Miao
University of California, Santa Barbara, USA

L. E. Moser
University of California, Santa Barbara, USA

P. M. Melliar-Smith
University of California, Santa Barbara, USA

ABSTRACT

In this chapter we describe a distributed e-healthcare system that uses service oriented architecture as a basis for designing, implementing, deploying, invoking and managing healthcare services. The e-healthcare system that we have developed provides support for patients, physicians, nurses, pharmacists and other healthcare professionals, as well as for medical monitoring devices, such as blood pressure monitors. The system transmits e-prescriptions from physicians to pharmacists over the Internet. It offers multimedia input and output, including text, images and speech, to provide a human-friendly interface, with the computers and networks hidden from the user.

INTRODUCTION

According to Carmen Catizone of the National Association of Boards of Pharmacy (Catizone, 2002), there are as many as 7,000 deaths from incorrect prescriptions in the United States each year. A Washington Post article (Weiss, 1999) indicates that as many as 5% of the 3 billion prescriptions filled each year are incorrect. In the United States Institute of Medicine report, To Err is Human: Building a Safer Health System, Kohn et al. (USIOM, 2000) discuss human errors in the workplace:

Human beings, in all lines of work, make errors. Errors can be prevented by designing systems that make it hard for people to do the wrong thing and easy for people to do the right thing.

The report sees the need to improve the quality of healthcare systems, ease the access to healthcare and healthcare information, and reduce the cost of delivery of healthcare. The Healthgrid review (Healthgrid Association & Cisco Systems, 2004) concludes that large healthcare systems have difficulties in managing personal data, standardizing the data, extracting content-based knowledge, and federating databases.

Computing and networking technology can contribute greatly to the quality of healthcare. The slow adoption of such technology in healthcare is caused in part by the highly decentralized nature of healthcare and in part because healthcare professionals are often uncomfortable with computers and networks, and feel that such technology is not central to their healthcare mission, even though they acknowledge that accurate record keeping and communication are essential to good healthcare.

In this chapter we present a distributed e-healthcare system that we have developed. The system is intended for use by patients, physicians, nurses, pharmacists and other healthcare professionals, as well as by medical monitoring devices. It aims to provide user interfaces that busy healthcare professionals and fearful patients find attractive and convenient to use, as well as more effective and efficient communication between them.

A patient can make an appointment with his/her primary care physician on the Web. The physician can refer the patient to a specialist electronically, if he/she is unable to treat the patient. When the physician prescribes medication, the system communicates an e-prescription over the Internet from the physician to the pharmacy, decreasing the probability of incorrect or lost information. The patient can check his/her prescription status on the Web and arrange for pickup or delivery of the medication.

BACKGROUND

Extensive work has been undertaken on the development of electronic healthcare information systems. Much of the work on such systems has focused on record keeping and databases based on the notion of the electronic medical record (Bourke, 1994; USIOM, 1997; Taylor et al., 2004; Tsiknakis et al., 1997). Work has also been done on access and security (Anderson, 1996; Andersen et al., 2001), as well as on social implications of recording and communicating healthcare information (Bloomfield, 1991). Less work has been done on human-computer interfaces and usability by healthcare professionals and patients, which our e-healthcare system aims to address.

Governmental and private organizations have promoted the use of electronic technology for healthcare, but these organizations typically incline towards centralized or centrally administered systems (Andersen et al., 2001; Detmer, 2003). Because of the fragmented nature of healthcare in the United States and the increasingly international nature of healthcare services and patients, more distributed and interoperable e-healthcare systems based on open international standards are needed (Grimson et al., 2000).

Beyer et al. (2004) discuss the limitations and challenges of developing an architecture for an integrated healthcare network. They identify flexibility, adaptability, robustness, integration of existing systems and standards, semantic compatibility, security and process orientation as key issues in developing a healthcare network. Song et al. (2006) present a survey of computer-aided healthcare workflow. They define workflow properties and provide a summary of requirements for common healthcare practices.

Omar and Taleb-Bendiab (2006) have utilized the service oriented architecture, in conjunction with grid computing technology, for a sensor and actuator framework that monitors the health status of a patient and provides feedback. Our e-healthcare system provides more extensive services that involve patients, physicians, nurses and pharmacists, as well as medical monitoring devices, whereas their system focuses specifically on the use of medical monitoring devices.

Care2x (2007) is an open-source, Web-based university project that implements a modern hospital information system for training medical students and healthcare engineering students. It includes a central data server and a health exchange protocol, and is implemented using the Apache Web server, the PHP scripting language and the mySQL database system. Our e-healthcare system focuses on the interactions between patients, physicians, nurses, pharmacists and medical monitoring devices outside the hospital setting, rather than on a health research data network or healthcare training for the hospital environment.

Subramanian et al. (2006) have developed a model for patient-centered healthcare services using a mobile device to push/pull data to/from a data analysis engine based on the service oriented architecture. Also relevant is the work of Budgen et al. (2007), who have developed a data integration broker for healthcare systems that uses a software service model to collect and integrate data from autonomous healthcare agencies.

THE DISTRIBUTED E-HEALTHCARE SYSTEM

Design

The distributed e-healthcare system that we have developed is based on the service oriented architecture (Srinivasan & Treadwell, 2005), and uses both Web servers and Web services (W3C, 2004) and also Atom/RSS (Bray, 2005). The service oriented architecture is an appropriate model for developing a distributed e-healthcare system, because it supports an open, networked ecosystem of multiple providers and users. Web servers and Web services support collaboration and enable interactions over the Internet by using standard protocols and conventional interfaces to facilitate access to the application logic and information. Atom/RSS provides syndication of content over the Web and enables synchronization of data in different databases.

Our distributed e-healthcare system comprises a Patient module, a Clinic module and a Pharmacy module. It uses desktop/server computers, hand-held mobile devices such as PDAs and smart cell phones, and medical monitoring devices such as blood pressure monitors. To provide more convenient input and output for healthcare professionals, the system employs various multimedia technologies, such as speech software for speech recognition (SRI, 2007) and speech synthesis (AT&T, 2007).

The Patient, Clinic and Pharmacy modules use security and privacy mechanisms to protect the patients' information in the e-healthcare system. Personal healthcare information is confidential, so access to that information must be restricted to authorized users. Users of the system are authenticated, and session information is kept in a log of service calls. Resources in the system are attached to the resource creator, and privileged users can view/modify the data in the system. For applications deployed on devices like PDAs/smart cell phones, authentication and session management are strictly enforced.

Patient Module

The Patient interface of our e-healthcare system, shown in Figure 1, allows a patient to request an appointment with a physician for a specific

Figure 1. Patient interface

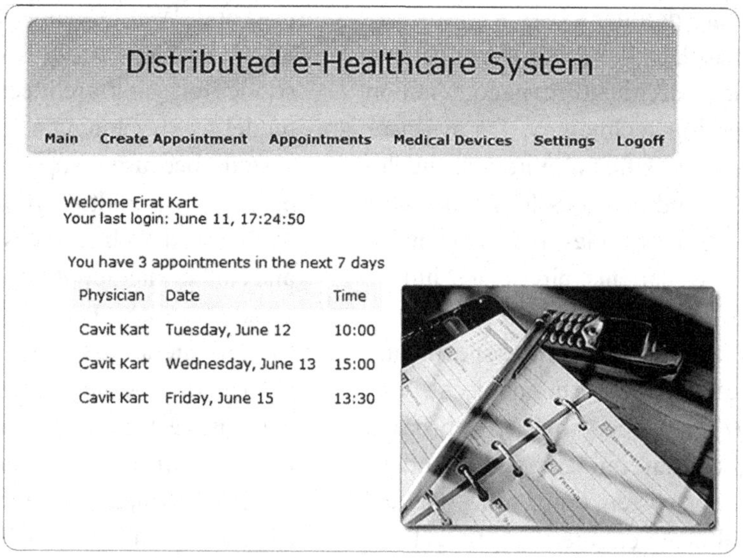

date/time, by communicating with the clinic Web service. Initially, a patient must make an appointment with his/her primary physician. The primary physician can refer the patient to a specialist, and the patient can arrange an appointment with the specialist.

The patient can see his/her previous appointments, and check the status of a prescription associated with an appointment. The e-healthcare system sends reminders about appointments with the physician, the status of prescriptions at the pharmacy, and messages from the physician or the pharmacist to the patient.

Medical monitoring devices, deployed with wired or wireless network support, are used to report periodically, or in an emergency, the status of the patient. Such devices do not send any patient-identifying information. Information is transmitted along with the serial number of the device, and the association with the particular patient is made by the clinic Web service. Unless the patient registers the device on the medical

Figure 2. Clinic module

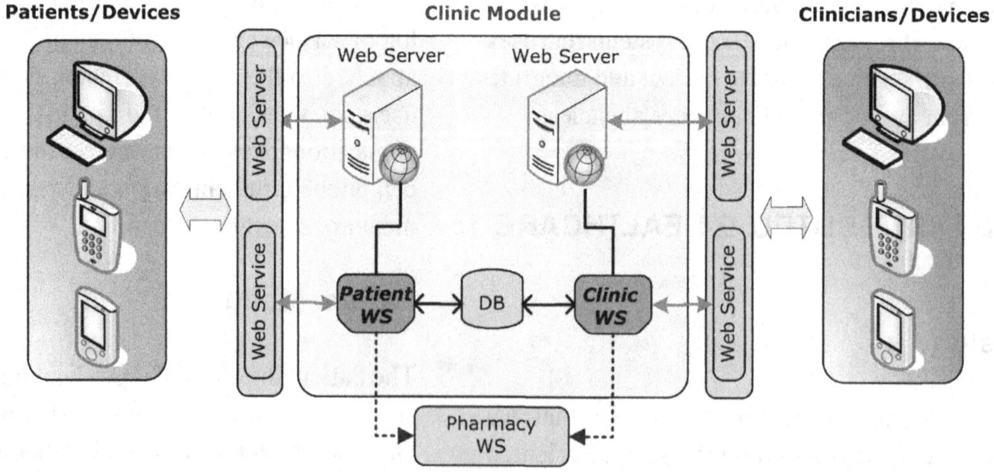

devices Web page, information from the device is discarded.

In our e-healthcare system, the Patient interface is Bluetooth-enabled to a blood pressure monitoring device, which transmits information from the patient to the patient's laptop or desktop computer. That information is communicated over the Internet to the clinic Web service for examination by the physician. The physician and the patient can see the historical data from the blood pressure monitor as a list and/or in a chart.

Clinic Module

The Clinic module, shown in Figure 2 provides support for routine activities of the healthcare professionals at the clinic. It maintains healthcare-related information, such as the physician's appointments, the patients that he/she has examined, notes related to the patients, etc. Access to a patient's private information is restricted and secured, as discussed previously.

The Clinic module exposes Web server and Web service interfaces for the clinic staff, the patients and the medical monitoring devices. The Web server interface is intended for users who prefer to use a Web browser to access the e-healthcare services at the clinic. The Web service interface can be used by humans or devices to communicate with, and deliver information to, the e-healthcare system. Applications that are implemented in Java use the Web service to communicate with the Clinic module. The Web server uses the Web service to access the data.

The Clinic module allows a physician or a nurse to create and view a patient's profile, and to add, delete and edit information (height, weight, blood pressure reading, temperature, diagnosis, etc) about the patient associated with the particular patient profile. The clinic server application runs as a Java servlet and provides Web pages for the physician and the patient to access via the hypertext transfer protocol (HTTP) over the Internet. The patient information is stored in a database at the clinic, including the patient's profile, appointments related to the patient, and prescriptions related to the patient. The clinic Web service communicates with the database over a wired or wireless local-area network using Java database connectivity.

The Clinic client application runs on a handheld mobile device, such as a PDA or a smart cell phone, and exploits multimedia input and output, including speech software in order to provide a human-friendly interface for the physicians and nurses. The Clinic client application also allows the physician to create an e-prescription for the patient corresponding to a particular appointment.

The clinic Web service discovers information about the pharmacies in the area, augments the e-prescription with the name of the pharmacy to which the physician is to send the e-prescription, and sends the e-prescription for the particular patient to the particular pharmacy using the Pharmacy Web service. To locate the pharmacy closest to the patient's home or the clinic, the clinic Web service uses the Yahoo! LocalSearch (Yahoo, 2007) Web service.

The physician can use the Web Server interface to access the e-healthcare system using a browser from a desktop/laptop computer or a PDA/smart cell phone. The physician can use the PDA to enter/retrieve information about the patient during/after an appointment and access this information any time, any where. The use of a PDA with a small keyboard makes it difficult for the physician to input information about the patient. Consequently, in addition to the graphical interface, we have enabled the PDA with speech software. Speech recognition software (SRI, 2007) allows the physician to enter/retrieve information by speaking. Feedback to the physician is provided by means of speech synthesis software (AT&T, 2007). Such speech software eases the task of the physician in completing tasks and encourages the use of the PDA.

Pharmacy Module

The Pharmacy module, shown in Figure 3, exposes Web server and Web service interfaces. The Web server interface allows the users to access the e-healthcare system at the pharmacy using a Web browser. The Web service interface provides access for applications deployed at the pharmacy and can also be used by humans and devices. The Pharmacy module provides services to the pharmacists, patients and devices used at the pharmacy.

The Pharmacy module allows a pharmacist to view the outstanding e-prescriptions from the physicians and to view the e-prescriptions for a particular patient. The Pharmacy server application runs as a Java servlet and provides Web pages for the pharmacist, the physician and the patient to access via the hypertext transfer protocol (HTTP) over the Internet. The e-prescriptions for the patient are stored in a database at the pharmacy for the pharmacist's and the patient's reference. The pharmacy Web service communicates with the database over a wired or wireless local-area network using Java database connectivity.

When the physician submits a new e-prescription to the pharmacy, the Clinic module communicates directly with the Pharmacy module over the Internet. Removing human intervention from the communication between the physician and the pharmacist, and maintaining the information electronically, reduces the possibility of human errors.

The pharmacist can view the outstanding e-prescriptions for the patients, as the Pharmacy module receives them from the physicians. The Pharmacy Web service updates the status of the e-prescriptions as the pharmacist fills them.

When the pharmacist has filled an e-prescription, the Pharmacy Web service sends a notification to the Patient Web service. The patient can also determine, via the Web Server or Web service, whether an e-prescription has been filled and is ready for pick up or delivery. When the patient has collected the medication, the Pharmacy module sends an acknowledgement to the Clinic module, so that the physician knows that the patient now has the medication.

According to the National Community Pharmacists Association, a pharmacy in the United States dispenses an average of 204 prescriptions per day (Alexandria, 2006). Most of these prescriptions are renewals of existing prescriptions. Therefore, the Patient interface also has access to services that provide renewals of existing prescriptions, custom alerts, etc.

Figure 3. Pharmacy module

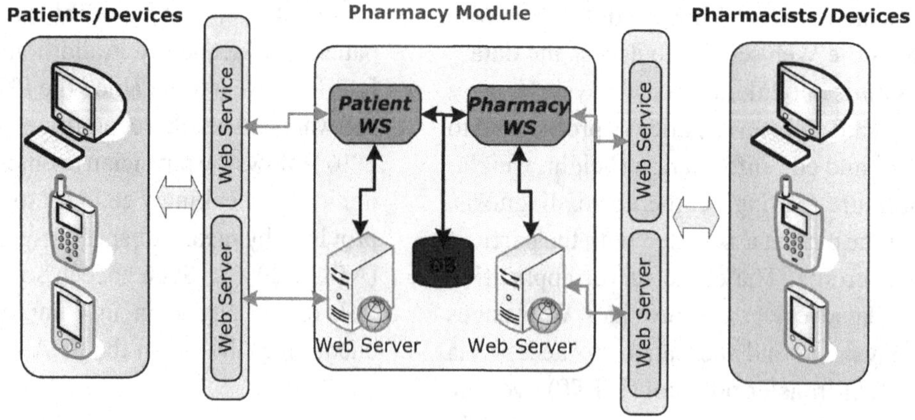

Implementation

We have deployed the Web servers and Web services of our distributed e-healthcare system on 3 GHz computers with 2 GB memory. We have deployed the client applications on 2 GHz computers with 2 GB memory. The client applications communicate with the Web servers or Web services over the wide-area Internet.

For the PDA we used the OQO device, which is a full-featured 3" x 5" personal computer. The OQO device is powered by a 1 GHz Transmeta Crusoe processor, which is powerful enough to run both an embedded speech recognition engine and our clinic client application for the physician. The device features a 800 x 480 resolution screen that is capable of providing the physician with detailed graphical information. The PDA can communicate with a desktop or server computer using wireless (WiFi) communication. The PDA displaying the e-prescription manager and a list of medications is shown in Figure 4.

While it is possible to use any programming and/or scripting language to implement a service oriented architecture or a distributed e-healthcare system, we decided to use the Java programming language for its ability to be deployed on small wireless devices as well as on powerful server computers.

In the following subsections we discuss the particular software technologies that we employed in our distributed e-healthcare system and the considerations that we used in making these choices.

Figure 4. Physician's PDA displaying the e-prescription manager and a list of medications

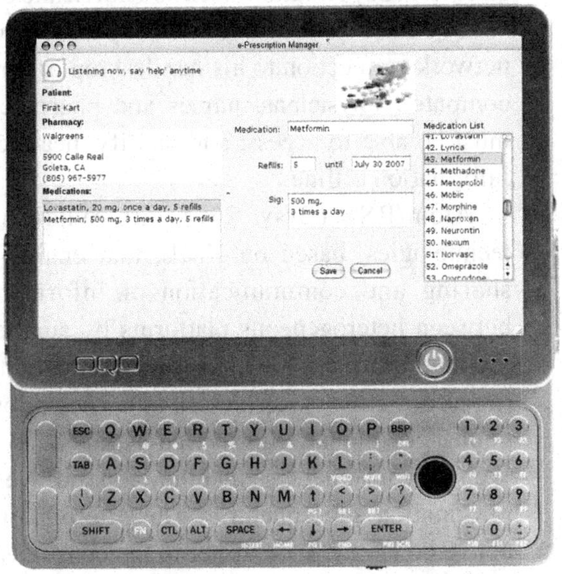

Web Services

Our Web services use the Apache Axis2 Framework (which is the core engine for Web services built on Apache Axiom) and the Apache Tomcat server (Apache, 2007).

Most developers using Web services need to work with data in the form of Java objects, rather than XML documents. Last-generation frameworks, such as Axis and JAX-RPC, implemented their own forms of data binding to convert between XML and Java objects, which was a limited solution for developers. Axis2 is designed to support plug-in data binding using a wide-range of data binding frameworks. To ease the development and debugging of our distributed e-healthcare system, we used plain old Java objects (POJO), based on the Spring Framework (SpringF, 2007).

The data binding support uses customized extensions to the Axis2 WSDL2Java tool. This tool generates Axis2 linkage code based on WSDL service descriptions in the form of stubs on the client-side and message receivers on the server-side. The client-side stub acts as a proxy for making calls to the Web service, defining method calls that implement the Web service operations. The server-side message receiver acts as a proxy for the client, by calling the actual user-defined Web service method. The client applications use the auto-generated stubs to make Web service calls and create/parse the XML representations of the Java objects.

Speech Software

Our e-healthcare system uses speech software for speech recognition and speech synthesis, as described below.

The e-healthcare system uses the DynaSpeak speech recognition engine from SRI (2007). DynaSpeak supports multiple languages, adapts to different accents, and does not require training by the user prior to use. It incorporates a hidden Markov model (HMM) for separating speech from interfering signals with different statistical characteristics. DynaSpeak is ideal for embedded platforms, because of its small footprint (less than 2 MB of memory) and its low computing requirements (66 MHz Intel x86 or 200 MHz Strong Arm processor). DynaSpeak can be used with either a finite-state grammar or a free-form grammar. We chose to use the finite-state grammar, because it offers greater control over parsed phrases than the free-form grammar does.

The e-healthcare system also uses the Natural Voices speech synthesis engine from AT&T (2007). Natural Voices provides a simple and efficient way to produce natural sounding device-to-human voice interaction. It can accurately and naturally pronounce words, and speak in sentences that are clear and easy-to-understand, without the feeling that a computer is talking to the human. Natural Voices supports many languages, male and female voices, and the SAPI, VoiceXML and JSAPI interface standards. Using Natural Voices, we created text-to-speech software for the prototype device that runs in the background and accepts messages in VoiceXML format.

Medical Monitoring Devices

Our distributed e-healthcare system supports the use of medical monitoring devices, deployed with wired or wireless network support, to report periodically, or in an emergency, the status of the patient. Such medical monitoring devices can include networked electronic blood pressure monitors, glucose monitors, weighing scales, pillboxes, etc.

Currently, our e-healthcare system is enabled with the A&D blood pressure monitor device (A&D, 2007), which transmits readings using a Bluetooth radio. After pairing the Bluetooth device with a Bluetooth adapter on a laptop or desktop computer, the blood pressure monitor transmits data to the specific service. Having received this information, the Client application uploads the readings to the Clinic module for storage and enables access to this information by healthcare professionals and patients.

The output from the blood pressure monitoring device on a patient's laptop or desktop computer is shown at the top of Figure 5. The blood pressure history of the patient as a clinic Web service is shown at the bottom of Figure 5.

Atom/RSS

Enabling physicians, nurses and pharmacists to use PDAs or smart cell phones requires those devices to be able to communicate with the Clinic and Pharmacy modules on their desktop or server computers using a wireless or wired network. It is possible that, at certain times and places, network communication is not available. For example, in an emergency situation, such as a hurricane or an earthquake, a physician cannot expect to have a network connection to his/her desktop or server computer. Physicians, nurses and pharmacists must be able to access, and modify, healthcare information offline.

Atom/RSS (Bray, 2005) are syndication technologies, based on XML, that enable the sharing and communication of information between heterogeneous platforms by augmenting that information with meta-data tags so that the information is self-describing. They allow a publisher to make information available on the Web for consumers, so that they can retrieve the information subsequently. The information is delivered from the publisher to the consumer as an XML file, called an Atom/RSS feed.

Figure 5. At the top, output from the blood pressure monitor on a patient's computer. At the bottom, the blood pressure history of the patient as a clinic Web service

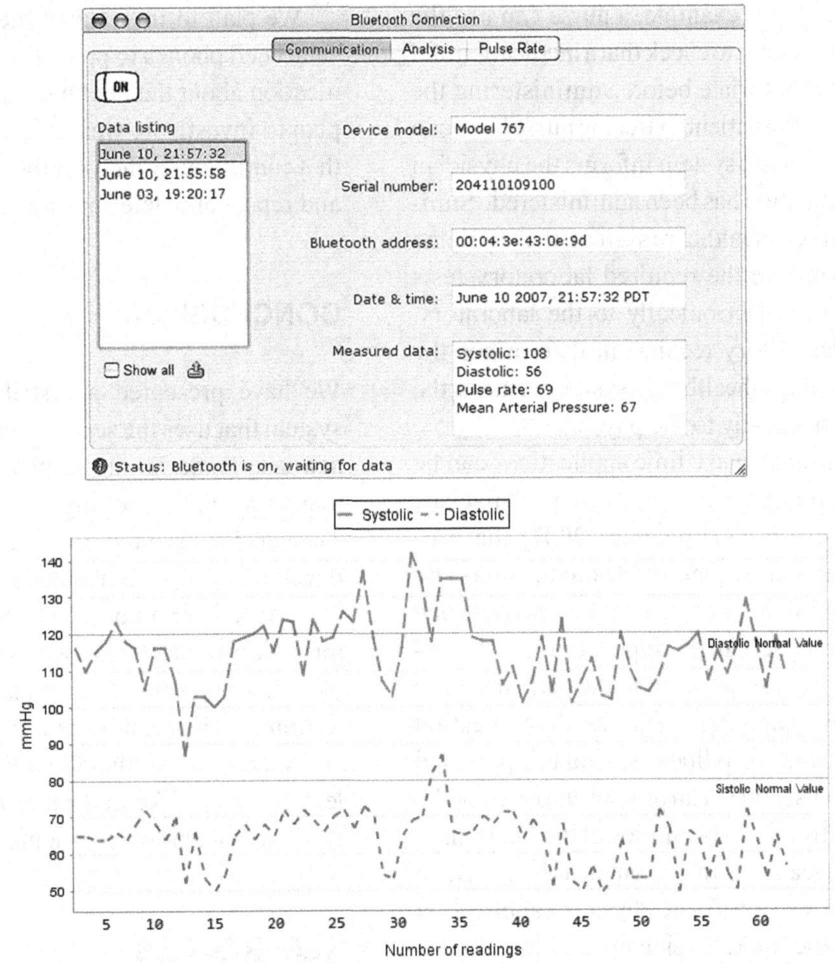

We have developed a Consistent Data Replication and Reliable Data Distribution infrastructure (Kart, Moser & Melliar-Smith, 2007) that replicates information from one computer to another computer. We can use that infrastructure to replicate information from the physician's desktop or server computer to his/her PDA, thus allowing the physician to view that information when it is offline.

In our infrastructure, Atom feeds are used to synchronize the information on the physician's PDA with that on his/her desktop or server computer. At the start of the day, our software on the PDA retrieves the necessary updates from the clinic Web service on the desktop or server computer via a wired or wireless network. Any modifications to the information on the PDA are stored locally on the PDA. At the end of the day, our software on the PDA generates an update feed for the clinic Web service on the desktop or server computer to read.

FUTURE WORK

Our distributed e-healthcare system currently focuses on the relationships between patients, physicians, nurses and pharmacists. We plan to extend the technology to provide other healthcare services and to accommodate other healthcare professionals. For example, a nurse can use the e-healthcare system to check that a medication and dosage are appropriate before administering the medication to the patient. After the nurse has done so, the e-healthcare system informs the physician that the medication has been administered. Similarly, using the e-healthcare system, the physician can communicate the required laboratory tests for the patient electronically to the laboratory. After the laboratory technician determines the test results, the e-healthcare system returns the results electronically to the physician.

The Pharmacy and Clinic applications can be interfaced to applications used by pharmacists, such as Epocrates Rx (Epocrates, 2007), that provide information on appropriate medications and dosages, and that warn of interactions between medications. The Patient application can be extended to provide reminders to the patient to take medications at appropriate times. A medication dispensing device (e-pillbox), such as that provided by MedSignals (2007), can prompt and monitor the regular and timely consumption of medications, a significant weakness in current healthcare. Such a device can also notify the Physician application when the patient has taken a medication.

Communication between the physician and the patient between the patient's visits to the clinic is also lacking in current healthcare systems. Our distributed e-healthcare system can be extended to provide such communication, so that the physician can monitor the progress of the patient and the patient can report symptoms or receive reassurances. This sort of monitoring can reduce the number of unnecessary visits of the patient to the clinic and can increase the number of patients that should have been, but were not, seen by the physician. If physicians lack communication with patients, hospitals are in even worse shape because they have little contact with patients once they have been discharged. Our distributed e-healthcare system can enable hospitals to remain in communication with their discharged patients and to monitor the progress of their recovery.

We plan to investigate the use of PDAs and smart cell phones to provide continuing communication about the health of the patient. We also plan to investigate wearable monitoring devices that continuously monitor the health of the patient and report any deterioration.

CONCLUSION

We have presented a distributed e-healthcare system that uses the service oriented architecture as a basis for designing, implementing, deploying, managing and invoking e-healthcare services. The service oriented architecture facilitates the development of a distributed e-healthcare system by supporting an open, networked ecosystem of multiple providers and users who can collaborate, using Web servers, Web services and Atom/RSS. Multimedia input and output, particularly graphics and speech, make the e-healthcare system seem less computer-like and more attractive to users who are not computer-oriented.

REFERENCES

A&D. (2007). *Blood pressure monitor.* Retrieved from http://www.lifesourceonline.com

Alexandria, V. (2006). *Number of independent pharmacies on the rise, impact of medicare part D looms on the horizon.* Retrieved from http://www.ncpanet.org/media/releases/2006/~number_of_independent_pharmacies_on_the_04-28-2006.php.

Andersen, R., Rice, T.H. & Kominski, G.F. (2001). *Changing the U.S. health care system: Key Issues in health services, policy and management.* Josswey-Bass.

Anderson, R.J. (1996). *Security in clinical information systems.* British Medical Association.

Apache. (2007). *Axis2, Axiom, Tomcat*. Retrieved from http://ws.apache.org/

AT&T. (2007). Natural Voices speech synthesis software. Retrieved from http://www.research.att.com/ ~ttsweb/tts/

Beyer, M., Kuhn, K.A., Meiler, C., Jablonski, S. and Lenz, R. (2004). Towards a flexible, process-oriented IT architecture for an integrated healthcare network. *Proceedings of the 2004 ACM Symposium on Applied Computing*. Nicosia, Cyprus (pp. 264-271).

Bloomfield, B.P. (1991). The role of information systems in the UK National Health Service: Action at a distance and the fetish of calculation. *Social Studies of Science 21*, 701-734.

Bourke, M.K. (1994). *Strategy and architecture of health care information systems*. Springer.

Bray, T. (2005). *RSS 2.0 and Atom 1.0 compared*. Retrieved http://www.tbray.org/atom/RSS-and-Atom.

Budgen, D., Rigby, M., Brereton, P. and Turner, M. (2007). *A data integration broker for healthcare systems. IEEE Computer 40*(4), 34-41.

Care2x. (2007). *Hospital information system*. Retrieved from http://www.care2x.org

Catizone, C. (2002). Colorado state board of pharmacy news. Retrieved fromhttp://www.nabp.net

Detmer, D.E. (2003). Building the national health information infrastructure for personal health, health care services, public health and research. *BMC Medical Informatics and Decision Making 3*, 1-40.

Epocrates. (2007). *Prescription software*. Retrieved from http://www.epocrates.com

Grimson, J., Grimson, W. & Hasselbring, W. (2000). The SI challenge in health care. *Communications of the ACM, 43*(6), 48-55.

Healthgrid Association & Cisco Systems. (2004). *Healthgrid whitepaper*. Retrieved from http://whitepaper.healthgrid.org.

Kart, F., Moser, L.E. & Melliar-Smith, P.M. (2007). Reliable data distribution and consistent data replication using the atom syndication technology. *Proceedings of the International Conference on Internet Computing*. Las Vegas, NV, (pp. 124-132).

MedSignals. (2007). *Electronic pillbox*. Retrieved from http://www.medsignals.com.

Omar, W.M. & Taleb-Bendiab, A. (2006). Service oriented architecture for e-health support services based on grid computing. *Proceedings of the IEEE International Conference on services oriented Computing,* Chicago, IL (pp. 135-142).

Song, X., Hwong, B., Matos, G., Rudorfer, A., Nelson, C., Han, M. & Girenkov, A. (2006). Understanding requirements for computer-aided healthcare workflows: Experiences and challenges. *Proceedings of the 28th International Conference on software engineering*. Shanghai, China, (pp. 930-934).

Spring Framework. (2007). Retrieved from http://www.springframework.org/

SRI. (2007). *DynaSpeak speech recognition software*. Retrieved from http://www.sri.com/

Srinivasan, L. & Treadwell, J. (2005). *An overview of service oriented architecture, Web services and grid computing*. Retrieved from http://h71028.www7.hp.com/ERC/downloads/SOA-Grid-HP-WhitePaper.pdf

Subramanian, M., Ali, A.S., Rana, O., Hardisty, A. & Conley, E.C. (2006). Healthcare@Home: Research models for patient-centered healthcare services. *Proceedings of the 2006 International Symposium on Modern Computing* (pp.107-113).

Taylor, K.L., Colton, C.M., Baxter, R., Sparks, R., Srinivasen, U., Cameron, M.A. & Lefort,

L. (2004). A service oriented architecture for a health research data network. *Proceedings of the International Conference on Scientific and Statistical Database Management,* Santorini, Greece (pp. 443-444).

Tsiknakis, M., Chronaki, C.E., Kapidakis, S., Nikolaou, C. & Orphanoudakis, S.C. (1997). An integrated architecture for the provision of health telematic services based on digital library technologies. *International Journal of Digital Libraries 1*(3), 257-277.

U.S. Institute of Medicine. Dick, R.S., Steen, E.B. & Detmer, D.E. (eds.) (1997). *The computer-based patient record - an essential technology for health care*. National Academy Press.

U.S. Institute of Medicine. Kohn, L.T., Corrigan, J.M. & Donaldson, M. (eds.). (2000). To *err is human: Building a safer health* system. National Academy Press.

Weiss, R. (1999). Medical errors blamed for many deaths: As many as 98,000 a year in U.S. linked to mistakes. *The Washington Post.*

World Wide Web Consortium (W3C) (2004). *Web services architecture*. Retrieved from http:// www.w3.org/TR/ws-arch.

Yahoo! (2007). *LocalSearchAPIs*. Retrieved from http://developer.yahoo.com/search/local/.

KEY TERMS

Atom/RSS: Two different, but related, families of feed formats that are used to publish frequently updated digital content on the Web. Both feed formats are based on the eXtensible Markup Language (XML).

E-Healthcare System: A healthcare system based on the application of information and communication technologies that provides a wide range of healthcare services to its users including physicians, nurses, pharmacists and patients. Typically, these services are provided over the Internet.

Electronic Medical Record (EMR): A medical record in digital format.

E-Prescription: Electronic transfer of a medical prescription in digital format from an physician to a pharmacist, in contrast to the current paper-based method.

Service Oriented Architecture (SOA): A software architecture that uses loosely coupled services to support the requirements of business processes and users. Resources on the Internet are made available as services that can be accessed without knowledge of their underlying platform implementation.

Speech Recognition: The process of interpreting human speech for transcription, or as a method of interacting with a computer or device, using a source of speech input, such as a microphone.

Speech Synthesis: The artificial production of human speech. Speech synthesis technology is also called text-to-speech technology because of its ability to convert text into speech.

Web Server: A computer or computer program that accepts hypertext transfer protocol (HTTP) requests from clients (Web browsers), and that serves them HTTP responses along with optional data content, typically Web pages such as HyperText Markup Language (HTML) documents and linked objects, such as images.

Web Service: A software service that executes typically on a remote computer and that can be accessed by clients over the Internet. A Web service is based on standards such as the eXtensible Markup Language (XML) and the Simple Object Access Protocol (SOAP) and, thus, provides interoperable interactions over the network.

Chapter VIII
Telepsychiatry Within European E-Health

Davor Mucic
Psychiatric Centre Little Prince, Denmark

ABSTRACT

In this chapter the author gives the short review over wide range of telepsychiatry applications. Furthermore, describes completely new and innovative approach regarding assessment and/or treatment of asylum seekers, refugees and migrants in Europe. Experiences from both Danish telepsychiatry survey and the first international telepsychiatry collaboration in Europe ever, will be reviewed in this chapter. Numbers of benefits within mental health care systems all over the European Union can be achieved by establishing of an International European Telepsychiatry Network. The chapter ends by suggestions for future development within mental health services in EU.

INTRODUCTION

The term "telepsychiatry" in this chapter refers to audio-video conferencing in real time.Telepsychiatry connects patients and mental health professionals, permitting effective diagnosis, treatment, education, transfer of medical data and other activities related to mental health care. Overall, studies confirm the notion that telepsychiatry assessments can produce reliable results, telepsychiatric services can lead to improved clinical status, and patients and clinicians are satisfied with treatment delivered via telepsychiatry (Simpson et al. 2001; Kopel et al., 2001; Bose et al., 2001; Bishop et al., 2002).

There are quite considerable possibilities that telepsychiatry presents to health care system, practitioners and patients. There is a number of published surveys on wide range of telepsychiatry applications such as:

1. Assessment and/or treatment of diverse psychiatric disorders (Deitsch et al.2000; Hilty et al. 2000; Alessi 2002 ; Ruskin et al. 2004;)
2. Supervision and education of clinicians and staff (Gammon et al. 1998)
3. Forensic psychiatry (Zaylor et al. 2000; Brodey et al. 2000)
4. Psychology (Koocher et al. 2000: Capner, 2000)
5. Socialwork (McCarty et al. 2002)
6. Military psychiatry *
7. Geriatry (Tang et al. 2001; Yoshino et al. 2001)
8. Cultural psychiatry (Mucic, 2007)
9. Mental health service of individuals with hearing disabilities (Afrin et al. 1997)

Nevertheless, telepsychiatry can be cost-effective by reducing costs of transport for both clinicians/staff and the patient respectively (Hyler et al.2003).

However, the potential for 'linking' patients and clinicians by using video conferencing has not been explored in Europe in the same degree as in USA, Canada and Australia. The main explanation for minor telepsychiatry activities is higher accessibility to mental health services in Europe then in rural areas in Australia or Canada where telepsychiatry has been developed since 1959. European telepsychiatry pioneers are in Norway where rural areas' need for specialists' expertise has been partly satisfied via telepsychiatry. Aside from Norway, most recent telepsychiatry activities in Europe took/take place in England (McLaren et al. 2002),Finland (Sorvaniemi et al. 2005), Canary Islands (Cuevas C.et al. 2003), Sweden and Denmark (Mucic, 2007).

DANISH TELEPSYCHIATRY MODEL

Since early nineties, Denmark faced significant barriers in providing mental health care service towards refugees and migrants on their mother tongue. In the country with only few clinicians of other ethnic origin then Danish, the most of the treatment of refugees and migrants is provided via translators. Psychiatric Centre Little Prince in Copenhagen is the first and so far the only place in Denmark that use telepsychiatry in order to assess and/or treat asylum seekers, refugees and migrants via their own mother tongue (www.denlilleprins.org).

The first telepsychiatry project in Denmark initiated and realized by clinicians affiliated to the Centre increased the access to appropriate cross-cultural clinical, educational and consultation service. The project started in 2004. runs over three years and is supposed to grow in to a sustainable telepsychiatry service. The survey so far involved 60 patients from 8 countries speaking 6 different languages. There were 100% admission to both assessment and continuously treatment under the survey period. All patients were asked to complete the 10-items questionnaire after end of the telepsychiatry-contact in order to determine satisfactory level, advantages and disadvantages by using telepsychiatry.

Patients` response to telepsychiatry in Danish survey has been very positive regardless degree of mental illness. Key predictor of patient satisfaction in the survey was possibility to communicate on mother tongue. Both, participants with or without previous experience by translator provided mental health care prefer remote contact on mother tongue rather then contact via translator.

Several publications and international presentations followed the developing of the survey (see www.denlilleprins.org). Furthermore, the methodology, guidelines and clinical experiences have been developed in order to improve mental health service towards asylum seekers, refugees and migrants in Denmark.

Encouraged by the success, Psychiatric Centre Little Prince expanded the activities across the boundaries of Denmark. Not so far away, in Malmö, Sweden, the first international telepsychiatry collaboration in Europe was initiated in spring 2006. Sweden is a country with much longer immigrating tradition then Denmark and consequently far more clinicians of other ethnic origin then we could find in Denmark. It was obvious to try built the bridge and "borrow" the resources from neighbour country. Consequently, the clinicians that speak Arabic, Polish, Kurdish and ex-Yugoslavian languages are now placed in Sweden while the patients are in Denmark.

IT network in Sweden is compatible and as well developed as in Denmark. The same equipment was used and the results of the trial were as positive as in Danish survey.

Technical Set Up

Video-conferencing equipment connect Psychiatric centre Little Prince in Copenhagen with two hospitals, one asylum seekers centre, and one social institution. The distance from Psychiatric Centre Little Prince is from 145-200 km, respectively.

Dansk Telemedicin A/S provided technical support (www.telemed.dk). Wherever possible, commercial off-the-shelf equipment was used. Different systems were tested before deciding on standalone medium-level video conferencing units connected to LCD TV-screens. Using a medium-level system resulted in a better image and sound quality than the cheaper entry-level systems available. Stand-alone (TV-based) units proved user-friendlier and more stable than Windows computer based system. The equipment had built-in support for AES encryption (Advanced Encryption Standard). All installations used Pan-Tilt-Zoom cameras, allowing the psychiatrists to remote control patient-side cameras. Until recently, ISDN (H.320) has been the videoconference technology of choice in both Europe and the rest of the world where telepsychiatry services have been established. There are, however, certain disadvantages to using ISDN. These include limited bandwidth, high installation costs, high traffic costs and limited availability. To overcome these issues, IP-based units were

Figure 1. Videoconferencing in real-time enables psychiatric assessment without translators

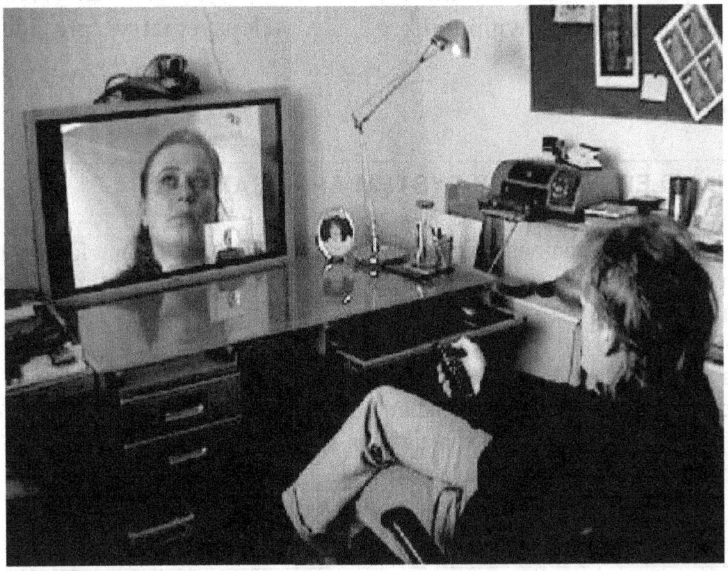

used (H.323/H.264). In Denmark the clinics were connected by 2 Mbit/s SHDSL connections (Symmetric high-speed digital subscriber line). Even though symmetric lines were used, the bandwidth was limited by the upstream speed. Available bandwidth was often substantially lower, typically in the 768-1.500 kBit/s range.

In Sweden 10 Mbit/s fibre connections were used, as high-speed connections are cheaper and more readily available in Sweden. Due to the packet-based nature of IP data traffic, IP-based videoconference (H.323) systems are more sensitive to network delays than circuit based ISDN solutions. The latency (network delay) was low, generally less than 100 ms. This resulted in an acceptable quality, with less than 1% dropped frames.

RECENT CHALLENGES IN EUROPE - INNOVATIVE THINKING

According to international published researches there was only one international telepsychiatry trial between Australia and New Zealand (Samuels A., 1999). Such trial has never been done in Europe before. Results and experiences from the first European telepsychiatry collaboration raise some interesting questions regarding future development of mental health care within EU.

The enlargement of the European Union brings together a diverse group of new members. Free movement of EU citizens increases the claims towards mental health care systems in each European country. At the same time, the number of refugees from Africa, Middle east and Balkan is already growing problem in mental health care systems all over the Europe. Shortages of resources with cross cultural expertise and "cross-cultural background" make psychiatric assessment and/or treatment more time consuming and expensive. There is a number of research describing difficulties in dealing with cross-cultural patients. The most of patients speak only mother tongue, which makes the use of translators unavoidable. The use of a third person in per definition confidential relationship may affect patients` compliance.

One solution to this growing problem in Europe is to bring "cultural expertise" to the patient by using telepsychiatry.

In a field such as assessment and treatment of migrants/refugees, often torture survivors, who are significantly underserved on their own language, telepsychiatry enables access to appropriate speciality service. There are no doubts that direct contact with the patient is preferable in almost all settings within psychiatry/psychology/psychotherapy. However, the Danish survey confirms the postulate that the patients prioritize telepsychiatry- provided contact via mother

Table 1.

POTENTIAL TELEPSYCHIATRY SYSTEM APPLICATIONS
• Conduct treatment team with select skills- sign language and many foreign languages staff
• Acute psychiatric assessments
• Discharge planning
• Follow up service
• Access to child, adult, geriatric, forensic and deaf services specialty staff
• Second opinion service between mental health professionals and GP`s
• Distance supervision and staff consultation
• Psycho education of family members
• Distance learning via case conferencing and best practice demonstration
• Consultations to other countries within EU

tongue rather then direct contact via translator. The results of the survey may contribute to positive changes in policy and routines within mental health service, not only in Denmark but also hopefully all over Europe.

At the same time, telepsychiatry provide opportunities for participation of other individuals involved in work with the patient (family members, social worker, GP, stuff on psychiatric department etc.).

A "second opinion service" toward GP`s provided via telepsychiatry, can decrease the number of inappropriate admissions, long stays and readmissions into the acute sector. In near future, we may incorporate telepsychiatry in chronic disease management and support patient self-management. This means that the equipment may be installed at patients' own homes with possibility to access the psychiatric expertise whenever it is needed.

A vision for the future may be developing of a *European Telepsychiatry Network* with capability to link clinicians and patients from different European countries and consequently maximize access to expert skill resources within EU. However, every National Telepsychiatry Network should develop own telepsychiatry applications as suggested in table 1. Developing of such national and especially international networks needs clear legal, regulatory, and ethical guidelines.

On the other hand, the advantages in potential European telepsychiatry network are many which may justify the future efforts in order to develop such network (Table 2.).

CONCLUSION

According to brief described results and experiences with telepsychiatry survey initiated in Denmark, one may see considerable possibilities in future developing within European mental e-health. Numbers of applications and reliable benefits are not negligible even for high-developed social societies such as Scandinavian. Mental health care towards asylum seekers, refugees and migrants is only one of many potential telepsychiatry applications. Threatening resource shortage in whole Scandinavia forces us to think innovative and use technology in order to reduce limitations within mental health service towards domestic population.

Used as a supplement to existing mental health care system, telepsychiatry brings professional mental health expertise to especially outlying areas with resource shortage but also to any other areas with limited access to relevant mental health care. Telepsychiatry is the tool for improvement of mental health care limitations such as cultural, educational, linguistically and nevertheless economical. Telepsychiatry can

Table 2.

ADVANTAGES IN POTENTIAL (EUROPEAN) TELEPSYCHIATRY NETWORK
• Increase access to sign language and many foreign languages staff
• Increase speed and accuracy of diagnosis and treatment
• Increase access to child, adult, geriatric, forensic and deaf services specialty staff
• Increase collaboration among GP`s, staff within primary care service and mental health service
• Increase continuity of care and professional contact
• Improve education
• Increase efficiency and effectiveness through improved performance
• Reduce staff costs: travel time, staff time
• Decrease the number of inappropriate admissions and readmissions into the acute sector

increase the international exchange of resources and contribute to developing of European mental e-health by building the bridges over cross-cultural barriers in mental health service systems all over the EU.

Finally, the successful integration of telepsychiatry could improve the quality of mental health service towards domestic European citizens as well as asylum seekers, refugees and migrants within EU community.

REFERENCES

Afrin J. A., Whittemore KR (1997). A telemedicine success story. *Carolina Health Services Review, 4*, 225-231.

Alessi, N. (2002).Telepsychiatric care for a depressed adolescent. *Journal of the American Academy of Child & Adolescent Psychiatry, 41*(8), 894-895.

Bishop J. E., O'Reilly R. L., Maddox K., et al.(2002). Client satisfaction in a feasibility study comparing face-to-face interviews with telepsychiatry. *J Telemed Telecare 8*, 217–221.

Bose U., McLaren P., Riley A., et al.(2001). The use of telepsychiatry in the brief counseling of non-psychotic patients from an inner-London general practice. *J Telemed Telecare 7*(suppl. 1), 8–10.

Brodey B. B., Claypoole K. H., Brodey I. S., et al.(2000): Satisfaction of forensic psychiatric patients with remote telepsychiatric evaluations. *Psychiatric Services 51*, 1305–1307.

Brown F. W. (1998). Rural telepsychiatry. *Psychiatr Serv; 49*, 963-964.

Capner M. (2000). Videoconferencing in the provision of psychological services at a distance. *J Telemed Telecare 6*, 311–319.

Cuevas C. et al. (2003).Telepsychiatry in Canary Islands: user acceptance and satisfaction. *J Telemed Telecare, 9*, 221-224.

Deitsch S. E., Frueh B. C., Santos A. B. (2000). Telepsychiatry for post-traumatic stress disorder. *J Telemed Telecare 6*, 184-186.

Gammon D., Sorlie T., Bergvik S., Hoifodt T. S. (1998). Psychotherapy supervision conducted by videoconferencing: a qualitative study of users experiences. *J Telemed Telecare, 4*(suppl. 1),33 5.

Hilty D. M., Sison J. I., Nesbitt T. S., Hales R. E. (2000). Telepsychiatric consultation for ADHD in the primary care setting (letter). *J Am Acad Child Adolesc Psychiatry 39*, 15-16

Hyler S. E., Gangure D. P. (2003). A review of the costs of telepsychiatry. *Psychiatr Serv, 54*, 976-980.

Koocher G. P., Morray E. (2000). Regulation of telepsychology: a survey of state attorneys general. *Professional Psychology, Research, and Practice 31*, 503–508.

Kopel H., Nunn K., Dossetor D.(2001). Evaluating satisfaction with a child and adolescent psychological telemedicine outreach service. *J Telemed Telecare, 7*(suppl 2), 35–40.

McCarty D., Clancy C (2002). Telehealth: implications for social work practice. *Social Work 47*,153–161.

McLaren P. et al. (2002). North Lewisham telepsychiatry project, *J Telemed Telecare, 8*,(2), 100.

Mucic D. (2007). Telepsychiatry pilot-project in Denmark. WCPRR Jan : 3-9.

Naval telemedicine (1998). Fleet lines up to provide live teleconsulting; telepsychiatry saves time and money on the high seas. *Telemedicine and Virtual Reality 3*(4), 40 - 47.

Simpson J., Doze S., Urness D., Hailey D., Jacobs P.(2001).Telepsychiatry as a routine service -the perspective of the patient. J *Telemed Telecare; 7*, 155-60.

Ruskin P. E., Silver-Aylaian M., Kling M. A., et al.(2004). Treatment outcomes in depression: comparison of remote treatment through telepsychiatry to in-person treatment. *American Journal of Psychiatry, 161*(8), 1471-1476.

Samuels A.(1999). International telepsychiatry: A link between New Zealand and Australia. *Aust N Z J Psychiatry, 33*(2), 284-6.

Sorvaniemi M., Ojanen E., Santamaki O. (2005). Telepsychiatry in emergency consultations: A follow-up study of sixty patients. *Telemed J E Health 11*(4),439-41.(ISSN: 1530-5627).

Tang W. K., Chiu H., Woo J., et al.(2001). Telepsychiatry in psychogeriatric service: A pilot study. *International Journal of Geriatric Psychiatry 16*, 88–93.

Yoshino A., Shigemura J., Kobayashi Y., et al. (2001).Telepsychiatry: assessment of televideo psychiatric interview reliability with present- and next-generation internet infrastructures. *Acta Psychiatrica Scandinavica 104*, 223–226.

Zaylor C., Whitten P., Kingsley C. (2000). Telemedicine services to a county jail. *J Telemed Telecare 6*(suppl 1), S93-S95.

KEY TERMS

AES (Advanced Encryption Standard): Is a block cipher (a method for encrypting information) adopted as an encryption standard by the U.S. Government. AES has been analyzed extensively and is now used widely worldwide. In June 2003, the US Government announced that AES is secure enough to be used for classified, top secret information.

Encryption: Is the process of transforming information to make it unreadable to anyone except those possessing a special key. Encryption has long been used by militaries and governments to facilitate secret communication. Encryption is now used in protecting information within many kinds of civilian systems, such as computers, networks, mobile telephones, and bank automatic teller machines.

European Telepsychiatry Network: Network based on telepsychiatry provided exchange of professional resources, clinical and theoretical psycho-education and supervision of clinicians and stuff members. Furthermore, the network should be used in order to assess and/or treat wide range of psychiatric disorders in different patient population groups such as: asylum seekers, refugees and migrants; deaf individuals; individuals with diverse movement disabilities that results in transport limitations etc.

ISDN (Integrated Services Digital Network): Is a circuit-switched telephone network system, designed to allow digital transmission of voice and data over ordinary telephone copper wires, resulting in better quality and higher speeds than that is available with the PSTN system. More broadly, ISDN is a set of protocols for establishing and breaking circuit switched connections, and for advanced call features for the user. In a videoconference, ISDN provides simultaneous voice, video, and text transmission between individual desktop videoconferencing systems and group (room) videoconferencing systems.

Mental Health: The successful performance of mental function, resulting in productive activities, fulfilling relationships with other people and the ability to adapt to change and cope with adversity. Also the psychological state of someone who is functioning at a satisfactory level of emotional and behavioural adjustment

Mental Health Care: Individual or group care by credentialed or licensed psychiatrists, psychologists, social workers, or other counsellors related to the mental health of the individual.

SDSL (Symmetric Digital Subscriber Lineis): A network connection with data rates between 72 and 2320 kbit/s. It runs over one pair of copper wires, with a maximum range of about 3 kilometres. The main difference between ADSL and SDSL is that SDSL has the same upstream data transfer rate as downstream (symmetrical), whereas ADSL always has smaller upstream bandwidth (asymmetrical). However, unlike ADSL, it can't co-exist with a conventional voice service on the same pair as it takes over the entire bandwidth.

Telepsychiatry: The use of telecommunication technologies with the aim of providing psychiatric services from a distance (Brown, 1998). By "telecommunication technologies" means the use of radio, TV, e-mail and finally videoconferencing. The most advanced form of telepsychiatry is video conferencing in real time. This means that the patient and the psychiatrist can both see and hear each other at the same time. Videoconferencing can be provided either via ISDN or via broadband internet.

Chapter IX
Pitfalls and Successes of a Web-Based Wellness Program

Azizah Omar
Universiti Sains Malaysia, Malaysia

ABSTRACT

In this chapter the author discusses several marketing principles and issues related to pitfalls and successes of Telehealth application in the case of a Web -based wellness program called Wellness Online Program (WOLP). WOLP takes a holistic approach to health or 'wellness' and runs for six weeks. It aims to help individuals to manage and improve their own wellbeing regardless of geographical location. Two groups have been recruited, doctor-referred group (DRG) and self-referred group (SRG). The acceptance of WOLP between the two groups was measured by using the technology acceptance model (TAM) at midway (Week 3) and study exit (Week 6). Findings show that the creation of WOLP to deliver wellness among individuals outside the primary healthcare environment is possibly cheaper, convenient, and more accessible than in the primary healthcare setting. However, issues regarding Web -based wellness program implementation are very important and it is crucial for service providers to thoroughly analyse as this will determine the success of the program.

OVERVIEW

Rapid changes in today's lifestyles resulting from industrialisation, urban and economic development, as well as market globalisation have led to a significant impact on our lifestyle. There is no doubt that the changes have the potential to improve and enhance the standard of living and provide greater access to services (such as transportation, education, communication and healthcare). However, there are also significant negative consequences on our overall health and wellbeing where people are becoming more sedentary and have poorer eating habits due to lack of time and overwork. Physical inactivity and diet disorders for instance, are associated with the development of many chronic diseases, such as coronary heart disease, diabetes, hypertension, and cancer in both developing and developed countries. It has been reported in a projection study of future mortality and disability worldwide that non-communicable disease mortality could increase from 28.1 million deaths in 1990 to 49.7 million in 2020 (Murray & Lopez, 1997). Death from injury may increase from 5.1 million to 8.4 million. The leading causes of disability-adjusted life years (DALYS) are predicted to be heart disease, unipolar depression, road-traffic accidents, cancer, hypertension, and HIV. Deaths from substance exposure, such as tobacco-attributable mortality, would increase from 3.0 million deaths in 1990 to 8.4 million deaths in 2020. Promoting an appropriate holistic approach to a "*healthy lifestyle*" may therefore play an important role in health and wellbeing.

The advent of new information, and communication technology (ICT) applications, especially the Internet and the World Wide Web (WWW), facilitates health information transfer, providing opportunities for programs that may bring changes in behaviour. Such programs potentially enhance the health and wellness of individuals both inside and outside the healthcare industry and across different cultures (Omar, 2005). The integration of ICT in the healthcare industry is referred to as *telehealth.* Telehealth is not just a technology; it is an IT-based innovation that has the potential to support and enhance physician-patient care as well as improve healthcare organisations' competitiveness (Hu et al., 1999). The critical factor is a long-term, ongoing interaction between new ICT based programs and the individual patient.

WHY CHOOSE WOLP

Over the years, the concept of health is no longer viewed as treating or curing patients of diseases. Rather the paradigm has shifted towards the prevention or elimination of diseases through the concept of *wellness* (Hettler, 1984). It involves a philosophy of self-respect and self-care that can be accessed by different persons in different ways, then nurtured and extended into other areas of their lives. Wellness is proactive rather than reactive process of making choices towards enhancing overall wellbeing through practices of *healthy lifestyle.* Healthy lifestyle refers to an individual's health behaviour which aims, not only in reducing risk of disease and injury, but also achieving optimal wellness components of each individual namely; physical, emotional, social, intellectual, occupational and spiritual health. None of these wellness components works in isolation. For instance, poor physical health would lead to an imbalance in emotional health or spiritual health. Similarly, lack of social health can lead to poor intellectual as well as emotional health.

Encouraging evidence suggests that physicians can play a vital role in changing the physical activity habits of their patients. It has been reported that patients are more likely to engage in recommended levels of physical activity if they are asked by their doctors during their medical consultations. However, not all physicians are incorporating this awareness into their practices. Data from the US National Health Interview Survey (NHIS) in 1995 (Wee et al., 1999) showed that only 34% of 9,299 respondents reported counseling their patients about exercise at their last visit. The reasons for not integrating this approach into their practices included limited consultation time and fee, no proper training, work pressure, doubts about the effectiveness of preventive interventions and lack of patients' commitment to change. This situation would get even worse if patients also lose interest in having contact with their healthcare providers or could not see their physicians as often as they would like because of limited access to after-hours care, long travel and waiting time, or being uninsured (Forrest & Starfield, 1998). As a result, those, particularly the general public, opt to use the Internet as an alternative means to reach health information and stay abreast with their health needs.

It has been estimated that every year about 60 million patients turn to the Internet for healthcare information, and even physicians also increasingly use this technology whether they like it or not. Due to the ever growing demand for Internet use, many organisations have integrated such technology into their wellness programs, mainly targeting their employees with the aim to reduce the rate of absenteeism, generate lower healthcare expenditure and, in turn, produce higher profits (O'Connell, 2004).

According to Prince (2002), Web -based wellness programs are an effective way for companies to reduce their health expenditure. With these user-friendly and interactive of wellness programs, employers can offer various self-health management tools such as health assessment, immunisation, reminders, group discussions, diet programs, care and prevention recommendations to their employees. The implementation of in-house wellness and prevention programs can have a dramatic impact on a company's bottom line where workplace wellness programs are all about improving employee health and wellbeing and, at the same time strengthening the company's financial position in the marketplace (Gillette, 2001).

The goal of this new way of accessing health information is to empower and educate the consumers or patients for self health-management as well as to improve their quality of life. By having informed consumers or patients, the prevention of illness can be practiced at an early stage and enhance their wellness management. Therefore, research is needed that moves beyond traditional clinic-based models and explores other avenues for intervention with the goal of increasing the number of people attempting to change their lifestyle behaviour in order to benefit from the long-term effects on overall wellbeing.

Implementation of WOLP

Infrastructure

Owing to the diverse applicability of the Internet, it can be used as an alternative strategy to promote an awareness of healthy lifestyle, especially in the general public, as well as to improve health and wellbeing. A 6-week Web based wellness program called the *Wellness Online Program (WOLP)* was developed with the main objective to determine whether such a program would change the attitudes

Table 1. Summary of WOLP activities to be practised by WOLP users

WOLP activities	Week 1	Week 2	Week 3	Week 4	Week 5	Week 6
Physical						
• Fitness	✓	✓	✓	✓	✓	✓
• Nutrition	✓	✓	✓	✓	✓	✓
Social	✓	✓	✓	✓	✓	✓
Emotional				✓	✓	✓
Intellectual				✓	✓	✓
Occupational					✓	✓
Spiritual			✓	✓	✓	✓

and/or behaviour of individuals towards a better wellness performance. Unlike other programs, WOLP emphasises more about planning and motivating people to make positive changes to various aspects of their wellness management rather than just giving them information to read and leaving them to their own devices. It aims to bring the individual's attention to aspects of his or her lifestyle that may be contributing to feelings of "unwellness", and to encourage the pursuit of wellness as a lifelong behaviour pattern.

WOLP was delivered via the Internet to its users (i.e. participants) and it offers three major health-related components – health information, wellness activities that users are required to perform every week, and interactive health self-assessments. The program covers six domains of wellness; physical (fitness and diet), social, emotional, intellectual, occupational and spiritual wellbeing as (Hettler 1984) (Table 1).

Recruitment Procedure

Two groups of participants were recruited; doctor-referred group (DRG) and self-referred group (SRG). The DRG participants (n=50) refers to patients from a primary healthcare centre (Melbourne, Australia). They were recommended by their general practitioners to use WOLP according to the following selection criteria: being aged 18 or above, needing to improve nutritional habits, sedentary lifestyle, interested in health and wellness, seeking health information, likely to benefit from a lifestyle program, not being pregnant (female participants), not suffering from clinical depression, not being intellectually impaired and having access to the Internet.

The other group (SRG), consisting of 150 apparently healthy individuals, was recruited from the general public through the WOLP Web site. An advertisement about the program was placed on the WOLP Web site four weeks prior to the commencement of the study. No attempt was made to find out why the participants visited the Web site.

Assessment and Intervention Procedure

The success of WOLP was evaluated based on the predictive determinant factors of technology acceptance as postulated in the *technology acceptance model* (TAM) (Davis, 1989; Davis et al 1989). The participants were required to complete the TAM questionnaire to indicate the levels of WOLP acceptance at midway (Week 3) and study exit (Week 6). At the same time, they were asked to indicate the extent of agreement or disagreement (using 7 Likert-point of closed-end statements) of their perceptions or beliefs about using WOLP. Altogether a total 39 items, which can be categorised into seven groups of parameters namely, perceived usefulness (PU), perceived ease of use (PEOU), subjective norms (SN), training (T), attitude (A), intention (I) and

Table 2. Characteristics of wellness program intervention

Doctor-Referred Group	Self-Referred Group
Face-to-face training by WOLP trainer (extensive)	Online or virtual training (minimal contact)
Scheduled and personalised regular follow-up visits with WOLP trainer	Standard weekly online follow-up reminders
Standard and personalised weekly on-line reminder plus phone calls by WOLP trainer	E-mail communications with the WOLP trainer (kept to minimum)
WOLP trainer always available for communication (in-person and phone)	

usage behaviour (UB) were constructed as WOLP acceptance parameters.

Both groups were exposed to the same WOLP program. As the main objective of this study is to evaluate the acceptance of WOLP within and outside the primary healthcare environment, two different procedures were applied on these two groups of participants (Table 2). The DRG participants were asked to attend a face-to-face training session conducted at the healthcare centre at study entry (Week 0), and two follow up sessions at midway and study exit. Each session took about 45 minutes. The SRG participants, on the other hand, were required to strictly follow the self-instruction procedures for WOLP available on the Web site. They were asked to familiarise themselves with WOLP, its background, content and its navigation. This was considered to be a "virtual" or "on-line" training. Communication with the researchers via email was kept to a minimum and only related to WOLP procedures.

THE PITFALLS AND THE SUCCESSES OF WOLP

The application of telehealth in healthcare delivery especially in clinical specialties (e.g. teleradiology, teledermatology and telecardiology) is demonstrably more feasible, compared to a normal traditional face-to-face approach for patients' care management. For instance, in a case of emergencies due to geographical location or remoteness such as the Antarctic, on ships, in airplanes or on the battlefield where difficulties may arise in getting a doctor to the patients for treatment in time, the telehealth application such as telephone, wireless satellite, and teleconsultation has a valuable role in the healthcare delivery (Balas et al., 1997). Such distance medical care enables greater continuity of care by improving access, efficiency and supporting the coordination of activities between clinicians and patients. Despite the numerous benefits telehealth can bring to us, the pitfalls and challenges are still there. In addition to skyrocketing costs of infrastructure (e.g. network cabling, hardware, and software) and maintenance, it has been identified that the lack of user acceptance of this new ICT is one of the critical factors in the success of this system (Agarwal & Prasad, 1999; Davis, 1993).

The Technology Acceptance Model (TAM)

According to TAM, higher system utilisation would result in better acceptance of the system which in turn would promote greater productivity and performance (Agarwal & Prasad, 1999; Davis, 1989; 1993). Extensive literature on technology acceptance has emphasised that two specific users' behavioural beliefs, *perceived usefulness* and *perceived ease of use*, can influence the acceptance of a system (Chau, 2001; Davis, 1989; Davis et al, 1989). These beliefs are postulated to have a direct effect on users' *attitude* and *intention*, which in turn would influence users' usage behaviour in using a given system. However, these acceptance parameters can also be influenced by other external factors such as individual differences (Agarwal & Prasad, 1999), training, subjective norms or support from management, colleagues or friends (Davis et al., 1992) or the system characteristics itself (Davis, 1993).

TAM is an intention-based model that is developed specifically for explaining and/or predicting the acceptance of computer technology among users, from their intention to use it in the future. Originally, TAM was adapted from the Theory Reason Action (TRA), which indicates that beliefs influence attitudes, which in turn lead to intentions, which subsequently guide or generate behaviours or actions. TAM has been used extensively as a fundamental technology framework of measuring any system's success across various fields and environments that involve technology implementation. It was considered a very good, compatible and reliable tool due to its generalisability, robustness, parsimony, IT specificity and cost effectiveness (Agarwal & Prasad, 1997; Davis, 1993; Hu et al, 1999).

As noted by Davis (1993) that, given the large investments at stake when developing new systems, it is desirable to forecast user acceptance as early as possible in the design process. The understanding and the creating of the conditions under which information systems will be embraced by human organisations must remain a high-priority research issue as sufficient predicability of future user acceptance could reduce the risk of user rejection. It is therefore, considerably very important for a new program like WOLP to be assessed on a small scale before bigger deployment is carried out.

Acceptance Parameters of WOLP

In a context of WOLP study, the acceptance parameter(s) can be classified into two categories:

i. **Modifiable by systems:** the acceptance parameters that can be improved and/or influenced by increasing or enhancing the characteristics of the program itself (such as content, instructions, write-up, design, or simplicity) and are largely under control of information systems designers, developers, selectors or managers (Davis, 1993). *Perceived usefulness* and *perceived ease of use* parameters are categorised under this group and usually associated with systems characteristics. Higher perceived ease of use to operate a system would result in greater perceived usefulness among users and, in turn, increased acceptance of the system.
ii. **Modifiable by users:** the acceptance parameters that can be improved and/or influenced through users' behaviour toward using a given system. Parameters included in this category are *attitude* and *intention* towards adopting a given system or program.

These two parameters are often the pivotal factor determining the success or failure of a technology information system or program (Davis, 1989). The more the users form positive intentions and attitudes to use the system/program, the better the program acceptance will be.

However, according to Davis and colleagues (1992), each of these parameters, either modifiable by systems or modifiable by users, can also be influenced by external parameters of technology acceptance such as *subjective norms* (support from doctor/WOLP trainer) and *training* (online/face-to-face).

User Acceptance of WOLP

Demographic Characteristics

Of the 200 participants recruited, only 20 in DRG (40%) and 89 in SRG (59.3%) completed the WOLP program over the six-week period. The majority of these participants in both groups were female (76%), aged between 30-49 years (53%), and had a university or college degree or higher (53%). About 91% of the WOLP population considered themselves as 'health conscious', and 74% did not subscribe to any health-related materials (including journals, magazines, or newsletters). The Internet was found as their main source of health information, especially for the individuals in the SRG, and the most popular information obtained from the Internet was about health and nutrition.

Acceptance of WOLP for Completed Users

Both perceived usefulness and perceived ease of use parameters were better predictors of WOLP acceptance than any other acceptance parameters investigated in this study, especially among the users in SRG. However, the DRG users placed greater emphasis as compared to the SRG users on the subjective norms (support from doctor or WOLP trainer) as well as the training (face-to-face) parameters in order to enhance the adoption of the Web -based wellness program. This in turn had higher implications in term of healthcare cost, accessibility, coverage and personalisation.

Perceived Usefulness and Perceived Ease of Use

In general, this study confirms that perceived usefulness, and perceived ease of use factors are primarily important acceptance parameters that can influence the acceptance of WOLP over the 6-week period regardless of the study group setting. Users in both DRG and SRG seemed to be relatively "pragmatic" and tended to focus on usefulness and ease of use when coming to deal with Web -based programs that are delivered through the Internet. These findings appear to support other studies on TAM that perceived usefulness and perceived ease of use are the strongest predictor of users' technology acceptance as well as antecedent to users' attitude, subjective norms and perceived behavioural control (Agarwal & Prasad, 1999; Davis, 1989; Davis, 1993; Davis et al., 1992; Hu et al., 1999; Mathieson, 2001).

These two beliefs were postulated to affect users' technology usage due to the reinforcement value of outcomes such as increased job performance, rewards, or other benefits gained (Davis, 1989). Judgments about a system's usefulness are affected by an individual's cognitive matching of their job goals with the consequences of system use (or job relevance), and that output quality takes on greater importance in proportion to a system's job relevance (Venkatesh & Davis, 2000). In the context of the present study, users' usage behaviour in accepting WOLP is largely dependent on the users' perception or beliefs that their health and wellbeing would improve as a result of using WOLP. Alternatively, if users do not believe that WOLP can help or assist them to improve their health, then, this would lead to program rejection. Therefore, systems or applications that are easy to use, not difficult or complicated to understand, and by their use will increase users' performance or productivity, are positively associated with positive attitude and intention to utilise the applications. However, the influence of perceived usefulness and perceived ease of use factors on users' attitude and intention as well as subsequent behaviour would be higher for experienced users compared to the inexperienced users. In other word, users who have had previous experiences or exposure to similar technology facilities such as the Internet are more likely to have positive perceptions about the Internet application than to inexperienced users.

Results from this study also indicate that, despite no significant difference in these acceptance parameters between these two groups, the acceptance of WOLP among the DRG participants tended to be more dependent or influenced by the "modifiable by users" factors *(attitude and intention)* and other "external" factors *(support from doctor/WOLP trainer and face-to-face training)* compared to the SRG participants. Most often inexperienced or unfamiliar users of a given object are influenced by external control factors rather than internal control factors (Ajzen & Fishbein, 1980). *Internal control* factors refer to characteristics of the user or individual, such as skill and will power. In contrast, *external control* factors depend on the situation, such as time, opportunity, cooperation and support from others or superiors. Therefore, findings from the present study appear to support the notion above that the Internet-established users (or Self-referred group) are more likely to rely on their previous computer or technical skill to operate similar applications via the Internet, and on self-interest or will power to motivate themselves to improve their health and wellbeing. However, DRG participants might not have the technical experience to operate such applications via the Internet and thus, they are more likely to rely on support from doctors and/or WOLP trainers, and face-to-face training.

Attitude

Results also show that users' attitudes toward future fee charges for using WOLP and intention to use WOLP for future usage are significantly more greatly influenced in DRG than the SRG. A similar response was observed where more than 80.0% of users in DRG "agreed" that their acceptance of WOLP over a 6-week period of study was significantly influenced by their future intention to use WOLP.

These findings also suggest that the internet users in SRG had less concern about the future cost of WOLP as long as the benefits gained from WOLP to improve their health was achievable. As Davis and colleagues (1989) suggested, in established technology users, the perceived usefulness factor has a direct effect on behavioural intentions to use the technology over and above its influence via attitude. Alternatively, external variables such as hands-on training and support from management or suppliers provide the bridge between internal beliefs, attitudes and intentions among the inexperienced-users. In essence, the SRG participants are more likely to focus on the current usefulness of WOLP to improve their wellness and make a decision later whether to continue or discontinue the program (i.e. future intention of using WOLP).

It is however conceivable that users in DRG may have had underestimated the potential benefits gained from WOLP, rather than focused on the cost of the program for future usage. One explanation of this effect could be the concern about the existing medical expenses. They may have thought this would burden them with extra health costs which they already had to pay for medical consultations, and costs for medications and existing prescribed treatments. Thus, having an extra wellness program like WOLP may influence their attitude in accepting the program and future intention to use WOLP. Another possible explanation is that DRG participants may not need further general health advice or a wellness program as they have easy access to their doctor during the follow-up treatments.

It has been suggested that if a system is not perceived as useful or will not offer any benefits to the individuals and possibly disadvantages in performing their work, it may inhibit their ability to perform their job and obtain rewards (Davis et al., 1989). Thus, in this study, the chances of the DRG participants rejecting WOLP were higher than the SRG participants as they believed that WOLP would not give any further benefits to improve their health. In fact, they might perceive that using WOLP would minimise the direct communication and interaction with their doctor. This is one of the most important reasons why patients would prefer to go to the primary healthcare centre, not only for the physical examination procedure, but also to have direct contact with the doctor.

Support from Doctor or WOLP Trainer and "Face-to-Face" Training

Results also indicate that the higher proportions of users in DRG "agreed" that "support from doctors and/or WOLP trainer" and a face-to-face training facility were significantly important factors in influencing the acceptance of WOLP over the 6-week period than that in the SRG. They also agreed that that the face-to-face training facility offered by the WOLP trainer had significantly influenced their acceptance of WOLP. Around 82.0% of the DRG participants "agreed" that the face-to-face training had influenced the acceptance of WOLP. On the other hand, only 44.0% of the SRG participants "agreed" that the "online" training had influenced the acceptance of WOLP over the 6-week period of the study.

These findings suggest that the DRG participants are driven to accept WOLP primarily on the basis of support from their doctor and the face-to-face training facility offered by the WOLP trainer, which in turn increases their perceived usefulness and perceived ease of use to operate the program via the Internet. These findings appear to support other studies that the relative influence of subjective norms (support from others) on intentions is expected to be stronger for potential users with no prior experience with the technology since they are more likely to rely on the reactions of others in forming their intentions (Agarwal & Prasad, 1999). Generally, users who have a lack of computer knowledge or have inadequate hardware and software need to rely heavily on outside resources and technical support from the management or supplier in order to enhance the technology adoption. Thus, results from this study confirm that the acceptance of WOLP among the SRG participants (established-Internet users) are more likely to be influenced by perceived usefulness and perceived ease of use beliefs than among the DRG participants. In contrast, the acceptance of WOLP among the DRG participants is more likely to be influenced by the support from the doctor and WOLP trainer, and the face-to-face training.

In a computer usage context, the direct compliance-based effect of subjective norms on intention over and above perceived usefulness, and perceived ease of use will occur in mandatory, but not voluntary system usage settings (Venkatesh & Davis, 2000). In other words, people may choose to perform a behaviour, even if they are not themselves favourable toward the behaviour or its consequences, if they believe one or more important referents think they should, and they are sufficiently motivated to comply with the referents. On the other hand, in the situation of voluntary setting, subjective norms can influence users' intention indirectly through the internalisation process of perceived usefulness. *Internalisation* refers to a process in which a user comes to believe that a particular system is actually useful, and in turn forms an intention to use it as a result of suggested social information from his or her superior, friends, colleagues or other sources (Venkatesh & Davis, 2000). The initial usage of a system may be influenced by perceptions of superior mandate, but people will continue to use the system only if they are able to view its benefits unequivocally (Agarwal & Prasad, 1997). Hence, in respect to the SRG participants, the perceptions about WOLP usefulness may still increase due to the persuasive wellness information exposure from various sources (such as friends, health journals, magazines, television, radio or billboards). This, in turn, enhances users' acceptance to use WOLP even without any mandatory instructions to use the program.

Overall Acceptance of WOLP

These findings demonstrate that for a better acceptance of WOLP among the SRG participants, *perceived ease of use* and *perceived usefulness* factors of the program should be given highest priority in WOLP future development. On the other hand, the users in the primary healthcare setting environment tend to rely heavily on support from doctor and/or WOLP trainer, and the face-to-face training facility in order to enhance the adoption process of WOLP. Conceivably, the Internet-established users, like the SRG, can assimilate new technology quickly and become familiar with its operation without such intense training as might be necessary for the DRG participants (Hu et al., 1999). This shows that the interactive and user-friendly program instructions and procedures provided in WOLP are sufficient to provide virtual technical support for SRG participants compared to the DRG participants. The creation of Web -based wellness programs like WOLP would lead to enormous cost-saving, accessibility, and a convenient means to deliver and promote primary healthcare messages among the established Internet users, especially in the public domain compared to the primary healthcare setting. This will have considerable implications for our healthcare system.

For example, Web -based programs delivered in primary healthcare settings will require intensive training and support from doctors or health trainers. This will increase health expenditure as hiring technical experts will be too costly and time consuming for training sessions with participating doctors, health trainers and patients. There are other possible limitations of WOLP if the program can only be accessed in a primary healthcare setting, such as space or location of the health centre and patient convenience (including travelling time and cost) for follow-up sessions. It is likely this will reduce the adoption process of such applications.

Accessibility and coverage issues of WOLP to be delivered in primary healthcare are other possible anticipated problems. Accessibility refers to "more than mere physical access and it is comprised of physical, interface and informational dimensions" (Agarwal & Prasad, 1997). Thus, if WOLP can only be accessed through the primary healthcare setting, then not every individual will have the opportunity to access the program at anytime and anywhere and thus the objective of "Health for All" is unattainable. In other words, how can we educate and deliver the primary healthcare messages and information to every individual if the access to such facilities is controlled and limited? Having controlled technology innovations will not generate any further advantages, not only to the potential adopters and investors, but also to the community by and large.

Another anticipated problem that may arise if WOLP can only be accessed in a primary healthcare setting, is a risk that acceptance failure will be higher due to inharmonious relationships between WOLP trainers and patients. Most technology acceptance failure among the potential non-experienced users is due to unrealistic expectations of technical support, training, and harmonious working relationships (Chau, 2001). In reality, the supplier or management would always expect the users to make an effort and be proactive in accepting the technology innovation for better performance. Similarly, in this present study, the doctor would also expect the patients to make some effort and be motivated to improve their wellness by learning from various resources. Alternatively, patients would expect their doctor to play a major role in providing them with support and motivation to improve their health and wellbeing. This can create "communication misunderstanding" or tension in patient-doctor relationships that, in turn, lead to users' dissatisfaction and program rejection.

It has been suggested that the trainer behaviour represents an important factor that is associated not only with the organisation of course materials, exercises, and explanation of key concepts, but also with the encouragement of appropriate behaviour formation from the trainees (Agarwal & Prasad, 1999). This implies that users' learning ability may not be solely dependent on a training method, but also on the approach used by effective trainers. However, hiring good and effective trainers or IT consultants (in particular for the face-to-face training) is always related to an enormous investment in cost and time. Therefore, this study appears to support the notion that WOLP is far more economical, is highly accessible and has a higher coverage in promoting wellness in a large scale environment (SRG participants) than the primary healthcare setting (DRG participants).

Acceptance of WOLP Between the Completed and Drop-Out Users in the Self-Referred Group

It is proposed that users may be persuaded to use a new system early in the implementation process but the benefits from system usage may never be derived in the absence of continued, sustained usage (Chau, 2001). Thus, it is explicitly important to identify the determinant factors of system rejection within the desired target group. Results from this study show that there was no significant difference of WOLP acceptance between the "drop out" users and "completed" users in almost every determinant factor of WOLP acceptance, except in attitude towards future fee charges for WOLP. A greater proportion of the SRG participants were reported to drop out from the program due to their attitude toward fee charges for future usage of WOLP than that of completed users (36.1% vs. 12.4%). This suggests that future "cost" or "price" charges for product or services offered in WOLP will be a major contributor to program rejection over and above any other acceptance factors among the SRG participants.

This study appears to confirm other findings that individuals will be less likely to experiment with new technologies if they perceive a significant risk associated with such exploration (Agarwal & Prasad, 1997). "Online browsers" (those who browse the Web but do not shop online) are different from "online buyers" from the perspective of users' online shopping behavioural attitude (Lepkowsaka-White, 2004). The online browsers have more negative perceptions towards some aspects of online shopping than online buyers. For instance, prices, fear of using computers, less skill at using the Web , less time pressure to purchase the products somewhere else and higher value of social interaction with suppliers are among the reasons why they probably do not appreciate the existence of such facilities. Primarily, the online users are more interested in lower prices than the online buyers when it comes to buying decisions which are usually associated with system rejection.

In contrast, the online buyers always perceive that the online shopping facility provides them with greater product varieties, uniqueness, choices, convenience, and time saving over and above the price factor. Thus, in the context of the present study, it is obvious that the "drop out" users have greater concern with the extra "cost" or "charges" they might have to pay for future usage of WOLP. Perhaps in their mind, WOLP is similar to other online merchandising that offers a wide range of health services or products which requires users to pay a certain amount as a result of utilising the services.

Another possible explanation of this effect is that the users might equate the cost of utilising the online wellness program and benefits gained with "bricks and mortar" wellness centres such as gymnasiums, or seeing a doctor. The "drop out" users may think that WOLP only provides them with wellness information and activities to improve their health and wellbeing. However, WOLP would not provide them with any fitness equipment or a personal trainer and thus they would be paying only for health information which already exists and is accessible in abundance on health Web sites. Besides, the "drop out" users may perceive that WOLP may lead them to unnecessary extra medical expenditure as they are advised to see their doctor if any health problem arises during their participation in the program. These factors may overcome their perceived benefits gained from WOLP. As a result, users would discontinue the program. On the other hand, the completed users may have a strong positive perception about WOLP.

FUTURE CHALLENGES AND DEVELOPMENT

When considering the impact of WOLP in promoting wellness among the SRG users (general public) as compared to the DRG users (primary healthcare), several limitations must be kept in mind.

i.. The behavioural outcome measures employed in this study are based on self-perceptions that could not be verified as individuals' perceptions are very subjective and different from each other.

ii. The 6-week period covered by this study was not long enough to understand fully the long-term benefits of WOLP, as no follow-up arrangements were made after the users completed the wellness online program. Besides the positive results shown in most of the existing intervention studies, a very limited number reported a focus on lifestyle interventions in respect to a holistic approach to health, such as WOLP. Thus, periods of performance in regard to lifestyle or behavioural modification in future research should be explored (e.g. perhaps 24 months observation or more so).

iii. This study only measured the impact of behavioural outcomes on users in relation to WOLP adherence. Thus, results cannot be generalised to biomedical outcomes such as body weight, cholesterol, hypertension, or other health-related disease. Clinical studies might be useful in future exploration.

Future studies, researchers or developers of Web -based wellness programs should incorporate the application of SWOT analysis for WOLP (strengths, opportunities, threats and weaknesses) as it identifies useful determinant factors that may influence program acceptance. Table 3 indicates possible indicators of WOLP's strengths, opportunities, threats and weaknesses to promote wellness, especially among the general public.

Recommendation for Future Studies

The majority of the WOLP users were women, suggesting that the program may be more ame-

Table 3. SWOT analysis of WOLP

Strength features	DRG	SRG
1. WOLP has the potential to generate healthy individuals and, in turn, enhance the development of healthy communities	✓	✓
2. WOLP can deliver health education in a larger community regardless of geographical location and time		✓
3. WOLP provides interactive, holistic, continuous, and up-to-date support in terms of knowledge and information on wellness	✓	✓
Weakness features		
1. WOLP provides information about health and wellness that is too generic. Sometimes, this may cause confusion among users that have different health needs.	✓	✓
2. WOLP requires intensive "face-to-face" training in primary healthcare-setting. This can be costly, time consuming and inconvenience for patients and doctors/WOLP trainers.	✓	
3. Follow up scheduled and personalised weekly reminders and phone calls to users in primary healthcare setting can be costly, time consuming and inconvenience.	✓	
Opportunity features		
1. WOLP is a potential tool/platform in assisting doctors/health providers to explain to their patients or individuals certain health conditions that require lifestyle modifications in improving their health.	✓	✓
2. WOLP can collaborate with various sectors such as pharmaceutical, insurance, food and beverages manufacturers, education, public health and IT departments.	✓	✓
3. WOLP can be further improved to cater for various target groups with different population backgrounds, cultures, ethnicity, languages, IT experience, age and sex.		✓
Threat features		
1. Issues of confidentiality or privacy of users' information can be jeopardised by unreliable and unscrupulous service providers. These providers may sell users' health information to other companies such as pharmaceutical or insurance companies.		✓
2. WOLP can be costly if not properly designed and implemented. Since it involves IT, maintenance costs, IT experts (programmers) and other costs are usually high.	✓	✓
3. WOLP may be seen as a "substitute doctor" for some individuals or patients. This can pose a threat to individuals in treating themselves without proper observation or examination by doctors.	✓	✓

nable to these individuals. Therefore future studies may need to develop wellness programs that appeal to men and younger individuals. Besides, WOLP seems to attract highly educated, higher income and professional users rather than the lower socioeconomic status users. It is advisable that future research should thus consider the socioeconomic status as one of the main criteria for Web -based program development.

Despite the potential benefits of enhancing individuals' overall wellness through Web-based programs to reach a wider population regardless of their locations, issues of Internet accessibility will still remain as a barrier for certain groups of people who have no access to the technology. As WOLP can only be accessed online, we recommend that future research should integrate with various avenues, strategies or collaborations that can provide more Internet access to these people.

The WOLP study indicates that an on-line program can be more effective and can benefit users in a Self-Referred Group rather than those who are in a Doctor-Referred Group. Therefore, it may be useful for future research to integrate WOLP with personalised wellness activities that are tailored to the specific needs of various groups' characteristics by age, gender, or health conditions.

Future research should also explore potential program modifications that might enhance the effectiveness of the program among users. WOLP could be modified to allow users to manipulate wellness areas in which they think they need most help to improve their overall wellbeing. For example, users could choose any wellness domains that they want to begin with in the first week of the program and so on, depending on the overall scores obtained for each wellness domain at baseline. Otherwise, users could just adhere to the designated WOLP. It is likely that users could have some control and choice in changing their behaviour to enhance overall wellness.

CONCLUSION

This present study confirms that the integration of technology (the Internet) outside and within primary healthcare can promote wellness in the public domain. It leads to the conclusion that a primary healthcare doctor may not always be required for the acceptance of such a program. This study also proves that telehealth has a worthwhile impact of telehealth on wellness. Other issues that relate to the acceptance of the technology integration in developing Web -based program such as WOLP, in particular, are necessary to be taken into consideration.

REFERENCES

Ajzen, I. and Fishbein, M. (1980). *Understanding attitudes and predicting social behavior,* Englewood Cliffs: Prentice Hall, New Jersey.

Agarwal, R. and Prasad, J. (1999). Are individual differences germane to the acceptance of new information technologies? *Decision Sciences, 30*(2), 361-375.

Balas, E.A., Jaffrey, F., Kuperman, G.J., Boren, S.A., Brown, G.D., Pinciroli, F. and Mitchell, J.A. (1997). Electronic communication with patients: evaluation of distance medicine technology. *JAMA, 278*(2), 152-159.

Chau, P.Y.K. (2001). Influence of computer attitude and self-efficacy on IT usage behaviour. *Journal of End User Computing, 13*(1), 26-33.

Davis, F.D. (1989). Perceived usefulness, perceived ease of use, and user acceptance of information technology. *MIS Quarterly, 13*(1), 319-340.

Davis, F.D. (1993). User acceptance of information technology: system characteristics, user perceptions and behavioral impacts, *Int J Man-Machine Studies, 38*, 475-487.

Davis, F.D., Bagozzi, R.P. and Warshaw, P.R. (1989). User acceptance of computer technology: a comparison of two theoretical models. *Management Science, 35*(8), 982-1003.

Davis, F.D., Bagozzi, R.P. and Warshaw, P.R. (1992). Extrinsic and intrinsic motivation to use computers in the workplace. *Journal of Applied Social Psychology, 22*(14), 1111-1132.

Forrest, C.B. and Starfield, B. (1998). Entry into primary care and continuity: the effects of access. *Am J Public Health, 88*(9), 1330-1336.

Gillette, B. (2001). Promoting wellness programs results in a healthier bottom line. *Managed Health care Executive, 11*(2), 45-46.

Hettler, B. (1984). Wellness: encouraging a lifetime pursuit of excellence. *Health Values, 8*(4), 13-17.

Hu, P.J., Chau, P.Y.K., Sheng, O.R.L. and Tam, K.Y. (1999). Examining the technology acceptance model using physician acceptance of telemedicine technology. *Journal of Management Information Systems,* 16(2), 91-112.

Lepkowska-White, E. (2004). Online store perceptions: how to turn browsers into buyers? *Journal of Marketing Theory and Practice, 12*(3), 36-47.

Mathieson, K., Peacock, E. and Chin, W.W. (2001). Extending the technology acceptance model: the influence of perceived user resources. *Information Systems, 32*(3), 86-112.

Murray, C.J.L. and Lopez, A.D. (1997). Alternative projections of mortality and disability by cause 1990-2020: global burden of disease study. *The Lancet, 349*(9064), 1498-1504.

O'Connell, B. (2004). Corporate wellness programs. *Biopharm International, 17*(10), 16-17.

Omar, A., Wahlqvist, M.L., Kouris-Blazos, A. and Vicziany, M. (2005). Wellness management through Web -based programmes. *Journal of Telemedicine and Telecare, 11*(S1), S8-11.

Prince, M. (2002). Altering lifestyle through Internet fitness monitoring. *Business Insurance, 36*(14), T6 - T7.

Venkatesh, V. and Davis, F.D. (2000). A theoretical extension of the technology acceptance model: four longitudinal field studies. *Management Science. 46*(2), 186-204.

Wee, C.C., McCarthy, E.P., Davis, R.B. and Phillips, R.S. (1999). Physician counseling about exercise. *JAMA. 282*(2), 1583-1588.

KEY TERMS

Perceived Usefulness: The degree to which a person believes that using a particular system would enhance his or her job performance. It reflects a person's beliefs or expectations about outcomes (Davis, F.D., 1989).

Perceived Ease of Use: The degree to which a person believes that using a particular system would be free of effort. It encapsulates the extent of which a potential user considers usage of the target technology to be relatively free of the effort to perform specific tasks using a given systems (Davis, F.D., 1989).

TAM: Abbreviation of technology acceptance model.

Technology Acceptance Model: A theoretical framework model developed by Davis in 1989 to investigate the acceptance levels of new technologies. It is an intention-based model that is developed specifically for explaining and/or predicting the acceptance of computer technology among users, from their intention to use it in the future. The intention for future use can be explained in terms of their perceived usefulness, perceived ease of use, attitude and other external factors.

Wellness: A holistic approach to health that focuses on an individual's consciousness and making choices that are actively involved in enhancing wellbeing. It consists of six domains or dimensions of health namely physical (fitness and diet), social, occupational, intellectual, emotional, and spiritual.

Wellness Online Program: An interactive Web based wellness program that is accessible via online (the Internet) for its users. It offers various health information, health self-assessments, and health activities. It emphasises more about planning and motivating users to improve their overall wellbeing.

WOLP: Abbreviation of Wellness Online Program.

Chapter X
A Web-Based Application to Exchange Electronic Health Records and Medical Images in Ophthalmology

Isabel de la Torre Díez
University of Valladolid, Spain

Roberto Hornero Sánchez
University of Valladolid, Spain

Miguel López Coronado
University of Valladolid, Spain

Jesús Poza Crespo
University of Valladolid, Spain

María Isabel López Gálvez
University of Valladolid, Spain

ABSTRACT

This chapter describes a Web -based application to store and exchange Electronic Health Records (EHR) and medical images in Ophthalmology: TeleOftalWeb 3.2. The Web -based system has been built on Java Servlet and Java Server Pages (JSP) technologies. Its architecture is a typical three-layered with two databases. The user and authentication information is stored in a relational database: MySQL 5.0. The patient records and fundus images are achieved in an Extensible Markup Language (XML) native database: dbXML 2.0. The application uses XML-based technologies and Health Level Seven/Clinical Document Architecture (HL7/CDA) specifications. The EHR standardization is carried out. The main application object is the universal access to the diabetic patients EHR by physicians wherever they are.

INTRODUCTION

Healthcare computing or medical informatics is one of the fastest growing areas of information and communication technology (ICT) application. Electronic records in health fall under the purview of health informatics. It is a combination of computation, computer science and medical record keeping. Recent technological advances have enabled the introduction of a great number of telemedicine applications in healthcare computing (Hung, K, Zhang, Y, 2003). The information systems are a necessary part of the telemedicine services. They provide storage, retrieval, connection and evaluation of the medical information. One of these systems is the Electronic Patient Record (EPR). They store and administrate all the medical data about a patient (Horsch, A, Balbach, T, 1999). An EPR is a fundamental part of health information technology and its use is growing quickly. It is indicative of the advances in medical informatics and facilitates the doctor-patient relationship. It can be organized either on a document-based backbone, or on a structured database system. An EPR transmitted through the Internet is especially important. It contains a private material of medical information for a patient.

In most European countries, the National Health Service (NHS) is investing large amounts in information technology (IT) (Mocanu, M.L, et al., 2004). In this context, the idea of electronic health records (EHR) has been around for a decade or more (Ferreira, A, et al., 2004). The EHR is a secure, real-time, point-of-care and patient-centric information resource for physicians. The EHR must enable the communication of healthcare information to support shared patient care, improved quality of care and effective resource utilisation. EHR may contain data about medical referrals, medical treatments, medications and their application, demographic information and other non-clinical administrative information. Some benefits of the EHR systems are their universal access, coding efficiency and efficacy, easier and quicker navigation through the patient record another (Smith, D, Newell, L.M, 2002). In spite of the advantages of EHR, there are several barriers to their adoption such as training, costs, complexity and lack of a national standard for interoperability (Gans, D, et al., 2006).

Many EHR-related initiatives have been announced in Canada. In May 2006, the government of British Columbia announced spending of $150 million towards the creation of online computerized medical records for doctors (Canadian Institute for Health Information, 2006). EHR-related initiatives are under way and each addresses a specific part of health care, primary, acute and community care. For example, the Ontario Primary Care Network in Canada is a pilot project involving approximately 40 physicians and 300.000 patients. Individual physicians are implementing office systems for the capture of patient information and support office administration. Community care providers are piloting projects to improve the delivery of services to their customers (Office of Health and the Information, 2001).

Nowadays, telemedicine applications often involve many institutions using different systems and technologies. This complicates the necessary technical standardization (Holle, R, Zahlmann, G, 1999). International and national institutions and organizations are concerned with standardization of EHR systems such as ISO Health Informatics Standards Technical Committee (ISO/TC 215), CEN Technical Committee (CEN/TC) 251, openEHR, Health Level 7 (HL7), Integrating the Healthcare Enterprise (IHE), Digital Imaging and Communication in Medicine (DICOM) to name but a few (Bott, O.J, 2004).

ISO/TC 215 has defined the EHR and also produced a technical specification ISO 18308 describing the requirements for EHR Architectures. It provides standardization in the field of information for health. It ensures compatibility of data for comparative statistical purposes and to reduce duplication of effort and redundancies.

CEN/TC 251 is the body within Europe mandated to develop standards for Health Informatics. It is a workgroup within the European Union working on standardization in the field of Health ICT. The goal is to achieve compatibility and interoperability between independent systems and to enable modularity in EHR systems.

OpenEHR is the next generation public specifications and implementations for EHR systems and communication, based on a complete separation of software and clinical models. It is dedicated to the development of an open, interoperable health computing platform, where a major component is clinically effective and interoperable EHR. It does this by researching clinical requirements, and creating specifications and implementations.

HL7 is a not-for-profit organization involved in development of international healthcare standards. It is used for many different medical environments. HL7 Document is intended to be the basic unit of a document-oriented EPR. The patient medical record is represented as a collection of documents. The HL7 standard defines the message, segment, field, etc. The HL7 Clinical Document Architecture (CDA) is an XML-based document markup standard that specifies the structure and semantics of clinical documents for the purpose of exchange.

IHE is an initiative to integrate existing standards into a comprehensive best-practice solution. It does not create new standards, but rather drives the adoption of standards to address specific clinical needs.

DICOM is a cooperative standard. It was developed from 1990 to 1996, mainly by the American College of Radiology (ACR) National Electrical Manufacturers Association (NEMA) committee in the United States, with contributions from European standardization organizations, the Japanese Industry Radiology Apparatus (JIRA), the IEEE, HL7 and ANSI as well as from European manufacturers and societies. The goal of the DICOM Standard is to achieve compatibility and improve workflow efficiency between imaging systems and other information systems in healthcare environments worldwide. This standard allows the exchange of medical images and related information between systems from different manufacturers. One of the DICOM advantages is that only a part of the defined keys are specified (Neri, E, et al., 1998).

In order to HL7 standard, there are mobile clinical information systems by using HL7 to integrate the patient data (Choi, J, et al., 2006), EHR applications in different medicine areas such as oncology (James, A, et al., 2001) and emergency departments (Amouh, T, et al., 2005).

In ophthalmology, the diabetic retinopathy is one of the major causes of blindness among the people. According to World Health Organization (WHO), diabetic retinopathy is considered to be the result of vascular changes in the retinal circulation. In the early stages vascular occlusion and dilations occur. It progresses into a proliferative retinopathy with the growth of new blood vessels. Many approaches are proposed by the authors to automate and detect the presence of diabetic retinopathy in fundus images (Satyarthi, D, 2006). The evaluation of digital images allows the diabetic retinopathy to diagnose. In this chapter, we present a Web -based application, TeleOftalWeb 3.2, to store and exchange ophthalmology EHR and fundus images by using XML and Java technologies. We employ EHR systems specifications as HL7/CDA and ISO/TC 215. Thanks to the use of XML-based technologies and HL7 specifications, this application allows the EHR standardization. It ensures interoperability among different applications and institutions. We worked in the application development with ophthalmologists from the Instituto Universitario de Oftalmobiología Aplicada (IOBA), Spain. TeleOftalWeb 3.2 provides a telemedicine service, electronic medical records and fundus images in different formats. It manages a database with information about patients and their eyes fundus photographs. Moreover, it allows the images visualization and processing. Any specialist may access their records immediately and see medical images.

SYSTEM OVERVIEW

TeleOftalWeb 3.2 has been built on Java Servlet and Java Server Pages (JSP) technologies. The EHR and medical images are stored in the native XML database. Its architecture is a typical three-layered with two database servers (relational and native XML), one application server and a thin client. Figure 1 shows the application architecture. The client application consists of a interface based on JSPs running on the Web server. The server application communicates with the databases to retrieve data. The application is platform-independent thanks to use XML and Java Technologies. In communication with the native XML database, we used the languages XPath and XUpdate. XPath is employed to find information in an XML document. It models an XML document as a tree of nodes. There are different types of nodes, including element nodes, attribute nodes and text nodes. The primary purpose of XPath is to address parts of an XML document. XUpdate makes heavy use of XPath for selecting a set of nodes to modify or remove. XUpdate is a simple XML update language. You can use it to modify XML content by simply declaring what changes should be made in an XML syntax. XUpdate is a pure descriptive language that is designed with references to the definition of XSL Transformations (XSLT).

The development environment was NetBeans IDE 4.1 of Sun Microsystems. The IDE runs on many platforms including Windows, Linux, Solaris, and the MacOS. Java was the basis application programming language. We included all tools and Application Programming Interface (API) as Javascript, JSP, Java Servlets and Java Database Connectivity (JDBC). Combining Java and XML leads to the attractive dual portability of code and data. Wherever Java programs can run, they can also access XML information. This enables Java and XML information to interoperate efficiently and effectively on different platforms (Fan, R, 2005). We used Tomcat 5.5.9 to process the requests, JSP and Java Servlets.

The users can access and retrieve medical information and images through Web browsers as Mozilla Firefox, Microsoft Internet Explorer and others. The EHR can be displayed in the following formats: portable document format (PDF), hypertext markup language (HTML) and XML. The medical records and the images can be viewed in this portable format. The users can view and store joint photographic experts group (JPEG), DICOM and other type of images in the user module. For security, all data transmissions were carried over encrypted Internet connections such as secure sockets layer (SSL) and hypertext transfer protocol over SSL (HTTPS).

Figure 1. Application architecture

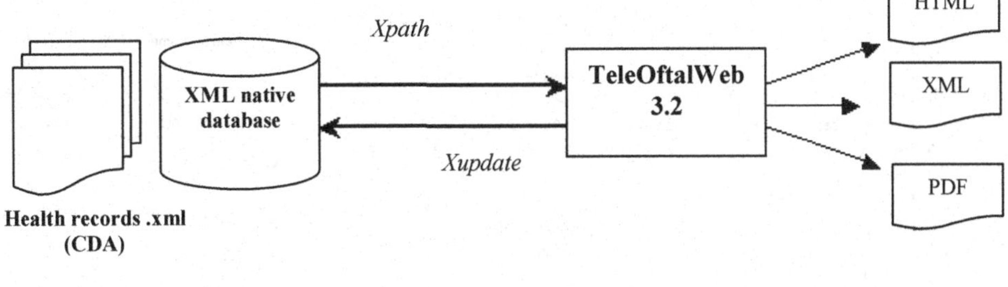

DATA MODELLING

We chose free open-source database servers. For the manager module, we used a relational database to store the personal and authentication data. The database manager was MySQL Server 5.0 with the Connector/J-3.1.11. MySQL is a multithreaded, multi-user and SQL relational database Server (RDBMS). In the MySQL database, we stored all the user data and access information to Web application. It has two tables: "users" and "permissions". The table "users" contains personal user data. The user identification, user name, password and user type appear in table "permissions". The primary key is the same in both tables (identification number). The data modelling in the MySQL database is shown in Figure 2.

An XML database is a data persistence software system that allows data to be imported, accessed and exported in the XML format. There are two XML databases classes: XML-enabled and native XML. The first one maps all XML to a traditional database (such as a relational database), accepting XML as input and rendering XML as output. The native XML database has an internal model that depends on XML and uses XML documents as the fundamental unit of storage.

Table 1. Levels of document granularity in CDA; Release one and release two

CDA Release One	CDA Release Two
CDA Level One	Unconstrained CD specification
CDA Level Two	CDA specification with section-level templates applied
CDA Level Three	CDA specification with entry-level templates applied

We applied a native open-source XML database, dbXML 2.0, to manage and store the EHR and medical images. The Java servlet inserts the record into the dbXML database. It stores and indexes collections of XML documents in both native and mapped forms for highly efficient querying, transformation, and retrieval. The EHR are stored in the native XML database according to the ANSI/HL7 CDA R1.0-2000 template. CDA distinguishes three different levels of granularity as shown in Table 1, where each level iteratively adds more markup to clinical documents, although the clinical content remains constant at all levels (Eichelberg, M, et. al, 2006).

There is only one CDA level one document type definition (DTD) for all types of clinical

Figure 2. User data modelling in MySQL database

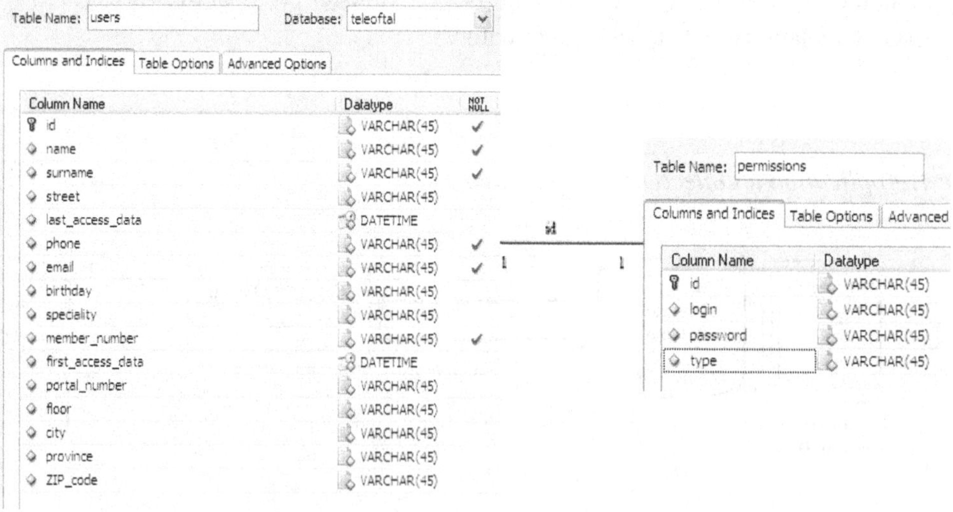

documents. CDA Level One is specified by three components: the CDA Header, the CDA level one body and reference information model (RIM) data type DTD. The CDA Level One Body is specified in the CDA Level One DTD and is derived from document analysis. RIM data type DTD is an XML implementation of the abstract data type specification. It used by both the CDA and the HL7 Version 3 message specifications. A **HL7/CDA** document is comprised of a header, referred to as the "CDA Header", and a body, which at CDA Level One is referred to as the "CDA level one body". The CDA header identifies and classifies the document and provides information on authentication, the encounter, the patient, and the provider. The body contains the clinical-related information that we want to exchange.

The CDA specification prescribes XML markup for CDA documents: CDA instances must valid against the CDA schema and may be subject to additional validation. The CDA schema is shown in Figure 3.

The CDA level one body is comprised of nested containers. There are four types of containers: sections, paragraphs, lists, and tables. Containers have contents and optional captions. Contents include plain text, links, and multimedia. CDA document is a defined and complete information object that can exist outside of a messaging context and/or can be a MIME-encoded payload within an HL7 message. The CDA is only the first example of HL7's commitment to the advancement of XML-based e-healthcare technologies within the clinical, patient care domain. The scope of the CDA is the standardization of clinical documents for exchange. A HL7/CDA structure may include texts, sounds, pictures and all kind of multimedia contents. It can refer to external documents, procedures, observations, and acts. It includes information about authors, authenticators, custodians, participants, patients, and so on (Treins, M, et al., 2006).

The XML-based architecture described in the CDA v1.0 standard has been used to define the health information format. Thanks to the use of XML-based technologies and HL7 specifications, our application fulfils the EHR standards. Its development methodology is a continuously evolving process that seeks to carry out specifications that facilitate interoperability between healthcare systems. In Figure 4 we can also see

Figure 3. CDA schema

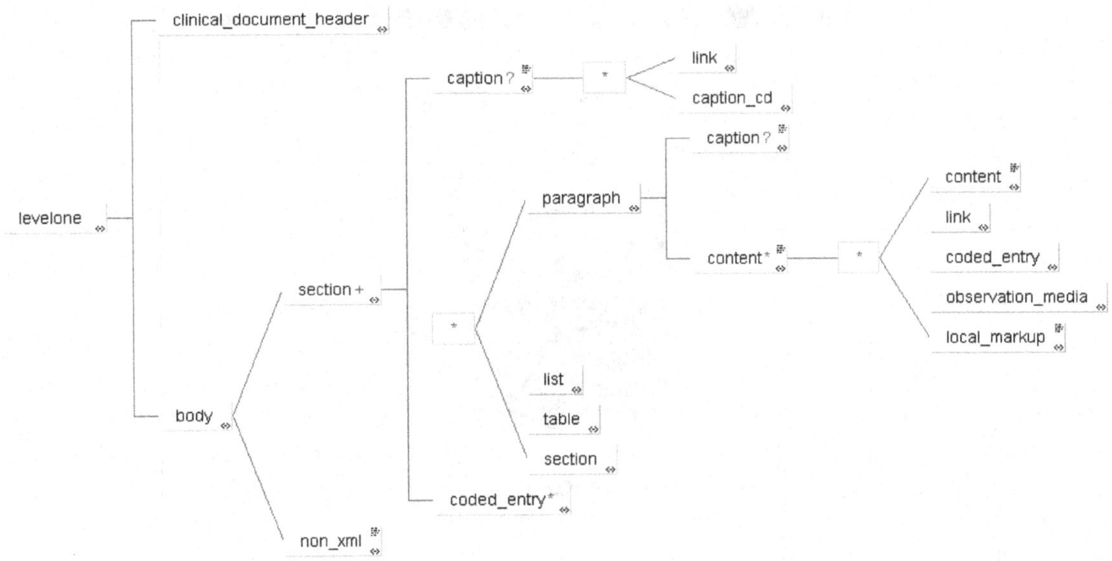

Figure 4. Manager interface in the dbXML database

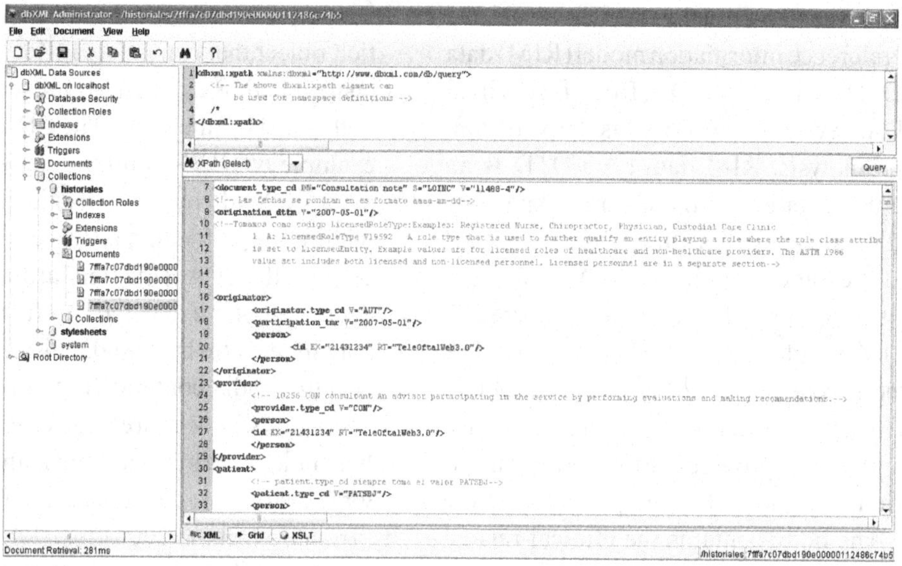

the CDA level one DTD in the XML native database, dbXML 2.0.

APPLICATION MANAGER MODULE

The manager module interface is shown in Figure 5. The manager can access to the Web platform. He/She has to introduce the login and password.

Figure 6 shows the application users. The two user roles are: manager and user. The application manager can do the following actions:

- Create users. The manager has to introduce the following compulsory information: surname, name, identification number, member

Figure 5. TeleOftalWeb 3.2 (manager module)

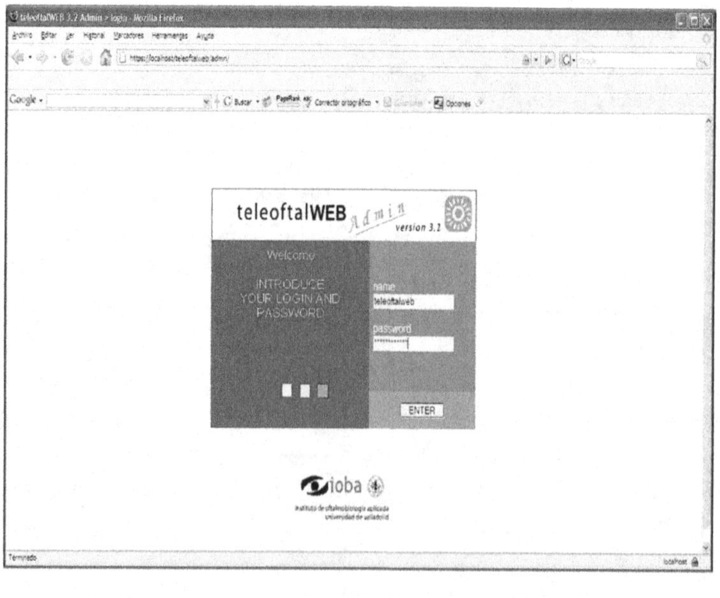

Figure 6. Application users

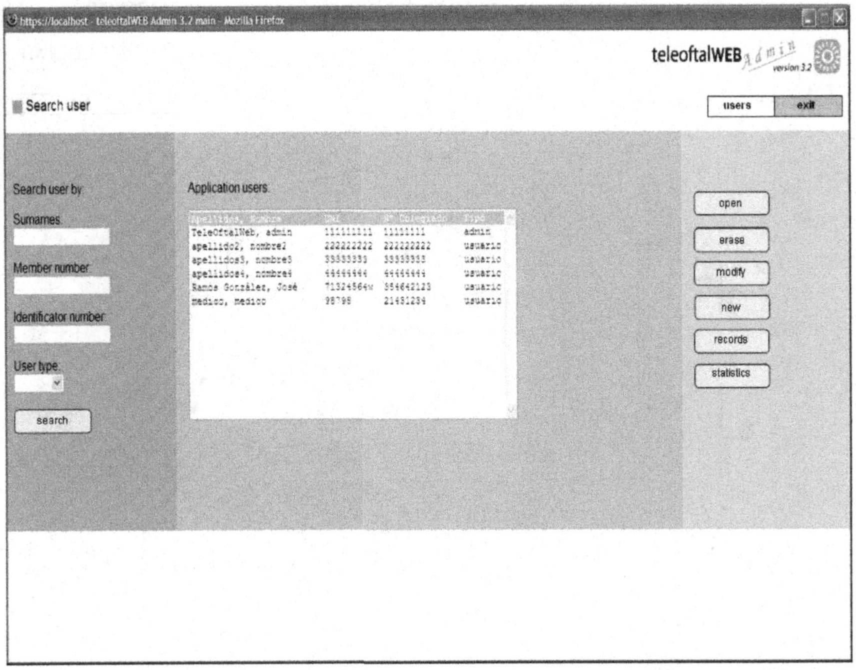

number, phone, e-mail, specialty, user type, login and password.

- Show records. A list of patients is displayed.
- Erase users.
- Modify and show the user information.
- Show the user statistics. It is shown the total number of records by users.
- Search users by different criteria such as surname, identification number, type of user and member number.

APPLICATION USER MODULE

The authorized users can access to this module. They have their login and password. The users can do the following actions:

- Create new records (see Figure 7). They have to introduce the necessary data: patient affiliation information, patient precedents, medical exploration and diagnostic. The affiliation information is always necessary to complete the record.
- Erase records.
- Search revisions.
- Create new revisions in a record.
- Search records by different criteria: patient's surname, patient's identification number, record creation date and record origin. The user can share the records with other application users.
- Erase revisions.
- Edit images.
- Add new images (JPEG, DICOM and others formats) in different records. Figure 8 shows this action. The images editor allows to show images and to change their shape and colour, to make them bigger or smaller. The images can be changed in other colours (red, green, blue) and the users can add comments. The reset option allows the users to see the original image. The users can keep

Figure 7. Create a new record

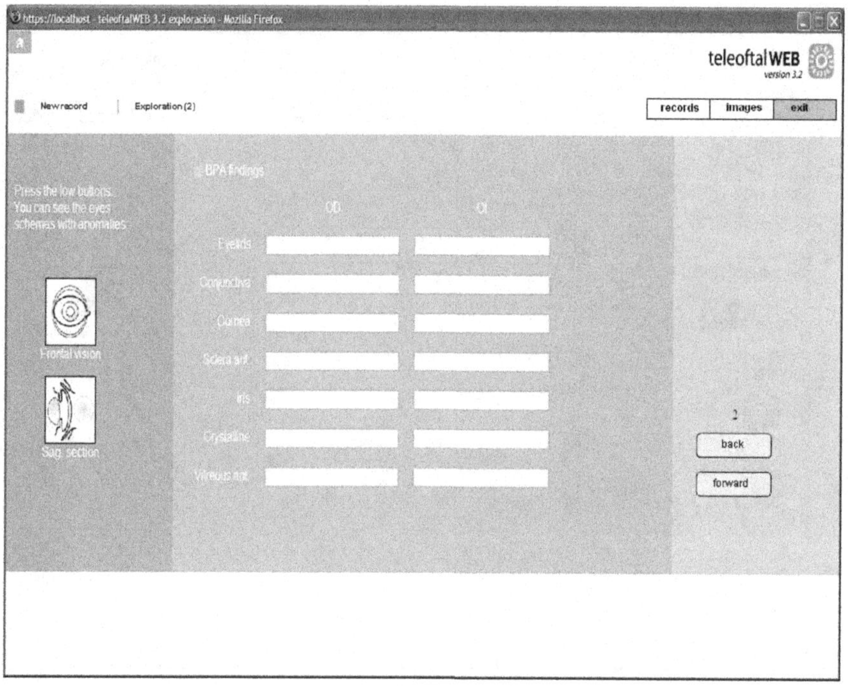

Figure 8. Images editor

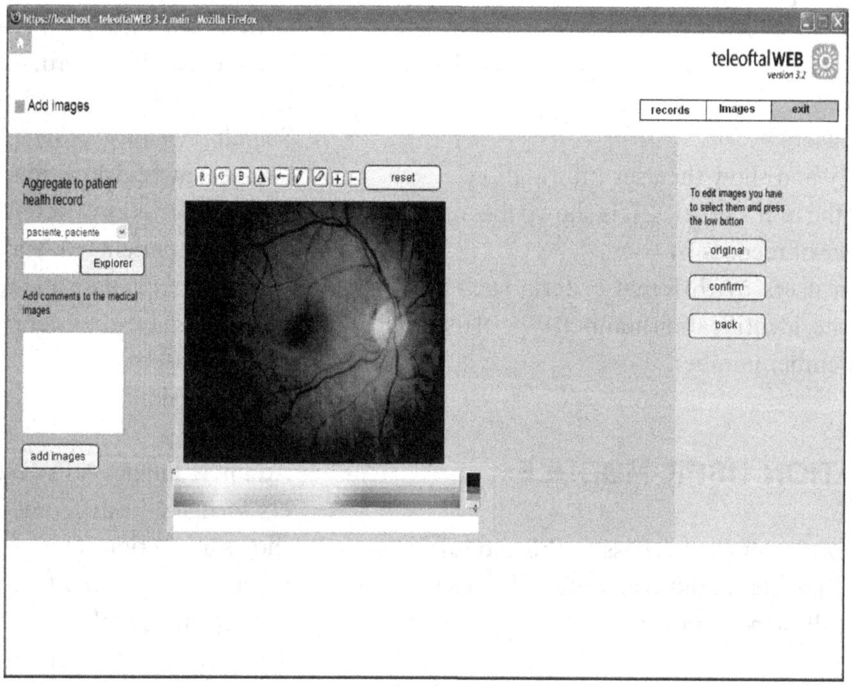

the modified images in the XML native database.

- Erase images in the records.
- Search images in different formats according to the following criteria: image identification number, surnames, image creation date and comments.

DISCUSSIONS AND CONCLUSION

A Web -based application has been developed to store and exchange EHR and medical images in Ophthalmology using HL7/CDA and XML technologies. The EHR system facilitates new interfaces between care and research environments, leading to great improvements in the scope and efficiency of research. The EHR in our application contains information about patient affiliation information, patient precedents, medical exploration and diagnostic.

We apply XML and Java technologies to interoperate efficiently and effectively on different Web platforms. The extensive use of HL7/CDA standard is desirable, not only in cardiology environment but also for all fields present in medicine (Marcheschi, P, et al., 2004). We apply it in an ophthalmology application. There are several EHR applications in different medicine areas such as oncology and emergency departments. In the telematic system for oncology (James, A, et. al., 2001), they use a data warehouse as EPR server. The authors do not present a standardization process for the EHR. In our application, we applied EHR standards. The information system designed for emergency department (Amouh, T, et al., 2205) has been implemented by prototyping a Web-based. It is a multiplatform and multiuser system, using the Java programming language. There are few standards for modern day electronic records systems as a whole, there are many standards relating to specific aspects of EHR. The standards differ in the progress achieved in the standardization process each of the content formats seems to be suitable for implementing EHR.

There are important barriers in the EHR adoption such as the lack of national information standards and code sets. Moreover, the lack of available funding and interoperability can be presented. We treat to solve some of these problems to the EHR adoption in Ophthalmology.

The main advantages of this application are: its adaptation to the standard HL7/CDA, facilitates the interoperability between institutions and applications. Moreover, the transactions are secure. The Web -based applications allow to improve data access for patient data management. The physicians can analyze the patient records in everywhere. They only need a computer with Internet.

We use Base64 encoding and decoding. The application allows to store and display DICOM, JPEG images and other formats. The ophthalmologists can detect one of the most important eye diseases between diabetic people, the diabetic retinopathy.

DICOM is also used in other image related medical fields, such as pathology, endoscopy, dentistry, ophthalmology and dermatology. Its wide availability is central for implementing the EHR (Noumeir, R, 2003). The DICOM structured report (SR) is the diagnostic report that encodes the interpretation and the impressions of the physician. The information contained in a SR is grouped into nine information modules. Those modules contain all the information needed to identify the patient, the study, and the series in which the document is contained.

REFERENCES

Amouh, T., Gemo, M., Macq, B., Vanderdonckt, J., Wahed, A., Reynaert, M.S., Stamatakis, L., Thys, F. (2005). Versatile clinical information system design for emergency departments. *IEEE Transactions on Information Technology in Biomedicine, 9*(2), 174-183.

Bott, O. J. (2004). Electronic health record: Standardization and implementation, 2nd. *OpenECG Workshop*. Berlin, Germany, pp. 57-60.

Canadian Institute for Health Information (2006). Understanding family physician usage of electronic health records in Canada. *Results From the 2004 National Physician Survey*, (pp. 1-11).

Choi, J., Yoo, S., Park, H., Chun, J. (2006). MobileMed: A PDA-based mobile clinical information system. *IEEE Transactions on Information Technology in Biomedicine*, 10(3), 627-635.

Eichelberg, M., Aden T., Riesmeier J., Dogac A., Laleci G. (2006). Electronic health record standards – a brief overview. In *Proceedings of the 4th International Conference on Information and Communications Technology (ICICT 2006)*. Cairo, Egypt.

Fan, R. Ceded, L., Toser, O. (2005). Java plus XML: a powerful new combination for SCADA systems. *Computing & Control Engineering Journal, 16*(5), 27-30.

Ferreira, A., Correia, R., Antunes, L., Palhares, E., Marques, P., Costa, P., da Costa Pereira, A. (2004). Integrity for electronic patient record reports. *Proceedings of the 17th IEEE Symposium on Computer-Based Medical Systems (CBMS'04)*, (pp. 4-9).

Gans, D., Kralewski, J., Hammons, T., Dowd B. (2006). Medical groups' adoption of electronic health records and information systems. *Health affairs (Project Hope), 24*(5), 1323-1333.

Holle, R., Zahlmann, G. (1999). Evaluation of telemedical services. *IEEE Transactions on Information Technology in Biomedicine, 3*(2), 84-91.

Horsch, A., Balbach, T. (1999). Telemedical Information Systems. *IEEE Transactions on Information Technology in Biomedicine, 3*(3), 166-175.

Hung, K., Zhang, Y. (2003). Implementation of a WAP-based telemedicine system for patient monitoring. *IEEE Transactions on Information Technology in Biomedicine, 7*(2), 101-107.

James, A., Wilcox, Y., Naguib, R.N.G. (2001). A telematic system for oncology based on electronic health and patient records. *IEEE Transactions on Information Technology in Biomedicine, 5*(1), 16-17.

Marcheschi, P., Mazzarisi, A., Dalmiani, S., Benassi, A. (2004). HL7 clinical document architecture to share cardiological images and structured data in next generation. *Computers in Cardiology*, 617-620.

Mocanu, M.L., Dorobantu, M., Mocanu C., Burdescu, D. (2004). A distributed database system for glaucoma monitoring. *European Journal for Biomedical Informatics*, 50-58.

Neri, E., Thiran, J., Caramella, D., Petri, C., Bartolozzi, C., Piscaglia, B., Macq. B., Duprez, T., Cosnard, G., Maldague, B., De Pauw, J. (1998). Interactive DICOM image transmission and telediagnosis over theEuropean ATM network, *IEEE Transactions on Information Technology in Biomedicine, 2*(1), 35-38.

Noumeir, R. (2003). DICOM structured report document type definition. *IEEE Transactions on Information Technology in Biomedicine, 7*(4), 318-328.

Office of Health and the Information (2001). Toward electronic health records. *Highway Health*. Canada.

Satyarthi, D., Raju, B.A.N, Dandapat, S. (2006). Detection of diabetic retinopathy in fundus images using vector quantization technique. In *Proceedings of the Annual India Conference*, (pp. 1-4).

Smith, D., Newell, L.M. (2002). A Physician's perspective: Deploying the EMR. *Journal of Healthcare Information Management, 16*(2), 71-79.

Treins, M., Curé, O., Salzano, G. (2006). On the interest of using HL7 CDA release 2 for the exchange of annotated medical documents. *Proceedings of the 19th IEEE Symposium on Computer-Based Medical Systems (CBMS'06)*, (pp. 524-532).

KEY TERMS

Base64: It is a positional notation using a base of 64. It is the largest power-of-two base that can be represented using only printable ASCII characters. This has led to its use as a transfer encoding for e-mail among other things. It uses the characters A–Z, a–z, and 0–9 in that order for the first 62 digits but the symbols chosen for the last two digits vary considerably between different systems.

Extensible Style Language Transformation (XSLT): The language used in XSL style sheets to transform XML documents into other XML documents. An XSL processor reads the XML document and follows the instructions in the XSL style sheet, then it outputs a new XML document or XML-document fragment.

Document Type Definition (DTD): DTD is primarily used for the expression of a schema via a set of declarations that conform to a particular markup syntax and that describe a class, or type, of SGML or XML documents, in terms of constraints on the structure of those documents. A DTD may also declare constructs that are not always required to establish document structure, but that may affect the interpretation of some documents.

HyperText Transport Protocol Secure (HTTPS): It is the protocol for accessing a secure Web server. Using HTTPS in the URL instead of HTTP directs the message to a secure port number rather than the default Web port number of 80.

International Standardization Organization (ISO): It is a worldwide federation of national standards bodies. The work of preparing International Standards is normally carried out through ISO technical committees. Each member body interested in a subject for which a technical committee has been established has the right to be represented on that committee. International organizations, governmental and non-governmental, in liaison with ISO, also take part in the work.

Java: It is an object-oriented applications programming language developed by Sun Microsystems in the early 1990s. Java applications are typically compiled to bytecode, although compilation to native machine code is also possible. The language itself derives much of its syntax from C and C++ but has a simpler object model and fewer low-level facilities.

Java Database Connectivity (JDBC): It is an API for the Java programming language that defines how a client may access a database. It provides methods for querying and updating data in a database.

Joint Photographic Experts Group (JPEG): JPEG is a *lossy compression* technique for color images. Although it can reduce files sizes to about 5% of their normal size, some detail is lost in the compression

Java Server Pages (JSP): It is a Java technology that allows software developers to dynamically generate HTML, XML or other types of documents in response to a Web client request. The JSP syntax adds additional XML-like tags, called JSP actions, to be used to invoke the functionality. It lets you separate the dynamic part of your pages from the static HTML.

Portable Document Format (PDF): It is a file format developed by Adobe Systems. PDF captures formatting information from a variety of desktop publishing applications, making it possible to send formatted documents and have them appear on the recipient's monitor or printer as they were intended. To view a file in PDF format, you need Adobe Reader, a free application distributed by Adobe Systems.

Reference Information Model (RIM): It specifies the grammar of HL7 messages and, specifically, the basic building blocks of the language and their permitted relationships. The RIM is not a model of healthcare, although it is healthcare specific, nor is it a model of any message, although it is used in messages. At first site the RIM is quite simple.

Secure Sockets Layer (SSL): A protocol developed by Netscape for transmitting private documents via the Internet. SSL uses a cryptographic system that uses two keys to encrypt data, a public key known to everyone and a private or secret key known only to the recipient of the message.

Chapter XI
Clinical and Biomolecular Ontologies for E-Health

Mario Ceresa
Politecnico di Milano, Italy

Marco Masseroli
Politecnico di Milano, Italy

ABSTRACT

This chapter mainly focuses on biomedical knowledge representation and its use in biomedicine. It first illustrates the existent more relevant bioinformatics resources and why they need to be better integrated. Then it describes what the main problems that machines can encounter in processing the factual biomedical knowledge are, what terminologies, classifications and ontologies are, and why they could help in better organizing and exploiting the bioinformatics resources available online. The authors hope that a concise perspective of the field and a list of selected resources, commented with their scope and usability, may help interested people in quickly understanding the main principles of knowledge representation in biomedicine and its high relevance for modern biomedical research and e-health.

INTRODUCTION

In the current post-genomic era, molecular medicine is increasingly gaining relevance both in health care research and practice. Availability of the complete sequence of the human genome and of new nanotechnology approaches in molecular biology allows quickly and simultaneously studying thousands of genes and their expression levels. Advancements in information technologies and biomedical informatics are providing tools and techniques to manage the amount of data produced, and are making more easily accessible several different databanks of biomolecular information and many methods for their analysis. With the increasing biomolecular and biomedical informatics progresses, many healthcare sites are progressively more offering several genetics tests at relatively low costs. In the near future, biomolecular tests and screenings are expected to revolutionize the diagnosis of inherited diseases in a similar way as imaging tests from different techniques (e.g. computer tomography (CT), magnetic resonance (MR), positron emission tomography (PET), single photon emission computer tomography (SPECT), ultra sounds (US)) have transformed the diagnostic practice of several illnesses and the diagnostic services offered by healthcare providers.

Although genetics tests can now be easily and routinely performed thanks to the automatic or semiautomatic procedures developed, management and interpretation of the data they produce, in particular of the results of more advanced biomolecular exams, still present a number of issues. In fact, they generate a great amount of data that need to be efficiently stored and statistically analyzed in order to identify, among all genes or proteins studied in each test, those significantly altered in the tested conditions. Moreover, to correctly interpret such test results, the known structural, functional, and phenotypic information about the identified genes and protein products need to be further analyzed. Such information - which include presence of specific sequence characteristics and protein domains; cytogenetic localization; expression in different cellular tissues and organs; and involvement in particular biological processes, molecular functions, biochemical pathways, genetic diseases or phenotypes - are increasingly available within numerous distributed databanks, generally easily accessible also through Web interfaces. However, some issues hamper their effective and comprehensive use for the simultaneous analysis of the several hundreds of relevant genes and proteins identified in each biomolecular test. Such difficulties include: spreading of the required information among many heterogeneous databanks, the way most databanks provide these information (i.e. within unstructured HTML pages, one page for each gene or protein entry with all the information in the databank about the entry), and still lack of usage of common terminologies and bio-ontologies to describe biomolecular structural and functional characteristics of genes and their protein products and their phenotypic manifestations.

THE NEED FOR ONTOLOGIES

Bioinformatics research is heavily based on distributed resources spread across the Web. These resources can either be data sources such as genomic or proteomic databanks, or algorithmic sources. This last are collectively known as *Web Services* and usually perform some complex or resource demanding algorithm on uploaded data. A very typical bioinformatics Web service is a *sequence similarity analyzer* that receives a nucleic or amino acidic sequence as input and tries to find all the similar sequences among those within the selected database/s. All of these Web services are invaluable resources for the researcher, but when one finds himself using more and more Web resources, he/she can find quite awkward to switch back and forth from one to another to make multiple step articulated analyses. Moreover, these resources often differ in the data format for input or output. Thus, one eventually finds himself to desire better automatized tools that can take care of converting from one data format to another or automatically picking up data from several databanks, using them with distinct online resources and filtering only the relevant results. To make it short, users would really enjoy more automatized tools. The main problem for their implementation is that the Web is actually highly optimized for human users, not for machines: software programs that try to gather data and promote integration between services are uneasy with natural language and its highly ambiguous semantics. Moreover, the large amount of data and information that have been collected in medical and biological domains often suffers from the lack of common terminologies and standardization, as the same concepts are referred to in different manners across distinct resources. While in more formalized domains, like Physics and Math, a vast amount of knowledge is encoded in both numbers and mathematical formulas and it is easily manipulated by computers, Biologists and Clinicians mainly collect information and knowledge about facts, and these are difficulty handled by computer systems. As discussed in Stevens et al. (2000b), if machines are to compute with factual knowledge as they compute with continuous mathematics and strings, the semantic has to be precisely defined and standardized. Three of the instruments used to reach this goal of defining a precise and standardized semantic are (from the least to the most powerful): terminologies, classifications and ontologies. Though the first ones are simple collections of the names of the entities involved in a domain, they can be tremendously useful as they define a common vocabulary that can be shared among the application of that domain. Classifications stand a step further from terminologies: they include a common controlled vocabulary for the domain of interest and cluster each concept or entity of the domain in one or more categories, each of them can have subcategories as well. Last but far the most powerful technologies for knowledge representation are ontologies. These describe a piece of reality: a collection of classes of entities and the relationships among them. They contain a controlled vocabulary or terminology, plus a semantic network that encodes the relationships between each term of the vocabulary. They are often used to represent and share knowledge about a domain, by modelling classes of entities pertaining to the domain and the relationships among them.

In order to shorten the distance between human and machine knowledge representation, the World Wide Web Consortium (W3C) published some standard proposals. Some of the most impacting were: the eXtended markup language (XML) standard that is both easily extendible and machine readable, the resource description framework (RDF) that encodes statements in machine readable format, and the Web ontology language (OWL) that enables knowledge representation and sharing. This latter standard is the *de facto* standard for building ontologies for the Web. OWL exists in three different versions, with increasing expressivity and computational complexity:

- *OWL-Lite* is the simplest version, in which one can express only simple relationships
- *OWL-DL* is probably the most widely used as it meets a balance between the need for an expressive language and computational complexity
- *OWL-Full* has the strongest expressivity power, but makes no guarantees on computational properties.

Each version of the language includes and extends the preceding one. In other words, each OWL-Lite ontology is also a valid OWL-DL ontology (the contrary does not holds); and each OWL-DL ontology can also be expressed in OWL-Full (again the contrary does not holds). These W3C standards emerged as more and more people put great effort in extending the actual Web structure to support machine based processing, giving rise to the *Semantic Web*. By complying with these standards, machines still would not be able to truly understand any information, yet software programs would be able to process it in a much more efficient way (Lussier and Bodenreider, 2007).

Knowledge is usually encoded to make a meaningful use of it. To this aim, there are a lot of *reasoning services* in the Semantic Web. A reasoning service is simply a program that can import knowledge and use some deductive process to derive new knowledge from the previously imported one. The really important point is that the more the language used to encode the desired knowledge is expressive, the more difficult the reasoning with that language is. This problem deeply roots in mathematics and logics. For each formal system one could define the properties of **correctness** and **completeness**. A system is correct if one can prove **only** true facts, that is the system is not contradictory. A system is complete if one can prove **all** facts that logically derive from the considered axiom. In a system that is both complete and correct, one can prove **all and only** the true facts, which is quite a useful property. Unfortunately, all logic systems that are expressive enough to be useful in everyday applications are somewhat incomplete, that is there are some true facts that are not provable within the system. But what would happen if a reasoner is asked to prove an improvable formula? As it can not *decide* whether the asked property is true or false, it simply never ends searching for a solution, no matter how long it would take. This behaviour is also known as *the indecidability problem*, and strongly limits the power of the language we can choose to represent our knowledge. For this reason, Semantic Web applications (and most of the ontologies) will use OWL-DL instead of the more comfortable and powerful OWL-Full, which however gives no guarantees on computational properties.

Having a good language both to express an ontology and to reason with it in a sound way, which are the ontology key factors that make it a good and useful one? A good ontology should at least have a consistent use of terms, supported by logically coherent (non-circular) definitions, in both human-readable and computable formats and support making inference both within itself and across other ontologies. In the past few years a great scientific effort has been made in building robust and large ontologies about different domains. Nevertheless, presently in the biomedical and biomolecular domains only few of them are widely used (Bodenreider and Stevens, 2006). The most important are described below.

The Open Biomedical Ontologies (OBO) Foundry (http://obofoundry.org/)

It is a collaborative experiment to produce well-structured vocabularies for shared use across different biological and medical domains. The OBO Foundry introduces a new paradigm for biomedical ontology development by the establishment of gold standard reference ontologies for individual domains of inquiry. All the ontologies that are accepted in the OBO standard must distinguish:

- Continuants (cells, molecules, organisms, ...)
- Occurrents (events, processes)
- Dependent entities (qualities, functions, ...)
- Independent entities (their bearers)
- Universals (types, kinds)
- Instances (tokens)

Examples of different types of relationships that are included in OBO, and thus that are com-

Table 1. Examples of common OBO relationships

Foundational	is_a part_of
Spatial	located_in contained_in adjacent_to
Temporal	transformation_of derives_from preceded_by
Participation	has_participant has_agent

mon to all the ontologies that share its standard, are shown in Table 1.

Foundational Model of Anatomy (FMA) (http://sig.biostr.washington.edu/projects/fm/) (Rosse and Mejino, 2003)

It is an evolving computer-based knowledge source for bioinformatics that is concerned with the representation of classes and relationships necessary for the symbolic modelling of the structure of the human body in a form that is understandable to humans and is also navigable, parsable, and interpretable by machine-based systems. Specifically, the FMA is a domain ontology that represents a coherent body of explicit declarative knowledge about human anatomy, although its ontological framework can be applied and extended to all other species. The FMA ontology has four interrelated components:

1. **Anatomy taxonomy (AT)**, which classifies anatomical entities according to the characteristics they share and by which they can be distinguished from one another
2. **Anatomical structural abstraction (ASA),** which specifies the part-whole and spatial relationships that exist between the entities represented in AT;
3. **Anatomical transformation abstraction (ATA),** which specifies the morphological transformation of the entities represented in AT during prenatal development and postnatal life cycle
4. **MetaKnowledge (MK),** which specifies the principles, rules and definitions according to which classes and relationships in the other three components of FMA are represented.

Gene Ontology (GO) (http://www.geneontology.org/) (Ashburner et al., 2000)

It is a very important effort, started in November 1999, addressing the need for an integrated resource that provides consistent descriptions of gene products in different biomolecular genomic resource. The main aim of GO is promoting consistent annotation of gene products with the following three major functional categories and their subcategories:

- Biological processes
- Cellular components
- Molecular functions

The first describes biological processes such as metabolism or signal transduction. The second one helps specifying where a biological process takes place. The last one describes the biochemical activity independently from a precise cellular localization or a precise biological process.

The semantic structure of GO is a direct acyclic graph (DAG), i.e. a graph composed of nodes and edges. Each node represents a single concept, a GO category, described by a term of the controlled vocabulary. Edges, which link together two nodes, represent relationships between the concepts, and hence between the vocabulary terms. At present, in the gene ontology only two kinds of relations exist: *specification* (i.e. the "*IS_A*" relation) and *membership* (i.e. the "*PART_OF*" relation). Through them, either very general terms or very precise terms can be represented. A DAG is very similar to a hierarchical tree structure because no cycles exist between nodes, and edges have a one-way meaning. Nevertheless, a DAG differs from a hierarchy in that a 'child' (i.e. a more specialized concept or term) can have many "parents" (i.e. more generic concepts or terms) and may have different types of relations with its different parents.

Despite its broad definition and wide use in the biomolecular domain, GO has some problems, mainly due to its still short life, its uneven growing complexity, and the fast increasing knowledge of the domain it represents. At present, the main GO problems are:

- Presence of only two relations, which somewhat limits the amount of information expressible besides possibly leading to metonymy. In fact, there are cases in which neither of the only two possible types of relations that can be assigned between two categories is correct according to the definition given to the related categories. Thus, although introducing a new type of relation would correctly express the semantic of the relationship, the only chance to correct these cases is to change the definition of at least one of the two related categories, i.e. to define better terms to represent them.
- Although GO nodes should not contain species-specific definitions, many molecular functions, biological processes, and cellular components included in the GO are not common to all life forms but apply to only a few taxonomic class of organisms. The problem concerns the need for species-specific terms to describe molecular functions, biological processes, and cellular components in individual groups of organisms. As more and more species-specific terms are added to the GO vocabularies, it becomes difficult to maintain both the global interspecies relations for which GO strives, and the precise terms required for intraspecies gene annotation.
- When a GO node has multiple parents, multiple paths are established from the node to the ontology root node. Besides making the resulting DAG confusing, this might lead to interpretation errors when two father nodes have incompatible biological characteristics (for instance in different species). This is because a child node inherits the biological characteristics of all its father nodes. However, such a problem can be solved by defining different *contexts* for the given child node with multiple parents, each *context* with a unique path to the ontology root.
- Sometimes presence of circularity, as in the term GO:O19836: "*Haemolysis: The processes by which an organism effects haemolysis*". Circularity is a bad characteristic because neither humans nor machines can use the definition to understand what the term means.

Despite such and other problems, the GO remains a very useful instrument to connect at best several annotations concerning individual biological concepts but related to different species, or simply sparsely stored in heterogeneous databases. Therefore, it allows automatically performing controlled searches and semantic clustering of diverse gene annotations, which is very useful in many genomic analyses (e.g. high-throughput gene expression) to group genes and gene products to some high level concept/term. Besides helping in better interpreting results of such experimental analyses, this ability is fundamental also in the characterization of less known genes. In fact, if in the same cellular component an uncharacterized gene is co-expressed with well-characterized genes annotated to some GO process, one can infer that the "unknown" gene's product is likely to act in the same process. In Masseroli and Pinciroli (2006) the interested reader can find a more in depth discussion and a comparison among tools that can be used to perform analysis and semantic clustering of genes based on GO annotations.

Unified Medical Language System (UMLS) (http://umlsinfo.nlm.nih.gov/) (Bodenreider, 2004)

The National Library of Medicine (NLM) Unified Medical Language System project facilitates the development of computer systems that behave as if they "understand" the meaning of the language of biomedicine and health. To that end, NLM produces and distributes the UMLS knowledge sources (databases) and associated software tools (programs) for use by system developers in building or enhancing electronic information systems that create, process, retrieve, integrate, and/or aggregate biomedical and health data and information, as well as in informatics research. By design, the UMLS knowledge sources are multi-purpose. They are not optimized for particular applications, but can be applied in systems that perform a range of functions involving one or more types of information (e.g. patient records, scientific literature, guidelines, public health data). The associated UMLS software tools assist developers in customizing or using the UMLS knowledge sources for particular purposes. Researchers can use the UMLS products in investigating knowledge representation and retrieval questions. Among UMLS key points there are a broad coverage of medical terms and the absence of multiple inheritance (i.e. each term has only a parent).

Others Ontological Resources

The list of the other biomedical and biomolecular ontological resources presently available could be quite long. Those that are attracting interests and are increasingly used are listed below in alphabetical order.

- **BioPax** (http://www.biopax.org/): A fully-featured ontology describing biological pathways. It currently covers metabolic pathways, molecular interactions and protein post-translational modifications. In the near future it will be expanded to support signaling pathways, gene regulatory networks and genetic interactions.
- **eVOC** (http://www.evocontology.org/): A set of ontologies that describes gene expression features (e.g. the organism anatomical system and cell type where, the developmental stage when, and the pathological condition in which a gene is expressed) and facilitates a link between genome sequence and expression phenotype information. These sets are mutually orthogonal, i.e. each of them provides a different view on the domain, untangled from the others. This helps in querying the provided information, as one can easily combine the different views to build up complex queries.
- **ImMunoGeneTics (IMGT) Ontology** (http://imgt.cines.fr/): A high-quality integrated knowledge resource specialized in immunoglobulins, T cell receptors, major histocompatibility complex, immunoglobulin superfamily, major histocompatibility complex superfamily and related proteins of the immune system of humans and other vertebrate species. IMGT consists of sequence databases (IMGT/LIGM-DB, IMGT/MHC-DB, IMGT/PRIMER-DB), genome database (IMGT/GENE-DB), and structure database (IMGT/3Dstructure-DB).
- **MGED vocabulary** (http://www.cbil.upenn.edu/Ontology/MGED_ontology.html): It is conceived for describing a biological sample, the treatment that it receives, and the microarray chip technology used in a high-throughput biomolecular experiment.
- **Molecular Biology Ontology** (http://www.cs.man.ac.uk/~stevensr/onto/node8.html): A general reference ontology for molecular biology that represents an attempt to provide clarity and communication within the molecular biology database community.
- **Pharmacogenetics and Pharmacogenomics Knowledge Base (PharmGKB)** (http://www.pharmgkb.org/): It curates information that establish knowledge about the relationships among drugs, diseases and genes, including their variations and gene products.

- **RiboWeb** (http://smi-web.stanford.edu/projects/helix/riboweb.html): An ontology describing ribosomal components, their associated data and the computations for processing them.

MAIN DISTRIBUTED BIOMEDICAL RESOURCES AVAILABLE ONLINE

Among the most interesting online biomedical resources there are several databanks that store genomic or proteomic data. These databanks constitute a cross referenced environment used to manage a great amount of data and able to provide heterogeneous structural, functional and phenotypic information on genes and proteins. As illustrated in Maffezzoli and Masseroli (2006), these biomolecular databanks can be classified in **primary databanks**, which store only the essential information regarding nucleic or amino acidic sequences, and **derivative** or **specialized databanks** that enrich the primary descriptions with annotations from several heterogeneous sources. The primary databanks can be subdivided in:

- **DNA databanks:**
  - GenBank at the National Center for Biotechnology Information (NCBI) (US) (http://www.ncbi.nlm.nih.gov/).
  - European Molecular Biology Laboratory (EMBL) data library at the European Bioinformatics Institute (EBI) (UK) (http://www.ebi.ac.uk/embl.html).
  - DNA Data Bank of Japan (DDBJ) (Japan) (http://www.ddbj.nig.ac.jp/).
- **Protein databanks:**
  - Swiss-Prot/TrEMBL (http://www.expasy.org/sprot/). which provides a high level of annotations.
  - UniProt (Unified Protein Resource) (http://www.pir.uniprot.org/), the world's most comprehensive catalog of information on proteins. It is a central repository of protein sequences and functions created by joining the information contained in Swiss-Prot, TrEMBL, and PIR databanks.

Among the derivative databanks a few well known examples are:

- **UniGene** (http://www.ncbi.nlm.nih.gov/sites/entrez?db=unigene): Each UniGene entry is a set of transcript sequences that appears to come from the same transcription locus (gene or expressed pseudogene), together with information on protein similarities, gene expression, cDNA clone reagents, and genomic location.
- **Entrez Gene** (http://www.ncbi.nlm.nih.gov/sites/entrez?db=gene): It is a databanks for gene-specific information, which includes records from genomes that have been completely sequenced, that have an active research community to contribute gene-specific information or that are scheduled for intense sequence analysis. The content of Entrez Gene represents the result of both curation and automated integration of data from NCBI's Reference Sequence project (RefSeq – http://www.ncbi.nlm.nih.gov/RefSeq/), from collaborating model organism databanks and from other databanks within NCBI.
- **Online Mendelian Inheritance in Man (OMIM)** (http://www.ncbi.nlm.nih.gov/sites/entrez?db=OMIM): A comprehensive, authoritative and timely knowledgebase of human genes and genetic disorders compiled to support human genetics research and education and the practice of clinical genetics. Each OMIM entry has a full-text summary of a genetically determined phenotype and/or gene and has numerous links to other genetic databanks.

- **InterPro** (http://www.ebi.ac.uk/interpro/): It provides integrated access to annotations about protein families, domains, and functional sites in which identifiable features found in known proteins can be applied to unknown protein sequences. It integrates several protein signature databanks including PROSITE, PRINTS, ProDom, Pfam, SMART, TIGRFAMs, PIRSF, SUPERFAMILY, Gene3D and PANTHER.

A lot of other resources are available as well on the Internet for use in genomic and proteomic experiment analysis, also in the form of *Web Services*. Some of the most interesting are:

- **FASTA** (http://www.ebi.ac.uk/fasta/): It is a heuristic algorithm that calculates possible suboptimal similarities between nucleotide or protein sequences. It uses dynamic programming methods to find a set of subsequence alignments, called "*hot spot*", that are combined in order to approximate the alignments of a longer sequence and obtain better global inter-similarities. The name stands for FAST-All, reflecting the fact that this algorithm implementation can be used for a fast comparison. It achieves a high level of sensitivity for similarity searching at high speed, which is attained by trying to identify potential matches before attempting the more time consuming optimised search. It provides a good balance between accuracy and execution time.
- **BLAST** (http://www.ncbi.nlm.nih.gov/BLAST/): The Basic Local Alignment Search Tool implements another heuristic approach that tries to find suboptimal inter-similarity matches between nucleotide or protein sequences. It uses rules more strict to find better, although less numerous, *hot spot* alignments. Its strategy is finding high inter-similarity regions in alignments without "*gaps*", i.e. without any element deletions o insertions in none of the two compared sequences, although alignments with *gaps* can be created by connecting the most similar regions found. Built on the FASTA algorithm, it is widely used because it is quicker and can output a whole range of possible matches, each annotated with a statistical estimate of similarity.
- **ELM** (http://elm.eu.org/): A computational biology resource for investigating candidate functional sites in eukaryotic proteins. The current version of the ELM server provides core functionality including filtering by cell compartment, phylogeny and globular domain overlap (using the SMART/Pfam databases). In addition, both the known ELM instances and any positionally conserved matches in sequences similar to ELM instance sequences are identified and displayed.
- **Harvester** (http://harvester.fzk.de/harvester/): It crawls and cross links many bioinformatics sites, providing a single Web page access point to a great amount of aggregated resources and genomic databanks. Among the others: CDART, CDD, ensEMBL, Entrez, GenomeBrowser, gfp-cDNA, GoogleScholar, gopubmed, H-Inv, HomoloGene, Hwiki-Forum, iHOP, IPI, MapView, Mitocheck, OMIM, PolyMeta, PSORT II, RZPD, SMART, SOSUI, SOURCE, STRING, Unigene, UniprotKB.
- **SMART** (http://smart.embl-heidelberg.de/): The Simple Modular Architecture Research Tool allows identification and annotation of genetically mobile domains and performing analysis of domain architectures. These domains are extensively annotated with respect to phylogenetic distributions, functional classes, tertiary structures and functionally important residues. Each domain found in a non-redundant protein database, as well as search parameters and taxonomic information, are stored in a relational database

system. User interfaces to this database allow searches for proteins containing specific combinations of domains in defined taxonomies.

Most of all these resources were created mainly for human users, that is, they are not optimized for machine interoperability. Often they use different formats in input and output or, if they share some common informative resource such as GO, there is no guarantee they will ever use the same resource version. Yet, the possibility to compose the preceding services to reduce their shortcomings and increasing their strengths could be tremendously useful for the analysis of biomedical data. To this aim many efforts are being done in defining a common interface to integrate these services in a coherent and automatic way.

INTEGRATION AND USE OF BIOMEDICAL RESOURCES

The integration of the numerous biomedical resources available and their effective use to support biomedical knowledge discovery and better health care is currently one of the major goals of the bioinformatics and computational biology community. All efforts towards this goal are deeply influenced by the availability and extensive use of high-quality bio-ontologies describing the biomolecular and clinical domains. As building such sound ontologies is a difficult task, several international institutions are taking over and helping founding, coordinating and spreading bio-ontologies results. A good review of these efforts can be found in Bodenreider et al. (2005), the most relevant contributions of which we summarize here. The Institute for Formal Ontology and Medical Information Science (IFOMIS) primarily contributes to the introduction of ontologies in medicine and develops collaborations with developers of biomedical ontologies such as the GO Consortium and the Structural Informatics Group at the University of Washington. The National Center for Biomedical Ontologies (NCBO) is involved in the development of ontologies of the OBO family, and in the use and design of the Protege tool. This is probably the most used and widespread free ontology editor; it can be found at http://protege.stanford.edu/. Last but not least, since the W3C has announced the creation of the Health Care and Life Sciences Interest Group, several task forces started addressing the conversion of existing resources into the RDF/OWL format and the development of Semantic Web applications for health care. All these ontologies and resources foster the development of new bioinformatics applications for integration and use of the numerous biomedical knowledge sources available. Some relevant examples of applications developed for the effective use of biomedical knowledge expressed through ontologies and controlled vocabularies are:

- **GoMiner** (http://discover.nci.nih.gov/gominer/) (Zeeberg et al., 2003): It is a tool for biological interpretation of 'omic' data, including data from gene expression microarrays. Omic experiments often generate lists of dozens or hundreds of genes that differ in expression between samples. GoMiner leverages the gene ontology to identify the biological processes, functions and components represented in these lists. Instead of analyzing microarray results with a gene-by-gene approach, GoMiner classifies the genes into biologically coherent categories and assesses these categories. The insights gained through GoMiner can generate hypotheses to guide additional research.
- **GFINDer** (http://www.bioinformatics.polimi.it/GFINDer/) (Masseroli et al., 2004; Masseroli et al., 2005; Masseroli et al., 2007): The Genome Function INtegrated Discoverer is a Web tool for effective using genomic information available in many

heterogeneous databanks accessible via the Internet that allows performing statistical analyses and data mining of functional and phenotypic annotations of gene sets, for instance identified in high-throughput biomolecular experiments. It automatically retrieves annotations of several functional and phenotypic categories from many different public sources, identifies the categories enriched in each class of a user-classified gene list and calculates statistical significance values for each category. GFINDer also enables gene classification according to functional categories and the statistical analysis of obtained results. It therefore permits better understanding of high-throughput experiment results and mining hidden biomedical knowledge by examining user nucleotide sequence ID lists and applying clustering and statistical analysis methods to their currently available genomic annotations retrieved from several databanks. The annotations considered in GFINDer include biological processes, cellular components, and molecular functions provided by the gene ontology, Biochemical Pathways supplied by the Kyoto Encyclopaedia of Genes and Genomes (KEGG) databank (http://www.genome.jp/kegg/), Protein Families and Domains from Pfam (http://www.sanger.ac.uk/Software/Pfam/) and InterPro databanks, and clinical and phenotypic information (i.e. Phenotypes and Phenotype Locations associated with inherited disorders or genetic loci) provided by the OMIM databank.

- **DAVID Bioinformatics Resources 2007** (http://david.abcc.ncifcrf.gov/home.jsp) (Huang et al., 2007): The Database for Annotation, Visualization and Integrated Discovery resources aim to provide functional interpretation of large lists of genes derived from genomic studies. Besides many integrated annotations from several public resources, DAVID provides tools and functions for gene-term enrichment analysis and to allow users to quickly group functionally related genes and terms into a manageable number of functional biological modules to more efficiently interpret genome-scale datasets. The main provided functionalities are:
  - Identification of enriched biological themes, particularly GO terms
  - Discovering of enriched functional-related gene groups
  - Clustering of redundant annotation terms
  - Visualization of genes on BioCarta and KEGG pathway maps
  - Display of related many-genes-to-many-terms on 2-D view
  - Search for other functionally related genes not in the list
  - Highlight of protein functional domains and motifs
  - Listing of interacting proteins
  - Linking of gene-disease associations
  - Exploration of gene names in batch
  - Conversion of gene identifiers from one type to another
  - Redirection to related literature

All these applications are very important to identify the roles played by the genes considered in functional genomic experiments and help translating the massive gene expression and protein data produced into biological knowledge (Al-Shahrour and Dopazo, 2005).

Among the developed applications that use ontologies to enable sharing complex biological information and integrating heterogeneous databases it is important to mention the following:

- **Transparent Access to Multiple Bioinformatics Information Sources (TAMBIS)** (http://www4.wiwiss.fu-berlin.de/dblp/page/record/journals/bioinformatics/StevensBBNJPGB00) (Stevens et al., 2000a)): It uses an ontology, the TAMBIS ontology (TaO), to enable biologists to ask questions over multiple external databases using a common query interface. The TaO describes a wide range of bioinformatics tasks and resources without containing any instances. It only contains knowledge about bioinformatics and molecular biology concepts and their relationships; the instances they represent still reside in external databases.

- **Biozon** (http://biozon.org/doc/) (Birkland and Yona, 2006): It addresses the growing need to corroborate and integrate data from different resources and aspects of biological systems for effective analysis of new genes and other biological entities. It aims at creating a unified biological knowledge resource with emphasis on protein and DNA characterization and classification.
- **BioMoby** (http://biomoby.org/) (Wilkinson and Links, 2002): It defines an ontology-based messaging standard through which a client can automatically discover and interact with task-appropriate biological data and analytical service providers without requiring manual manipulation of data formats as data flows from one provider to the next.
- **Taverna** (http://taverna.sourceforge.net/) (Hull et al., 2006): It is an open source tool that tries to enable users to easily connect multiple services in a visual manner, mapping the outputs of a service with the inputs of another. Once the mapping has been established, one can run all the different Web services in a row and gathers or exports the results.
- **MOWServer** (http://www.inab.org/MOWServ/) (Navas-Delgado et al., 2006): Based on semantic interconnection of different BioMoby services, it is able to integrate different data collection and Web services. It is compatible with Taverna and provides user-to-service interfaces automatically generated on top of the BioMOBY standard.

As better ontological resources are developed, all these applications will also increasingly enable complex reasoning about biomedical knowledge, hopefully unveiling additional knowledge useful to improve patient health care.

CONCLUSION

Research in bioinformatics heavily relies on online databanks and Web Services that are spread all over the Internet. While all of these resources can be extraordinary useful to researchers, they have not revolutionized the way scientists follow their experiment yet. There is still a lack of integration and common standards among them: different data formats, different interfaces and conventions are all common issues in this scenario. These problems make it difficult, if not impossible, to automate common, tedious, or error prone tasks, and slow the interconnection of the resources. Among all available technologies to tackle such issues, ontologies are the most promising ones for studying newer approaches that could help in integrating such resources together. They actually allow for a coherent and comprehensive hierarchy of concepts (and of the terms that describe them), and restrict the semantic to such a level that automatic reasoning is made possible. Moreover, ontologies can also be used as high level interfaces to access the vast amount of information that result from functional genomics research, support their integration and computational analysis, and foster translational research towards health care practice. On top of that, improved clinical ontologies and terminologies allow a homogeneous description of the articulated observations and prescriptions collected in clinical databases. This is very useful to permit their subsequent evaluation for comparative or epidemiological studies. The few biomedical ontology based approaches lately proposed for integrating the biomolecular and clinical information stored in distributed heterogeneous databases are greatly supporting investigations of genetic aetiology of diseases. All these endeavours are providing new and stronger knowledge bases and biomedical informatics applications to the modern medical procedures and patient health care and e-health.

REFERENCES

Al-Shahrour, F., Dopazo J. (2005). Ontologies and functional genomics. In *Data Analysis and Visualization in Genomics and Proteomics.* Azuaje, F., Dopazo J. (Eds.). New York, NY: John Wiley & Sons, pp. 99-112.

Ashburner, M., Ball, C.A., Blake, J.A., Botstein, D., Butler, H., Cherry, J.M., Davis, A.P., Dolinski, K., Dwight, S.S., Eppig, J.T., Harris, M.A., Hill, D.P., Issel-Tarver, L., Kasarskis, A., Lewis, S., Matese, J.C., Richardson, J.E., Ringwald, M., Rubin, G.M., Sherlock, G. (2000) Gene ontology: tool for the unification of biology. The Gene Ontology Consortium. *Nature Genetics, 25*(1), 25-29.

Birkland, A., Yona, G. (2006). BIOZON: a hub of heterogeneous biological data. *Nucleic Acids Research, 34*(Database issue), D235-D242.

Bodenreider, O. (2004). The Unified Medical Language System (UMLS): integrating biomedical terminology. *Nucleic Acids Research, 32*(Database issue), D267- D270.

Bodenreider, O., Mitchell, J.A., McCray, A.T. (2005). Biomedical Ontologies. In: Altman, R.B., Dunker, A.K., Hunter, L., Jung, T.A., Klein, T.E. (Eds.). *Proceedings Pacific Symposium on Biocomputing 2005.* Hackensack, NJ: World Scientific Publishing Co., Inc., pp. 76-78.

Bodenreider, O., Stevens, R. (2006). Bio-ontologies: current trends and future directions. *Briefings in Bioinformatics, 7*(3), 256-274.

Huang, D.W., Sherman, B.T., Tan, Q., Kir, J., Liu, D., Bryant, D., Guo, Y., Stephens, R., Baseler, M.W., Lane, H.C., Lempicki, R.A. (2007). DAVID Bioinformatics Resources: Expanded annotation database and novel algorithms to better extract biology from large gene lists. *Nucleic Acids Research, 35*(Web Server issue), pp. 1-7, Epub ahead of print.

Hull, D., Wolstencroft, K., Stevens, R., Goble, C., Pocock, M.R., Li, P., Oinn, T. (2006). Taverna: a tool for building and running workflows of services. *Nucleic Acids Research, 34*(Web Server issue), W729-W732.

Lussier, Y.A., Bodenreider, O. (2007). Clinical ontologies for discovery applications. In: Baker, C.J.O., Cheung, K.H. (Eds.). *Semantic Web: Revolutioning knowledge discovery in the life sciences.* New York, NY: Springer, pp. 101-119.

Maffezzoli, A., Masseroli, M. (2006). Chapter XLV: Genomic databanks for biomedical informatics. In: Lazakidou, A.A. (Ed.). *Handbook of Research on Informatics in Healthcare and Biomedicine.* Hershey, PA: Idea Group Inc., pp. 357-366.

Masseroli, M., Bellistri, E., Franceschini, A., Pinciroli, F. (2007). Statistical analysis of genomic protein family and domain controlled annotations for functional investigation of classified gene lists. *BMC Bioinformatics, 8*(Suppl 1), S14, pp. 1-10.

Masseroli, M., Galati, O., Pinciroli, F. (2005). GFINDer: genetic disease and phenotype location statistical analysis and mining of dynamically annotated gene lists. *Nucleic Acids Research, 33(Web Server issue), W717-W723.*

Masseroli, M., Martucci, D., Pinciroli, F. (2004). GFINDer: Genome Function INtegrated Discoverer through dynamic annotation, statistical analysis, and mining. *Nucleic Acids Research, 32(Web Server issue), W293-W300.*

Masseroli, M., Pinciroli, F. *(2006).* Using Gene Ontology and genomic controlled vocabularies to analyze high-throughput gene lists: three tool comparison. *Computers in Biology and Medicine, 36*(7-8), 731-747.

Navas-Delgado, I., Rojano-Munoz, M. del M., Ramirez, S., Perez, A.J., Andres Leon, E., Aldana-Montes, J.F., Trelles, O. *(2006)*. Intelligent client for integrating bioinformatics services. *Bioinformatics, 22*(1), 106-111.

Rosse, C., Mejino, J.L.V.Jr. (2003). A reference ontology for biomedical informatics: the Foundational Model of Anatomy. *Journal of Biomedical Informatics, 36*(6), 478-500.

Stevens, R., Baker, P., Bechhofer, S., Ng, G., Jacoby, A., Paton, N.W., Goble, C.A., Brass, A. (2000a). TAMBIS: Transparent Access to Multiple Bioinformatics Information Sources. *Bioinformatics, 16*(2), 184-185.

Stevens, R., Goble, C.A., Bechhofer, S. (2000b). Ontology-based knowledge representation for bioinformatics. *Briefings in Bioinformatics, 1*(4), 398-416.

Zeeberg, B.R., Feng, W., Wang, G., Wang, M.D., Fojo, A.T., Sunshine, M., Narasimhan, S., Kane, D.W., Reinhold, W.C., Lababidi, S., Bussey, K.J., Riss, J., Barrett, J.C., Weinstein, J.N. (2003). GoMiner: a resource for biological interpretation of genomic and proteomic data. *Genome Biology, 4*(4), R28, 1-8.

Wilkinson, M.D., Links, M. (2002). BioMOBY: an open source biological Web services proposal. *Briefings in bioinformatics, 3*(4), 331-341.

KEY TERMS

Bioinformatics: A join branch of biology and informatics concerned with the development of techniques for the collection and manipulation of biological data, and the use of such data to make biological discoveries or predictions. It comprehends all computational methods and theories applicable to molecular biology and the computer-based techniques for solving biological problems, including manipulation of models and datasets.

Biomedical Informatics: The discipline that studies biomedical information and knowledge, focusing in particular on their structure, acquisition, integration, management, and optimal use. It adopts and applies results from a variety of other disciplines including Information Science, Computer Science, Cognitive Science, Statistics and Biometrics, Mathematics, Artificial Intelligence, Operations Research, and basic and clinical Health Sciences.

Biomolecular or Genomic Databank: A structured repository of biomolecular, genomic or proteomic data, often integrated with their related biological, medical, clinical, or experimental information. Generally it also provides interfaces and tools for browsing, querying, and sometime analyzing the data it contains.

Classification: A collection of terms organized in categories. Thus, it includes only the *is-a* relationship between terms. This enables machines to group together bottom level terms up to their higher level ancestor, e.g. grouping all "*lipidic methabolism*" related terms under the upper term "*metabolism*".

Controlled Vocabulary: A collection of precise and universally understandable terms that define and identify the concepts of a domain in a unique and unequivocal way, e.g. the anatomical terminology. Such a vocabulary is said *controlled* because it is defined and maintained updated by people, the *curators*, who are expert of the domain the vocabulary refers to. Controlled vocabularies are very useful in extended and complex domains, such as Medicine and Biology, where distinct concepts must be identified with high precision in order to codify, analyze, and communicate the domain knowledge. Though they are similar to terminologies, the difference is that a terminology does not guarantee that its terms are precise, accurate and unequivocal, but it is rather a list of used terms for a specific domain.

Genomics: The systematic identification and study of Genomes, each of them including all the whole genetic material of a living organism.

Ontology: A semantic structure useful to standardize and provide rigorous definitions of the terminology used in a domain and to describe the knowledge of the domain. It is composed of a controlled vocabulary, which describes the concepts of the considered domain, and a semantic network, which describes the relations among such concepts. Each concept is connected to other concepts of the domain through semantic relations that specify the knowledge of the domain. A general concept can be described by several terms that can be synonyms or characteristic of different domains in which the concept exists. For this reason the ontologies tend to have a hierarchical structure, with generic concepts/terms at the higher levels of the hierarchy and specific concepts/terms at the lover levels, connected by different types of relations.

Proteomics: The study of the whole of all possible proteins (amino acid sequences) of an organism, translated from different transcripts (mRNA sequences transcripted from a nucleotide sequence).

Semantic Network: A graph structure useful to represent the knowledge of a domain. It is composed of a set of objects, the graph nodes, which represent the concepts of the domain, and relations among such objects, the graph arches, which represent the domain knowledge. The semantic networks are also a reasoning tool as it is possible to find relations among the concepts of a semantic network that do not have a direct relation among them. To this aim, it is enough "to follow the arrows" of the network arches that exit from the considered nodes and find in which node the paths meet.

Terminology: A collection of names of the entities involved in a domain. It simply states which are the principal terms used in the domain without any further information. Though it is a quite simplistic approach, yet it is extremely useful because helps computer programs to recognize the relevant terms and concentrate only on them. Although sometimes could be difficult to understand the difference between a terminology and a controlled vocabulary, the former is just a list of the terms used in a domain, while the latter guarantees that its terms are precise, accurate and unequivocal.

Chapter XII
Distributed Medical Volume Registration

Roger Tait
Nottingham Trent University, UK

Gerald Schaefer
Aston University, UK

ABSTRACT

The registration of corresponding patient volumes is often a pre-requisite for medical imaging tasks. Accurate alignment, however, usually results in high computational complexity and can hence take a considerable amount of time. This is particularly true with 3-D volume data which adds another dimension to the registration process. One possibility of keeping registration times feasible is to distribute computation among several processors so that it maybe accomplished in parallel. This chapter provides a short survey of parallel registration approaches which have been proposed together with some recent research adopting a blackboard architecture for distributed high performance image and volume registration purposes.

INTRODUCTION

The ability to visualise hidden structures in detail using 3-D volume data has become a valuable resource in medical imaging applications (Maintz & Viergever, 1998). Importantly, the alignment of volumes enables the combination of different structural and functional information for diagnosis and planning purposes (Pluim, Maintz, & Viergever, 2003). Transform optimisation, re-sampling, and similarity calculation form the basic stages of a registration process (Zitova & Flusser, 2003). During transform optimisation, translation and rotation parameters which geometrically map points in the reference (fixed) volume to points in the sensed (moving) volume are estimated. Once estimated, voxel intensities which are mapped into non-discrete co-ordinates are interpolated during the re-sampling stage. After re-sampling, a metric is used for similarity calculation in which the degree of likeness between corresponding volumes is evaluated. Optimisation of the similarity measure is the goal of the registration process and is achieved by seeking the best transform. All possible transform parameters therefore define the search space. Due to the iterative nature of registration algorithms similarity calculation represent a considerable performance bottleneck which limits the speed of time critical clinical applications.

The use of parallel computing to overcome these time constraints has become an important research area (Nicolescu & Jonker, 2000). Conveniently, many of the similarity calculation strategies employed in medical registration are inherently parallel and therefore well suited to distribution. An important consideration when adopting a parallel processing approach is the architecture of the host system. In a computer constructed of multiple processors with shared-memory, data distribution is not required. These systems are viewed as tightly-coupled architectures. In contrast, a loosely-coupled architecture consists of multiple computers in different locations. Loosely-coupled architectures therefore require data distribution, communication, and accumulation mechanisms. Logically, the most effective distribution scheme will depend on the architecture of the host system (Seinstra, Koelma, & Geusebroek, 2002). The two contrasting architectures of host systems are illustrated in Figure 1.

BACKGROUND

In the context of parallel processing, registration of medical data has been achieved by Warfield *et al.* (Warfield, Jolesz, and Kikinis, 1998) who introduced a non-rigid algorithm based on the work-pile paradigm. Their goal was to develop an inter-patient registration algorithm which can be applied without operator intervention, to a database of several hundred scans. In an initial step, each scan is segmented using a statistical classification method. This pre-processing stage

Figure 1. Tightly vs. loosely-coupled architectures. Data is either fetched from main memory via a memory bus, or is transferred over a communications network.

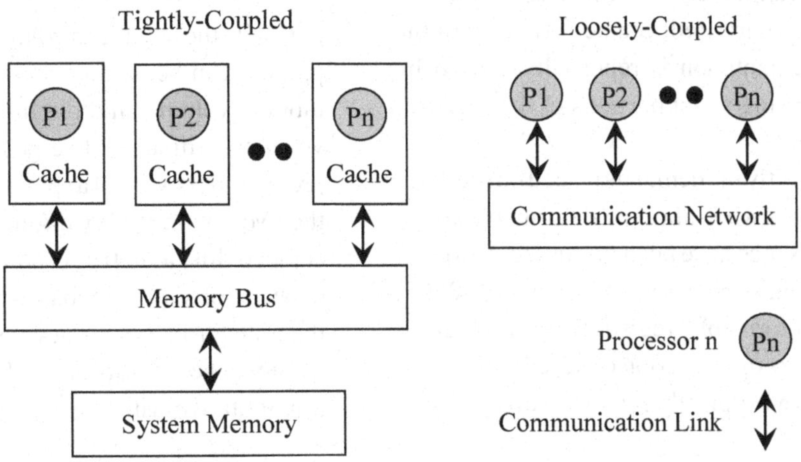

is used to identify different tissue types including skin, white matter, grey matter, and bone structure. Once segmented, a transform which brings these features into alignment is estimated. The system employs a message passing interface and cluster of symmetric multi-processors to execute parallel similarity calculation operations using multiple threads. Crucially, work is dynamically load balanced. Results published by the group show that successful registration of 256 × 256 × 52 voxel brain scans can been achieved in minutes rather than hours.

Christensen (1998) compares two non-threaded architectures, Multiple Instruction Multiple Data (MIMD) and Single Instruction Multiple Data (SIMD). The work presented raises implementation issues and timing analysis for the registration of 32 × 32 × 25, 64 × 64 × 50, and 128 × 128 × 100 voxel datasets. During each clock cycle, the SIMD implementation performs calculations in which all processors are performing the same operation. The MIMD implementation, in contrast, breaks an algorithm into independent parts which are solved simultaneously by separate processors. The movement of data in both shared-memory systems is unrestricted and during execution each processor has access to the whole memory. The main performance bottleneck associated with both approaches was reported as scalability of hardware with increasing numbers of processors. Crucially, the MIMD implementation is recorded as being approximately four times faster than its SIMD counterpart. Reduced performance of the SIMD implementation is reportedly caused by overheads during serial portions of the registration algorithm.

More recently the demands placed on registration algorithms when aligning deformable structures in 3-D space have been discussed. Salomon *et al.* (Salomon, Heitz, Perrin, & Armspach, 2005) introduce deformable registration of volumes which involves optimisation of several thousand parameters and typically requires several hours processing on a standard workstation. Based on simulation of stochastic differential equations and using simulated annealing, a parallel approach that yields processing times compatible with clinical routines is presented. The approach represents a hierarchical displacement vector field which is estimated by means of an energy function. The energy function is scaled in relation to the similarly measure and is re-evaluated at the end of each transform parameter optimisation cycle. The algorithm is reportedly suited to massively parallel implementation and has been successfully applied to the registration of 256 × 256 × 256 volumes. Again the results published demonstrate how alignment can be achieved in minutes rather than hours.

In the next section, a coarse-grained approach to parallelism is described which increases flexibility and allows the issues of fine-grained parallelism to be ignored. Building on a distributed blackboard architecture, the approach adopted supports multiple distributed agents organised in a worker/manager model. Crucially, the basic alignment steps are allocated to individual processors, the most computationally intensive of which being performed concurrently.

SIMILARITY CALCULATION USING A DISTRIBUTED BLACKBOARD ARCHITECTURE

Formally the inputs to a volume-based registration process can be defined as the fixed volume, the moving volume, and the transform used to map voxel co-ordinates. The goal of the registration process is recovery of a spatial mapping that brings the two volumes into alignment (Yoo, 2004). To achieve this, a metric is employed to generate a measure of similarity based on how well aligned the transformed moving volume is with the fixed volume. The measure of similarity produced forms a quantitative criterion which can be optimised in a search space defined by transform parameters (Penney *et al.*, 1998). Importantly, by employing a gradient-descend optimisation technique the metric can be used to produce derivatives of the similarity measure with respect to each transform parameter. Using the resulting derivatives, updated transform parameters can be estimated and evaluated.

To parallelise the registration process, both fixed and moving volumes require division into segments and distribution. The similarities between corresponding volume segments can then be estimated concurrently. To achieve this, transform parameters are propagated to all processing nodes in the distributed processing network. On receiving transform parameters, each node computes derivatives of the similarity measure for the segments allocated to it. The local derivatives computed are then accumulated and summed into a global derivative. This allows the transform parameters to be updated based upon the similarity of complete volumes. Convergence testing is then performed using the newly updated transform parameters. Depending on the success or failure of convergence testing, propagation of updated transform parameters and hence evaluation of new parameters can occur.

The iDARBS Framework

DARBS (Distributed Algorithmic and Rule-based Blackboard System) is a distributed blackboard architecture based on a client/server model (Nolle, Wong, & Hopgood, 2001). In DARBS the server functions as a blackboard and client modules as agents. Conveniently, each agent represents a structure in which rules and algorithms can be embodied. iDARBS (imaging DARBS) an underlying framework (Tait, Schaefer, & Hopgood, 2006a) on which registration algorithms can be hosted (Tait, Schaefer, & Hopgood, 2006b), consists of Distributor, Worker, and Manager Agent types:

- The Distributor Agent splits selected volumes into segments which are placed on the blackboard.
- Worker Agents take segments from the blackboard and perform local processing.
- The Manager Agent supervises Worker Agent activities.

The accumulation of local derivatives by the Manager Agent and the propagation of updated transform parameters to Worker Agents are illustrated in Figure 2.

Figure 2. The flow of local derivatives and current transform parameters between framework components.

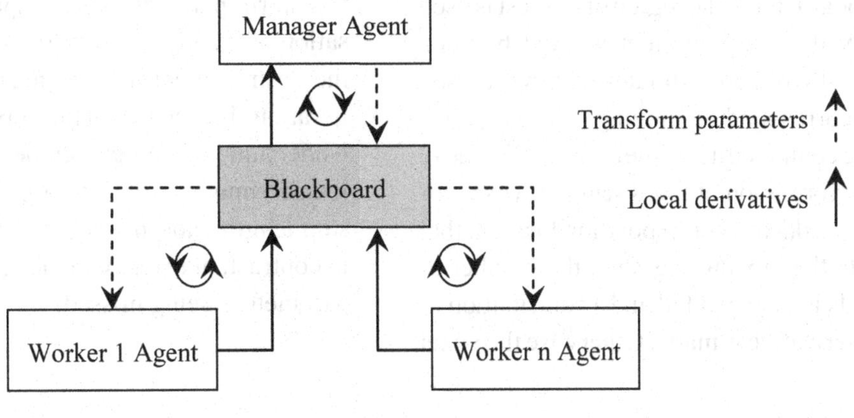

Initialisation of the Alignment Process

The Distributor Agent places predefined parameters associated with the optimisation process on the blackboard. The parameters include an initial step length, a minimum step length, and the maximum number of iterations to be performed. Logically, the initial step length is used to initialise the optimisation process. Convergence of optimisation and hence the selection of final transform parameters is controlled by the minimum step length.

To start the alignment process, the Distributor Agent calculates an initial centre of rotation and a translation. Employing both fixed and moving volumes, initial parameters are estimated using centres of mass computed from intensity levels. Once estimated, the fixed volume centre is set as the rotational centre of the initial transform. The translation component, in contrast, is set as the vector between the fixed and moving volume centres. To simplify calculation, no rotation is specified in the initial transform. Crucially, the use of centres of mass over geometrical volume centres results in a robust estimate of the initial transform.

Estimation of Local Derivatives

For similarity between segments to be calculated, the Worker *n* Agent employs a region of interest and current transform parameters retrieved from the blackboard. First, the region of interest is used to identify the fixed segment without borders. Then, for all voxel co-ordinates within the fixed segment, corresponding moving segment co-ordinates are computed using the current transform. If the transformation of fixed segment voxel co-ordinates results in a corresponding location that falls inside the moving segment, the number of valid voxels is incremented and a contribution to the local derivative is made. Otherwise the voxel is considered invalid and the next fixed segment voxel co-ordinates are processed. By evaluating all voxels, local derivatives of the similarity measure with respect to each transform parameter are generated.

The contribution to a local derivative represents a summation of intensities, from a moving segment gradient image, around the mapped voxel co-ordinates. Using a recursive Gaussian filter, a gradient image is created from the moving segment. The gradient image represents a vector field in which every vector points in the direction of its nearest edge, an edge being a rapid increase or decrease in neighbouring intensities. Each vector has a magnitude proportional to the second derivative of the intensity in the direction of the vector. Created once after retrieval of the moving segment, the gradient image is used for all iterations of the optimisation process.

Advancing the Transform Parameters

To update the current transform parameters, a gradient-descent optimisation scheme is employed to advances the current transform in the direction of the global derivative. If the direction of the global derivative abruptly changes, it is assumed that an optimum has been encountered and the step length is reduced by a half. Once the step length becomes smaller than the predefined minimum, the optimisation process is considered as having converged. This allows the precision of final transform parameters to be specified. If optimisation of the transform parameters fails to reach the desired precision, the maximum number of iterations is used to halt the optimisation process. Understandably, large numbers of iterations and long computational times result when the initial step length chosen is small. Large step lengths, in contrast, may result in the optimum transform parameters being missed.

EXPERIMENTAL TESTING

Efficiency tests are presented and demonstrate the performance increase of volume registration in non-distributed and distributed processing environments. To determine the accuracy of alignment between volumes a normalised correlation similarity metric was selected for testing purposes. Timing of an experiment started when the Manager Agent propagates transform parameters to all Worker Agents. Timing stopped when the Manager Agent places the final transform parameters on the blackboard. A sequential algorithm, constructed of the same components was used as a performance benchmark for comparison. The datasets used for testing, two MRI T1 volumes of an anatomically normal male head (Stark & Bradley, 1999), contain 180×218×180 voxels with a known translation and rotation. The volume pair was registered three times and average processing times calculated.

Computed using all voxels, normalised correlation calculates the cross-correlation of the volumes to be registered. Once calculated, the cross-correlation is normalised by the square root of the autocorrelation of each volume. Suited to volumes of the same modality, appealing properties of the metric include the production of a search space containing sharp peaks and well defined troughs. The accurate alignment of volumes, results in values near one being produced by the metric. Misalignment, in contrast, produces values of less than one. The distributed normalised correlation measure of similarity $S(F,M,T)$ is defined as (see Box 1.) where F and M are fixed and moving segment intensity functions respectively, T is a spatial

Box 1.

$$\frac{\partial S}{\partial p} = -\frac{\sum_{i=1}^{R}\left[\sum_{j=1}^{Q_i}\left(F(x_{ij})\frac{\partial M(T(x_{ij},p))}{\partial p}\right) - b\sum_{j=1}^{Q_i}\left(M(T(x_{ij},p))\frac{\partial M(T(x_{ij},p))}{\partial p}\right)\right]}{a}$$

Box 2.

$$= -\frac{\sum_{i=1}^{R}\left[\sum_{j=1}^{Q_i}\left(F(x_{ij})\frac{\partial M(T(x_{ij},p))}{\partial p}\right) - b\sum_{j=1}^{Q_i}\left(M(T(x_{ij},p))\frac{\partial M(y)}{\partial y}\bigg|_{y=T(x_{ij},p)}\frac{\partial T(x_{ij},p)}{\partial p}\right)\right]}{a}$$

with

$$a = \sqrt{\sum_{i=1}^{R}\left[\sum_{j=1}^{Q_i}F^2(x_{ij})\sum_{j=1}^{Q_i}M^2(T(x_{ij},p))\right]}$$

and

$$b = \frac{\sum_{i=1}^{R}\left[\sum_{j=1}^{Q_i}F(x_{ij})M(T(x_{ij},p))\right]}{\sum_{i=1}^{R}\left[\sum_{j=1}^{Q_i}M^2(T(x_{ij},p))\right]}$$

Figure 3. Sequential vs. distributed processing speed of volume registration using normalised correlation as a similarity metric.

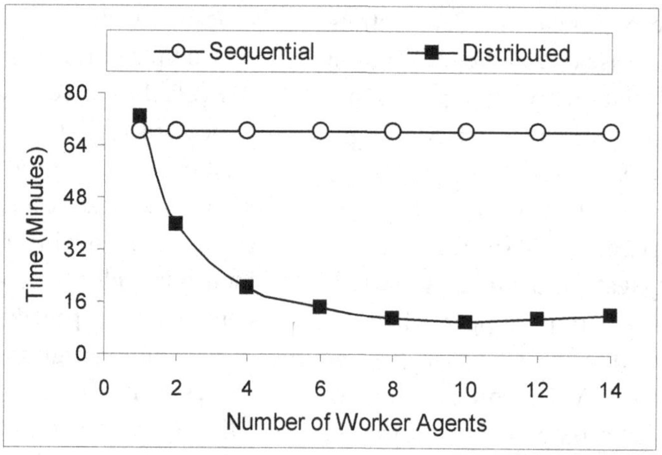

transform, and x_{ij} is the jth voxel of segment i from the fixed volume. R is the number of segment a volume is divided into and Q_i is the number of valid voxels mapped between segments identified by i. The derivative of the distributed similarity metric with respect to transform parameter p is computed as (see Box 2.) where $M(T(x_{ij},p))$ represents a discrete input which has been interpolated using a B-spline interpolation scheme. $\partial T(x_{ij},p)/\partial p$ is the transform Jacobian which is used to estimate variations in the mapped voxel co-ordinates with respect to transform parameter p. When a voxel location that maps outside of the moving segment is encountered, its contribution to the local derivative is discarded.

Figure 3 shows results, plotted as time against number of Worker Agents, obtained whilst performing volume registration with normalised correlation as a similarity metric. As can be seen, average processing time of registration was reduced from 68 minutes to approximately ten minutes when ten Worker Agents were employed. The distributed algorithm was observed to converge after 54 iterations with transform parameters which matched those computed by the sequential algorithm.

FUTURE TRENDS

Deformable registration is based on the assumption that an evenly spaced mesh of control points can be placed over fixed and moving volumes. A transform is then used to estimate the displacement necessary to map between corresponding control point locations. In order for registration to be performed, each control point plus underlying intensities are transformed and compared with their counterpart until an acceptable level of similarity is achieved. Such algorithms have recently emerged in distributed processing environments and are achieved by assigning subsets of control points to individual processing nodes. Conveniently, the use of free-form deformations permits the independent movement of control points and removes the need for processor-to-processor communications (Loeckx, Maes, Vandermeulen, & Suetens, 2004). Crucially, the resulting implementations are designed to address the computational burden associated with the estimation of transform parameters for locally deformed volumes.

CONCLUSION

Registration is an important step in medical analysis tasks where information is extracted from a combination of sources. Traditionally, volume registration algorithms have been implemented using single processor architectures which are limited by memory and speed constraints. Such limitations have a negative impact in clinical applications where real-time processing allows physicians to monitor the progress of treatment while a patient is present. Importantly, the most successful registration algorithms employ intensity-based correlation as a measure of similarity (Maintz & Viergever, 1998; Zitova & Flusser, 2003). Although a variety of similarity metrics have been developed, in practice they represent a considerable computational burden during the alignment process. The main reason for this is the high cost associated with multiple evaluations of a complex transform and the interpolation of non-discrete intensity co-ordinates. The surveyed literature makes clear that concurrent similarity calculation can be achieved and provides better performance than non-parallel approaches (Warfield, Jolesz, & Kikinis, 1998; Christensen, 1998; Salomon *et al.*, 2005). The large speedups reported are, however, difficult to obtain and only specialised hardware is capable of maintaining such efficiencies when scaled. As a consequence, the applications developed to address the problem of slow volume registration speeds are restricted to high-cost specialised architectures found predominantly in the research environment.

While various approaches to distribution have been employed, it is fine-grained parallelism that achieves the best results (Ourselin, Stefanescu, & Pennec, 2002; Hastings *et al.*, 2003; Rohlfing & Maurer, 2003). These methods are based on the low level decomposition of an algorithm within a tightly-coupled architecture. Understandably, such algorithms are difficult to implement and minimise computational expense by eliminating the exchange of data between processors. In this chapter, a novel coarse-grained approach to high performance intensity-based volume registration has been presented. The approach adopted has been shown to significantly improve processing speed, clearly outperforming sequential versions of the same algorithm. By employing an intensity-based algorithm the complicated segmentation of features fundamental to landmark-based registration methods have been avoided. As a consequence, the algorithm distributed does not require user intervention. Unlike other high performance volume registration applications, the decoupling of algorithm components allows transforms of any type to be incorporated. This explicit separation also permits different similarity calculation and transform parameter optimisation strategies to be employed, with only minor modifications to the existing framework.

REFERENCES

Christensen, G.E. (1998). MIMD vs SIMD parallel Processing: a case study in 3D medical image registration. *Parallel Computing, 24*, 1369-1383.

Hastings, S., Kurc, T., Langella, S., Catalyurek, U., Pan, T., & Saltz, J. (2003). Image processing for the grid: a toolkit for building grid-enabled image processing applications. In *Proceedings of the 3rd IEEE/ACM International Symposium on Cluster Computing and the Grid*. 36-43.

Loeckx, D., Maes, F., Vandermeulen, D., & Suetens, P. (2004). *Non-rigid image registration using free-form deformations with a local rigidity constraint*. Lecture Notes in Computer Science. 3216, 639-646.

Maintz, J.B.A., & Viergever, A. (1998). A survey of medical image registration. *Medical Image Analysis, 2*, 1-36.

Nicolescu, C., & Jonker, P. (2000). Parallel low-level image processing on a distributed memory system. In *Proceedings of the 15th Workshop on Parallel and Distributed Processing*, 226-233.

Nolle, L., Wong, K.C.P., & Hopgood, A.A. (2001). DARBS: a distributed blackboard system. *Research and Development in Intelligent Systems, 18*, 161-70.

Ourselin, S., Stefanescu, R., & Pennec, X. (2002). Robust registration of multi-modal images: towards real-time clinical applications. In *Proceedings of the 5th International Conference on Medical Image Computing and Computer-Assisted Intervention*, 140-147.

Penney, G.P., Weese, J., Little, J.A., Desmedt, P., Hill, D.L.G., & Hawkes, D.J. (1998). *A comparison of similarity measures for use in 2D-3D medical image registration. IEEE Transactions on Medical Imaging, 17*, 586-595.

Pluim, J.P., Maintz, J.B.A., & Viergever, M.A. (2003). *Mutual information-based registration of medical images: a survey. IEEE Transactions on Medical Imaging, 22*, 986-1004.

Rohlfing, T., & Maurer, C.R. (2003). Non-rigid image registration in shared-memory multi-processor environments with application to brains, breasts, and bees. *IEEE Transactions on Information Technology in Biomedicine, 7*, 16-25.

Salomon, M. Heitz, F. Perrin, G.R. & Armspach, J.P. (2005). A massively parallel approach to deformable matching of 3-D medical images via stochastic differential equations, *Parallel Computing 31*, 45-71.

Seinstra, F.J., Koelma, D., & Geusebroek, J.M. (2002). A software architecture for user transparent parallel image processing. *Parallel Computing. 28*, 967-993.

Stark, D.D., & Bradley, W.G. (1999). *Magnetic resonance imaging: third edition.* Mosby Publishing, USA.

Tait, R.J., Schaefer, G., & Hopgood, A.A. (2006a). iDARBS – A distributed blackboard system for image processing. In *Proceedings of the 13th International Conference on Systems, Signals and Image Processing*, 431-434.

Tait, R.J., Schaefer, G., & Hopgood, A.A. (2006b). Towards high performance image registration using intelligent agents. In *Proceedings of the 13th International Conference on Systems, Signals and Image Processing*, 435-438.

Warfield, S.K., Jolesz, F., & Kikinis, R. (1998). A high performance approach to the registration of medical imaging data. Parallel Computing. 24(9), 1345-1368.

Yoo, T.S. (2004). *Insight into images: Principles and practices for segmentation, registration, and image analysis.* A.K. Peters Ltd, USA.

Zitova, B., & Flusser, J. (2003). Image registration methods: a survey. *Image and Vision Computing. 21*, 977-1000.

KEY TERMS

Blackboard Architecture: An artificial intelligence application based on and analogous to a group of experts seated in a room with a large blackboard working as a team to solve a common problem.

Coarse-Grained Parallelism: A term used to describe an algorithm that has been divided into high-level components each of which can be hosted by a separate processor.

Distributed Agents: Software entities, designed to execute as independent threads and on distributed processors, capable of acting autonomously in order to achieve a pre-defined task.

Fine-Grained Parallelism: A term used to describe an algorithm that has been divided into low-level components each of which can be hosted by a separate processor.

Image Registration: The process whereby two images, differing by a spatial transformation, are brought into geometric alignment.

Parallel Processing: The concurrent execution of the same task, split into components, on multiple processors in order to achieve faster processing speeds.

Similarity Metric: A measure used to quantitatively judge how well a transformed sensed (moving) image fits a reference (fixed) image by comparing intensities.

Chapter XIII
Electronic Commerce for Health Products Services–Problems–Quality and Future

Bill Ag. Drougas
HATRLab, Greece & Higher Technological Institute of Epirus, Greece

ABSTRACT

Internet today is one of the most useful tools for information, education and business or entertainment. It is one of the modern technology tools giving us many applications world wide in various fields. One of the most important applications of the Internet is the e-commerce for quality health and medical products. There are an enormous number of Web sites offering health products with the method of E-commerce but still there are many problems with the quality of these products. To the other side many individuals are not able to choice and to know about the quality of these health products that offered today on line with the Internet companies. There are many serious proposals today in to the direction of the quality of the products in health. In this paper summarized many informations about the on line commerce for health products, some of the most popular products and the methodology to train individuals in to the direction to buy and choose quality products. In this paper also presented and analyzed the characteristics and criteria of one serious Internet health company and its Web site. Also how the different scientific organizations can help people and the electronic health commerce to be more effective in to various fields in the division of the popular health. This will be more effective after training and giving criteria and or educating Internet users for a serious choice in to their on line commerce with the E-Health Commerce Web Organizations.

INTRODUCTION

The Internet is changing today very fast how people may give and receive health information in various fields of the public health. All people who are able to use the Internet for health-related purposes-patients, health care professionals and administrators, researchers, those who create or may sell any health products or services, and other stakeholders-must join together to create a safe environment and enhance the value of the Internet for meeting health care needs.

Health products may be offered today from various accredited or not companies world wide. This is of course one of the problems existed today in the electronic health commerce. This problem is more usual and bigger today in the Internet with the appearance of many virtual commerce organizations and companies offering plenty of different health products without presenting an official level of quality. It is very easy today to contact with millions of health sites and offerings. Also millions of emails sent every day to every one with offering via Internet for various registered or not health products. This is a big problem because we are not able to know if these companies registered from an official health or any government organization.

Health related Web sites are now amongst the most frequently accessed sites on the Internet with current estimates indicating that there are now over 100,000 sites offering health related information (Eysenbach G, Sa ER, Diepgen TL. 1999) .

The data gathered from multiple stake holders in the health care delivery process provide relevant feedback on the design of an E-health site used to empower patients as the primary consumers of medical services (Payton F.C.-Lucas H. 2001)

There are four generally accepted types of e-commerce:

- Business to Business (B2B)
- Business to Consumer (B2C)
- Government to Business (G2B)
- Government to Citizen (G2C)

All the above types of the E-Commerce found in the E-Health Service (EHS)

BACKGROUND

The first step of the E-Health commerce began from the world wide affiliations of the international electronic commerce and the Internet population. Public and personal Health was always one of the big problems in the modern people. In to this direction the existed different problems till today with the new character of the public health and the national health systems make individuals to find new directions for their demands. One of these directions is the Internet information resources and e-commerce. Last years the health care industry –a $1 trillion a year market sector – is not, however, largely represented in current e-commerce research.

A recent study sponsored by Cisco Systems estimates that revenue derived solely from E-Commerce increased 127 percent from 1977 to 1998 (Barua, A and A.B. Whinston 1999). This tremendous growth of the E-Commerce can be attributed to a global population and changing demographics of the Internet users that are increasingly accessing the www. (Business Week, 2000) With the creation of the Web in around 1990 by the Englishman Tim Berners-Lee and the Belgian Robert Cailliau working at CERN in Geneva, Switzerland, anything was changed internationally and continues till today very fast giving many applications to individuals world wide especially in the field of personal or public health.

Slowly in the beginning but very fast today continues growing the E-Health commerce with many different offerings, products and applications. There are millions of Internet sites today offering different health products informations and the opportunity for access of an on line commerce in various products. But this is still a not so serious work.

ISSUES

There are various types of services offered from the health companies today through via an Internet connection. In the division of Health commerce there are still many problems existed with the quality and the official recognized products. There only a few officially recognized companies offered certified health products today. Many of these companies registered from official government organizations and have an accredited certificate of quality.

It is very simple today to begin an international e-company which will serve people through the Internet. But this is not that we want. There are many different emails from various Internet companies and individuals that have been sent to over one million of Internet users every one minute with special offers of various health products.

It is important to know if the health company owns an accredited certification of quality and or have been recognized from an official organization.

It is also important to create serious tools to search the informations presented through Internet resources in the Web today.

The aim of such tools is to assist individuals to sift through the mountains of information available so as to be better able to discern valid and reliable messages from those which are misleading or inaccurate (Eysenbach G, Sa ER, Diepgen TL. 1999) There are a lot of different services offered today from many serious Internet Health commerce organizations and companies.

Table 1

About Us (informations for the company)
Making and purchase
Shipping and handling
Delivery schedule
Back orders
Tax charges
Credit card security
Guarantee
Reaching us
Privacy policy
Returns policy

Table 2.

Cialis
Levitra
sildenafil Citrate
Tadalafil
Vardenafil
Viagra
Amino acids
Special formulas
Essential fatty acids
Multi vitamins & minerals
Vitamin supplements
Weight loss
Cleanse & detox
Proteins
Sports nutrition
Skin & hair care
Liquind nutrition
Teeth care
Detox foot pads
Acne treatment
Anti wrinkle cream
Anticandida
Baby skin care
Blisters
Face creams
Hair mineral analysis
Mouth ulcers
Nail Care
Skin rash
Blocked sinuses gymnastics machines
Hygienic products
Animal health
Animal Nutrition
Gymnastic products

In the following Table 1 summarized some of the services from these E-Health companies

About the types of different products offered today from various Internet companies we are able to know that the most usual products today are some of them summarized in the next TABLE 2. There are also many more different products but over 95% of the Internet companies today offer the products summarized in the following list.

Table 2 summarizes some of the products offered on line summarized

Similarly, the health care industry – a $1 trillion a year market sector – is not, however, largely represented in current e-commerce research.(Forester Research 1998) While there are Web sites that sell pharmaceutical drugs and give medical advice, there are limited numbers of market places that allow patients/consumers, employers, physicians, hospital administration and managed care organizations to conduct e-commerce transactions via WWW. (Payton F.C.-Lucas H. 2001)

Health is key to a quality lifestyle and the key to health is not just exercise but exercise on quality health equipments. Equipments that understand the endurance level of individuals and motivate them to achieve fitness Goals-safely.

In a survey of 180 people consisting of 46% females, 86,2% from the United States, median age of the U.S. participants being 29 and 85% of white ethnicity, the forum found that the leading determinant in predicting on-line buying in B2C domain was Product information (*http://ecom.wharton.upenn.edu*) (Bell,S.G.L Lohse and E.J. Johnson 1999) In the left figure given a typical discount offer on line which sent by email. The site offers informations about the name of the drug a picture of this the price and the URL of the official Web site.

Some sites present informations about the use of their products and info about the positives with the accreditation of various scientists collaborated with the company.

Virtual communities with the potential of convergence to B2C market have been designed and implemented to support B2C needs of patients (Timmers P. 1999).

Such convergence has been delivered via home-health networks that include four levels of functionality to patients: (1) Decision Support, (2) Electronic Mail, (3) Bulletin Board on a myriad of Health conditions, such as AIDS/HIV and Alzheimer's and (4) On –line encyclopedia.(Payton F.C. and P.F.Brenman 1999).

The next following advertise which received also by email gives informations about an official accredited organization for a certified on line Pharmacy 100% customer satisfaction as it claims.

TRADE HEALTH ORGANIZATIONS

There are many organizations today offering on line health informations and medical products.

In a special reports Issue of the Wall Street Journal offered an extensive analysis of health care and the future of care delivery. The journal provided a listing of top e-health sites including The New England Journal of Medicine, Mayo Clinic , Medline, Health Gate, Health on the Net, RxList, Health A to Z and the CancerNet etc.(The wall Street journal reports 1998). That is does the site engage in an "economic" transaction that would result in pricing goods and or services which facilitate electronic markets and exchange. (Grover, V. and Ramanlan 1999)

As a result of the wealth of information available and its apparent popularity, a number of organisations have begun to provide specific tools for searching, rating, and grading this information, while others have set up codes of conduct by which site providers can attest to their high quality services (Eysenbach G, Sa ER, Diepgen TL. 1999). Some of the registered trade organizations with a world wide service and quality certifications summarized in Table 3

Let's see what happens today with the quality criteria presented from the organizations?

Table 3.

American Herbal Products Association **http://www.ahpa.org**
Consumer Healthcare Products Association http://www.chpa-info.org
Council for Responsible Nutrition http://www.crnusa.org
Functional Foods for Health **http://www.ag.uiuc.edu/~ffh/ffh.html**
National Nutritional Foods Association http://www.nnfa.org
Natural Products Industry Center http://www.NPICenter.com

The set of quality criteria is based upon a broad consensus among specialists in this field, health authorities, and prospective users. It is now to be expected that national and regional health authorities, relevant professional associations, and private medical Web site owners will present.

1. Implement the Quality Criteria for Health Related Web sites in a manner appropriate to their Web site and consumers
2. Develop information campaigns to educate site developers and citizens about minimum quality standards for health related Web sites
3. Draw on the wide range of health information offered across the European Union and localise such information for the benefit of citizens (translation and cultural adaptation)
4. Exchange information and experience at European and the international level about how quality standards are being implemented. (Payton F.C. and P.F.Brenman 1999)

EDUCATING USERS

There are million of Internet users every day. Many of these users ask the Internet machine about one problem and a lot of them search for medical informations and products.

After contacting Web companies they must be able to choice what is accredited or not.

Individuals must be able to know about the quality certification and the accredited health organizations. We know today that just only a few of the Web users know how to use the accredited Internet informations. In their daily lives as consumers of information delivered via the traditional media, most people learn to use a wide range of assessment tools. Internet is a most useful tool for individuals today in any level of education.

In the world of Internet content, however, it is less evident what the relevant indicators of quality are. It is for this reason that quality marks and user guides have proliferated, namely to educate the consumer and to provide a recognisable "quality" label which site creators may use to promote their sites. This is most important for the future of the Internet. Accordingly, for such codes to be effective it is highly important that the public are informed about the existence of the Codes through public education campaigns.

There is a big problem today with the on line commerce especially in to the field of the medical and the health products. It is very difficult to know which one of the products is an original product and meets the qualities from health organization or from the local medicine organization. Every Internet user it is important to ask if the product is registered as an official laboratory product and meet all the scientific criteria. So it is important to establish criteria of quality medical products to protect different ages of individuals world wide during their e-commerce on line contacts.

Any offered seminars by local government organizations and or non profit medical organizations will help people to their choices. There are many products today, offered with a low cost but we are sure that there also so many products without any quality certification presented through the World Wide Web by e-companies.

Both consumers and businesses participate in naming their own prices for goods and services due to the introduction of e-auctions and e-market places.

Some of the criteria that must meet every Internet commerce user are:

- To ask for quality and high standards certified products
- To ask for simply medical products if he/she does not know if the company is a scientific laboratory or any scientific organization.
- To ask for any of the official product documents and the official guarantee from the company and to know if he pays for the official taxes.
- To search for any informations from various other scientific organizations about the product and to have cross informations about his/her choice.

Some of the key factors that ensure usability (J. Kaminski 2006):

- Ease of learning: Can users intuitively learn how to navigate the site without much effort?
- Efficiency of use: Once they have grasp the layout, can a user accomplish tasks quickly on the site. For instance, do they know where to click to contact you?
- Memorability: On a second or subsequent visit, will a user remember how to navigate the site easily?
- Error frequency and severity: How many errors do users make as they attempt to use the site? How serious are these errors? Is error recovery easy or difficult?
- Subjective satistfaction: How much does the user like using the site? Is it appealing and user-friendly?

The benefits of offering a comprehensive Web site for Health products to the public may include the follow:

- User empowerment
- Service access
- Meet regulations and criteria
- Save money
- Consistent information
- Clear policies and procedures

Any one may contact his personal doctor to take more informations about the product and will receive more scientific info than any other contact. When every information abut the product will be registered then will be able to buy the product with an on line service.

FUTURE TRENDS

The Internet is changing very fast today how people give and receive health information. This is very serious especially in the field of health. People who can use the different Internet health sites and services share a responsibility to help assure the value and integrity of the health Internet by exercising judgment in using sites, products, and services, and by providing meaningful feedback about online health information, products, and services.

Questions regarding security and confidentiality and quality issues are still hampering the development of e-health. National standardization bodies and international agencies should develop common standards, protocols and methodologies to establish criteria for the e-health applications. (Gurjit Kaur, Neena Gupta 2006)

While this work offers specific user-defined requirements in the e-health and e-commerce space, this study has several limitations.

The electronic commerce will continue in the future serving people around the world with a lot of quality products especially in the medical products will offer many new products for self and social health from serious organizations and companies.

E-Commerce will help people especially in the agricultural places or them who live alone without any other family members near them. People in every Nation will have access with the contemporary products and the medical informations by the www. This will make a global family especially in medicine serving people in different places and making a friendship to persons with various Nationalities under the same direction which is the personal and social health. People will have the opportunity to take serious quality and certified informations about health and new products from various e-commerce professional organizations and buy different products.

This will help also the National health promotion and education making more informed people in to the division of the contemporary health products and services. Large fortune 500 companies, such as Cisco Systems and Nortel Networks, have confronted this e-health challenge and the future of Ecommerce in Health (Payton F.C.-Lucas H. 2001). Many accredited organizations will help individuals in to the direction of quality health products today.

The future of the E-Health and the accredited health products is very good but still we have a long time to work in to the quality of health and in to the direction to protect the individuals and any accredited health product because this is the future of health services and applications worldwide..

REFERENCES

Barua, A and A.B. Whinston (1999). *Measuring the Internet Economy.* Center for E-Commerce Research, University of Texas at Austin, October 1999, pp 3.

Bell, S.G.L Lohse and E.J.Johnson (1999). *Predictors of Online Buying Behaviors, Communications of the ACM, 42*(12) December 1999, 32-38.

Business Week (2000). *The E.biz., 25,* May 15 2000, pp 44.

Drougas B. (2003). *Applications of Teleinformatics in Medicine.* ATEI of Epirus 2001.

Eysenbach G, Sa ER, Diepgen TL. (1999) *Cyber medicine.* Interview by Clare.

Forester Research, power ranking for top Consumer Sites (1999). Retrieved November 19, 1999 from http://www.forester.com

Forester Research (1998). *US Online Business Trade According to Forester Research,* Press release. December 17, 1998.

Grover, V. and Ramanlan (1999). Six Myths of Information and Markets: Information Technology Networks, Electronic Commerce and the Battle for Consumer Surplus. *MIS Quarterly 23*(4) December 1999.

Gurjit Kaur , Neena Gupta (2006). *Journal of Evolution and Technology, 15*(1), 23-35

Health and Medicine (1998). *The wall Street journal reports.* October 19, 1998.

Kaminski J. (2006). *Designing high quality health sites.* Retrieved from http://www.bellaonline.com

Koilias H, Kalafatoudis S, Mandila E. (2004). *Introduction in to informatics and the use of the computer. New technologies.* Kleidarithmos Publications Athens.

Lazakidou A., Lazakidou G.(2004). *New Applications and futures in to the information community* p.p 77-88. Kleidarithmos Publications, Athens.

Lazakidou A. Hatzimitsis D. Evaggelou I. (2004) .*Virtual World and New Technologies.* p.p 89-94. Kleidarithmos Publications, Athens.

Payton F.C, Lucas H. (2001). Health Care B2C Electronic Commerce. In *Proceedings of the 34th Hawaii International Conference on System Science,* 2001.

Payton F.C. and Brenman, P.F. (1999). .*How a community health information network is really used, communications of the ACM.* pp 85-89 December 1999

Timmers P (1999) *Electronic commerce Strategies and Models for Business-To-Business*. New York NY: John Willey and Sons, Inc.

KEY TERMS

E-Health Commerce: This is a division of the electronic commerce. This typically uses electronic communications technology of the World Wide Web , to promote the health products and or to serve local or international individuals in the area of the Social or personal health. Frequently depends on computer technologies other than the World Wide Web , such as databases, and e-mail, and on other non-computer technologies, such as transportation for physical goods sold via e-commerce. The basic tool for the E- health commerce is the Internet technologies.

Electronic Commerce: Is exactly analogous to a marketplace on the Internet. Electronic Commerce (also referred to as EC, e-commerce eCommerce or ecommerce) consists primarily of the distributing, buying, selling, marketing and servicing of products or services over electronic systems such as the Internet and other computer networks. The information technology industry might see it as an electronic business application aimed at commercial transactions; in this context, it can involve electronic funds transfer, supply chain management, e-marketing, online marketing, online transaction processing, electronic data interchange (EDI), automated inventory management systems, and automated data collection systems. Electronic commerce typically uses electronic communications technology of the World Wide Web , at some point in the transaction's lifecycle, although of course electronic commerce frequently depends on computer technologies other than the World Wide Web , such as databases, and e-mail, and on other non-computer technologies, such as transportation for physical goods sold via e-commerce.

Web Site: Is a collection of Web pages, images, videos and other digital assets and hosted on a particular domain or sub domain on the World Wide Web.

A Web page is a document, typically written in HTML, that is almost always accessible via HTTP, a protocol that transfers information from the Web site's server to display in the user's Web browser.

All publicly accessible Web sites are seen collectively as constituting the "World Wide Web ".

The pages of Web sites can usually be accessed from a common root URL called the homepage, and usually reside on the same physical server. The URLs of the pages organize them into a hierarchy, although the hyperlinks between them control how the reader perceives the overall structure and how the traffic flows between the different parts of the sites.

World Wide Web (or the "Web "): Is a system of interlinked, hypertext documents that runs over the Internet. With a Web browser, a user views Web pages that may contain text, images, and other multimedia and navigates between them using hyperlinks. The Web was created around 1990 by the Englishman Tim Berners-Lee and the Belgian Robert Cailliau working at CERN in Geneva, Switzerland. Since then, Berners-Lee has played an active role in guiding the development of Web standards (such as the markup languages in which Web pages are composed), and in recent years has advocated his vision of a Semantic Web.

Chapter XIV
Distributed Knowledge Management in Healthcare

Christos Bountis
Oxford Radcliffe Hospitals, UK

ABSTRACT

This chapter introduces and reviews the concept of distributed knowledge management within the Healthcare environment and between Healthcare and other partner organisations. As management should not be mistaken for control, distributed should not be identified with multicentered. Trade-offs between managerial centralism and social contextuality should be allowed. Although the core issues in knowledge management are not technological, tools that can support the central versus social dualism of knowledge management are critical to the effective and appropriate use of generated knowledge. Information tools can significantly affect the user experience and local social wiliness to participation and enhance the managerial trends that make use of knowledge networks and shared logistics. They include service-oriented architectures (SOA), artificial intelligence networks (AIN), multiple agent systems (MAS) and the contextual tools of Web 2.0. All of those tools feed their functionality on the semantic detail, the granularity and the trust levels enjoyed by their information sources.

The Working Nature of Knowledge

How much of an individual's knowledge is really personally developed and independent of its environment? Personal knowledge is guided by and in dynamic balance with other community or organisational knowledge. The definition of knowledge it self points to a higher degree of subjective elaboration of information and data originating in facts, procedures, concepts, interpretations, ideas, observations and judgements (Alavi & Leidner, 1999). We could consider organisations and communities as the subject in the aforementioned statement thought the internalisation and capture of knowledge by an individual relies strictly on cognitive elements, such as perspectives, believes, skills and expertise. Alavi and Leidner identify data and information as being of different nature to knowledge and suggest indeed that "knowledge is information processed in the mind of individuals: it is personalized information (which may not be new, unique, useful or accurate)". Tuomi (Hoffmann, Loser, Walter, & Herrmann, 1999) proposes an inverse hierarchy that requires knowledge to exist before data can be collected and information can be formulated; knowledge does not exist outside of a "knower" and when "articulated, verbalised and structured becomes information which, when assigned a fixed representation and standard interpretation, becomes data". The intercurrent theme in the aforementioned definitions is that all the components of what we commonly call knowledge, including information and data elements, have strong contextual attributes. Knowledge, information or data deprived of their contextuality are inevitably hampered by imprecision and loss of therefore their relevance and trustworthiness is directly dependent on the degree of contextual use.

For an organisation the process of knowledge capture and creation is an expression of formalisation of procedures that are well documented and which are usually crystallised in tandem with factual knowledge in a rather abstract manner. This organisational knowledge product is often generalised and involves some degree of abdication of the fine context from where the original information was obtained. The degree of context tolerance a knowledge base suffers is related to the aimed audience spread and it is proportional to the topic's contextual variability. For example, if for knowledge base we consider an operational manual of a blood gas analyser (devices mostly stationed in high dependency hospital wards), the relevance of the material will be higher to its audience if that manual is specifically written for specialist intensivists instead that when it is written for an audience that includes non specialist doctors and nurses. Similarly the manual will be more relevant if it is just written for a specific type and version of a blood gas analyser device and in the specific context of an adult medical intensive care unit in a specific hospital. In the contrary if the manual is abstracted to include all the types of blood gas analysers in any sort of high dependency unit in the country, its contextuality to machine and environment specifications is compromised and its relevance reduced. The latter type of organisational content abstraction although useful for the purpose of aim acquisition and standard level consolidation in procedures and outcomes it is fairly irrelevant to the end user both in terms of process and factual knowledge. That is why overarching guidelines and protocols are often reproduced and adapted to local applications, in an activity that can be compared to a vertical Delphi cycle. Closing this cycle, from the social stage to the central stage, is only possible by centripetal knowledge collection and comparison techniques, like audits, quality schemes or surveys.

Organisational Knowledge and Distribution

High-level consolidation of organisational knowledge and information is useful to the enterprise and the society. It can offer the basis for auditing, monitoring, comparisons and standardisation. This sort of collective knowledge is social, since sociality is the precondition for something to be a meaning (Bonifacio, Bouquet, & Traverso, 2002). Groups and people continuously negotiate common perspectives of local, contextual knowledge (perspective making) (Boland JR & Teknasi, 1999) and try to understand in each domain how the matter looks like from a different perspective (perspective taking) (Boland JR & Tenkasi, 1999), (also respectively called single and double loop learning (Argyris & Schoen, 1978)). High-level organisational knowledge therefore is a dynamic conglomeration of "local knowledges" in the attempt of the participating groups to share perspective and of the organisation it self to consolidate its knowledge capital.

Simon's (Simon, 1997) work on rationality as well as later managerial theories have confirmed that acquiring information is a financial activity that can be measured. It derives that knowledge management (KM) is a managerial task for every enterprise and that knowledge can be handled as a market good (Daveport). Because both procedural and bounded (factual) knowledge acquisition has a cost and a trade value, enterprises tend to increase the completeness of the offered knowledge and avoid localisms. Then the satisfaction of their target audience (knowledge customers) is pursued by the use of technologies that elaborate the vast repositories of information and externalised knowledge. Such information methods can include indexing and mapping, semantics and representations, search tools and data mining etc. In the other hand, the school of intellectual capital (Stewart, 1997) (Sveiby, 2004) offers a second common objectivist approach, which considers instead knowledge not so much for its potential market value but for its potential redeployment and reuse in similar situations within the enterprise it self. It focuses on how knowledge is a tangible asset that is part of people, structure and context of projects and activities and how that knowledge can be systematically replicated and communicated. In this latter approach knowledge and information is less abstracted and generalised and the greater its reuse the more the generated value. The core tools in this method are those of externalisation and codification, employed in a manner to specifically enhance clustering and similarity retrieval.

Organisational KM can also be seen from a subjectivist approach in line with the context centric general knowledge considerations mentioned before. In this light, March (March, 1991) describes organisational knowledge as mental model groups and the hosting organisations as "garbage cans"; containers of knowledge that attempt to make sense of processes and justify decisions. The context of knowledge in these circumstances is critical as it acts as an internal property of the organisation that is looking to enhance its decision taking both retrospectively and prospectively. Serge (Senge, 1992) and Argyris (Argyris & Schön, 1995) propose that organisational KM systems should capture and manage contextual schemas and structures in tandem with knowledge mental models as these can aid interpretation and encourage communication and sharing. For example, an elective speciality clinic organised by a healthcare unit or the availability of out of hours procedures and the related protocols are closely related to the skill mix at hand at any giving moment. Capturing this context of "skill mix" in association with the factual and procedural knowledge applied of those circumstances produces a transferable view of the care unit, for applicable use in the entire healthcare system. The sociality of knowledge is further enhanced when knowledge is mostly considered in its practical nature. Brown and Larve (Brown & Duguid, 1991) (Lave & Wenger, 1991) suggest that knowledge acquires significance from within group habits and in the context of social practices. The flow of organisational knowledge can then be considered to take place in a similar cyclic manner of externalisation-internalisation flow as the personal knowledge development does.

Nonaka (Nonaka, 1998) unifies the domains of personal and organisational knowledge in the aspect of sociality and proposes a process of explicitation, refinement and crystallisation. That effectively closes the gap between the abstract and social aspect of knowledge as seen in the subjective theories and the reusable, valuable knowledge as seen in the objectivist approaches. At the level of a complex organisational environment this process can easily become cumbersome and inflexible and might run the risk to generate outdated or non-applicable knowledge. Community based approaches of knowledge generation and exploitation seem to be more effective in supporting knowledge workers and complex environments, but they can contrast the central enterprise vision of consolidation and managerial control. On the other hand though, high degree of contextualisation and distribution of knowledge capture can lead to knowledge isolation due to high specificity and therefore to poor communication traits and poor transferability. Bonifacio et al propose a mental platform based on the characteristics of knowledge and its context, to be used when balancing the trade off between centralisation (the stable valuable and controllable environment paradigm) and distribution (the community and tolerant/dynamic paradigm). This platform can be used as means to create a balanced trade-off in KM that can both facilitate the crystallisation of explicit knowledge and the making and sharing of community-distributed knowledge.

The concept of distribution in KM has been widened by many experts to include partners of knowledge exchange (Hoffman, Hoelscher, & Sherif). The potential partners from within an organisational business space have mutual interest in sharing knowledge at an extra organisational level that is pertinent to the domain of business activity. In manufacturing for example, product state models are shared, so engineering and specification data is communicated, together with the manufacturing and logistics workflow information [Chinese top bicycle manufacturer]. In this way different phases of production can take place in a reliable and uninterrupted process, across different production units, across businesses (time and space independence of knowledge creation to knowledge use) (Kühn Pedersen & Holm Larsen, 2000). In the modern example of e-commerce and Internet business, partner knowledge sharing techniques include data feeds, web services, application level interfaces and content provision (Malhotra, 2002). Although the product of Internet business is very often just information, its relevance and its trade value are very dependent on the partner's knowledge sharing input. The generated value return in its turn is divided between the knowledge partners, which in isolation would not have been as successful. Business models that draw on distributed KM platforms promote specialisation, reward quality and usually enhance end user experience since both product generation and delivery opportunities are more flexible and multipartnered. Knowledge sharing between groups and particularly between organisations or enterprises relies on mutual trust, which entails confidentiality. The resulting inherited interdependency also implies mutual risk, that most of the times is not symmetrical. New economies and pure Knowledge-based economies (i.e. biotechnologies, high-tech, software industry) base their profitability and success on speed to market, virtualisation and globalisation (Raich, 2000). This is the era of the ubiquity of information retrieval and therefore of the ubiquity of the customer base. Enterprises need to connect to their customer base with information that is reliable, auditable but also localised and individualised. Information retrieval services like Google Maps for example, that overlays geography and related information, have already discovered the added value and the distinction localised domains of retrieval offer in today's world overwhelmed by competitive information. Knowledge and information service businesses have to shape their process models in manners that allow and offer distributed KM that can identify actuality, sociality, relevance and know-how.

Distributed Knowledge Management in the Health Care Domain

Healthcare is an environment rich with diversity of process and logic. Most of the IT implementations in the healthcare have resulted in systems that locally reflect the existent managerial structures and the legacy elements in use. As a result healthcare IT systems are fragmented, usually due to supplier imposed restrictions, and their configurations are not enhanced by tools of information exchange or other non proprietary expansion capabilities (Kendall 1998)(Medicaid 1999). Local and National Governments have identified the need for overarching communication in Healthcare and initiated projects that could allow effective data integration and common delivery entities (see eEurope 2005 Action Plan3, the Connecting for Health project in the UK and Connecting for Health business initiative in the USA). The core focus of most of these is the implementation of common datasets that can be used in communicating patient data and resource booking. Since homogenisation of focus and contextual abstraction of data takes place when ageing common datasets and "hard" interfaces, process and knowledge that are being included are very often forced to common denominators. IT systems at this scale tend to "factorise" those organisational models, as most of them do not allow structural data flexibility at a distributed level. As architecture of IT systems is an expression of local organisational models, centralism is a constraining force to acceptance, innovation and diversification (Gay, 1998).

Medical knowledge is created, transmitted and obtained very much at a local and practical level. A significant degree of contextuality to local community procedures and resources is needed to allocate actions and integrate information. What do I do with a diabetic patient presenting with consistent haematuria, or with a patient complaining of the worst ever headache (relevant to resource usage and referral policies)? What is the action protocol for a patient having a slightly deteriorated eGFR (estimated expression of renal function) and when is best to prescribe antibiotics in infant ottitis media case (contextual learning and structural knowledge needs)? The answers to these clinical scenarios might be different for the different roles or stakeholders of the healthcare process and depend on both the local process and the national or evidence based recommendations. Having a clinical practice that only complies with the latter guidelines might be unfit to local care pathways. Local level processes tend indeed to get structured on a pragmatic level, that is very similar to classic business paradigms, and reflects resource availability, service demand, local population (market) position and the local business targets. At a level below the care units involved the social interactions, the intentions, the skills and the interests of the members of these units are critical in shaping the departmental policies and the interactions with other units.

Social (contextual) capture of knowledge at a level that is less relevant for the organisation than the care unit level mentioned before are usually not pursued by higher-level management. Central organisational control tends to disregard local factors that produce social and contextual information, through conglomeration and abstraction, since this type of management concentrates into consolidation of processes and statements (perspectives) about activities. Vopel (2003) sustains this position by saying that it is not necessary or indeed relevant to obtain the true right knowledge since knowledge is only an organisational tool to reduce decisional ambiguity and justify actions. This might be a pragmatic desirable in some circumstances and the true core philosophy of public and political opinion stands in phenomena like the postcode lottery complaints in the United Kingdom (the National Health System's different approaches to treatment expenditure in the UK, according to patient residence location, have recently come under criticism that subsequently has lead political decision making). This sort of approach is based in the formalisation and uniformity of healthcare services in a consistent manner at every local level and at such degree that common knowledge systems can be applied. Such tactic although theoretically feasible, in practice is likely to affect job satisfaction and to find local resistance in application, due to a variety of personal and social environment issues.

Knowledge systems are for an organisation like a spoken language: certain standards are required for communication but inflexibility reduces incentive and satisfaction. It has been proven that inflexible systems can negatively affect performance and creativity. That can be translated to improper efficiency in providing local level healthcare or even loss of opportunities relating to service development and medical research. The UK's Human Tissue Act 2004 constrains provide a good example on how central strategy that safeguards common standards can introduce hurdles in practical terms.

The healthcare services are often characterised as a "cottage industry"; one that does not have to oblige to the rigid standardisation and quality levels the manufacturing industry has to comply with when certifying functions or products. Indeed no ISO standards exist for the treatment of tuberculosis or the intervention of an appendicectomy. Instead medical conduct is rather assessed in relation to common practice and performance targets set by a combination of audit outcomes and expert input on minimums and desirables. On a unit level, vertical assessments and social interactions produce adjustments and re-organisation. That of course is not to say that research, medical studies, evidence based practice, other technological advances or any political or overall managerial guideline and directive are not influencing the healthcare practice. The local units consider overall inputs and change practice either as a direct response to those sources of information or in response to changes in practice applied by peer units. There is therefore interaction between centrally introduced knowledge and knowledge from distributed healthcare communities and peer roles. The healthcare environment self organises in a complex space between simple centrally driven organisation and chaotic practice (Jadad 2006). Plseck and Greenhalgh introduce complex adaptive systems as model solution that can deal with the fuzziness of information and circumstances. The conventional managerial thinking of organisation clockwork, thoroughly planned and broken down is unlikely to be of practice in the healthcare industry. In healthcare, organisational goals are dealt in a non-linear manner from distributed actors that might be local managers, doctors or other health professionals. The uncertainty of benefits for the actors, the steep leaning curves, the diversity of skills, the importance of local systems, the nature of ownership, the concurrence of expertise and the importance of original schemas and limits to organisational change have all been blamed for failures in implementation of centrally driven information projects (Southon 1999). The advent of the Internet and the enhancement of information dissemination and social integration via technological tools are pushing the healthcare sector to adopt new practice rules and methods (Plsek 2001). Those tools have multiple effects on all levels of the organisation as well as wider elements like the public, the patients themselves, care partners and the associated industry. A lot of recent activity has focused onto patient centered systems (i.e. FP7 EU funded projects), but systems and organisations always seem to have the upper hand in setting deliverables. Human centered approaches that involve not only the tool-to-human interface but a wider consideration of functionality, system specifications and fundamental processes in a multi centered / distributed manner amongst stakeholders demonstrate the added value that this approach can have in knowledge and schedule intense environments (Rinkus 2005). Core elements of such approach are the human players of the processes that take place, which are often "advocated' by a single tool/computing entity which handles the interfaces to the other partners of the process in a distributed way. The design of such systems is based on reliability and relevance of contextually rich information shared amongst process partners and on the communication ability between partner / source systems.

Distributed KM & Health Care Process Integration

Managing the process of creating local knowledge within autonomous groups and exchange it across them is what we call distributed knowledge management (DKM) (Bonifacio 2002). Although autonomy and heterogeneity are intrinsic characteristics of knowledge creation, shared semantics and declared contextuality can facilitate interoperability, use and dissemination. Traditional conceptualisation of knowledge according to managerial or epistemological approach of centralisation is incompatible with the social and local semantics of knowledge and can drive users away from knowledge management systems that are sterile of context.

Knowledge and information handling sits on the basis of successful distribution and integration of services in the healthcare. The key to usage-enabling setup of knowledge systems is the degree of the fitness of content to the proposed use. And although generating customised and localised knowledge has always been practised extensively, our proliferative and competitive information society requires that two main issues are being addressed: the effective use of the highest level expert or evidence based advice and the successful adaptation of knowledge systems to localised know-how and with integration of appropriate procedural information.

The aim of this chapter is to explore the granularity and requirements that knowledge and the systems that generate it and handle it require so that efficient and flexible use is possible. To better demonstrate the implications and fine ramifications of the way the set up and granularity of knowledge handling systems affect process we will start with a common life scenario.

Scenario 1: A run to the airport. Just ordered your main course at a local bistro. Your simple task in this afternoon is to collect visitors from the nearby international airport, 35km away. They phoned on the same morning confirming their flight schedule is fine. You think that departing in about 45 minutes will provide you with sufficient time to welcome them at the arrival desk.

An extraordinary performance of human brain's data integration capabilities! You have combined your knowledge of the bistro's handling times, info on your car and driving attitudes, info on the route, parking and access to the arrivals location as well as an estimate on your visitors' timeframe from the plane to the exit gate. That is amazing indeed and surely anymore efficient than that would be probably stressful to carry out.

It would also be unlikely you would be enjoying additional assistance in planning this afternoon drive, as you are quite confident in your local environment. But would you like to know of a sudden delay in the flight schedule or a traffic jam on the motorway?

Some time later you have the similar task of getting your flight home from a distant ultra-modern place. Your new task assistant device says that you have plenty of time to enjoy your luxurious vanilla ice mountain dessert. Tap on that and you will see that is has structured, categorised and calculated a series of elements presented in classes with weighted probabilities attached to them. On top it says: overall likelihood 96%, sources validity grade 1A. Not only it has detected your voice order at the café, as an order was expected by your sensed presence at the location, but it has also interrogated the kitchen about the preparation time, taken into account the description of the order as to the time needed for an enjoyable consumption, checked with your rented vehicle about your usual driving attitudes for the type of the road, requested the amount of luggage in the trunk, and the petrol and tyre status. It has also verified with your GPS navigator distances, traffic info sourced from the live motorway control, weather conditions and predictions originated both from the weather service source and reviewed locally and it has double-checked with the emergency services for any actual or predicted anomalies. Obviously the latest info on your plane's schedule and traffic control has been incorporated. Average times for airplane preparation for your airline and expected waiting times have been accounted for. It is also alerting your rental service at the airport with a live estimate time of your arrival and it will check you and your language into the flight before your arrival so boarding passes and bag identifiers can be provided at your arrival at the rental station. Security control knows of your arrival so a short walk from the car to the exit gate provides all the necessary time for biometric scans to take place. Your chosen magazine is expecting you at the waiting lounge and your favourite drink will be served once sited in the plane!

Not far from utopia, you would think or perhaps not? This exiting scenario is based solely on the employment of existing technologies. The only assumption is that live integration of data and services is provided, allowed and accepted. Information services like the GPS Navigator, the Café's ordering system and the traffic and weather service make use of a complex and extensive series of data capture elements that can provide the integrative device with enough input for knowledge generation: the task assistant saying that "you have plenty of time". This is appropriate, contextual and at the same time uses a flexible statement so to increase acceptance (tap the clock icon and you will get the entire task algorithm breakdown).

It is likely that you'll desire to use the task assistant even at home where more routine trips are made. Indeed it works like a sensorial extension of your existing mental processes and it could significantly increase quality and effectiveness for your tasks. If need be, its overall integration could be bypassed and information sources used in isolation. Nevertheless though, it could be seen either as an enhancement or a threat to your commonsense intelligence. Management science has proven that at an organisational level the coordination of multiple commonsense, empirical practices is less effective in average than the coordination of formalised practices, which are calibrated and interrelated in synchronisation []. The level of effectiveness though usually archived using the latter approach is limited from the introduction of buffer elements (i.e. over- or under-booking resources) aimed to allocate flexibility to systems programmed at a high abstract level. At the personal level, an aiding system is more accepted when it is unobtrusive, flexible, and reliable and either adds significant capabilities or it improves quality of life (i.e.: the mobile phone paradigm).

In the aforementioned scenario the task assistant is not only improving your travel experience but is also assisting effectiveness and coordination of the car rental service, the airport services, the airline and even possibly of the road management systems and Café's order prioritisation algorithm. The bidirectional information exchange that takes place can allow those remote stakeholders of your travel to generate procedural knowledge themselves though their own task assistant integration. So the car rental service can plan the handling of the incoming vehicle, the boarding desk can focus on the missing passengers, the traffic control can allocate a runway slot and so on. We will refer to this higher level 'knowledge task assistant" entities as KIM, Knowledge Integrator Modules. The Information Feed Services (IFS) like the weather service or the traffic control are agglomerations of captured data and they are being used to provide intelligence information to the KIMs under specific conditions. The conditional use of the IFS by the KIM should be mostly based on simple logical rules that can be both programmed on a higher level and that can be understood by the KIM's user. The IFS are integral to complex systems of information provision and utilisation that run between computing units. Some of those units are just there to facilitate computation and communication (middleware) and some directly represent the interests of the involved KIMs. The cornerstone trait of these computing units is their autonomy to perform functions that might be diverse for the same unit depending on the task assignments. That is based on their ability to comprehend machine contextual language. Other than autonomy and the associated sociality necessary to archive understanding of their environment, those computational units should ideally be equipped with elements of reactiveness and proactiveness. In the trip to the airport scenario the task assistant KIM proactively interacts with the café and the airport facilities and successfully reacts to conditions of traffic, weather or car status.

Many programming languages and techniques have been applied to the creation of unit networks of these qualities: Boolean logic cascades, object-oriented architectures, data mining techniques crawling and meta-searching, advanced service oriented architectures (SOA), artificial intelligence networks (AIN) and multiple agent systems (MAS). AIN and MAS are the ones that satisfy most of the desirable criteria described previously. MAS is simpler to explain and program though its behaviour might not the more predictable of the two. Excessive training of the AIN system might make it inflexible to change and heavily weighted to predefined answers.

The airport run is an analogous task to an instance of an episode of care though the health system. Intentions, targets, KIMs, information sources, organisational constrains and outcomes are involved. But if the airport run scenario is hard to visualise as possible, a similar KIM based process in the Health Care sector is even harder. How difficult is to imagine that your Family Doctor proactively will inform you that with your next repeat prescription waiting for you at the supermarket's till it has included some anti-malaric medication for the eventual prophylaxis you might want to use before your trip to India in 2 weeks time (information links and source of data sharing also notified). Or that after your accident at the pitch, an x-ray slot has been timed to your arrival to the Trauma Unit (coordination of your GPS phone with the local A&E) and that you will not be asked three times the same demographic and allergy questions while being in terrific pain. Or even that during your hospital stay, your medication, care management and diagnostics have been coordinated to avoid any misfit and have used the best possible expert evidence and service coordination for your own benefit. Ironically imagination might not the only problem here, as those procedural flows will seem naturally pragmatic to lay peoples minds and rather expected.

Berners-Lee et al in their visionary paper in 2002 (Berners-Lee 2002) on Web 2.0 and the semantic technologies also use the particularly suited environment of healthcare with all its social and financial ramifications for a realistic use case scenario. For processes to work properly on a local contextual level, a volume of automated machine reasoning based on semantic communications and contextual understanding is necessary. Ontological [openGalen] and semantic vocabularies [MedWeb] as well as intelligent multidimensional clustering [UMLS, LoINC] have been employed to assist indexing, auditing and machine communications. Empowering the machine interactions are inference rules that are embedded in ontology systems (concept associations: is part, has, belongs) in tandem with any additional expression formatting. In parallel, broadcasting of electronic services and with their self-descriptions and performance data will allow effective service discovery so functions can be carried out with maximum effectiveness and minimum input. Providing structure and semantic context to resources makes them transparent more readily usable and can transform them into a business service. For example defining indications, scope and reference performance of pathology diagnostic services within the complicated healthcare domain can allow "value chain" requests for services and produce outcomes in a human centered fashion (requester-black box interaction, i.e. the user can use pathology services without specifically knowing of their existence). That provides the basis for both the healthcare user and the pathology service to focus in their core activity, the care of the patient and the provision of analysis respectively. Using machine reasoning can mean in this case that specific additional data relating to either the patient healthcare provision or to information required for appropriate provision of analysis can be exchanged at any stage of the request-report cycle without the need of human involvement (box-to-box interaction). Nevertheless the process can be human assisted or supervised on either side. If all the necessary procedures are put in place for the proper transit of specimens and communication of results, pathology investigations at this point become location independent. Successful cases of geographical expansion of private pathology services have indeed demonstrated that in healthcare economies of scale can be archived when organisations distribute their knowledge management. Such organisations do successfully operate in geographical spans of thousands of miles across (see the Australian "IBISWorld Australia Pathology Services Industry Market Research Report" or United States examples of Pathology providers market). These pathology providers guarantee the service terms while the location where the investigation takes place might even be concealed on unimportant to the requester.

If the product of healthcare is the provision of service to the patient, the aforementioned healthcare service model matches closely the industrial product model where the product state specifications are exchanged across businesses. Investigation-location independence is in wide use particularly for specialised or uncommon investigations. However, outside the private domain examples already mentioned, today the procedural knowledge (which investigation to send where) mostly resides in user groups or in listing portals where pathology service offerings are collected (see www.AssayFinder.com or www.EuroGenTest.org). Thus, the lack of self-descriptive models reduces the opportunity for expanded use and automation in investigation use and communication (see the issues that any Lab-to-Lab project has encountered). Implementing DKM to this exemplar domain within healthcare will bring structure and machine understanding of procedural knowledge. That in turn allows communication and sharing of information with resources rich in structural knowledge, which in turn can function as indication and interpretation pointers to investigations (i.e. LabTestsOnline initiatives and local KM projects like Oxford's Pathology eLABook). With knowledge exchange and contextuality declarations, services can be discovered, duplication can be avoided and resources can be saved. The coupling between the physical world subjects and objects and the machine understanding of the process (the human to box interactions) is done with the use of Universal Resource Identifiers (URIs). URIs, when extended to the physical world, produce clarity of process and tactile understanding of actions and aims to the human actors. Such processes, coupled with elements of automation and proactive acknowledgement do make the difference in process outcomes that are otherwise too complicated or too trivial to be performed accurately on a high target level (Staves 2007).

The DKM Granularity Dilemma

How much is enough and how much is too much? When this question is about knowledge granularity the answer is not easy and it does depend significantly on many system factors. Granularity is a property of knowledge classification and refers to the amount of refinement of its codification and of its attached semantics. Knowledge granularity can be seen 1) at a document level, that is documents with little information attached on the content other than the title and the container folder information (as in the case of paper documents and many document sharing portals now common); 2) at a document level but with additional descriptive elements to aid classification and discovery (as in scientific papers key terms, web pages header keywords and light semantic web content); 3) at sentence/paragraph/concept level, where semantics are either attached to the entry or the entry is placed in fixed semantically declared fields (as in rich semantic web projects or in database driven knowledge portals and system tools, ie Electronic Patient Records); 4) at an ontological semantic level that allows contextuality and meaning at any applicable part of the content (some wiki projects, social network knowledge & web 2.0 & 3.0, folksonolomy). Because granularity completeness is often related to user input, granularity can be both a threat and an opportunity for an information project. Granular context and semantics completeness require a progressive amount of effort the more advanced is the level of granularity required. That can constitute a significant hurdle for isolated projects with broad scope that rely on human input for their contextual completeness. Consider as an example the completion of a knowledge base for internal procedural operations in a Laboratory Unit. If we are building the resource from the ground up and we intend to include contextuality and semantics up to level 3 or 4 the effort required will be very significant. If other resources both within the Unit (i.e. semantic registers of materials and locations, etc) and from other similar laboratory units (i.e. contextualised structural knowledge on materials, feeds of standard procedures, etc) where available, the amount of effort requi red would be considerably reduced. The more social exchange and semantic information is available the easier is to complete the knowledge base. If the self-description of resources is to the degree of machine understanding, computing units can then complete (or assist the completion) of the procedural protocols. Providing machine meaning to the protocols can extend their use as sources of information for the management of materials and specimens and as service feeds to other services or to partner business units. For example, analytical material could be shared amongst laboratories within the same organisation and combined workload and procedural protocols feeds can allow automation when scheduling time on analytical platforms that are common. Also, laboratory units that accept referred specimens can permit a feed for discovery of the services they wish to provide. Similarly, other laboratory units can enhance their own offering of knowledge services by borrowing from the available feeds bounded and procedural knowledge with or without local contextual elements. The federation and self-discovery that will take place in this descriptive environment will create a dynamic self-assessed social marketplace for that type of service (see the eBay® paradigm). Different actors, roles and organisations will federate, balance and present their knowledge selection in their own particular manner (Bountis 2002).

Fine granularity semantics become easier the more resources are available. A critical mass of semantic resources within the same domain can set the scene for information tools to start interacting semi or completely automatically to accommodate process and produce information (as seen in scenario 1). Information services can be used in relation to their relevance and trust scores, enhancing so the social and interactive nature of knowledge. Trust is a highly social phenomenon, but computing units can handle trust indexes much more efficiently. In the other hand much is dependent on the characteristics of the system in use. Systems should self capture but also incite users to capture contextuality as a first step to traceability and organisational memory: i.e. who accompanied the patient to the investigation room, which instrument was used and by whom when an X-ray is done; what are the other contents of the cupboard where the drugs are kept, what was the staff health condition at the day this patient got admitted, who has the right to see what patient data, what services patients trust and when are they available, etc.

Computer Agents and Other Technologies

As already said, the structure of knowledge does not predict its function and the limitations in distributing knowledge management are not technological but organisational. In a wider sense how the resources are communicated and how the machine reasoning takes place is of little importance to the end user. The organisational and social change issues lie in understanding the knowledge externalisation and the contribution each actor of the system has. Nevertheless, sufficient granularity, appropriate context capture and easy-to-use experience can only be achieved with the use of systems architectures that can demonstrate properties of 1) autonomy of process, 2) tolerance of heterogeneity, 3) reusability of unit, 4) coordination between units and 5) that possess problem solving abilities. Sociality is a central feature of such architectures and comes in the form of negotiation, aggregation, discovery, declaration and initiative. Classic object-oriented (OO) architectures are able to satisfy a relative degree of autonomy, heterogeneity and reusability but are not able to sustain the complex social function required. The more modern semantic web services do possess some elements of sociality (like discovery, invocation, composition and monitoring) and can enhance the functions of OO systems. AI also demonstrates most of the needed elements and can indeed be successfully used in DKM. Its role though is rather partial because of limited sociality traits and issues like acquired inflexibility after repetitive task exposure. In many projects involving decision support in healthcare tasks AI has been used successfully either on it own or in concomitance with other logic systems. In the recent years the engineering paradigm for DKM systems is based on MAS. Healthcare in particular has a high degree of heterogeneity and many interdependencies. Heterogeneous agents systems constituted of autonomous agents and their groups enjoy of all the required properties of proactivity, autonomy and problem solving.

Agent technology is a computing field in rapid evolution. For agent is indeed intended a computing unit that satisfies the aforementioned property criteria, but its language model or constitutional elements are not strictly defined. The base technologies for current MAS are a series of established architectures and standards: Extensible Markup Language (XML), Resource Description Format (RDF), Web Srvices (SOAP, UDDI, WSDL) peer-to-peer computing, pervasive computing, service oriented computing, distributed object technologies, and others. Architecturally MAS use schemas related to semantic content communication and other specifically developed to aid agent system applications: web ontology language for services (OWL-S), web service modelling ontology (WSMO), agent-oriented software engineering, CommonKADS & DÉCOR methods. Transitional methods for the passage from the organisational to social and then to agent implementation models have also been devised (van Elst 2003).

Scenario 2: Poor growth with tummy problems. It only became obvious after his third birthday that Luke was poorly developing. Before that, his performance on the growth chart was just below average and that was mostly blamed to his poor appetite. His father worried as he was punched in his heath assistant KIM some additional details on Luke including signs of appetite, food intake and behaviour towards food. Luke was rather a low energy kid but with spells or erratic behaviour. Shortly after their General Practitioners' KIM was requesting permission to inform the doctor of the new status. When tapping the info button the screen relates to strong family history evidence of paediatric onset endocrine disease with similar manifestations. The history info reports data collection from the last three generations and across distant family members (many not in contact or even known to Luke's parents). The GP's KIM also suggested some additional details and an action plan. Luke could be seen after an overnight fast by the Paediatric Endocrinologist in a nearby hospital 45 miles away, on the morning after. The family accepted the invitation and choose the next day slot instead of a wait of three days for the local specialist slot. They kept reading the relative info pointed out by the GP's KIM as well as insights from other parents that found themselves in similar instances. They knew they should not prelude anything, as the probability of the inherited disease calculated for Luke was only 15%. They were though very worried since a diagnosis was not in place and some differential possibilities grave.

Luke had several diagnostic testing, including ultrasound, done the next morning. Some were performed in the clinic and other specimens where sent elsewhere. 24 hours later, coeliac disease (intolerance to gluten) in association with early stages of diabetes type I was diagnosed. In the afternoon the family was counselled on Luke's dietetic and supplement requirements. A care pathway that will lead to islet cell transplantation was applied. His parents accepted the plan and their healthcare KIM was updated with new targets, schedules and lead sources. A skin sensor will now monitor his sugar levels at frequent intervals and pass on readings to the family's health care assistant. The monitoring of his sugars, hypoglycaemic treatment and advice of his diet will now be a collective effort with feedback from the GP and the local paediatrician, all put together as needed and according to role taken with the help of their assistants. The family's KIM will coordinate and will assist in the selection of food via radio frequency identifiers in the products purchased. When out to a restaurant or friends the KIM proactively will again aid the selection of nutrients free of gluten.

In this scenario the social acceptance of the computer aid system is in place with high levels of confidence, trust and reputation. The system is seen rather as an alternative way to communicate with other humans (GP) or organisations (secondary care) or even machines (booking system, food RDIF). The system is dynamic and serves to integrate information before offering feedback. The linear guidance towards an action plan in a world of information overload is a parallelism of the knowledge system to the navigator example given in scenario 1. Once again also this scenario is technologically feasible and the mojor issues to be resolved are social and organisational. The knowledge integrator module (KIM) concept mostly behaves as a higher-level computer agent of the properties mentioned before.

Industrial and commercial models have already demonstrated the potential of such approaches. In healthcare examples of MAS systems are found in medical pharmacy systems , community care, patient scheduling, decision aid. Successful examples of agent based DKM in healthcare include finance administration systems, organ transplant systems assistance location and remote assistance systems (Moreno 2003).

Many European funded projects (EDAMOK, FRODO, KnowMore, Edutella, GroupLens, Let's Browse, etc) that have looked into DKM for business application purposes can well serve as lessons learnt and examples for the healthcare domain. The healthcare market is opening up to new opportunities, created by biomedical and information technology advances. Centralism does not seem to benefit the interests of the complex organisations and the relations that are required. DKM in healthcare should be stimulated and healthcare system designers should allow for this social dimension of knowledge to tap into their resources. DKM system applications should consider all the possible view points and stakeholders of the process, including patients, healthcare professionals, healthcare providers and policy makers.

Knowledge technologies together with nanotechnology are the next big technological revolutions waiting to happen. They will advance in a variable pace in dependence to proposed commercial applications and social acceptance. It is unlikely that few killer applications will produce a critical mass for extended use, but they will induce the needed social behavioural brewing. The success of knowledge technologies will heavily depend in the degree of machine understanding of the content, the context and the interoperability with other constitutional computing units. Although some issues will be dealt by programmatic brute force others will only be tackled by unit adaptation and the Universal Plug and Play concept. Healthcare with its size and importance can lead the distributed knowledge service market of the future for the benefit of the industry and its customers.

REFERENCES

Alavi, M., & Leidner, D. (1999). Knowledge Management Systems: Emerging Views and Practices from the Field. *Proceedings of the Thirty-second Annual Hawaii International Conference on System Sciences-Volume 7 - Volume 7*, 7009.

Argyris, C., & Schoen, D. (1978). *Organization learning: A theory of action research.* Reading, MA: Addision-Wesley.

Argyris, C., & Schön, D. A. (1995). Organizational Learning II: Theory. *Method and Practice (Reading, MA: Addison-Wesley).*

Berners-Lee T, Hendler J, Lassila O. The semantic web. *Scientific American*. April 2002.

Boland JR, R., & Teknasi, R. (1999). Perspective making and perspective taking in communities of knowing. *Shaping Organization Form: Communication, Connection, and Community.*

Bonifacio, M., Bouquet, P., & Traverso, P. (2002). Enabling distributed knowledge management. managerial and technological implications. *Novatica and Informatik/Informatique*, *3*, 23-29.

Bountis C, Kay J. An integrated knowledge management system for the clinical laboratories: an initial application of an architectural model. Health data in the Information Society. In *Proceedings of MIE 2002. IOS Press.* Amsterdam 2002; 562-567

Brown, J. S., & Duguid, P. (1991). Organizational learning and communities of practice. *Organization Science*, *2*, 40-57.

Daveport, T. *H, and Prusak, L Working Knowledge: How Organizations Manage What They Know.* Boston. MA: Harvard Business School Press.

van Elst L, Dignum V, Abecker A. (2003). Towards agent-mediated knowledge management. *Agent-Mediated Knowledge Management: International Symposium AMKM 2003.* Stanford, CA, USA, March 24-26, revised and invited papers.

Gay, E. G. (1998). A State's use of the electronic medical record: a means to address Arkansas' health care responsibilities to her children-promoting access to cost-effective care. *International Journal of Technology Management*, *15*, 458-469.

Hoffman, J. J., Hoelscher, M. L., & Sherif, K. *Social capital, knowledge management, and sustained superior performance.*

Hoffmann, M., Loser, K., Walter, T., & Herrmann, T. (1999). A design process for embedding knowledge management in everyday work. *Proceedings of the international ACM SIGGROUP conference on Supporting group work*, 296-305.

Jadad A, Enkin M, Glouberman S, Stern A. (2006). Are virtual communities good for our health? *BMJ, 32*(7547).

IBISWorld Australia Pathology Services Industry Market Research Report. Retrieved January 10, 2008, from http://www.ibisworld.com.au/industry/retail.aspx?indid=615&chid=1

DB Kendall, SR Levine. Perspective: Pursuing The Promise Of An Information-Age Health Care System. Health Affairs, USA 1998

Kühn Pedersen, M., & Holm Larsen, M. (2000). Inter-Organizational Systems and Distributed Knowledge Management in Electronic Commerce. *Proceedings of IRIS, 23.*

Lave, J., & Wenger, E. (1991). Situated Learning: Legitimate Peripheral Participation (Learning in Doing: Social, Cognitive and Computational Perspectives). *Cambridge University.*

Malhotra, Y. (2002). A Case for Knowledge Management: Rethinking management for the New world of Uncertainty and Risk. *BRINT Institute.*

March, J. G. (1991). How Decisions Happen in Organizations. *Human-Computer Interaction, 6,* 95-117.

Moreno A. (March 31 - April 1, 2003). Medical Applications of MultiAgent Systems. Workshop: Intelligent and Adaptive Systems in Medicine. Prague.

Nonaka, I. (1998). The Knowledge-Creating Company. *The Economic Impact of Knowledge.*

Plsek P., Greenhalgh T. (2001). Complexity science. *BMJ 323,* 625-628, .

Raich, M. *Human Capital and Knowldge Management In the New Economy.* Retrieved from http://www.raich.net/

Rinkus S., Waljia M., Johnson-Throop K. A., Malin J., Turley J., Smith J., Zhang J. (2005). Human-centered design of a distributed knowledge management system. *Journal of Biomedical Informatics, 38*(1),4-17

Senge, P. (1992). *The fifth discipline: The Art and practice of the learning organization.* London, Century Business.

Simon, H. A. (1997). *Models of Bounded Rationality.* MIT Press.

Southon G, Sauer C, Dampney K. (1999). Lessons from a failed information systems initiative: issues for complex organisations. *International Journal of Medical Informatics, 55*(1), Pages 33-46.

Staves J., Davies A., Kay J., Pearson O., Johnson T, Murphy M. F. (2007). Electronic remote blood issue: a combination of remote blood issue with a system for end-to-end electronic control of transfusion to provide a "total solution" for a safe and timely hospital blood transfusion service. *Transfusion,* 2007 Dec

Stewart, T. A. (1997). *Intellectual capital: the new wealth of organizations.* New York, NY, USA: Doubleday.

Sveiby, K. E. (2004). *Methods for measuring intangible assets.* Retrieved from http://www.sveiby. com/articles/IntangibleMethods. htm

Vopel, O. Knowledge as resource and problem: the case of knowledge-intensive firms. In *Proceedings of I-KNOW'03.* Graz, Austria, July 2-4, 2003, 2003.

KEY TERMS

Computer Agents: A program that performs some information gathering or processing task in the background. Typically, an agent is given a very small and well-defined task. Although the theory behind agents has been around for some time, agents have become more prominent with the growth of the Internet. Many companies now sell software that enables you to configure an agent to search the Internet for certain types of information.

Contextual Knowledge: Knowledge in context, information, and/or skills that have particular meaning because of the conditions that form part of their description.

Distributed Knowledge Management System (DKMS): A DKMS is a system that manages the integration of distributed objects into a functioning whole producing, maintaining, and enhancing a business knowledge base. A business knowledge base is the set of data, validated models, meta-models, and software used for manipulating these, pertaining to the enterprise, produced either by using a DKMS, or imported from other sources upon creation of a DKMS. A DKMS, in this view, requires a knowledge base to begin operation. But it enhances its own knowledge base with the passage of time because it is a self-correcting system, subject to testing against experience. The DKMS must not only manage data, but all of the objects, object models, process models, use case models, object interaction models, and dynamic models, used to process data and to interpret it to produce a business knowledge base.

Organisational Knowledge: The capability, which members of an organization developed, to draw distinctions in the process of carrying out their work, in particular concrete contexts, by enacting sets of generalisations whose application depends on historically evolved collective understanding.

Section IV
Wireless Telemedicine and Communications Technologies in Healthcare

Chapter XV
An Analysis of a Successful Emergency Telemedicine Venture

Jelena Vucetic
Alpha Mission, Inc., USA

ABSTRACT

This paper describes business and technological challenges and solutions for a successful emergency telemedicine venture called MediComm. Its objective is to provide a new generation of integrated information and communication systems, targeting medical and emergency care organizations. This system enables multi-directional transfer of information (including voice, data, fax, video) between the organization's central information system and its mobile fleet of ambulance vehicles. MediComm enables emergency care personnel to take a patient's vital measurements and personal information in an ambulance on the way to the hospital, send the information to the hospital, and receive from the hospital directions for the patient's treatment during transportation. When the patient arrives into the hospital, his/her information will be already updated in the information system, and the medical personnel will be ready to provide the necessary care immediately. Thus, time will be saved, which for many patients is of critical importance. The treatment of patients will be more effective and simplified, which will result in substantially lower cost of medical care.

INTRODUCTION

With advances in information systems, telecommunications, Web applications and medical equipment, ***telemedicine*** (providing health care service remotely) has become very popular in the last decade. Current telemedicine applications include: teleradiology, prison telemedicine, telecardiology, and telehome health care (Brown, 1995). However, emergency care has not extensively benefited from the advances in telemedicine and the underlying technology.

The demand for ***emergency telemedicine*** has been created by the following factors:

- The time and place of health emergencies are unpredictable, while they typically require immediate medical intervention. Here are several examples:
    - **Cardiac arrest:** Among patients older than 55, who die from cardiac arrest, 91% do so outside of the hospital (Kyriacou, 2003). In order to save the patient's life, the "Call to Needle" time (from the emergency call for help, until the help is provided) should be less than an hour. A 12-lead ECG during the patient's transportation to the hospital increases the available time to perform a thrombolytic therapy effectively. Potentially, mortality can be reduced by 48% if treatment is received within an hour of onset of symptoms (Keeling, 2003). The benefits diminish thereafter.
    - **Car accidents:** According to (Kyriacou, 2003), approximately 77% of fatal injuries in accidents happen far away from any competent health care institution, which results in long response times. The mortality of injured is very high (66%) during the first 24 hours. However, the mortality can be reduced by earlier medical intervention, starting as soon as the patient is admitted to the emergency vehicle on the way to a hospital.
    - **Stroke:** Morbidity and disability due to a stroke can be significantly reduced if appropriate thrombolytic therapy is given within a "golden" 3-hour period of symptom onset. Currently, only 3% of candidate patients receive thrombolytic therapy due to missing the therapeutic window (Gagliano, 1998).
- Insufficient number of intensivists (specialists in emergency/intensive health care) — Currently, there are less than 10,000 intensivists in the U.S., while 35,000 to 40,000 are needed (Wiebusch, 2001). Less than 15% of intensive care units (ICU) have dedicated intensivists on staff (COMPACCS, 2000).
- Telemedicine may provide a way of stretching the expertise of existing intensivists in the future. Using emergency telemedicine systems, death rates can be reduced by 68% and health complications – by 50% (Gagliano, 1998).

Currently, when an emergency team transports a patient in a critical condition to a hospital or emergency center, only a basic health care is provided to the patient in the emergency vehicle. The majority of measurements of vital functions (biosignals) and administrative procedures are taken after the patient arrives to the hospital, not in the vehicle during transportation. For many patients, reducing the waiting time for emergency care may make a difference between life and death. For health insurance organizations, it may provide a substantial reduction in medical expenses.

Logical objectives resulting from the current situation follow:

- Reduce mortality and health risk to patients by improving quality of emergency health care in terms of: a) reduced waiting time for emergency health care; b) immediate access to remote specialists; c) improved convenience of transportation to the medical facility
- Organize medical and administrative staff in a more efficient and effective way
- Reduce health care costs

Major Challenges for Emergency Telemedicine

Numerous challenges have accompanied initiatives to introduce emergency telemedicine in daily operations of health care organizations:

- **Lack of reimbursement:** has been a major obstacle to wider use of emergency telemedicine. Only radiology and interpretation of some transmitted medical test results (e.g. ECG, EEG, and echocardiograms) receive full reimbursement from Medicare. So far, only 15 states in the US reimburse for telemedicine services under Medicaid.
- **State licensure laws provide barriers for telemedicine services across state lines:** Doctors licensed in one state may not be allowed to provide medical help remotely, to patients located in another state.
- **Malpractice liability issues:** Emergency cases typically involve high risk of mortality or health complications. Due to the very litigious environment, many doctors have been reluctant to pursue a career where, in addition to the inherent medical risk, they need to deal with an additional risk related to an innovative, relatively unproven technology.
- **Physicians' reluctance to telemedicine:** Due to fear of losing patients, requirements to change their practice patterns, discomfort with the technology, as well as lack of reimbursement, telemedicine has not been very popular among doctors.
- **Confidentiality and privacy issues (HIPAA compliance:** In addition to existing requirements for HIPAA compliance (Wachter, 2001) imposed on health care organizations, emergency telemedicine introduces privacy and security challenges related to out-of-the-network patients (with or without existing electronic health records). Also, wireless communications environment increases risks of intrusion to and disclosure of patients' private information.
- **Inadequate information structure:** Establishing a universal electronic healthcare record (EHR) and automation of processes are among most critical efforts in modern healthcare industry. The EHR incorporates all provider records of encounters where the patient has received medical care (Upham, 2004), including the medical history, operational and financial data. While there is general industry consensus that an EHR is essential for healthcare advancement and effectiveness, a standardized EHR has not been defined yet. Consequently, healthcare information systems are largely diverse and not standardized, which represents a significant challenge for their integration and automation of processes across different organizations.
- **Technical issues:** Broadband wireless technologies have been advancing in the last decade, with the third generation (3G) mobile communications standards promising to provide a wide range of services, from voice to high-rate data (up to 2.048 Mbps). In 2001, Japanese carrier DoCoMo launched the first 3G service with streaming video at 384 Kbps. In the US, there are three incompatible standards (cdma2000, WCDMA and global W-CDMA) with maximum rates of only 384 Kbps (effectively – around 56Kbps). 2G networks are still used for voice, while video streaming is relatively slow and of poor quality. Designers of 3G networks have identified high interference levels, high collision rates and low data rates as major challenges. While 3G technology has not fully transitioned from its field-trials phase to a full commercial deployment, a new (4G) technology has been announced with promises to provide data rates of up to 100Mbps and new services. An alternative technology, WiMAX, was announced in 2004 by Intel

Co. which has launched a new, wireless broadband chip for long-distance (up to 30 miles), high-speed Internet streaming data and voice with speeds of up to 75 Mbps. According to Intel Co. (2004), WiMAX is superior to CDMA in performance, high quality of data service, high spectrum efficiency, and lower future equipment costs. While WCDMA has advantage for voice service, WiMAX offers more benefits for data applications.

Previous Work

So far, several emergency telemedicine projects have produced a very valuable insight into potential benefits from this relatively new discipline.

For example, ***EMERGENCY-112*** (Kyriacou, 2003) is a European project for handling emergency cases in ambulances, rural health centers or ships by using a mobile telemedicine unit at the emergency site and a base unit at the hospital-expert's site. This system allows transmission of a patient's vital biosignals and still images, but no video. The transmission is performed through GSM (9600 bps up to 43200 bps) or satellite (2400 bps up to 64000 bps) links, which represents a limitation for the system that should be able to transfer:

- The ECG and SpO2 or Co2 waveforms as continuous signals - ECG data are sampled at a rate of 200 samples/sec by 10 bits/sample or 12 bits/sample, which generates 2000 bits/sec or 2400 bits/sec, respectively, for one ECG channel. SpO2 and Co2 waveforms are sampled at a rate of 100 samples/sec by 10 bit/sample, which generates 1000 bits/sec for one channel.
- Trends for SpO2, HR, NIBP, BP, Temp and monitor data - These trends are updated once per second, which generates approximately up to 200 bits/sec.
- Still images with a 320 × 240 pixel resolution, JPEG-compressed, resulting in approximately 5–6 KB data/image.

Through its field trials, EMERGENCY-112 project has provided a significant knowledge base and emphasized still-existing technological and operational challenges, such as:

- An average time to establish the connection between the emergency unit and the hospital was relatively long (28 seconds).
- 10 images per test were successfully transmitted. The average transmission time for several image files was from 18 to 26 seconds. The first-time image transmission success rate was 93%, while the rest 7% had to be retransmitted due to a line failure.
- The first-time transmission success rate for a single ECG lead was 85%, while the rest 15% had to be retransmitted due to one or more interruptions of the connection.

Another ***pilot project based in Maryland*** (Gagliano, 1998) was focused on development of a system that enables transfer of video images, audio, and biosignals captured in a moving ambulance over a digital wireless telephone system to a hospital. The information was reviewed in real-time by intensivists at their office workstations. This project was primarily focusing on early treatment and monitoring of stroke patients. While it has provided very encouraging results, it has also revealed existing challenges:

- Due to the limited wireless bandwidth (20 Kbps), the images were transmitted in "slow scan" fashion at about 1 image every 2.5 seconds with resolution of 320 pixels x 240 lines x 24-bits. The technology enables two modes as a tradeoff between motion handling and resolution. The ambulance staff can select either high-resolution still images sent in a store-and-forward fashion, or low-

resolution images/video sent in almost real-time. Using LEO satellite communications or wideband terrestrial wireless system that provides several Mbps transmission rate would ensure a better quality of real-time video transmission
- The system was based on the Windows 95 operating system, which was not very stable in a mobile environment. With more advanced versions of the operating system, these problems should be eliminated.

Proposed Solution

The proposed system (MediComm) enables transfer of information (including voice, data, fax, video) between a medical organization's central information system and its mobile fleet of ambulance vehicles (Vucetic, 2003). MediComm enables emergency care personnel to take vital measurements (biosignals) and personal information from the patient in an ambulance on the way to the hospital, send the information to the hospital, and receive directions from the doctor on call regarding the patient's treatment during the transportation. When the patient arrives into the hospital, all his/her information is already updated in the information system, and the medical personnel is ready to provide the necessary care immediately.

MediComm's system requirements include:

- Reliable, secure, high-quality multimedia communications between the medical center and each emergency vehicle in its fleet
- Reliable, secure, high-quality multimedia communications among emergency vehicles in the fleet
- Variety of applications: online voice (VoIP), video and data collaboration, email, access to the center's information system (to upload the patient's personal and insurance data to the information system, and to download the patient's health history to the emergency vehicle and the doctor on call), online presentations, Web surfing, etc.
- Videoconferencing reliability - Each videoconferencing call connects the first time and stays connected, even under adverse network conditions.
- Fast, accurate, comprehensive patient data available to all authorized participants
- Integration of the MediComm system with existing health care and insurance information systems (Ability to easily share data)
- Information backup in each emergency vehicle
- Integration of the MediComm system with medical measurement, monitoring and diagnostic devices in emergency vehicles

The proposed MediComm solution primarily relies on the advances in the following technologies (Vucetic, 2003):

- **Third-Generation Wireless (Terrestrial and Satellite) Technologies:** These technologies are coming on strong largely due to federal deregulation and the opening of the 900 MHz spread-spectrum bandwidth that has facilitated wireless medical applications in the home, clinics, and for trauma care (between emergency vehicles in the field and physicians in the emergency center). In addition, a new spectrum in the GHz domain has also become available.
- **Internet and Web Applications:** The integration of personal digital assistants (PDAs) with next-generation medical instruments and tools over the Internet will increase centralized computing or thin-client network applications for medicine. In addition, Internet and World Wide Web have enabled worldwide reach and compatibility of telemedicine applications.
- **Digital Signal Processing (DSP):** Advances in DSP and encryption techniques ensure improved quality, security and accuracy of the transferred information.

- **Integrated Information Systems:** Advances in database technologies and applications enable integration of emergency telemedicine systems with traditional health and insurance information systems, as well as integration of electronic patient records, diagnostic images, measurements and other clinical data in the electronic form.

Figure 1 (Vucetic, 2003) represents an emergency telemedicine system configuration that includes a major hospital, a local medical center, an intensivist on call, and an emergency vehicle.

The following functional units are located in the major hospital:

- **Medical Equipment (ME):** Major hospitals provide the most comprehensive set of expertise and relevant medical equipment to support emergency and critical care, surgery, anesthesia, and neonatal care.
- **Central Information System (CIS):** The existing information system that is currently being used by hospitals, emergency centers and other health care providers.
- **Local Area Network (LAN):** Combined voice, text, graphics and video transfers may vary from 1 MB to 100 MB. In a large hospital configuration, a 100BASE-T Ethernet is recommended to ensure net data rates of up to 10 MBps.
- **Servers/Firewall (SRV/FW):** Supporting the network infrastructure, Internet, email hosting, file sharing, Web services, information security, load balancing, clustering, CIS interface and applications, messaging/groupware, applications requiring high performance, extensive I/O, and a high memory throughput.
- **Workstations (WS):** General-purpose computers, such as a 3.60GHz 1MB L3 Cache Intel Pentium 4, with Windows XP Pro operating system
- **T-3 line (43 Mbps):** For multimedia communications between the hospital and the local medical center (Norris, 2002)
- **Fixed Multimedia Device (FMD):** used for high-speed, wireless communication between the medical personnel in emergency centers and hospitals, and mobile ambulance fleets, in order to transfer the patient information to the center during transportation. WiMAX protocol is recommended to ensure data rates of up to 75 Mbps (Upham, 2004).

Similar functional units can be found in the local medical center, with the following differences:

- **Medical Equipment (ME):** May not contain all elements that are provided in a major hospital. For example, only a basic Intensive Care Unit (ICU) may be provided, where for more complex medical procedures the patient needs to be transferred to the major hospital.
- **Local Area Network (LAN):** A 10BASE-T or a 100BASE-T Ethernet is recommended assuming combined voice, text, graphics and video data transfer among a smaller number of workstations than in a major hospital. This LAN would ensure net data rates between 1 and 10 MBps (Bez, 2005).
- **Local Information System (LIS):** Integrated with the CIS in the major hospital.

The following functional units should be located in an emergency vehicle:

- **Mobile Multimedia Device (MMD):** The MMD integrates end-user devices that collect various kinds of biosignals, with a workstation (e.g. a general purpose computer, such as a 2.13 GHz Intel Pentium M 770 PC, with Windows XP Pro operating system), and a digital camera. Ideally, the camera should have 640 x 480 resolution (at least 320 x 240 x 24-bit resolution, in a JPEG format, 30% compressed) (Burgiss, 2004). The minimum size of image files should be between 2 and 12 KBytes. The following biosignals should be continuously measured on the patient: ECG (200 samples/second, 12 bits/sample), Oxygen Saturation (100 samples/second, 10 bits/sample), Heart Rate (HR), Non-Invasive Blood Pressure (NIBP), Invasive Blood Pressure (IP), Temperature (T), and Respiration (R).

a. *Server/Firewall (FW)*, supporting the network infrastructure, web applications, information security, remote locations, workgroup email, workgroup applications, file and print.
b. *Wireless Communications Subsystem (WCS)* – The WCS provides connection of the emergency vehicle with an emergency center or a hospital. The minimum data rate should be 384 Kbps, using WiMAX protocol.

An intensivist on call should have in his/her office:

- **Workstation (WS):** A general-purpose computer, such as a 3.60GHz 1MB L3 Cache Intel Pentium 4, with Windows XP or Vista Pro operating system
- **Server/Firewall (SRV/FW):** Supporting the network infrastructure, web applications, information security, remote locations, workgroup email, workgroup applications, file and print.
- **T-1 or a fractional T-1line:** For multimedia communications with the hospital or an emergency center. A full T-1 line (1.54

Figure 1. MediComm System Solution

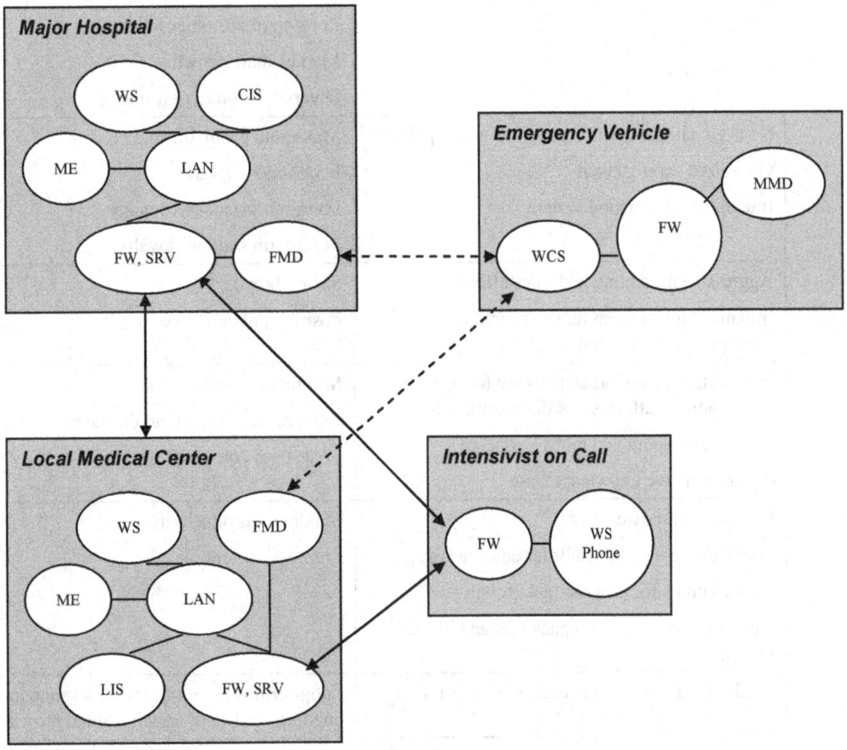

Mbps) would be recommended, as a leased line dedicated 24 hours a day. However, due to the cost constraints, a ½ T-1 (768Kbps) or a ¼ T-1 (384 Kbps) may be an acceptable alternative. Full T-1 and ½ T-1 lines enable transfer of high quality video images with 640 x 480 resolution. ¼ T-1 lines may provide acceptable still images with 640 x 480 resolution. However, the quality of motion video is compromised due to the lower bandwidth (Bez, 2005).

New Venture Management

MediComm is a new venture, requiring a highly competent and dedicated team. It includes:

- Top management with clearly defined vision, mission and strategy
- Middle management with strong project management, technological and communications skills
- Competent and motivated professional team members with strong commitment to the team and project responsibilities

Table 1 represents management strategies and objectives relevant to the success of the MediComm venture:

Cost-Benefit Analysis: For any new venture, a comprehensive cost-benefit analysis should be done in order to determine whether the venture should be pursued or not, based on the estimated Return-On-Investment (ROI) over its lifecycle.

Table 1.

Strategies	Objectives
Customer focus Establish strong relationships with customers High responsiveness Product quality Differentiation	Customer satisfaction High-quality system solutions that meet customer needs Long-term customer loyalty Market share growth Diversification to new markets
Strategic alliances with customers and suppliers Optimized supply chain Integrated information system	Maximum profitability Economies of scale Long-term customer loyalty Long-term supplier loyalty
Aggressive marketing and sales efforts Initiatives for the community benefit and environmental protection	Strong brand Positive public image
Use of state-of-the-art technology for the MediComm platforms and development tools Highly competent and motivated team Comprehensive knowledge base	Minimum time-to-market Capture maximum market share Long-term competitive edge
Employee empowerment Profit-and-loss responsibilities and rewards plan Opportunities for professional growth Attractive compensation packages and hiring incentives	Maximum productivity Employee retention
Establish strong relationships with investors	Long-term sources of funding to support ongoing R&D and organizational growth

Table 2.

Venture Stage	Top Management	Marketing	R & D	Operations	Sales	Administration	Deliverables
Market survey and analysis (8 weeks)	Strategic guidance, venture approval and support	Generate customer need, research current solutions and competitors	Generate technology and identify COTS platforms, technical concept evaluation	Generate process concepts, evaluate cost and feasibility	Create customer relations, pricing models	Financing, preliminary hiring of new team members, pricing, payroll, accounting	Product and process concept selected, specifications and Business Plan prepared
Product design, review and revision (7 weeks)	Approve Business Plan, form MediComm venture team	Validate performance specifications	Technical design, review and revision(s)	Preliminary process design	Gets customers feedback on specifications, pricing and field trial contracts	Financing, hiring, pricing, contracts, payroll, accounting	Venture team formed, product and process designed
Prototype development (15 days)	Authorize prototype development	Conduct market testing	Build prototype	Build process prototype	Gets customers feedback on specifications, pricing and field trial contracts	Financing, hiring, contracts, payroll, accounting	Product and process prototypes completed
Lab testing and revision (15 days)	Authorize testing	Conduct market testing	Technical prototype testing	Process testing	Field trial contracts, preliminary sales orders	Financing, hiring, contracts, payroll, accounting	Product and process tests completed
Pilot production and testing (15 days)	Authorize final design and pilot production	Finalize market plans, conduct test marketing	Final design	Final process design, pilot production and testing	Field trial contracts, preliminary sales orders	Financing, hiring, contracts, payroll, accounting	MediComm product and process ready for commercial launch
Field trials and customer feedback (4 weeks)	Authorize product launch and monitoring	Execute marketing plans and monitoring	Engineering services	Start to ramp-up to full production	Field trial contracts, preliminary sales orders	Financing, hiring, contracts, payroll, accounting	MediComm field trials with initial customers
Revision (2 weeks)	Review customer feedback and proposed revisions	Execute marketing plans and monitoring	Engineering services	Ramp-up to full production	Field trial contracts, preliminary sales orders	Financing, hiring, contracts, payroll, accounting	MediComm finalization based on customer feedback
Full production and testing (3 weeks)	Authorize full production	Execute marketing plans and monitoring	Reduced engineering services	Full production	Execute sales plans	Financing, hiring, contracts, payroll, accounting	Meet initial commercial objectives
Installation and customer training (20 days)	Identify new opportunities, monitor implementation of the Business Plan	Execute marketing plans and monitoring	Reduced engineering services	Full production	Execute sales plans	Financing, hiring, contracts, payroll, accounting	Meet initial commercial objectives
Customer support	Identify new opportunities, monitor implementation of the Business Plan	Identify new opportunities and customers	Reassignment to new projects	Full production	Execute sales plans	Financing, hiring, contracts, payroll, accounting	Meet initial commercial objectives and secure new opportunities

Table 2 presents functional responsibilities, a high-level schedule and deliverables for the MediComm venture (Maheu, 2001). Based on a more detailed schedule, work breakdown structure and required resources, non-recurring and recurring costs have been estimated for the whole lifecycle of the venture.

Non-recurring costs (Vucetic, 2003) are related to:

- Marketing research and specification of the system requirements
- Promotional efforts and brand strengthening
- System analysis and design (identification of off-the-shelf platforms, configuration management, application design)
- Application development (software design, development and testing)
- System integration and installation
- Lab (Alpha)-testing and modifications
- Field (Beta)-testing and modifications
- Financing activities (finding and securing the "seed" and first-round capital to support the non-recurring efforts before the sales are realized)
- Regular MediComm upgrades (design, development and testing of new system releases and applications)
- Administrative, legal and regulatory activities (human resources, intellectual property, certifications, licenses)

Recurring costs are related to the support of operations throughout the MediComm venture lifecycle:

- Purchasing off-the-shelf platforms
- Configuration management
- Installation and testing
- Customer training
- Customer support
- Sales and marketing activities
- Second-round financing activities (finding and securing capital for mass MediComm offering)

Profitability, long-term growth and competitive advantage are general ***financial benefits*** that any venture should provide. Therefore, the total market size, the annual growth rate of the market, as well as the market share that MediComm is expected to capture have been determined.

- The estimate of the total market size is based on a market survey that determined the overall number of emergency health care organizations (N), and an average number of emergency vehicles per organization (V). The total market size (M, in dollars) can be estimated as:

$$M = N \times V \times P$$

Where P denotes an average MediComm unit price in dollars.

- The estimate of the annual growth rate of the market is extrapolated from the average population growth rate, and the growth rate of emergency service organizations.
- The estimate of the MediComm market share (S) captured over its lifecycle of 4-5 years takes into consideration that a patent protection and the leadership in the market provide a level of exclusivity for a certain period of time. During this time, MediComm's market share is expected to grow with increased marketing and sales efforts in various market segments. However, after this period of time, new market entrants are expected to find their ways around MediComm patents and introduce their own alternative system solutions, thus causing a decline of the market share.
- Annual MediComm revenues are projected by multiplying the total market size (M)

with the market share (S) that MediComm is expected to capture. Starting from the market launch and for each subsequent year throughout MediComm's lifecycle, repeat the calculation using the total market size based on the projected growth for the year, the corresponding estimate of the MediComm market share, and the MediComm unit price.

FUTURE TRENDS

Future emergency telemedicine solutions will rely on advances in multimedia applications and transmission, as well as on the increased quality, reliability and security of information transfer. The following success factors are critical for wider acceptance and support of emergency telemedicine:

- Support by the major stakeholders (financial, organizational, government and regulators)
- Ability to integrate and share patient information across diverse, authorized health care organizations
- Improved wireless videoconferencing reliability
- High-quality data resolution
- Higher transmission rate (based on a wider bandwidth availability)
- Security and privacy
- Coverage of wider geographic areas
- Integration of emergency telemedicine with other medical disciplines

MediComm is initially positioned as a scalable telemedicine system, targeting emergency centers, ambulance, hospitals and other health care institutions with mobile fleets (e.g. helicopters, boats). The next step will be to explore expansion opportunities, such as (Vucetic, 2003):

- **Global Expansion:** This move involves customization of the initial system solution for various foreign markets (e.g. customization of the procedures, translation into the local language). This move is risky as any other international venture due to the insufficient information about foreign market needs. If we decide to implement this move, it would be necessary to establish a form of international business alliance with local partner(s) in each target country.
- **Expansion into different emergency and military organizations (DeMeis, 2002):** With new applications based on the initial system solution – This strategic move involves substantial risk because it includes both product and market diversification. We should undertake this move only if the previous ones do not provide sufficient profits over the long time period. In such a case, we should reevaluate why the previous moves have not met our expectations and whether we should make a radical change in our marketing approach.
- **Expansion into telepresence surgery:** Telepresence surgery is a technique by which a surgery may be conducted at one center while the expert (or a panel of doctors) is physically located at a remote location and yet is able to effectively guide, or consult with the surgeons who are actually performing the surgery. So far, telepresence surgery has been done by telebridging, where satellite communications are used to provide audio and video link in real time between two earth points almost exclusively. Such links are rather dependable and the results have been quite spectacular. For MediComm, a strategic move into telepresence surgery means radical modification of the initial system solution, and therefore involves
- **Expansion into telerobotics:** For MediComm venture, this would be the riskiest strategic move. Telerobotics surgery is a

technique where the main surgeon is physically located somewhere else but is able to operate on a patient using a telerobotic arm. Each one of the surgeon's movements performed at his/her geographic location are captured with the help of various sensors, and transferred (telemetered) across a telebridge to be accurately duplicated by robotic arms located by the patient. High-resolution video cameras precisely record and transmit in real time pictures of the operating area to the surgeon. He/she views the patient and all that he is doing, on the television screen or a computer display.

CONCLUSION

This paper presents technological and business challenges and solutions for an emergency telemedicine system that supports a wide variety of applications, including streaming video. So far, due to the limited wireless data rate (based on 2G and 2.5G standards), high-quality, high-reliability video streaming has not been possible. However, with recent advances in 3G wireless technologies (WiMAX, in particular), mobile multimedia applications have become a reality. The proposed MediComm solution announces a new generation of emergency telemedicine systems, which will hopefully become accepted by a wider healthcare industry (Costlow, 2004), including the homeland security and disaster recovery services. With more or less modified applications, MediComm may find numerous applications in other businesses that include mobile fleets, as well as in various international markets.

REFERENCES

Norris, A.C., (2002). *Essentials of telemedicine and Telecare*. Wiley.

Brown, N., (1995). *History of telemedicine, TIE*. Retrieved from http://tie.telemed.org/telemed101/topics/telemedicine_history.asp

Kyriacou, E. et al., (2003). Multi-purpose healthcare telemedicine systems with mobile communication link support, Biomed Eng Online. Retrieved from http://www.pubmedcentral.gov/articlerender.fcgi?tool=pmcentrez&artid=153497

Keeling, P. et al., (2003). Safety and feasibility of prehospital thrombolysis carried out by paramedics. *BMJ Publishing Group Ltd., 327*(7405): 27–28.

Gagliano, D., (1998). Wireless Ambulance Telemedicine May Lessen Stroke Morbidity. *Telemedicine Today,* 1998, *6*(1), 21.

Wiebusch, B., (2001), Telemedicine reduces mortality rate. *Design News*. Retrieved from http://www.designnews.com/article/CA83189.html?text=telemedicine.

COMPACCS Study (2000). *JAMA*, pp 284:2762.

Wachter, G., (2001). Implications of HIPAA's Privacy Rule For Telemedicine, TIE, http://tie.telemed.org/legal/issues/hippa2001.asp

Upham, R., (2004). The electronic health record: Will it become a reality?, Phoenix Health Systems, http://www.hipaadvisory.com/action/ehealth/EHR-reality.htm

Intel Co., (2004). Understanding WiMAX and 3G for portable/mobile broadband wireless. *White Paper* (305150-001US).

Vucetic, J., (2003). Telemedicine – the future of wireless internet applications. Invited Speaker, *Southeast US Wireless Symposium*. Winston-Salem, NC.

Bez, A., (2005). *Emergency medicine*. Retrieved from http://telehealth.hrsa.gov/pubs/tech/ems.htm

Maheu, M., Allen, A., Whitten, P., (2001). *Ehealth, telemedicine, and telehealth : A guide to startup and success.* Jossey-Bass.

Sam Burgiss, Rob Sprang, Joe Tracy, (2004). *Telehealth technology guidelines*. Retrieved from http://telehealth.hrsa.gov/pubs/tech/tech-home.htm

Costlow, D., (2004), Telehealth companies poised for market growth. *Design News*. Retrieved from http://www.designnews.com/article/CA404920.html?text=telemedicine

DeMeis, R., (2002), Hospitals to go. *Design News*. Retrieved from http://www.designnews.com/article/CA217944.html?text=telemedicine

KEY TERMS

Broadband Internet: A high data transmission rate Internet access, which ensures at least 200 kbit/s in one direction according to the FCC standard.

Digital Signal Processing (DSP): The processing of various kinds of signals by digital means. A signal is a stream of information representing anything from stock prices, radio or satellite transmissions, medical measurements to environmental measurements from remote sensors.

Electronic Healthcare Record (EHR): A record that incorporates all provider records of encounters where the patient has received medical care including the medical history, operational and financial data.

Emergency Telemedicine: Delivery of emergency medical services at a distance using advanced telecommunications, robotic and computer technology and their applications.

Health Insurance Portability and Accountability Act (HIPAA): A US law designed to provide privacy standards to protect patients' medical records and other health information provided to health plans, doctors, hospitals and other health care providers. Developed by the Department of Health and Human Services, these new standards provide patients with access to their medical records and more control over how their personal health information is used and disclosed.

Intensivist: A physician who specializes in the care of critically ill patients, usually in an intensive care unit (ICU).

Non-Recurring Costs: Costs that occur on a one-time basis, and are unlikely to occur again in the normal course of business. Non-recurring costs include: capital expenditures, unusual charges, design, development and investment costs, various kinds of losses, legal costs, and moving expenses.

Recurring Costs: Costs resulting from the ongoing, regular business operations, normal maintenance, and anticipated repair or replacement of components, systems or subsystems.

Telesurgery: Surgical procedures carried out at a distance using advanced telecommunications, robotic and computer technology and their applications.

Telerobotics Surgery: A technique where the main surgeon is physically located somewhere else but is able to operate on a patient using a telerobotic arm, while monitoring on a computer display the progress of the surgery.

Chapter XVI
Reconfigurable Embedded Medical Systems

Tammara Massey
University of California, USA

Foad Dabiri
University of California, USA

Roozbeh Jafari
University of Texas

Hyduke Noshadi
University of California, USA

Philip Brisk
Ecole Polytechnique Federale de Lausanne, Switzerland

Majid Sarrafzadeh
University of California, USA

ABSTRACT

This chapter introduces reconfigurable design techniques for light-weight medical systems. The research presented in this chapter demonstrates how the wise use of reconfiguration in small embedded systems is an approach that is beneficial in heterogeneous medical systems. By shrewdly designing embedded systems, one can make efficient use of limited resources through efficient and effective reconfiguration schemes that balance the tradeoffs between power consumption, memory consumption, and interoperability in heterogeneous environments. Furthermore, several reconfigurable architectures and algorithms presented in this chapter will assist researchers in designing efficient embedded systems that can be reconfigured after deployment, which is an essential feature in embedded medical systems.

INTRODUCTION

Moore's Law has allowed processor performance to double approximately every 18 months due to continuous breakthroughs in transistor technology. Although processor performance is paramount to high-performance computing, the world of embedded systems has other priorities: namely the minimization of power and silicon area. Moreover, embedded systems are specialized systems that often communicate via wireless networks with limited bandwidth and have limited communication and memory resources. The shrewd design of embedded systems, however, can make efficient use of limited resources through efficient reconfiguration schemes that balance the tradeoffs between power consumption, memory consumption, and interoperability in heterogeneous environments. Several of these projects are discussed here in the context of a reconfigurable fabric—literally, a wearable motherboard—as well as several customizable medical devices. Adaptive algorithms for communication throttling in response to dynamic environmental changes are also described. Lastly, we highlight the need to reprogram embedded systems following an extended period of time already employed in their respective environments. The architectures and algorithms presented demonstrate how well designed embedded systems can benefit from reconfigurability.

Moore's Law

In 1965 Gordon E. Moore, then R&D director at Fairchild Semiconductor, quantified the astounding growth of the new technology of semiconductors. Moore predicted that manufacturers would double the density of components per integrated circuit at approximately regular intervals (18 months), and would continue to do so until the molecular limits of silicon technology could be reached. This prediction—*Moore's Law*—has held steady for the past 40 years, although the semiconductor industry is beginning to reach the limits of what is physically achievable with silicon. Moore's Law, as applied to various processor families introduced by Intel (Schaller, 1999) is shown in Figure 1.

Figure 1. Number of transistors in Intel microprocessors almost has been doubled every two years.

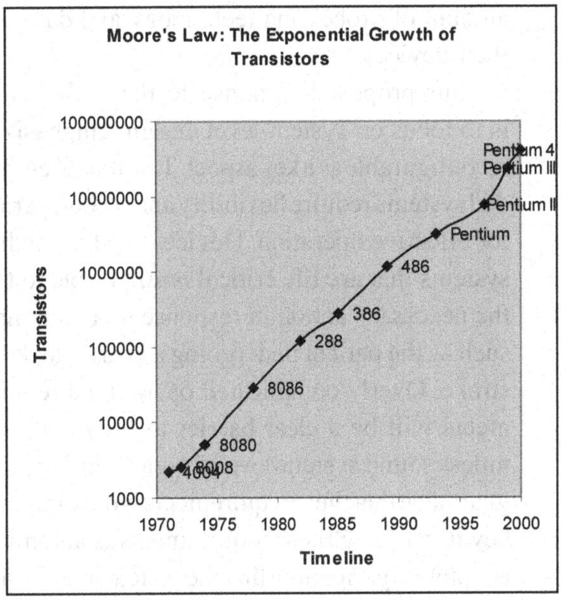

Until the past decade, circuit designers were afforded the luxury of neglecting the electrical performs of wires and metal interconnections beyond a cursory accounting of their parasitic capacitance. Effectively, they were able to increase transistor channel width to provide larger drive currents, thereby increasing transistor-level circuit performance. Unfortunately, transistors have shrunk to a point where interconnect latency and energy dissipation dominate overall transistor performance. On the other hand, wire and interconnect size is shrinking, effectively reaching its physical limit. Clearly, a wire cannot be narrower than an electron; and due to the effects of electro-migration, a significant number of electrons are dissipated during basic microelectronic communication. In short, the physical limits alluded to in Moore's Law are encroaching quickly, and embedded system designers must respond with new ways to pack an increasing amount of processing technology and data onto their devices.

Our proposed response to these challenges is to focus on system-level design, emphasizing reconfigurable as a key aspect. Traditional embedded systems require flexibility and reconfigurable for effective operation. Devices used in medical systems that are life critical *must* be able to take the necessary action in response to an anomaly, such as the patient undergoing a heart attack or a stroke. Overly complicated operational requirements will be a clear barrier to their adoption, unless sound system-level design techniques can guarantee that these requirements will be met. The key to meeting these requirements is automated adaptability, meaning that the system must be able to reconfigure itself in response the environment. Unfortunately, dynamic reconfiguration itself is non-negligible in terms of both performance and power consumption. Moreover, all reconfiguration in excess of changing a depleted battery places too much of a burden on the user, and will not be competitive economically.

Historically, the term *reconfigurable* in computer science has referred specifically to the *Field Programmable Gate Array (FPGA)*, a hardware platform that can implement any logic function. In terms of performance, area, and power consumption, the FPGA cannot compete with an *Application-specific Integrated Circuit (ASIC)*; however, it has other advantages. One advantage is the ability to reprogram the hardware design once a device is deployed in the field. Another advantage is that a system designer can simply purchase an FPGA without having to fabricate a custom circuit design; this is particularly important for device vendors who have relatively low volumes. In the context of this chapter, reconfiguration may include FPGAs, but does not require them.

Three different levels of reconfigurability are explored in this chapter. *Hardware reconfigurability*, for example, could refer to an FPGA or a hybrid system which includes an FPGA along with non-reconfigurable components. Hardware reconfigurability could also include the inclusion of new sensors to a system without having to reprogram it. *Software reconfigurability* is an approach whereby algorithms adapt to the environment and make the best possible use of the resources that are available; what makes this different from traditional operating systems research on preemptive scheduling. For example, hardware resources, process mix, and real-time requirements can all change arbitrarily. Lastly, *wireless reprogrammability* allows the system to be updated via a wireless network once it has been deployed in the field. This is particularly important for implantable medical devices, where any form of non-wireless reprogrammability implies an expensive surgical procedure; moreover packaging issues may render it impossible to reprogram the system by any other means.

Our preliminary work on reconfigurable systems employed hardware-based solutions, and was similar in principle to an FPGA with dedicated ASIC-like IP blocks called *Versatile Programmable Blocks (VPBs)* (Ogrenci et al, 2001a). Automated techniques were developed to generate and select an ideal set of VPBs for an application and to map the application onto the system (Ogrenci et al., 2001b) (Kastner et al., 2001). Integrating VPBs within an FPGA-like reconfigurable fabric minimizes reconfiguration time since the VPBs themselves are not reconfigured. On-chip memory blocks are also available for data storage, and the programmable interconnect provides an interface between the SPBs and other reconfigurable resources. However, the reconfiguration overhead was still quite high because of the cost of reprogramming hardware. Based on this experience, our more recent research efforts have focused on software-based reconfigurable architectures with reduced the (re)configuration and synthesis times.

Medical Motherboard

The term "motherboard" used in computer engineering reflects the idea of a platform that usually contains circuitry for at least one processor, interfaces to "plug in" peripherals such as a monitor and keyboard, and slots for accepting additional devices, such as network cards, sound cards, and video cards. Several different bus systems provide a communication interface among these various devices. In recent years, this term has become common in the commercial world of high-performance and desktop computing. In contrast, in the world of embedded systems, *Multiprocessor System-on-a-Chip (MPSoC)*, has provided the functionality that one would expect from a motherboard. MPSoC has various components that are connected via a *Network-on-a-Chip (NoC)* (Benini & DeMicheli, 2002) where the NOC itself provides similar functionality as a motherboard.

Our current research, in contrast, focuses on the development of a *Medical Motherboard*, which is much more closely related to the original motherboard paradigm rather than MPSoC/NoC. A medical motherboard is a platform that connects sensors to a collection of relatively small, low-powered processing units *(motes)*, and is intended for use in medical embedded systems. The medical motherboard is inherently reconfigurable because it automatically detects sensors as they are added and a lightweight software layer allows the system to adapt to the new sensors. Our work proposes a new architecture that will further reduce reconfiguration time. By fixing the number and communication structure between motes, the system remains flexible with respect to the inclusion of new sensors, but effectively minimizes the time required to reconfigure the system. At the same time, the system architecture is designed to tolerate the failure of one (or more) motes and/or potential loss of communication links between the motes. Our work also demonstrates how the wise use of reconfigurability in small embedded systems is an approach that is beneficial in heterogeneous medical systems.

RECONFIGURABILITY IN HARDWARE

The *plug-and-play (PnP)* paradigm allows the addition of new peripheral without manual installation of additional software. Although it was originally proposed for desktop operating systems such as Windows, PnP effectively describes what needs to take place for an embedded medical device to automatically adapt to the addition (or removal) of sensors during runtime.

CustoMed (Customizable Medical Devices)

CustoMed (Customizable Medical Devices) is a novel, fully-wearable architecture that reduces the customization and reconfiguration time for lightweight embedded systems. The most important component of CustoMed is the *Med Nodes* (Figure 2a), which are stand-alone components consisting of a processing unit, external sensor boards and a battery. Med Nodes support various types of sensors for physiological reading from the human body, including pressure sensors, piezoelectric sensors, accelerometers, and flex sensors. As such, they are effective building blocks that can be assembled to create a flexible system whose fixed basic structure allows quick reconfiguration. Moreover, the system is scalable and can easily support quick reconfiguration of a large number of Med Nodes (Jafari et. al, 2005b).

The primary role of the Med Nodes is to gather and transmit data. As discussed in the following paragraph, Med Nodes include a small mote for storage, but generally do not use it for complex processing tasks. Instead, processing is performed by a *portable base station*, such as a Pocket PC or a cellular phone. The Med Nodes gather data, which is then transmitted to the base station for

Figure 2. The CustoMed architecture (a) Med Nodes with flex and pressure sensors (b) components of CustoMed system deployed on a patient (c) an on-body terminal using med nodes.

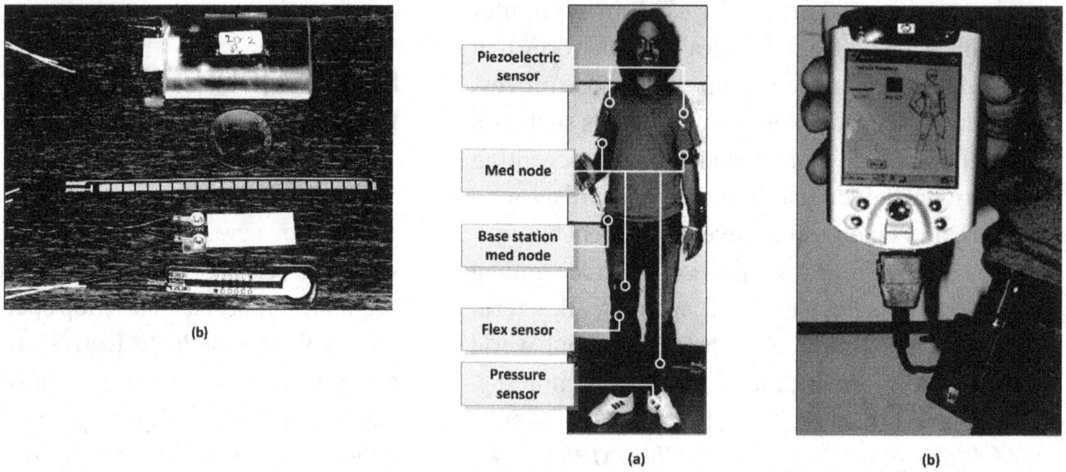

visualization and other processing through a wired network (Figure 2bc). Each Med Node currently uses a Mica2Dot or Mica2 mote, developed by Xbow, for storage. These motes have multiple interfaces that can support both wired and wireless communication as well as UART and I2C communication. The primary role of the motes in a Med Node is to aggregate data, which is then forwarded to the base station for processing. They can be reconfigured or programmed wireless to adaptively modify system specifications.

Using this architecture, a real-time monitoring system for human physiological and physical behavior was built for neurological applications (Jafari et al., 2006b). Wearable Med Nodes in Figure 3 quantitatively gauge the range and degree of motion in stroke patients during rehabilitation for physical therapy. Researchers also prototyped and evaluated a wireless, *in vivo* MEMS sensor for continuous measurement of the myotatic stretch reflex in traumatic brain injuries (LeMoyne et al, 2005).

RFAB – Reconfigurable Fabric

Recent research has explored the prototyping of advanced wearable platforms based on electronic textiles (DeVaal et al., 2003) (Marculescu, Mar-

Figure 3. The CustoMed architecture applied to a neurological applications (a) hand grip to quantitatively determine the range of motion of patients (b) interface to give doctors and patients feedback during rehabilitation.

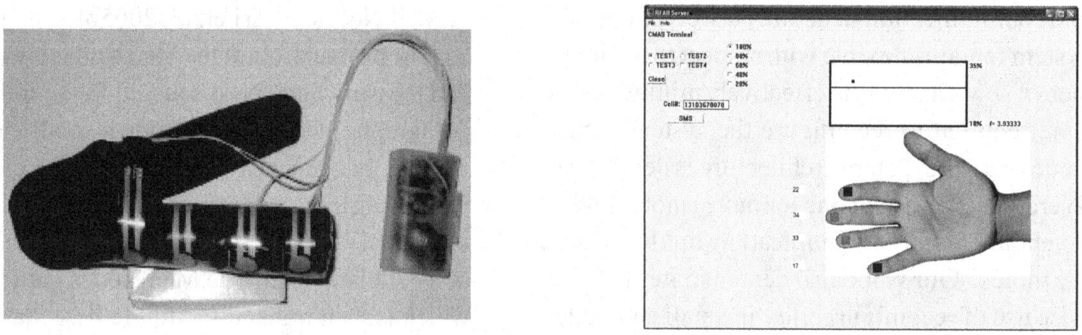

culescu, & Khosla, 2002) (Martin et al., 2003), resulting in the development of the first *RFab (Reconfigurable Fabric) Vest*, a pervasive medical monitoring jacket (Jafari et al., 2005a). What is significant about RFab is that the computation, storage, and communication modules of the system are woven directly into the fabric of the clothing itself. This "intelligent" fabric contains sensors in close proximity to the human body.

In RFab, reconfigurability is primarily used for robustness and fault tolerance rather than to increase performance. The fact of the matter is that all clothing, inevitably, will tear. This will sever communication links between motes and sensors and could possibly isolate certain components from the rest of the system depending on the severity of the tear. The reconfiguration capability allows RFab to rebuild interconnection pathways in response to a tear, thereby allowing the system to continue to operate. Moreover, there is also redundancy in the sensing, and control units embedded on the fabric. Therefore, if one unit becomes completely isolated, than a redundant clone can perform the same task in a manner that is wholly transparent to the user.

RFab employs an interconnect topology that is well-suited to specific tasks and effectively balances the computational load between motes. Specifically, the topology consists of wires organized into a mesh network. Redundancy was exploited in two approaches: *passive wiring* and *reconfigurable wiring*. In passive wiring, a Manhattan layout is used, providing diversity of paths between two points on the fabric. A relatively small tear along one path will not completely sever the communication link between the two points, because the other path remains in tact. The control units are attached at the junction crossings. This topology is similar to mesh topologies used for multiprocessor systems. Based on work in this area, a multihop packet routing protocol is used to perform communication. Routers are placed at the junction crossings along with the control units. In active wiring, simple switches and latches are used to control the state of routing resources in RFab. The switches are software-controlled electrical signal routers that are placed at junction crossings; these switches are dedicated to routing and perform no other functionality. The state of these switches is controlled by a distributed reconfiguration management service that allocates wiring resources according to traffic and fabric conditions (Jafari et. al, 2005a).

The envisioned application domain for the RFab vest is a sensor-driven personalized trans-dermal drug delivery clinical application. Low-latency fine-grained adaptation of drug dosage can be based on continuous physiological measurements from patients or in response to environmental and physiological measurements taken from the surrounding environment. Low latency is particularly important in hazardous

Figure 4. Architectural overview of RFab.

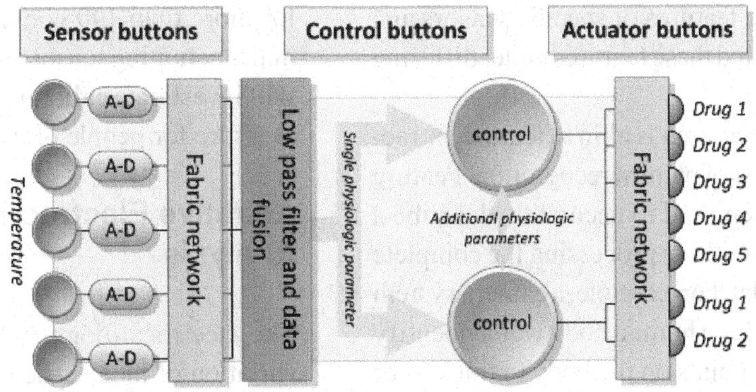

environments, such as industrial and military applications. The overall system architecture is shown in Figure 4. There are four main subsystems: computation/control, communication, sensing, and actuation. The last system, actuation, is responsible for drug delivery.

RECONFIGURABLE SOFTWARE

Reconfigurable software in heterogeneous embedded systems is essential for both usability and system performance. Software that can adapt to the environment in which it is deployed can effectively optimize the use of its resources. This is particularly important when it comes to issues related to power consumption and maximizing battery lifetime. Below, we describe an algorithm for CustoMed that dynamically recognizes the type of sensor that is attached to the device as well as an algorithm for adaptive electrocardiogram analysis.

Dynamic Sensor Detection

Dynamic sensor detection provides software support for the addition of a new sensor without requiring installation of additional software in the context of PnP. We investigated several different approaches. First, we analyzed complex signal processing algorithms, such as autocorrelation; however, the memory requirements of such algorithms were too large to fit into CustoMed. Instead, we opted for a simpler method that analyzed the unique features of specific sensors and accurately detected these features under differing circumstances.

This area of research is akin to feature extraction in the context of pattern recognition. Feature extraction is often used to accurately describe a large set of data without processing the complete data set in parallel. For example, a camera system that tracks a walking human body would identify a few important points on the body to track—for example, a few point on the head, torso, arms, legs, feet, and hands; of particular importance are joints, such as the knees, elbows and shoulders. An image processing application would then track these individual points rather than each pixel that comprises the image of the body. Feature extraction is essentially the process by which specific points to track are determined.

CustoMed uses a simple feature extraction algorithm that detects unique features. We analyzed two different types of sensors: pressure and flex sensors. The pressure sensor was place in a shoe and the flex sensor was placed on a patient's knee. The pressure sensor can determine the walking pattern of a patient, specifically by how much pressure is placed on different areas of the foot. A unique feature of the pressure sensor is that the sensor periodically drops to zero, which occurs whenever the foot is raised. Meanwhile, a flex sensor on the knee determines the angles at which a patient bends his or her knee over time. In contrast to the pressure sensor, the knee pressure disburses a constant pressure that changes continuously over time in dynamic sensor detection.

The Med Node could dynamically detect the type of sensor and run the approximate algorithm by detecting the unique features of the sensors. The experiments were done on sensor data collection by a person walking. During testing, a malfunctioning sensor could be detected based on whether data remained at a static number for long periods of time. Error checking was performed at regular intervals to determine static sensor readings. If the same value was repeatedly sent for more than 100 consecutive intervals, then a malfunctioning sensor was detected. Future work will investigate calibrating the average change in pressure for people of different weights.

Adaptive Electrocardiogram Analysis

The electrocardiogram (ECG) is the record of variation of bioelectric potential with respect to time as the human heart beats. Due to its ease of use and non-invasiveness, ECG plays an important role in patient monitoring and diagnosis. Multichannel ECG data provide cardiologists with essential information to diagnose heart disease in a patient. Our primary objective is to address the feasibility of implementing an ambulatory ECG analysis algorithm with real-time diagnosis functions for wearable computers.

ECG analysis algorithms have always been difficult tasks in the realization of computer aided ECG diagnosis. Implementation of such algorithms becomes even harder for small and mobile embedded systems that should meet the given latency requirements while minimizing overall energy dissipation for the system (Jafari et. al., 2006a).

Distributed architectures have been developed for cooperative detection, scalable data transport, and other capabilities and services that are essential to ECG analysis; however, the complexity of algorithms running on these systems has introduced a new set of challenges associated with resource constrained devices and their energy concerns. These obstacles may dramatically reduce the effectiveness of embedded distributed algorithms. Thus, a new distributed, embedded, computing attribute, dynamically reconfigurable architecture must be developed and provided to such systems. The capability of reconfiguration, in particular, may be of great advantage.

ECG analysis consists of preprocessing, pattern recognition, and classification. Reconfiguration can exploit new pattern recognition or feature extraction modules, whose development and implementation is a continuous and ongoing area of research. A component-based software reconfiguration will enable systems to overcome runtime issues associated with competition for limited resources by parallel tasks running on the same platform.

In pattern recognition, twenty-five features were extracted from ECG signal based on (Christov & Bortolan, 2004) and (De Chazal, O'Dwyer, & Reilly, 2004). Four features were derived from the RR interval (interval between two consecutive heartbeats). Five features were derived from heartbeat intervals. Six features were derived from geometric features. Eight normalized and non-normalized morphology features were extracted (Jafari et al., 2006a).

In the distributed algorithm, each detected feature was used in classification. The algorithm sought to have all simultaneously triggered features on the same processing unit to reduce transmission time between the distributed processors. This adaptable partitioning algorithm reconfigures how the features are distributed among the processing units to minimize communication. Based on various configurations (unique to each patient), modules can be added, modified or removed over the air using the Sensor Operating System (SOS) (Han et al., 2005) to reconfigure the system (Jafari et al., 2006a).

WIRELESS RECONFIGURABILITY

Wireless reconfiguration is important for networked embedded devices. Often, it is unrealistic or infeasible for a human to access the device to reconfigure it. Reconfiguration must therefore be initiated over a wireless network. Here, we describe an architecture for dynamic reconfigurable security in life-critical networked embedded systems.

Dynamic Security

Security is of legally-mandated importance to the health care industry. For example, the Health Insurance Portability and Accountability Act (HIPAA) mandates that a healthcare provider who "maintains or transmits health information shall maintain reasonable and appropriate administrative, technical, and physical safeguards to protect against any reasonably anticipated threats or hazards to the security or integrity of the information; and unauthorized uses or disclosures of the information." ("Health Insurance Portability", 1996)

However, security is challenging for embedded systems for many reasons. Cryptographic algorithms, one of the backbones of security, typically require a significant amount of processing and require large amounts of data storage (due to S-boxes). Since motes in embedded systems have limited processing and storage capabilities, implementing effective cryptography on such systems is a challenge.

We have designed and implemented a software architecture to meet the security and power utilization needs of the next generation of networked embedded system. The proposed architecture allows an embedded system sufficient flexibility to adapt to changing system requirements and to reprogram an embedded device with new applications using the wireless network.

The Dynamic Security System (DYNASEC) (Massey et al., 2007) is a software architecture that allows a centralized node to program other nodes with different levels of security. In particular, when the environment imposes stringent timing constraints on the system (for example, a patient suffers a heart attack and requires near-immediate drug delivery), then the strength of the cryptographic algorithm can be lowered to increase throughput. Modifying the system is necessary when the cost of security processing impedes the ability of the system to meet real-time constraints.

It is easy to see that DYNASEC fits within the requirements mandated by the HIPAA. Lowering the security level in response to real-time constraints imposed by life-critical anomalies should clearly fall within the "reasonable" clause of the act; moreover, it is quite obvious that the physical well-being of the patient who suffers from the anomaly should take precedence over the physical safeguards of the transmitted data.

Security protocols that exist today have been designed for the Internet—specifically, the wired, high-speed Internet, where nodes are assumed to be desktop processors or high-performance servers. As such, they assume that the nodes involved in a communication have unlimited computational abilities, unlimited power consumption, memory, and no real-time constraints imposed upon them. Embedded networks, in contrast, exist in a paradigm for which the exact opposite of each of these assumptions is true; computational power is limited, battery lifetime is a precious resource, memory is scarce, and real-time constraints are abundant.

Prior research on security protocols for embedded systems has focused on the analysis of energy consumption under various levels of security. (Ganesan et al., 2003) (Watro et al., 2004) (Malan et al., 2004) (Gura et al., 2004) (Perrig et al., 2002) (Karlof, Sastry, & Wagner, 2004) (Potlapally, 2003); however, flexibility and the possibility of reconfiguration have not been addressed (Schaumont et al., 2001) (Ravi et al., 1995) (Potlapally et al., 2003). This work has not considered the role of real-time constraints that occur in reaction to external events and/or changing environmental conditions.

Since embedded systems have limited resources to perform tasks, it is important to optimize the different components on the system in order to increase its lifetime and meet the system's deadlines. A lightweight security protocol dynamically maximizes security settings to meet timing and/or power constraints. This optimal security protocol contains integrity to verify that the message has not changed in transit and authentication information so that the receiver can confirm the identity of the sender. Encryption then ensures that only authorized nodes can read the information.

DYNASEC can switch between four different levels of security either statically or dynamically depending on timing and/or power constraints that are imposed by the system. Power constraints may account for battery lifetime or simply the desired lifetime of the system. The first level of security is plaintext, meaning no encryption. The second level includes authentication and cipher block chaining (CBC) which validates the integrity of the message. The third level adds encryption using the Skipjack protocol (Brickell et al, 1993). The fourth level also employs encryption, but replaces Skipjack with the stronger, but more computationally intensive, RC5 algorithm (Rivest, 1995).

In the absence of constraints, the fourth level of security is always used, since the strongest possible security is always deemed beneficial. If timing or power consumption constraints are imposed on the system, then DYNASEC must determine the highest level of security that will allow the system to meet its constraints. If the system cannot meet the constraints at the first level of security, then the situation is deemed to be infeasible.

In order to quantitatively analyze the delay, the code was run in the Avrora simulation environment (Titzer, Lee, & Palsberg, 2005). The processing delay for the four levels of security at the different payloads (100 bytes, 50 bytes, and 1 byte) was measured for normalized time periods. As the security levels or packet sizes increased, the processing delay increased. From our results changing the waveform of payload of 100 bytes to a heart rate extraction algorithm of 1 byte greatly reduced the number of packets that could be sent out into the network by approximately 75 fold.

The ability for code migration is important because it will allow DYNASEC to seamlessly incorporate new cryptographic protocols. For example, if a new cryptographic algorithm is invented in the next year, DYNASEC can use code migration to program all of the motes in the network with the new algorithm. Such an algorithm can either replace one of the existing security levels, or add a fifth level of security.

Sensor Operating Systems (SOS) is an operating system that provides code migration between different embedded systems (Han et al., 2005). Code migration occurs when one embedded system can download a program or module to be executed on another embedded system. Code migration is essential in creating systems that can be reconfigured after deployment. After the system is deployed, the software may need to be modified. SOS severs the ties between the core operating system and individual applications or modules. A module can be loaded or removed at run time without interrupting the core operating system. A lightweight medical processor can transmit a program or module to be executed on the processor. Code updates are essential in creating a system that can be reconfigured after deployment.

CONCLUSION AND FUTURE DIRECTIONS

The architectures and algorithms presented demonstrate how well designed embedded systems benefit from reconfigurability. Limited resources can be optimized through efficient and effective reconfiguration schemes that balance the tradeoffs between power consumption, memory consumption, and interoperability in heterogeneous environments. Reconfigurable hardware and software have the desirable feature of allowing design flaws to be fixed after deployment, which is an essential feature in embedded medical systems.

Several challenges that must be overcome when designing reconfigurable architectures for heterogeneous embedded systems are listed below.

- Limited Memory
- Limited Power
- Security
- Lack of Standardization to support Plug-and-Play

First and foremost, memory is limited. One problem with in-situ biological sensing is the extensive variation in morphology of bio-signals of different individuals and under varying conditions. Because of the large quantity of data produced by the sensors, the algorithms used to analyze and classify the bio-signals demand significant amounts of storage. Therefore, it is crucial to optimize the memory usage of such algorithms by employing adaptive and efficient methods for pattern classification.

Another challenge that needs to be addressed is the privacy of data transmitted by the embedded systems. HIPAA demands that patient data be stored securely. We presented a method for managing security in an embedded system, but future research needs to investigate better lightweight cryptographic algorithms for small embedded systems.

Standardization of communication and hardware in embedded medical systems is a virtual necessity. Standards will be necessary to support PnP among embedded medical devices. These standards should include communication protocols between sensors and hardware. Moreover, standardized communication protocols for embedded medical systems will aid connectivity, interoperability, and the quality of wireless medical devices.

REFERENCES

Benini, L. and DeMicheli, G. (2002). Networks on Chips: A New Paradigm for Component-Based MPSoC Design. *IEEE Computer.*

Brickell, E., Denning, D., Kent, S., Mahler, D. and Tuchman, W. (1993). SKIPJACK Review. *Interim Report.*

Christov, I. and Bortolan, G. (2004). Ranking of pattern recognition parameters for premature ventricular contractions classification by Neural Networks. *Physiological Measurement, 25*(5), 1281-1290.

De Chazal, P., O'Dwyer, M. and Reilly, R. (2004). Automatic classification of heartbeats using ECG morphology and heartbeat interval features. *IEEE Trans. Biomedical Eng., 51*(7), 1196-1206.

DeVaul, R., Sung, M., Gips, J, and Pentland, A. (2003). Mithril 2003: Applications and architecture. *Seventh IEEE Symposium on IEEE Wearable Computers*, pp 4-11.

Ganesan, P., Venugopalan, R., Peddabachagari, P., Dean, A., Mueller, F., and Sichitiu, M. (2003). Analyzing and modeling encryption overhead for sensor network nodes. *Wireless Sensor Networks and Applications (WSNA 2004).* San Diego, CA.

Gura, N., Patel, A., Wander, A., Eberle, H., and Shantz, S. (2004). Comparing elliptic curve cryptography and RSA on 8-bit CPUs. *Workshop on Cryptographic Hardware and Embedded Systems (CHES 2004).* Cambridge, MA.

Han, C., Rengaswamy, R., Shea, R., Kohler, E., and Srivastava, M. (2005). SOS: A dynamic operating system for sensor networks. *Third International Conference on Mobile Systems, Applications, and Services (Mobisys 2005).* Seattle, WA.

Health Insurance Portability and Accountability Act of 1996 (HIPAA) (1996). P.L. 104-191 Enacted H.R. 3103, August 21, 1996 110 Stat. 1936, codified 42 U.S.C. 1320.

Jafari, R., Dabiri, F., Brisk, P., and Sarrafzadeh, M. (2005a). Adaptive and fault tolerant medical vest for life critical medical monitoring. *20th ACM Symposium on Applied Computing (SAC 2005)*, March 2005. Santa Fe, NM.

Jafari, R., Dabiri, F., Sarrafzadeh, M. (2005b). CustoMed: A power optimized customizable and mobile medical monitoring and analysis system. *ACM HCI Challenges in Health Assessment Workshop in conjunction with CHI 2005.* Portland, OR.

Jafari, R., Noshadi, H., Ghiasi, S., Sarrafzadeh, M. (2006a). Adaptive electrocardiogram feature extraction on distributed embedded systems. *IEEE Transactions on Parallel and Distributed Systems special issue on High Performance Computational Biology (TPDS),* 17, (8), 1-11.

Jafari, R., Jindrich, D., Edgerton, V., Sarrafzadeh, M. (2006b). CMAS: Clinical movement assessment system for neuromotor disorders, *IEEE Biomedical Circuits and Systems Conference (BioCAS)*, London, UK.

Karlof, C., Sastry, N., and Wagner, D. (2004). TinySec: A Link Layer Security Architecture for Wireless Sensor Networks. *Second ACM Conference on Embedded Networked Sensor Systems (SenSys 2004).* Baltimore, MD.

Kastner, R., Ogrenci, S., Bozorgzadeh, E., Sarrafzadeh, M. (2001) Instruction generation for hybrid reconfigurable systems. *IEEE/ACM Intl Conf Computer-Aided Design (ICCAD)..*

LeMoyne, R., Jafari, R., Jea, D., Srivastava, M., Sarrafzadeh, M. (2005) Fully quantified evaluation of myotatic stretch reflex. *Symp Neuroscience,* 2005.

Malan, D.J., Welsh, M., and Smith, M.D. (2004) A public-key infrastructure for key distribution in tinyos based on elliptic curve cryptography. *First IEEE International Conference on Sensor and Ad Hoc Communications and Networks,* Santa Clara, California.

Marculescu, D., Marculescu, R., Khosla, P. (2002). challenges and opportunities in electronic textiles modeling and optimization. *Design Automation Conference*, pp 175-180.

Martin, T., Jones, M., Edmison, J, and Shenoy, R. (2003). Towards a design framework for wearable electronic textiles. *Seventh IEEE International Symposium on Wearable Computers*, pp.190-199.

Massey, T., Brisk, P., Dabiri, F., Sarrafzadeh, M. (2007). Delay aware, reconfigurable security for embedded systems. *Second International Conference on Body Area Networks (BodyNets 2007).* Florence, Italy.

Ogrenci S, Bozorgzadeh E, Kastner R, Sarrafzadeh M. (2001a) A super-scheduler for embedded reconfigurable systems. *IEEE/ACM Intl Conf Computer-Aided Design (ICCAD).*

Ogrenci S, Bozorgzadeh E., Kastner R., Sarrafzadeh M. (2001b). SPS: A strategically programmable system. *Reconfigurable Architectures Workshop (RAW).*

Perrig, A., Canetti, R. Tygar, J. D. and Song, D. (2002) The TESLA broadcast authentication protocol. *RSA Cryptobytes.*

Potlapally, N. Ravi, S., Raghunathan, A., Jha, N. (2003). Analyzing the energy consumption of security protocols. *International Symposium on Low Power Electronics and Design (ISLPED 2003).* Seoul Korea.

Ravi, S., Raghunathan, A., Kocher, P., and Hattangady, S. (2004). Security in embedded systems: design challenges. *ACM Transactions on Embedded Computing Systems. 3*,(3), 461-491.

Rivest, R. (1995) The RC5 encryption algorithm. *1994 Leuven Workshop on Fast Software Encryption,* pp. 86-96.

Schaller, R. R. (1999). Moore's Law: past, present, and future. *IEEE Spectrum. 34*(6), 52-59.

Schaumont, P., Verbauwhede, I., Sarrafzadeh, M., and Keutzer, K. (2001). A quick safari through the reconfiguration jungle. *Design Automation Conference (DAC 2001).* Las Vegas, CA.

Titzer, B., Lee D., and Palsberg, J. (2005). Avrora: scalable sensor network simulation with precise timing. *International Symposium on Information Processing in Sensor Networks (IPSN).* Los Angeles, California.

Watro, R., Kong, D., Cuti, S., Gardiner, C., Lynn, C., and Kruus, P. (2004). TinyPK: Securing sensor networks with public key technology. *2nd ACM Workshop on Security of Ad Hoc and Sensor Networks (SASN 2004).* Washington, D.C.

KEY TERMS

Algorithm: A well-defined procedure that usually takes some input, carries out a number of finite steps, and produces an output.

Architecture: The overall structure and organization of a computer system, in particular the hardware or software of the system.

Circuit: A hardware component that consists of resistors, capacitors, diodes, and transistors are formed directly onto the surface of a silicon crystal; several circuits form a microcomputer chip used in many computers

Code Migration: When one embedded system downloads a program or module to be executed on another embedded system.

Health Insurance Portability and Accountability Act (HIPAA): Mandates that a healthcare provider who "maintains or transmits health information shall maintain reasonable and appropriate administrative, technical, and physical safeguards to protect against any reasonably anticipated threats or hazards to the security or integrity of the information; and unauthorized uses or disclosures of the information." ("Health Insurance Portability", 1996).

Electrocardiogram: A recording of the electrical signal of the heart through electrodes placed on the heart or limbs of a patient; it is used to diagnose different medical conditions of the heart.

Embedded Medical Systems: A light-weight special purpose system that uses medical sensors to detect the vital signs of an entity.

Embedded Systems: A special purpose system that usually has limited resources (memory, computational power, and bandwidth) and is usually dedicated to a specific task.

Medical Motherboard: A platform that connects sensors to a collection of relatively small, low-powered processing units *(motes)*, and is intended for use in medical embedded systems.

Med Nodes: Stand-alone components consisting of a processing unit, external sensor boards and a battery that support various types of sensors for physiological reading from the human body.

Moore's Law – processor performance to double approximately every 18 months due to continuous breakthroughs in transistor technology.

Network: A group of computing devices that communicate with one another wirelessly or through a wired connection.

Operating System: Software that manages and coordinates the hardware resources on a computer.

Plug and Play: A paradigm allows the addition of new peripheral without manual installation of additional software.

Protocol: The rules governing communication in hardware and/or software.

Reconfigurability: The ability to rearrange components; in the context of embedded systems, it is the ability to dynamically being able to change the hardware or software after the system has been deployed without manually reprogramming it.

Security: The ability of a system to protect information and system resources in order to ensure confidentiality, integrity, and availability of the data.

Chapter XVII
Third Generation (3G) Cellular Networks in Telemedicine:
Technological Overview, Applications, and Limitations

Konstantinos Perakis
National Technical University of Athens, Greece

Dimitris Koutsouris
National Technical University of Athens, Greece

ABSTRACT

The evolutions in the field of telecommunications technologies, with the robustness and the fidelity these new systems provide, have significantly contributed in the advancement and development in the field of medicine, and they have also brought forth the need for their utilisation in the healthcare sector. Thus, telemedicine and e-Health have clearly started to become an important issue for implementation, operational deployment of services and a promising market for industry. Recognizing this trend, its importance in the lives of citizens all around the globe and its contribution in the daily healthcare delivery by all actors involved in the procedure, the authors of this chapter attempt to familiarize the readers with the impact that high broadband wireless networks have upon telemedicine services and with the way they facilitate the secure transmission of vital information stemming from bandwidth demanding applications in real time. After providing the readers with an overview of telemedical services and commenting on how they can offer added value to existing healthcare services, they provide an analysis of the wireless infrastructure that has facilitated telemedical services over the years, and point out the significant role that the third generation telecommunications systems can play in the field. After that, follows an analysis of the range of new applications that can be supported by the 3G telecommunications infrastructure, and the related research that has taken place in the European level regarding the utilization of 3G networks for telemedical applications. However, 3G networks are not a panacea; for this reason the limitations of this infrastructure is also stressed out. The authors conclude by discussing whether 3G networks can prove to be an attractive solution for telemedical services to healthcare providers.

INTRODUCTION

The evolutions in the field of telecommunications technologies, with the robustness and the fidelity these new systems provide, have significantly contributed in the advancement and development in the field of medicine; they have also brought forth the need for their utilisation in the healthcare sector, a sector that is information intensive and knowledge demanding. Thus, e-Health solutions are of crucial importance (Olsson & Lymberis & Whitehouse, 2004, p.312); telemedicine and e-Health have clearly started to become an important issue for implementation, operational deployment of services and a promising market for industry (Wooton, 1999) ("EU2004a", 2004). As had been forecasted a decade ago, healthcare institutions make extensive use of computer networks, mass storage devices, and sophisticated workstations at which humans and machines interact, assisted by advanced information processing tools and techniques of knowledge engineering, to achieve integration of multimodality multimedia, diagnostic data and expert medical knowledge (Orphanoudakis & Kaldoudi & Tsiknakis, 1996, 210). However, telemedicine is not a brand new service. On the contrary, telemedicine has been described from as early as as 1906, when W.Einthoven described the possibility of transmitting cardiogram information via telephone lines. This description became a reality in 1910 when S.G. Brown did actually transmit hearing sounds in London. In addition, a few years later, and more specifically in 1920, wireless communications were utilized in order to provide medical advice support in boats from the Norwegian hospital Haukeland.

Since 2004, the term eHealth aroused, defined by Eysenbach as: "eHealth is an emerging field in the intersection of medical informatics, public health and business, referring to health services and information delivered or enhanced through the Internet and related technologies. In a broader sense, the term characterises not only a technical development, but also a state-of-mind, a way of thinking, an attitude, and a commitment for networked, global thinking, to improve healthcare locally, regionally and worldwide by using information and communication technology"(Eysenbach, 2001, e20), (Pagliari et al, 2005, e9). The term eHealth is supposed to be an overall term, or even better an "umbrella" term, including all aspects of Health Telematics.

Telemedicine is one of the areas canopied under the umbrella-term – eHealth. The term 'telemedicine' derives from the Greek 'tele' meaning *'at a distance'* and the present word 'medicine' which itself derives from the Latin 'mederi' meaning *'healing'*. However, even though this service has been attributed many terms, there is not actually a standardized definition of it. On the contrary, various organizations have come up with different definitions of the term telemedicine. Thus for example, the World Health Organisation defines telemedicine as the delivery of healthcare services, where distance is a critical factor, by healthcare professionals using information and communications technologies for the exchange of valid information for diagnosis, treatment and prevention of disease and injuries, research and evaluation, and for the continuing education of healthcare providers, all in the interest of advancing the health of individuals and their communities (W.H.O., 1998). The Norwegian Center of Telemedicine on the other hand defines telemedicine as the research, the follow-up and the management of patients, as well as the education of patients and personnel, making use of systems that allows the direct access in patient data and the advisory services of experts, anywhere they might be located (Norwegian Centre for Telemedicine 2007). Furthermore, the Journal of Telemedicine & Telecare defines telemedicine as the medicine practiced from a distance, and as such, encompasses not only the diagnosis but the treatment, as well and in addition the medical education (Journal of Telemedicine and Telecare 2007). Even though not clearly defined however, telemedicine targets towards the qualitative healthcare provision for all citizens, trying to diminish and if possible eliminate geographical and/or economical barriers.

TELEMEDICINE SERVICES

Telemedicine services are currently employed to support various aspects of healthcare delivery, such as remote consultation (physician-physician or patient-physician) for diagnostic purposes, remote guidance and performance of a variety of therapeutic and surgical procedures thus making expertise available at remote sites (e.g. site-of-an accident, geographically isolated places, on board ships and planes, sea-plants, battle-fields, hazardous environments, space stations, etc), real-time access to educational material and statistical information on a global basis and remote use of distributed complementary facilities for medical information processing. Furthermore, an important goal of telemedicine is to guarantee continuity of care, rendering the medical history of a patient readily, timely and transparently available wherever and whenever needed.

Telemedicine/telehealth consists of a set of added-value telematic services, implemented over an advanced telecommunications infrastructure and supported by different information technologies and related applications. Its main goal is to provide different levels of support for remote monitoring, preventive, diagnostic and therapeutic medical procedures. Therefore, telemedicine can be considered as an extended virtual healthcare institution that encompasses available physical and human resources over a wide region in order to support remote medical procedures and patient management.

The emerging environment in which healthcare telematics services can be provided has a layered structure (Orphanoudakis & Kaldoudi & Tsiknakis, 1996, 210). The top layer corresponds to the actual services provided, such as tele-diagnosis, tele-monitoring, tele-consultation, tele-management, and other added-value services. The second layer consists of all computer applications that provide the necessary communications and computer supported cooperative working environment for telemedicine services to be realized. Such applications include electronic mail, multimedia conferencing, synchronous and asynchronous consultation, immersive environments and tele-presence, interactive image analysis and visualization of multimedia medical data, tools for querying geographically distributed medical databases, and a variety of other applications that facilitate added-value information services. The bottom layer corresponds to the hardware and software infrastructure that supports the aforementioned applications and consists primarily of medical equipment, distributed workstations, the telecommunications network, and tools for the management of network and other resources.

The primary goal of telemedicine is to provide support for remote expert consultation based on locally acquired medical data and remote guid-

Figure 1. Layered structure of healthcare services environment

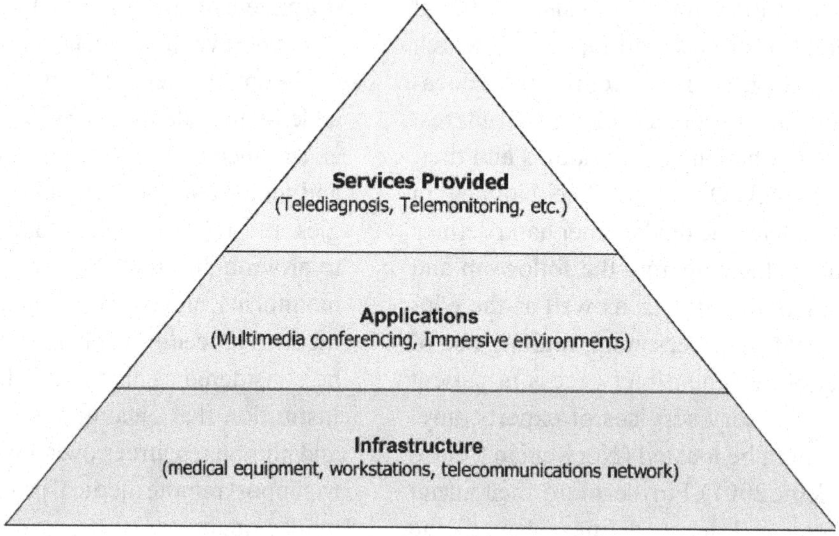

ance for locally performed medical procedures. Thus, telemedicine can cover a wide variety of medical needs, including provision of healthcare in remote areas, in transportation means, emergency telemedicine, homecare, tele-education, homogenisation of medical services and others. Different services are described as follows, based on the specific objectives of each telemedicine session.

Tele-Diagnosis

Typically, this service involves asynchronous point-to-point communication and requires relatively simple applications and a minimum infrastructure. In response to a request by a remote site, which transmits all or selected data of a diagnostic examination, specialists at a referral medical center review these data and return a diagnostic report to the requesting site. Tele-diagnosis is particularly useful for rural and other areas that are not well served by specialized medical personnel.

Tele-Monitoring

Video sequences of the examination room and the patient are transmitted to the expert, who monitors the procedure and interacts with the examination site through an image and voice data link. This service may also include transmission of vital biosignals and other related data, as in the case of home care telemedicine services. However, the requirement for real-time multimedia communication imposes additional technological demands on the available infrastructure.

Tele-Consultation

Providing a shared workspace among remotely located medical experts is one of the main functions of the tele-consultation service. This service requires the synchronous viewing and manipulation of the same set of medical multimedia data, as well as the real-time exchange of comments among all parties involved in the session. It is evident that the synchronization of the media and procedures involved in a tele-consultation session requires various types of complex transactions and resource management mechanisms, thus imposing serious demands on the underlying applications. Furthermore, the real-time nature of the service and the volume of multimedia data exchanged require a technologically advanced infrastructure.

Tele-Management

The combination of advanced tele-monitoring and tele-consultation services, with remote resource sharing, offers the possibility for the telematic management of diagnostic and therapeutic procedures. This service is gaining momentum together with parallel developments in the areas of broadband conventional and mobile communications, virtual reality and tele-presence (Kalawsky, 1993). Advances in computer assisted medical interventions, automatic surgical tools, and various forms of remote sensing, have already paved the way towards advanced telemedicine services in endoscopy and surgery.

Tele-Education

Distant learning in telemedicine can also be accomplished by special interactive tele-education sessions and the distribution of specially prepared educational material, such as hypermedia diagnostic imaging textbooks. Medical training has a lot to benefit from the development of wide area, medical education environments over high-speed networks.

Added-Value Services

Telemedicine is not limited to communication and collaboration among experts. Of increasing importance are added-value telemedicine services, which enable the sharing of a variety of other resources necessary for extending and improving the quality of healthcare procedures. For example, telemedicine can provide access to high-performance computing centers for advanced medical image processing and 3D visualization. Other added-value telemedicine services involve the retrieval of reference material from remote databases, such as on-line medical publications and digital atlases of the human anatomy. The sharing of such information is a valuable medical decision support tool and promotes the continuing education of medical personnel.

Thus, it is more than obvious that telemedicine can offer a plethora of advantages. If we were to summarize these advantages, we could say that telemedicine could offer:

- Equal rights of access in the services of health for the all citizens.
- High quality services of health to citizens of remote regions.
- Solution for management and organization problems to remote, underserved and with few resources primary point-of-care units
- Modernization of work environment
- Cross-check diagnosis
- Diffusion of medical information
- Smart management of medical resources
- Cost reduction
- Reduction of pointless travel

TECHNOLOGICAL INFRASTRUCTURE

It is therefore obvious that as the request for telemedical services is constantly rising and becoming even more demanding, the bottom layer of the structure, namely the infrastructure layer should become equally capable of providing such services. One such demand is the available bandwidth of the telecommunications networks. In the following paragraphs, the significant role that the third generation telecommunications systems - that are only recently being deployed in Europe - can play, as regards telemedical applications, is pointed out. The transition from 2G and 2.5G to 3G telecommunications systems could prove to be crucial, especially in relation to emergency telemedicine.

GSM

It is beyond doubt as well that the great outburst in mobile communications occurred in the mid 1980s, with the appearance of GSM (GSMWorld: GSM, 2007). During the early 1980s, analog cellular telephone systems were experiencing rapid growth in Europe, particularly in Scandinavia and the United Kingdom, but also in France and Germany. Each country developed its own system, which was incompatible with everyone else's in equipment and operation. This was an undesirable situation, because not only was the mobile equipment limited to operation within national boundaries but there was also a very limited market for each type of equipment. Thus, in 1982 the Conference of European Posts and Telegraphs (CEPT) formed a study group called the Groupe Spécial Mobile (GSM) to study and develop a pan-European public land mobile system. In 1989, GSM responsibility was transferred to the European Telecommunication Standards Institute (ETSI), and phase I of the GSM specifications were published in 1990. Commercial service was started in mid-1991, and by October 1997 GSM subscribers had grown to more than 55 million. GSM is not only a European standard. Over 200 GSM networks (including DCS1800 and PCS1900) are operational in 110 countries around the world.

As allocated by the ITU, GSM 900 utilizes the 890 – 915 MHz for the uplink and the 935 – 960 MHz for the downlink, GSM 1800 utilises the 1710 – 1785 MHz for the uplink and the 1805 – 1880 MHz for the downlink and GSM 1900 utilises the 1850 – 1910 MHz for the uplink and the 1930 – 1990 MHz for the downlink. GSM services are not limited to telephony but include asynchronous and synchronous data services (2.4/4.8/9.6 Kbps), value-added features (SMS, fax) and more (Dechaux & Scheller, 1993). As with all other communications, speech is digitally encoded and transmitted through the GSM network as a digital stream. GSM users can send and receive data, at rates up to 9600 bps, to users on POTS, ISDN, Packet Switched Public Data Networks, and Circuit Switched Public Data Networks using a variety of access methods and protocols (Dubendorf, 2003).

The network behind the GSM system seen by the customer is large and complicated in order to provide all of the services which are required:

- The Base Station Subsystem (the base stations and their controllers).
- The Network and Switching Subsystem (the part of the network most similar to a fixed network). This is sometimes also just called the core network.
- The GPRS Core Network (the optional part which allows packet based Internet connections).

All of the elements in the system combine to produce many GSM services such as voice calls and SMS.

The method chosen by GSM to divide up the bandwidth among as many users as possible is a combination of Time- and Frequency-Division Multiple Access (TDMA/FDMA). The FDMA part involves the division by frequency of the (maximum) 25 MHz bandwidth into 124 carrier frequencies spaced 200 kHz apart. One or more carrier frequencies are assigned to each base station. Each of these carrier frequencies is then divided in time, using a TDMA scheme. The fundamental unit of time in this TDMA scheme is called a burst period and lasts 15/26 ms (or approx. 0.577 ms). Eight burst periods are grouped into a TDMA frame (120/26 ms, or approx. 4.615 ms) (Dubendorf, 2003).

From the point of view of the consumers, the key advantage of GSM systems has been higher

Figure 2. The structure of a GSM network (WikiPedia: GSM 2007)

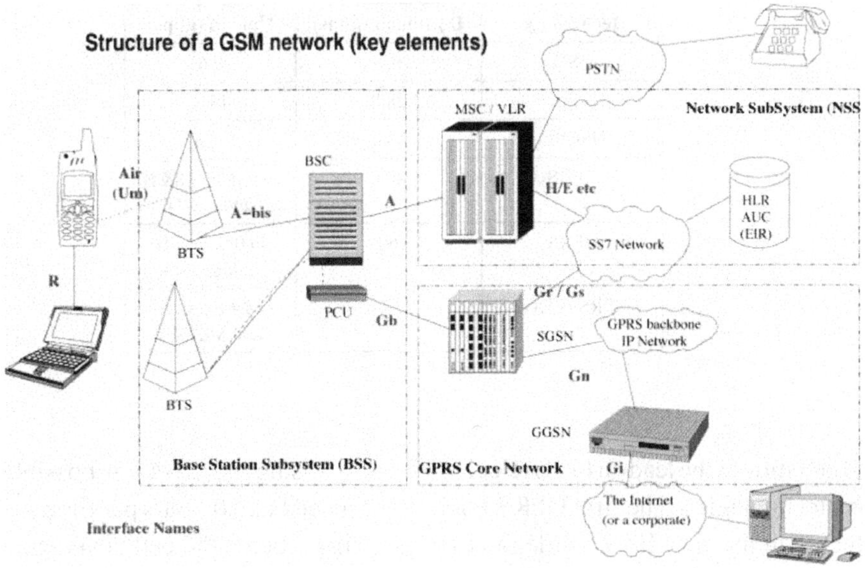

digital voice quality and low cost alternatives to making calls such as the Short Message Service (SMS). The advantage for network operators has been the ability to deploy equipment from different vendors because the open standard allows easy inter-operability. Like other cellular standards GSM allows network operators to offer roaming services which mean subscribers can use their phones all over the world.

GPRS

GPRS (short for general packet radio service) was recently introduced as the packet-mode extension

Table 1. GPRS Multislot Classes

Multislot Class	Downlink Slots	Uplink Slots	Active Slots
1	1	1	2
2	2	1	3
3	2	2	3
4	3	1	4
5	2	2	4
6	3	2	4
7	3	3	4
8	4	1	5
9	3	2	5
10	4	2	5
11	4	3	5
12	4	4	5
32	5	3	6

Table 2. GPRS upload & download rate per technology

Technology	Download (kbps)	Upload (kbps)
CSD	9.6	9.6
HSCSD	28.8	14.4
HSCSD	43.2	14.4
GPRS	80.0	20.0 (Class 8&10 and CS-4)
GPRS	60	40.0 (Class 10 and CS-4)
EGPRS (EDGE)	177.6	118.4 (Class 10 and MCS-9)

to GSM and constitutes the lead-in to 3G telecommunications technologies. The first GPRS trials were conducted in the year 1999, while the first GPRS networks rolled out in the year 2000, the same year the first GPRS terminals were released (GSMWorld: GPRS, 2007).

GPRS is a new non-voice, value added, high-speed, packet-switching technology for GSM networks. It facilitates sending and receiving small bursts of data, such as email and web browsing, as well as large volumes of data over a mobile telephone network. Its main innovations are that it is packet based, it increases data transmission speeds, and extends the Internet connection all the way to the mobile PC – the user no longer needs to dial up to a separate ISP (Dubendorf, 2003). GPRS users are considered to be always connected. Packet switching means that GPRS radio resources are used only when users are actually sending or receiving data.

GPRS speed is a direct function of the number of TDMA time slots assigned, which is the lesser of (a) what the particular cell supports and (b) the maximum capability of the mobile device expressed as a GPRS Multislot Class. Transfer speed depends also on the channel encoding used. The least robust (but fastest) coding scheme (CS-4) is available near the Base Transceiver Station (BTS) while the most robust coding scheme (CS-1) is used when the Mobile Station (MS) is further away from the BTS (WikiPedia: GPRS, 2007).

Using the CS-4 it is possible to achieve a user speed of 20.0 kbit/s per time slot. However, using this scheme the cell coverage is 25% of normal. CS-1 can achieve a user speed of only 8.0 kbit/s per time slot, but has 98% of normal coverage. Newer network equipment can adapt the transfer speed automatically depending on the mobile location. Theoretically, a GPRS connection can provide a data transmission speed of up to 171.2 Kbps (approximately three times as fast as the data transmission speeds of fixed telecommunications networks and ten times as fast as the current GSM network services) if eight slots are used. However, it is unlikely that network operators will allow a single user use up all the time slots. Therefore, maximum GPRS speeds should be compared against constraints in the GPRS terminals and networks. Nevertheless, bit rates up to 56 Kbps are achievable. The fewer the timeslots provided per user, the lower the data transmission speed.

UMTS

UMTS stands for Universal Mobile Telecommunication System and constitutes Europe's implementation of the 3G Telecommunications Systems. These new systems are a significant innovation over 2G and 2.5G systems because of their high operating flexibility, their ability to provide a wide range of applications and generally extend the services now provided to fixed networks users to mobile customers. 2G systems provide limited capabilities for real-time transmission of data and are limited in terms of maximum data rate. 3G mobile and wireless networks provide 144 kbps for full mobility applications, 384 kbps for limited mobility applications in macro and micro cellular environments and 2 Mbps for low mobility applications, particularly in the micro and pico-cellular environments (Muratore, 2001).

Contrary to the current GSM systems, UMTS allows for broadband data communication to mobile units, packet-based transmission of text, digitized voice, video, and multimedia, offering a set of services to mobile computer and phone users no matter where they are located in the world. The World Administrative Radio Conference that is responsible for assigning radio frequencies on a worldwide basis assigned a band between 1885 and 2025 MHz as well as between 2110 and 2200 MHz to 3G systems (Mandyam & Lai, 2002). In Europe, the first 15 MHz of the band coincided with part of the band currently used by the DECT system. The remaining portion of the spectrum for the terrestrial segment has been divided into a "paired" part (from 1920 to 1980 MHz for the uplink and from 2110 to 2170 MHz for the downlink) and an "unpaired" part (35 MHz, from 1900 to 1920 MHz and from 2010 to 2025 MHz) where there is no a-priori distinction between the portions assigned to the up-link and down-link, respectively (Holma & Toskala, 2000).

In order to maximize the number of users served per cell UMTS utilizes the CDMA technique (Code Division Multiple Access) which belongs to the family of spread spectrum techniques (Castro, 2001). Systems with CDMA access techniques enable users to transmit at the same frequency simultaneously, thus giving the ability to superimpose several signals on the same radio channel. In CDMA networks, all terminals use the same radio frequency. In networks with TDMA or FDMA access such as GSM, the terminal engaged in a call continuously measures the level and the quality of the signal received from the cells adjacent to the cell where it is currently located, as well as the radio channel carrying the call in progress (Muratore, 2001). This measurement is sent to the network on a channel associated with the one which is active between the network and the terminal. CDMA systems can provide fully asynchronous hand-over functions as well as the means for active connection maintenance between the mobile terminal and the network, over several radio links, which can also be activated through different radio base stations. In the channel changing stage, typical of the hand-over process, connection continuity is guaranteed through the multiple paths set up between the mobile terminal and the "controlling point" in the network, whereas in GSM for example, channel changing takes place by means of a "hop" between the radio channels of the two cells involved in the process, and hence through an "interruption" whose duration must necessarily be limited. In other words, in order to improve communication quality, the mobile terminal does not limit itself on remaining connected to a single Base Station but involves all Base Stations from which it receives a sufficiently good reference signal in the communication. The process of activating and releasing parallel links is carried out as a function of the quality of the signal received by the mobile terminal as it moves in the network.

Since 2006, UMTS networks in many countries have been or are in the process of being upgraded with High Speed Downlink Packet Access (HSDPA), sometimes known as 3.5G. Currently, HSDPA enables downlink transfer speeds of up to 3.6 Mbit/s. Work is also progressing on improving the uplink transfer speed with the High-Speed Uplink Packet Access (HSUPA). Longer term, the 3GPP Long Term Evolution project plans to move UMTS to 4G speeds of 100 Mbit/s down and 50 Mbit/s up, using a next generation air interface technology based upon OFDM.

As regards market launch, the first UMTS network in Europe was launched by Manx Telecom on the Isle of Man (a large island in the Irish sea) in 2001. Manx Telecom is part of the O2 group, which is now a subsidiary of Telefonica. O2 used the island as a testbed for 3G technology. The 3G service was launched in the UK and Italy in March 2003. To meet this early date, this was a soft-launch with limited coverage of the UK initially available. In February 2004, Vodafone began a wide-scale UMTS launch in several European markets, including the UK, Ireland, Germany, The Netherlands and Sweden, while Greece became a part of this market by mid-2004.

APPLICATIONS

The deployment of the third generation cellular networks has opened up many new horizons for over-the-air communication and more specifically for distant health care delivery. 3G systems can support higher data rates, thus allowing for a range of new applications. The integration of third generation telecommunication technologies in medicine could prove to be crucial in many aspects of remote provision of healthcare, which communication technologies used to-date (such as GSM or even GPRS) cannot support. Such systems can be used for tele-diagnosis, tele-monitoring and tele-consultation in various fields of medicine.

Thus for example, one of the most important fields of medicine that renders the use of broadband services imperative for modern healthcare provision is that of Emergency Telemedicine; paramedics that attend to accidents don't have the expertise to handle emergency situations. Real time transmission of various physiological parameters of the patients, such as ECG leads, oxygen saturation and blood pressure, between the paramedics of an ambulance and a specialized doctor, either inside a hospital / medical centre or on the move, constitute a significant aid to the doctors in order to guide the paramedics through the process of heart recovery and/or drug provision to the patients (Pavlopoulos & Kyriakou & Berler & Koutsouris, 1998). Apart from the transmission of the physiological parameters of the patients, the paramedics can also acquire and send to the specialized doctors still images or video of the patient. The visual contact is of crucial importance since the doctor obtains a thorough clinical image of the patient. Thus, a specialised doctor can telematically "move" to the patient's site and instruct unspecialized personnel when handling an emergency or telemonitoring case. Third generation cellular networks do not only guarantee the necessary bandwidth for the data transmission, they also guarantee the stability of the flow of the transmitted data. This is achieved due to the "soft hand-over" process, during which the mobile terminal switches from one cell to another in such a way that there is a point in time that it communicates with both cells.

Navarro et al have presented the architecture of a multi-collaborative mobile telemedicine system optimized to operate over 3G mobile networks, with the evaluation results showing a reliable performance over IPv4 UMTS access (Navarro et al, 2005). Encouraging are also the results of the experimental evaluation in terms of various performance metrics such as frame delay, jitter, frame delivery ratio and interframe interval, of a mobile tele-trauma system, capable of simultaneously transmitting video, medical images and ECG signals over real 3G network conditions (Chu & Ganz, 2004). Other scientific approaches that could be enhanced through the use of 3G cellular networks as regards emergency telemedicine include the wireless telemedicine project from the University of Maryland (Gagliano, 1998), the European Union's Ambulance (Pavlopoulos et al, 1998) as well as the British Lancashire Ambulance (Curry & Harrop, 1998), which all utilized the GSM cellular network. The same applies for the scientific approach of Xiao et al regarding the design of a telemedical system for ambulance support (Xiao et al, 2000). In addition, other telemedical approaches that are not however bandwidth demanding, can also benefit from the advanced features of the 3G cellular systems. Such are for example the cases of Karlsten et al, Anantharaman et al, Rodriguez et al and Istepanian et al (Karlsten & Sjoqvist, 2000) (Anantharaman & Han, 2001) (Rodriguez et al, 2001) (Istepanian et al, 1999).

Apart from emergency telemedicine scenario, 3G telecommunication networks can ease tele-consultation in fields of medicine requiring transmission of high definition still images, such as dermatological Images, X-Ray Images, Magnetic Resonance Images, Ultrasound Images and Computed Tomography; scenarios comprising transmission of still images include tele-radiology, tele-ophthalmology, tele-dermatology, tele-dentistry and more. It is a known fact that the high resolution of these images produces heavy payloads of data when they are to be transmitted. For doctors inside or outside of the hospital area (among doctors of the same hospital or doctors situated in hospitals scattered wherever 3G communications are available), the knowledge sharing and distribution amongst them as regards diagnosis is significantly helpful.

Studies have proved how time-saving and thus effective the utilization of 3G networks (as compared to GSM and GPRS) can be, in terms of transmission time, throughput and network utilization (Perakis et al, 2005). GSM and GPRS networks, due to their lack of broad bandwidth availability, render the transmission of such payloads inefficient, almost impossible. Yet, 3G cellular networks have minimized the time required for the transmission of such images, reducing them up to a ratio of 8 times. Nevertheless, the GSM network has been utilized for the transmission of medical images. Such is the case of the transmission of CT images for tele-consultation proposed by Reponen et al (Reponen et al, 2000). 3G networks can also substitute satellite systems, as the ones proposed by Stewart et al, Takizawa et al and Yogesan et al for the transmission of medical images in the fields of tele-radiology and tele-ophthalmology (Stewart et al, 1999) (Takizawa et al, 2001) (Yogesan et al, 2000).

Nevertheless, it is in some occasions imperative that real time video needs to be transmitted. This situation is very common – and yet crucial – in cases of accidents where the patient's body has been heavily injured, and the conveyance of the patient from the place of the accident to the ambulance and respectively to the hospital requires delicate movements. It is obvious that real time audio-visual communication with the expert doctor is imperative. The visual contact is of vital importance since the transportation of the patients can lead to severe nerve injuries that can – and should - be avoided. It is a known fact that only specialized medical personnel should be in charge of accident victims' transportations. In the case the specialized doctor is inside the hospital, the tele-consultation takes place via fixed (high speed internet, xDSL or hospital LAN) or wireless networks (hotspots inside the hospital). In the case the specialized doctor is on the move, 3G cellular networks can be utilized by both parties. It is obvious that this can put extra strain to the network, yet the bandwidth is sufficient for bi-directional videoconferencing. This video-conferencing capability could also be very helpful in the case of an echography examination, as proposed by Ribeiro et al in 1999 (Ribeiro et. Al, 1999). Video-conferencing over 3G networks and more specifically transmission of ultrasound medical streams over 3G networks have also been evaluated during the OTELO project, as analyzed in the forthcoming paragraphs (Garawi et al, 2006). 3G networks do not only grant users with the necessary bandwidth for the video-conferencing (studies have concluded that for acceptable video-conferencing sessions, at least 2 ISDN lines which equal 128 kbps are required), but they also diminish frame losses due to the "soft hand-over" process.

Last but certainly not least, another field of medicine that requires continuous monitoring of patients, which can be enhanced by 3G broadband services but are not nevertheless critical in this situation is that of homecare. For patients with

Figure 3a. Emergency Telemedicine Scenario

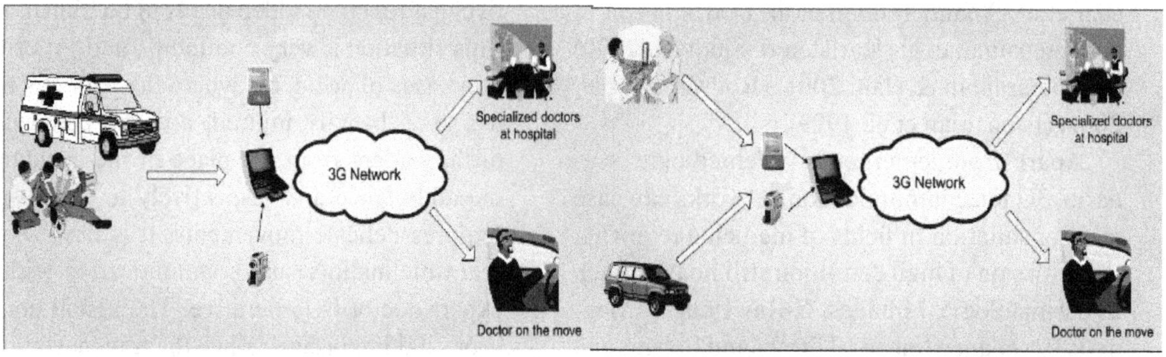

chronic diseases, continuous monitoring of critical data (Glucose measurements, Invasive and Non-Invasive Heart Rate (instances of hypertension), Saturation of Oxygen and other arithmetic data) can be both life-saving and self-assuring for the patients. Even in the cases of pregnant women, the continuous remote monitoring of both the mother's as well as the baby's medical data are crucial. Patients that are being monitored on a daily basis can be granted with complete freedom of movement and can pursue a normal everyday life. With continuous monitoring, the treating doctors have more and timely information as regards the patients' conditions and are able to provide better advice and suggest better treatment.

Several research approaches regarding homecare have been considered. Woodward et al have proposed the use of a telemedical system comprising a mobile telephone with sensors for patient monitoring, with the modular design of the system enabling telemedicine providers to adapt future mobile 3G standards (Woodward & Istepanian & Richards, 2001) (Istepanian, & Woodward & Richards, 2001). He has also described the modular design of an interface and processor for the transmission of multichannel biomedical signals over a Bluetooth to GPRS-based mobile cellular networks (Woodward & Rasid, 2005). Johnson et al have proposed the use of a wireless cardio-respiratory telemonitoring system for in-home use, while Mendoza et al and Elena at al have provided for heart-failure patients (Johnson et al, 2001) (Mendoza & Tran, 2002) (Elena et al, 2002). All these attempts could significantly boost their capabilities and services with the use of 3G cellular systems.

It is obvious that third generation communication systems are not only useful among paramedics and specialized doctors. They can be applied in a number of other incidents. Thus, they can be applied in organized extreme sport events, sports medicine and much more. After all, the market for para-health services and applications such as physical state monitoring during sports training is becoming increasingly common. Two scenarios, graphically illustrating the aforementioned mentioned scenarios are depicted in figures 3a and 3b. Figure 3a illustrates the emergency telemedicine scenario, where the paramedics can utilize a laptop combined with a 3G PCMCIA network card and a digital camera (or even a mobile phone with a high resolution VGA camera) in order to establish video-conferencing sessions with the specialized doctors and/or send images of the patients as well as screenshots of the medical equipment connected to the patient. Figure 3b illustrates the scenario of homecare and chronic disease management scenario.

RELATED RESEARCH

A plethora of research projects have either utilized and evaluated the 3G cellular networks, or have provided for their utilization. Apart from those however, various other projects could benefit from the advanced characteristics of 3G networks. For example, the **WardInHand** project (IST-1999-10479) allowed the management of key clinical information while providing decision support to mobile medical staff (Virtuoso, 2006). It provided a tool for workgroup collaboration and wireless access to the patients' clinical records. Thus, the medical stuff of a medical ward could make use of the system through the hospital WLAN, whereas during home visits fast and secure access could be granted via the 3G cellular networks.

The **TELEMEDICARE** (IST-1999-10754) incorporated advanced and reliable sensors on the body that supplied high quality medical data which were sent to the patient's computer through wireless communication (CORDIS: TELEMEDICARE, 2007) (TELEMEDICARE, 2007); the prize-winning **TeleInVivo** project (European Commission Telematics Technologies Program Project #HC4021) aimed at setting up a transportable telemedicine workstation, integrating in one custom-made device a portable PC with telecommunication capabilities and a light, portable 3D ultrasound station (TeleInVivo, 2007) (Kontaxakis & Sakas & Walter, 2006).

The **DOCMEM** project (IST-2000-25318) targeted ambulatory and in-hospital medical doctors and offered them an advanced interactive environment for getting a ubiquitous, permanent and intelligent access to patients' medical files. The work performed aimed at ensuring that the DOCMEM services were accessible through E-GPRS and would be scalable to UMTS networks (Eddabbeh & Drion, 2006).

The **Mobi-Dev** project (IST-2000-26402) constituted a European effort which addressed the increasingly demanding need of health professionals to effectively, accurately, securely, from anywhere, anytime and in a user-friendly way communicate with patients' databases located within hospitals, private offices, laboratories or pharmacies (CORDIS : Mobi-Dev, 2007). The Web Mobi-Dev, one of the outcomes of the project, consisting in an Internet-based wireless mobile system with speech understanding capabilities, corresponded to the project's original objectives, with the exception of UMTS support, that was not fully tested since this technology was still in a pre-commercial stage at the end of the project lifetime. Nevertheless, the supported UMTS connection permits the use of the system for transmitting large amounts of data (Mobi-Dev, 2007).

The **Healthmate** project (IST-2000-26154) contributed to the definition of a new generation of GPRS/UMTS portable personal systems (CORDIS : HealthMate, 2007). The project developed four tele-care innovative platforms to cope with a large number of potential client groups and health needs, also providing for UMTS interoperability, even though the UMTS networks were not available at the beginning of the project. Among the project objectives was to prioritize the continuity of care using the roaming capacity of GPRS and UMTS to move seamless from home cells to macro cells adjusting data rate on demand. As conceived, high bandwidth would permit to accomplish some features that were not possible with 2nd generation mobile telephony services (HealthMate, 2007).

The **AMON** project (IST-2000-25239) aimed to research, develop and validate an advanced, wearable personal health system that would monitor and evaluate human vital signs using advanced bio-sensors. The system gathered and analyzed vital information - including HR, 2-lead ECG, BP, SpO2, skin perspiration and body temperature - and transmitted the data to a remote telemedicine centre, for further analysis and emergency care, using GSM/UMTS cellular infrastructure (CORDIS : AMON, 2007). While first prototypes had problems with achieving the required medical accuracy on all the measurement, the tests have provided a clear indication of the feasibility of the concepts and validity of the solutions adapted by the project (AMON, 2007).

The **MobiHealth** project (IST-2001-36006) aimed at introducing new mobile value added services in the area of health, based on 2.5G and 3G technologies, through the integration of sensors and actuators to a Wireless Body Area Network (CORDIS : MobiHealth, 2007). These sensors and actuators would continuously measure and transmit vital constants along with audio and/or video to health service providers and brokers. A first objective of the MobiHealth project was to prove the advantages, the usefulness and the feasibility of the use of 2.5G and 3G infrastructures in e-health. Evaluation testing in 2003 showed the stability and effectiveness of the MobiHealth system as well as the feasibility of it being used in a wide range of medical fields (MobiHealth, 2007).

The **MOEBIUS** (Mobile Extranet Based Integrated User Services) project was an FP5 European Funded project, the objective of which was to develop a platform for remote access to intranet services using mobile access technology and investigate its performance characteristics to demonstrate the advantages for health care and business applications (MOEBIUS, 2007).

The **WEALTHY** "Wearable Healthcare System" system integrated computing techniques, smart sensors, portable devices and telecommunications, together with local intelligence and decision support system (WEALTHY, 2007). The system would assist patients during rehabilitation or subjects working in extreme stressful environment conditions ensure continuous intelligent monitoring. Smart material in fibber and yarn form endowed with a wide range of electro physical properties (conducting, piezoresistive, etc) were integrated and used as basic elements to be woven or knitted in fabric form. The simultaneous recording of vital signs would allow parameters extrapolation and inter-signal elaboration that contribute to make alert messages and synoptic patient table. The main objective of WEALTHY was to set up a wearable healthcare system that would improve patient or user autonomy and safety.

The **OTELO** project (IST-2001-32516) proposed the study and development of a fully integrated end-to-end mobile tele-echography system for population groups that were either temporarily or permanently not served locally by medical experts (CORDIS : OTELO, 2007). OTELO was a portable ultrasound probe holder robotic system, supported by mobile communications technologies, that reproduced the expert's hand movements during an ultrasound examination. The authors concluded that such advanced robotic m-health systems can successfully perform using commercial 3G networks [30]. In addition, 3G wireless communication technology can provide a cheaper and more convenient mobile medical service for the OTELO system.

The eTEN project **C-Monitor** (eTen-C27256) aimed at market validating a telecommunications platform for monitoring non-hospitalized patients, through which the patient could actively participate in his disease treatment and the doctors could monitor the disease condition of the patients more convenient, more flexible and change the treatment plan quickly based on the information acquired from the patients (CORDIS: C-MONITOR, 2007). Mobile patients and mobile physicians could interconnect through mobile networks, and be granted with the ubiquitous advantages, roaming capacity and seamless communication the UMTS could provide, along with higher data rates (C-MONITOR , 2007).

Furthermore, the eTEN project **LinkCare** (eTEN-C517435) aimed to market validate competitive services with a view to link health professionals in emerging care environments, incorporating 3 pilots, namely HCPB in Spain, CNRHA in Norway, and LITO in Cyprus (CORDIS: LinkCare, 2007) (LinkCare , 2007). The Cypriot pilot was based upon the project DITIS and is an Internet (web) based Group Collaboration system with secure fixed and mobile (GPRS/GSM/WAP) connectivity, that can greatly benefit from the 3G cellular networks. The system supported the dynamic creation, management and co-ordination of virtual collaborative medical teams, for the continuous treatment of patients with chronic diseases at home and specialist healthcare centers (Pitsillides et al, 2005). The Spanish pilot on the other hand was based on the Chronic Disease Management Model for COPD patients. The system integrated two main elements, the Chronic Patient Management Center and the Remote Access Units (DeToledo, 2002) (Del Pozo 2006). The RAU used by the medical staff during home visits (Mobile Home Visit Units) supported among others ubiquitous access to the chronic patient information database, and in order to communicate with the CPMC they utilized wireless networks (GSM/GPRS).

Other concluded projects that could also benefit from the use of 3G networks include the **MOMEDA**, the **Cardiology-On-The-Move** and the **EMERGENCY-112** projects, which had not provided for the use of broadband cellular networks since they were not available at the time.

LIMITATIONS

Third generations cellular networks however are not a panacea. According to the findings of Bults et al, services requiring fast, high capacities networks may be hindered by the restrictions imposed by the 3G network's goodput bottleneck and the asymmetric transmission capacity (Bults et al, 2005). The downlink capacity in 3G networks is much higher than that of the uplink, while the reverse is required in monitoring services, since the end-user (e.g. the patient) is the producer of information, transmitting high quantities of data. Val Jones et al conclude that we still suffer from limited bandwidth for some applications, such as those which require serving many simultaneous users with conversational applications requiring high-quality two-way audio and video, or generation of 3D animation in real time (Jones et al 2006). These networks also appear to have drawbacks and limitations, especially as regards their adaptation in the healthcare industry. The high cost of the communications links nearly precludes their use in everyday constant monitoring. Furthermore, the healthcare sector is a very complex industry, difficult to change, while the currently available telemedicine equipment can sometimes be difficult to handle, and thus meet the medical personnel's negative disposition in adopting them (Istepanian & Lacal, 2003). In addition, there is a lack of integration between mobile telemedicine systems and other information systems, while there are not enough numbers of demonstration projects that show mobile telemedicine's real savings potential (Istepanian & Jovanov & Zhang, 2004). Further issues that need to be further evaluated and resolved include the development of even more efficient modulation techniques, the allocation of new spectrum, the provision of personalized services as well as user acceptance issues (Nicopolitidis, 2002).

BENEFITS

According to the previously stated, we can conclude that the third generation telecommunications systems can can constitute a significant player as regards tele-medical applications. A great benefit to all users will be a more efficient management of medical resources and far greater independence. 3G cellular systems grant the users with flexible and swift access to expert opinion, as well as provide rapid responses to critical medical care regardless of geographical barriers. 3G cellular networks can improve on the one side the life of patients, as well as allow the introduction of new value-added services in the areas of disease prevention. The potential benefits of integrated wireless telemedicine based on 3G cellular networks can be summarized as follows (Tachakra et al, 2003):

1. It provides rapid response to critical medical care regardless of geographic barriers. Hence, severely injured patients can be managed locally and access to a trauma specialist obtained by wireless telemedicine.
2. Flexible and swift access to expert opinion and advice at the point of care without delay and better management of medical resources.
3. Interactive medical consultation and communication links of medical images and video data such as the videophones over Internet links in complete mobility and in global coverage and connectivity.
4. Increased empowerment and management of medical expertise especially in rural and underserved areas could be improved using these technologies.
5. The local hospitals usually do not share care or staff with larger hospitals. Consequently, some may suffer from weak medical and nursing staff who may be uncomfortable managing seriously ill patients.
6. Swift medical care can be made available in emergency and management of medical data in catastrophes or natural disasters where conventional communication links may be disrupted.

DISCUSSION

Utilization of 3G networks achieve a significant reduction as regards the time required for the transmission of data (biosignals, images and video of the patients) from the side of the patient to the side of the expert. Furthermore, the support of the "soft hand-over" process guarantees the stability of the flow of the transmitted data. Impermanent losses of signals may not be crucial in many real time applications, yet is crucial in cases where healthcare delivery is concerned and human lives are at risk. Nobody can doubt the fact that so far these third generation networks have not met the expectations they were supposed to meet when they were originally conceived. Nevertheless, since the number of 3G cells within every European country will keep increasing much like 2G cells did in the past, utilization of such broadband networks are bound to have an increasingly high field of application and a guaranteed success as more and more areas are covered by UMTS. And since the minimization of the time required for a patient to receive primary care has always been one of the utmost concerns of hospitals, health centers as well as ministries of health, the reduction of this time achieved by such networks is bound to make them an attractive solution.

REFERENCES

Benini, L. and DeMicheli, G. (2002). Networks on chips: a new paradigm for component-based MPSoC Design. *IEEE Computer*.

Brickell, E., Denning, D., Kent, S., Mahler, D. and Tuchman, W. (1993). SKIPJACK Review. *Interim Report*.

Christov, I. and Bortolan, G. (2004). Ranking of pattern recognition parameters for premature ventricular contractions classification by neural networks. *Physiological Measurement*, *25*(5), 1281-1290.

De Chazal, P., O'Dwyer, M. and Reilly, R. (2004). Automatic classification of heartbeats using ECG morphology and heartbeat interval features. *IEEE Trans. Biomedical Eng.*, *51*(7), 1196-1206.

DeVaul, R., Sung, M., Gips, J, and Pentland, A. (2003). Mithril 2003: Applications and architecture. *Seventh IEEE Symposium on IEEE Wearable Computers*. pp 4-11.

Ganesan, P., Venugopalan, R., Peddabachagari, P., Dean, A., Mueller, F., and Sichitiu, M. (2003). Analyzing and Modeling Encryption Overhead for Sensor Network Nodes. *Wireless Sensor*

Networks and Applications (WSNA 2004). San Diego, CA.

Gura, N., Patel, A., Wander, A., Eberle, H., and Shantz, S. (2004). Comparing elliptic curve cryptography and RSA on 8-bit CPUs. *Workshop on Cryptographic Hardware and Embedded Systems (CHES 2004).* Cambridge, MA.

Han, C., Rengaswamy, R., Shea, R., Kohler, E., and Srivastava, M. (2005). SOS: A Dynamic Operating System for Sensor Networks. *Third International Conference on Mobile Systems, Applications, and Services (Mobisys 2005).* Seattle, WA.

Health Insurance Portability and Accountability Act of 1996 (HIPAA) (1996). P.L. 104-191 Enacted H.R. 3103, August 21, 1996 110 Stat. 1936, codified 42 U.S.C. 1320.

Jafari, R., Dabiri, F., Brisk, P., and Sarrafzadeh, M. (2005a). Adaptive and fault tolerant medical vest for life critical medical monitoring. *20th ACM Symposium on Applied Computing (SAC 2005)*, March 2005. Santa Fe, NM.

Jafari, R., Dabiri, F., Sarrafzadeh, M. (2005b) .CustoMed: A power optimized customizable and mobile medical monitoring and analysis system. *ACM HCI Challenges in Health Assessment Workshop in conjunction with CHI 2005.* Portland, OR.

Jafari, R., Noshadi, H., Ghiasi, S., Sarrafzadeh, M. (2006a). Adaptive electrocardiogram feature extraction on distributed embedded systems. *IEEE Transactions on Parallel and Distributed Systems special issue on High Performance Computational Biology (TPDS), 17*(8), 1-11.

Jafari, R., Jindrich, D., Edgerton, V., Sarrafzadeh, M. (2006b). CMAS: Clinical Movement Assessment System for Neuromotor Disorders, *IEEE Biomedical Circuits and Systems Conference (BioCAS).* London, UK.

Karlof, C., Sastry, N., and Wagner, D. (2004). TinySec: A link layer security architecture for wireless sensor networks. *Second ACM Conference on Embedded Networked Sensor Systems (SenSys 2004).* Baltimore, MD.

Kastner, R., Ogrenci, S., Bozorgzadeh, E., Sarrafzadeh, M. (2001). Instruction generation for hybrid reconfigurable systems. *IEEE/ACM Intl Conf Computer-Aided Design (ICCAD).*

LeMoyne, R., Jafari, R., Jea, D., Srivastava, M., Sarrafzadeh, M. (2005). Fully quantified evaluation of myotatic stretch reflex. *Symp Neuroscience,* 2005.

Malan, D.J., Welsh, M., and Smith, M. D., (2004) A public-key infrastructure for key distribution in tinyos based on elliptic curve cryptography. *First IEEE International Conference on Sensor and Ad Hoc Communications and Networks,* Santa Clara, California.

Marculescu, D., Marculescu, R., Khosla, P. (2002). Challenges and opportunities in electronic textiles modeling and optimization. *Design Automation Conference*, pp 175-180.

Martin, T., Jones, M., Edmison, J, and Shenoy, R. (2003). Towards a design framework for wearable electronic textiles. *Seventh IEEE International Symposium on Wearable Computers,* pp 190-199.

Massey, T., Brisk, P., Dabiri, F., Sarrafzadeh, M. (2007). Delay aware, reconfigurable security for embedded systems. *Second International Conference on Body Area Networks (BodyNets 2007).* Florence, Italy.

Ogrenci S, Bozorgzadeh E, Kastner R, Sarrafzadeh M. (2001a). A super-scheduler for embedded reconfigurable systems. *IEEE/ACM Intl Conf Computer-Aided Design (ICCAD).*

Ogrenci S, Bozorgzadeh E, Kastner R, Sarrafzadeh M. (2001b). SPS: A strategically programmable system. *Reconfigurable Architectures Workshop (RAW).*

Perrig, A., Canetti, R. Tygar, J.D. and Song, D. (2002). The TESLA broadcast authentication protocol. *RSA Cryptobytes.*

Potlapally, N. Ravi, S., Raghunathan, A., Jha, N. (2003). Analyzing the energy consumption of security protocols. *International Symposium on Low Power Electronics and Design (ISLPED 2003).* Seoul Korea.

Ravi, S., Raghunathan, A., Kocher, P., and Hattangady, S. (2004). Security in Embedded Systems: Design Challenges. *ACM Transactions on Embedded Computing Systems, 3*(3), 461-491.

Rivest, R. (1995). The RC5 encryption algorithm. *1994 Leuven Workshop on Fast Software Encryption.* pp. 86-96.

Schaller, R. R. (1999). Moore's law: Past, present, and future. *IEEE Spectrum, 34*(6), 52-59.

Schaumont, P., Verbauwhede, I., Sarrafzadeh, M., and Keutzer, K. (2001). A quick safari through the reconfiguration jungle. *Design Automation Conference (DAC 2001).* Las Vegas, CA.

Titzer, B., Lee D., and Palsberg, J. (2005). Avrora: Scalable sensor network simulation with precise timing. *International Symposium on Information Processing in Sensor Networks (IPSN).* Los Angeles, California.

Watro, R., Kong, D., Cuti, S., Gardiner, C., Lynn, C., and Kruus, P. (2004). TinyPK : Securing sensor networks with public key technology. *2nd ACM Workshop on Security of Ad Hoc and Sensor Networks (SASN 2004).* Washington, D.C.

KEY TERMS

3G Systems: 3G systems can support higher data rates, thus allowing for a range of new applications. The integration of third generation telecommunication technologies in medicine could prove to be crucial in many aspects of remote provision of healthcare, which communication technologies used to-date (such as GSM or even GPRS) cannot support. Such systems can be used for tele-diagnosis, tele-monitoring and tele-consultation in various fields of medicine.

Cellular Networks: A cellular network is a radio network made up of a number of radio cells (or just cells) each served by a fixed transmitter, known as a cell site or base station. These cells are used to cover different areas in order to provide radio coverage over a wider area than the area of one cell. Cellular networks are inherently asymmetric with a set of fixed main transceivers each serving a cell and a set of distributed (generally, but not always, mobile) transceivers which provide services to the network's users. Cellular networks offer a number of advantages over alternative solutions like increased capacity, reduced power usage and better coverage.

GPRS: GPRS (short for general packet radio service) is a new non-voice, value added, high-speed, packet-switching technology for GSM networks. It facilitates sending and receiving small bursts of data, such as email and web browsing, as well as large volumes of data over a mobile telephone network. Its main innovations are that it is packet based, it increases data transmission speeds, and extends the Internet connection all the way to the mobile PC – the user no longer needs to dial up to a separate Internet Service Provider.

GSM: Global system for mobile communications (GSM) is the most popular standard for mobile phones in the world. Its promoter, the GSM Association, estimates that 82% of the global mobile market uses the standard. GSM is used by over 2 billion people across more than 212 countries and territories.Its ubiquity makes international roaming very common between mobile phone operators, enabling subscribers to use their phones in many parts of the world. GSM differs from its predecessors in that both signalling and speech channels are digital call quality, and thus is considered a *second generation* (2G) mobile phone system. This has also meant that data communication was easy to build into the system.

Telemedicine: Telemedicine is a rapidly developing application of clinical medicine where medical information is transferred via telephone, the Internet or other networks for the purpose of consulting, and sometimes remote medical procedures or examinations. Telemedicine may be as simple as two health professionals discussing a case over the telephone, or as complex as using satellite technology and video-conferencing equipment to conduct a real-time consultation between medical specialists in two different countries. Telemedicine generally refers to the use of communications and information technologies for the delivery of clinical care.

UMTS: UMTS stands for universal mobile telecommunication System and constitutes Europe's implementation of the 3G Telecommunications Systems. These new systems are a significant innovation over 2G and 2.5G systems because of their high operating flexibility, their ability to provide a wide range of applications and generally extend the services now provided to fixed networks users to mobile customers. Contrary to the current GSM systems, UMTS allows for broadband data communication to mobile units, packet-based transmission of text, digitized voice, video, and multimedia, offering a set of services to mobile computer and phone users no matter where they are located in the world.

Chapter XVIII
Telemedicine Consultations in Daily Clinical Practice:
Systems, Organisation, Efficiency

Anton V. Vladzymyrskyy
Association for Ukrainian Telemedicine and eHealth Development & Donetsk R&D Institute of Traumatology and Orthopedics, Ukraine

ABSTRACT

This chapter introduces usage of telemedicine consultations in daily clinical practice. Author has describe process of teleconsultation, sample schemes of systems, parties of this process and its roles. Also, main steps of clinical teleconsultation (determination of necessity for teleconsultation, preparation of medical information, observance of ethics and law conditions, preparation of conclusion) are shown. Special part is dedicated to efficiency of teleconsultation – author has propose own complex method for estimation of it. Furthermore, the authors hope that understanding of teleconsultations' process will make it more accessible and easy-to-use for medical practitioners.

INTRODUCTION

In this chapter the author describe approaches to usage of telemedicine consultation in daily clinical practice. First teleconsultations described at 1910s (published in JTT, 1997). Since that time telemedicine is use wide range of technologies – TV, satellite, Internet, cellular etc – for discussion of serious clinical cases at distance (Bashshur et al,1997, Kamaev et al, 2001, Nerlich et al,1999, Vladzymyrskyy,2004). Annually in the world are spent thousands teleconsultations. It is possible to say that this procedure is most wide spread telemedicine service.

Teleconsultation (telemedicine, remote consultation) – remote discussion of the clinical case via special computer information and telecommunication system to get answers to precisely formulated questions for the help in clinical decisions (Vladzymyrskyy,2003).

Author has propose classification of teleconsultation by 3 main classes: terms of teleconsultation leading, sort (kind) of organisation and technical platform.

1. **By term:**
   - **Synchronous:** All parties use the same telemedicine system in the same time (in real time);
   - **Asynchronous:** All parties use the same telemedicine system with time delay (sequential use).

2. **By sort:**
   - **Formal:** Two or more organizations were involved under a previously signed contract/protocol/agreement;
   - **Informal:** Free discussions of clinical cases in professional Internet societies (via mailing lists, Web-forums);
   - **Second opinion:** Teleconsultations for patients who contacted a medical organization by email or via a special online form/forum.

3. **By technical basis:**
   - Systems at the base of Internet and its services (e-mails, Web-platforms, mailing lists, IP-phones, IP-videoconferences, chats, messengers etc);
   - Systems at the base of special links (satellite, ISDN, ftn-protocol, computer health networks etc);

Systems at the base of cellular phoniness and its services (mobile Internet, SMS, MMS, voice etc).

SYSTEMS OF TELECONSULTATION

As we can see in Figure 1, there are 4 main participants of teleconsultation process (Vladzymyrskyy,2003):

Figure 1. Sample scheme of teleconsultation

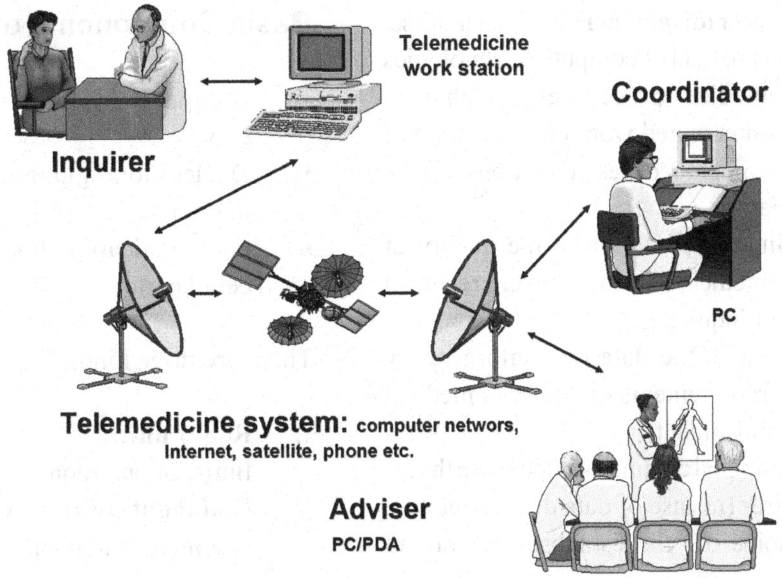

1. **Inquirer:** Legal or physical person representing a clinical case for the teleconsultation. Most frequently inquirer is the "face-to-face" physician/nurse, also - patient or relatives (in case of self-reference for teleconsultation, "second opinion"). Functions of the Inquirer:
   - Granting of the clinical case for teleconsultation, formulation of questions;
   - Registration of the medical documents according to the requirements of the adviser (digitalization, translation into foreign language etc.);
   - Granting the additional information by inquiry of the adviser;
   - Participation in synchronous procedures.

2. **Adviser:** Expert or group of the experts considering the clinical case which was presented for the teleconsultation. Functions of the Adviser:
   - Consideration and consultation of the clinical case in the stipulated terms;
   - Granting the conclusion with use of the standard medical terminology;
   - Participation in synchronous procedures.

3. **Coordinator (dispatcher):** Physician/nurse, expert in the field of computer technologies and telemedical procedures, which provides uninterrupted work on realization of telemedical procedures. Functions of the Coordinator:
   - Primary estimation of the quality of the medical data which were received from inquirer;
   - Check of the data on conformity by the requirements of adviser's medical establishment;
   - Additional communications with the inquirer (in case of data discrepancy);
   - Choice of the establishment or/and personal adviser for the teleconsultation;
   - Sending electronic case history to the adviser or/and in other telemedical centre;
   - Decision of organizational and financial questions of the telemedical network.
4. **Assistant:** Technical expert serving telemedical system. Functions of the Assistant:
   - Maintenance of technical readiness for telemedical system;
   - Elimination of technical failures and malfunctions;
   - Technical support and consultation of other participants of the telemedical procedure.

Technically teleconsultations realized by use of telemedicine work stations which linked by any telecommunication protocol.

Telemedicine work station (TWS) – complex of the hardware and software (multitask workplace) with opportunities of digitalization, input, processing, transformation, conclusion, classification and archiving of the any kinds of the medical information and realization of telemedical procedures (teleconsultation) (Vladzymyrskyy,2003).

Basic Components of Clinical TWS :

- Computer (PC, notebook, tablet, PDA etc);
- Devices for digitalisation of medical information;
- Communication line (Internet, satellite, cellular etc).

There are three kinds of clinical TWS:

1. **Room unit:** Not moving TWS within the limits of one room (office).
2. **Rollabout unit:** Moving version of TWS mounted on a mobile table. Such TWS can

easily be moved from one room to another (from physician's office to patients' yard etc).

3. **Mobile unit:** Moving TWS for outside/out-hospital telemedical procedures.

In daily clinical practice practitioners most often use next systems for teleconsultations:

1. TWS+Internet/Satellite/ISDN link.
2. TWS+special digital diagnostic equipment+Internet/Satellite/ISDN link.
3. TWS+special digital diagnostic equipment+kit for wide format videoconf erences+Internet/Satellite/ISDN link.
4. TWS at the base of cellular phone/ communicator+Mobile Internet /MMS link.

As an example of decision for clinical teleconsultation system author can propose own Best practice model, which was recognized by International Society for Telemedicine and eHealth (ISfTeH) in 2005.

Best Practice Model for Telemedical Equipment

Background: for any kind of telemedical procedures it's necessary: (1) to create an effective telemedical work station (TWS) with adequate free or/and licensed software, (2) connect TWS to some kind of telecommunication line.

The basic requirements for telemedical equipment: an opportunity of processing of any kind of the medical information, cheapness, standardisation, availability, simplicity and reliability of use, technical and information safety.

Main goals:

- Equipment for telemedical work station,
- Telecommunication lines,
- Software.

Decisions

We are propose a few sets for telemedicine work station.

Classical set for TWS: basis PC, SVGA monitor, multimedia equipment, CDROM/CDRW/ DVD, network adapter, high quality scanner, digital photocamera, digital videocamera, Web-camera, high quality colour printer, microphone, dynamics, modem, connector to hospital information system, sets of special digital equipment for diagnostic and treatment, auxiliary equipment.

Clinical set for TWS: basis PC, SVGA monitor, multimedia equipment, CDROM, network adapter, digital photocamera, printer, modem, auxiliary equipment.

Minimal set for TWS: basis PC, SVGA monitor, high quality scanner or digital photocamera, modem.

Optimal clinical set for TWS: basis PC, SVGA monitor, multimedia equipment, CDROM or CDRW, high quality scanner, digital photocamera, Web-camera, printer, modem, auxiliary equipment.

Example: in daily clinical practice we use TWS: PC (1000 Mhz and more) with multimedia equipment, scanner (1200 dpi and more), digital photocamera (1,3-3 mpx), printer (laser, 600x600 dpi and more), film-viewer, Web-camera.

Telecommunication lines - best ways:

- Direct and dial-up Internet lines for any kind of telemedical procedures;
- Mobile phones services for emergency teleconsultations.

Direct Internet lines (256 Kb and more, for videoconferences 512 Kb at least) intercity, interregional communications, communications between big regional hospitals and medical universities. Dial-up Internet lines (56 Kb and more) – for intraregional, intracity, rural-city communications. SMS/MMS services – for any kind of emergency teleconsultations.

Software

Its possible to use special or non-special software for telemedical procedures. We prefer:

- Standard licensed software from Microsoft™;
- Web-application designed with open code (optimal for medical establishments with low financial support);
- Special telemedical application on the base on Internet (for example, "Regional Telemedical System" ™).

Thus, in general any system for teleconsultation consist from telemedicine work stations, telecommunication lines and human factors (Inquirer, Adviser, Coordinator, Assistant). Gathering of work stations and selection of communication kind should be evidence-based and can be grounded at best practice models of worldwide eHealth organizations.

ORGANISATION OF TELECONSULTATION

Teleconsultation is the process, which consist of two main points:

1. Sending remote expert digital medical information about patients with *maximal* high diagnostic accuracy and with *minimal* volume.
2. Organization of an effective feedback.

In Figure 2, you can see the main steps of teleconsultation: digitalization of medical information, information exchange, notification about results.

As we can understand that for making medical information digital we are need equipment (some telemedicine work station); for digital information exchange we are need telecommunication

Figure 2. Main steps of sample teleconsultation

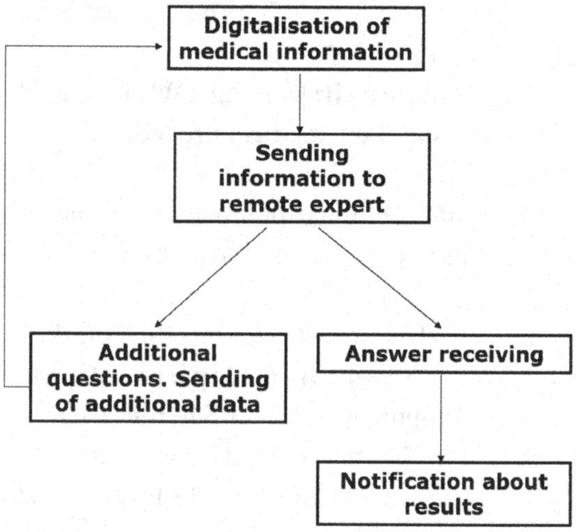

(some data bearer); and for notification about results of teleconsultation we are need methods for estimation of efficiency. Thus, it is possible to use almost any computer and telecommunication technology/tool for teleconsultation. Only one condition: this technology/tool should support digitalization, data transfer and feedback. So, there are 4 main steps for choice of the most effective technology (Figure.3).

Figure 3. Main steps for choice of the most effective technology for teleconsultation

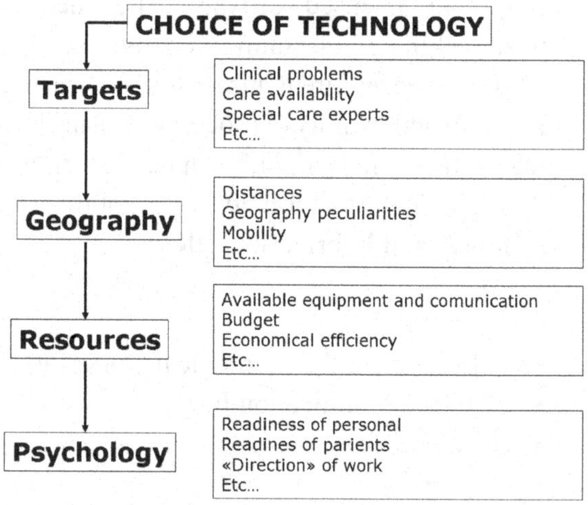

Figure 4. Algorithm for choice of the telemedical technology

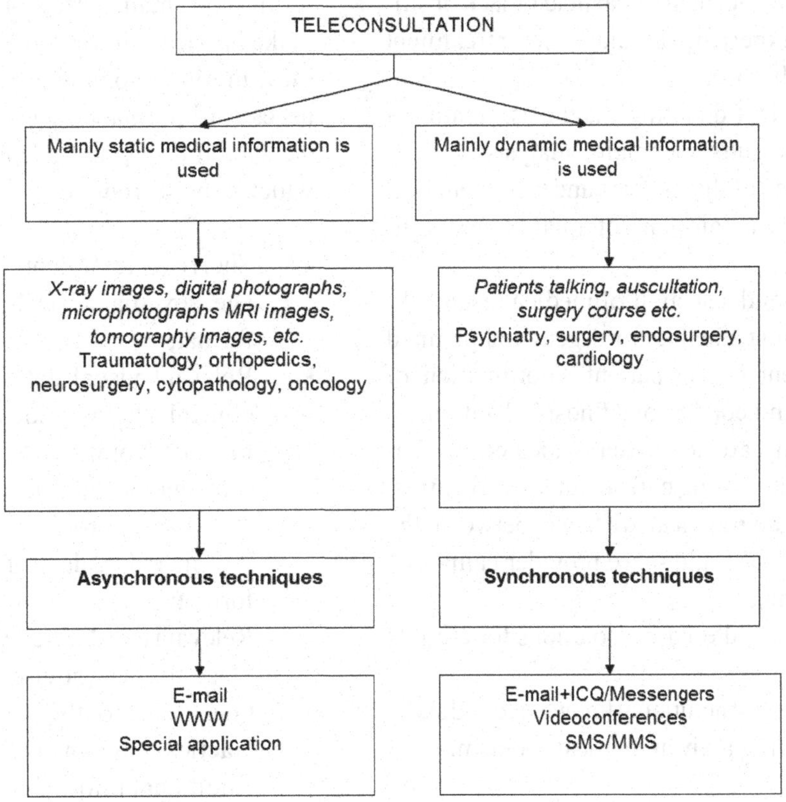

For example, early author had developed the algorithm which enables quick choice of the most suitable telemedical technique for a present clinical situation (Figure 4) (Vladzymyrskyy,2005). Synchronous teleconsultations are most suitable where dynamic types of medical information prevail, e.g. in psychiatry (direct communication between physician and the patient is of importance) and emergency surgery. Asynchronous teleconsultations are most suitable where static types of medical information prevail, e.g. trauma surgery, orthopaedics, dermatology, cytology, pathology.

In clinical practice teleconsultation include four main steps:

1. Determination of necessity for teleconsultation.
2. Preparation of medical information.
3. Observance of ethics and law conditions.
4. Preparation of conclusion.

For determination of necessity for teleconsultation it is possible to use list of iindications for teleconsultation in daily clinical practice (Vladzymyrskyy,2005):

- Determination (confirmation) of diagnosis;
- Determination (confirmation) of treatment;
- Determination of diagnosis and treatment of rare, severe diseases or diseases with a non-typical course;
- Determination of complication prevention methods;
- Need for a new and/or infrequent surgery (for treatment or diagnosis) or procedure;

- Lack of immediate specialists in the necessary or adjacent medical field or lack of sufficient experience for diagnosis or treatment of the disease;
- The patient doubting diagnosis, treatment and its results, complaint analysis;
- Decrease of diagnostics and treatment cost without impairment of quality and efficiency;
- Search and selection of medical establishment most suitable for urgent and planned treatment of the patient, coordination of terms and conditions of hospitalization;
- Medical care for patients located at considerable distance from medical centres, when geographical distance between the patient and health-care provider cannot be overcome;
- Search for alternative solutions for clinical tasks;
- Obtaining of additional knowledge and skills concerning a given medical problem.

For preparation of medical information practitioner needs equipment and rules for telemedicine case records. As you can see before telemedicine work station is use for digitalisation and exchanging of relevant medical information. Digitalisation could be done by to ways:

- Initial reception of medical data in the digital kind (from special computer aided/digital diagnostic equipment);
- "Manual digitalization" of medical data (by cameras, scanners, digitizers etc).

In clinical practice digital photo/video cameras, scanners, document cameras and film digitizers are widely adopted for preparation of medical information for teleconsultation.

After digitalization special processing should be perform, which include: elimination of not informative areas; reduction of volume without loss of diagnostic value; correction of images without loss of diagnostic value; anonymity.

In short, main targets of such processing – to make medical information with: maximal accuracy, minimal volume, safe. When we have all necessary information about patient in digital form we should to prepare telemedicine case record, which consist from:

- Short case text (identifier of the patient, date, age, sex, diagnosis, brief anamnesis) - text format;
- Relevant visual data (x-rays, CTs, MRIs, clinical photos, videoclips etc) - graphic files or dicom;
- Explanation data (accompanying text, anatomic area, projection, method of colouring, increase, date of research etc.) - text format;
- Relevant text data (clinical tests, opinions of "face-to-face" advisers etc) - text format;
- Questions to the adviser ("diagnosis?", "tactics of treatment?" etc) - text format;
- Additional information - any format.

The basic requirements for the telemedicine case record:

- Information and methodical conformity of the standard paper/electronic case record;
- As it is possible the smaller size of files with minimal losses of diagnostic value;
- Conformity to standards;
- Flexibility (an opportunity of use at any technological decisions);
- Safety.

3. Observance of ethics and law conditions could be done in frame of telemedicine deontology.

Telemedicine Deontology is a professional etiquette and a complex of moral requirements for the persons practising a telemedicine, principles of behaviour for medical, technical and support personnel.

Main problems of telemedicine deontology:

1. Observance of laws and ethical norms
2. Preservation of Medical Information
3. Attitudes — doctor-patient-information system"
5. Attitudes—inquirer-coordinator-adviser", "doctor-technician"
6. Physical and information safety of telemedicine systems
7. Standardisation and documentation
8. Information consent

For teleconsultation practice we should understand and adopt next rules:

1. Teleconsultation is used for the help in acceptance of the clinical decision.
2. Last decision must be accepted by the attending physician (inquirer).
3. The attending "face-to-face" physician should bear all responsibility for the patient due to using or not using of recommendations of the distant expert.
4. Information consent and signed agreement of patient should be best practice.
5. Main ways for teleconsultation safety: patients consent, anonymisation, login/password access for all telemedical work stations, digital signature system.

So, after remote discussion expert should prepare formal conclusion, which consist from:

1. General part (identifier of the patient, date and time of inquiry, date and time of conclusion, advisers' full name, place of work, degrees, posts) - text format.
2. Conclusion (answers to questions of the inquirer, additional information) - text format
3. Appendix (explaining Figures, example of the similar clinical case, the references to the literature and Internet etc.) - any format (text, graphic files, video etc).

Note that the Appendix is most important part, because opinion of expert should have evidence-based background.

Thus, choice of technology for teleconsultation (e-mail, IP-phone, videoconference etc) should be first of all grounded at medical targets, available recourses and clinical situation. Author has propose approaches and decisions for main steps of daily clinical telemedicine, include indications for teleconsultation, ways and methods for digitalisation of medical information, ethical rules, telemedicine case record description.

EFFICIENCY OF TELECONSULTATION

Usually researchers consider financial benefits (Bergmo,1997, PalaninathaRaja,2006), changes of clinical parameters (Chan,2000, Lambrecht,1997, Vladzymyrskyy,2004), moral, technical aspects and management improvements (Aoki,2003, Rosser,2000, Siden,1998, Rendina,1998) of teleconsultations. The complex estimation of quality of telemedical consultation is extremely actual question. Such method should be reliable, simple and accessible for any researcher (scientists, medical doctor, decision maker etc.). It should be the set of objective criteria which it would be possible to use for statistical processing with the purpose of comparison, studying of different kinds of telemedical consultations etc.

Author has propose three groups of parameters: relevance, economic feasibility, quality indicators.

Relevance. In some sources for the characteristic of efficiency of telemedicine the term "relevance" is used. In modern informatics relevance in information retrieval, measures a

Table 1. Scale for objective judgment of teleconsultation's relevance

1. Terms. Teleconsultation is lead:		
	Before the necessary terms	3
	In the necessary terms	3
	After necessary terms	2
	In terms of full loss of the urgency	1
2. Conformity of answers:		
	Full conformity	3
	Incomplete conformity of answers to questions, an illegibility of formulations and recommendations	2
	Discrepancy of answers to questions	1
3. Presence of the additional confirming information (articles, links, references, similar clinical cases etc), evidence-based recommendations:		
	Yes	3
	No	1
4. Influence on the clinical tactics:		
	Tactics of the adviser is completely accepted	3
	Essential change of own tactics	2
	Acknowledgement of own tactics	2
	Refusal of adviser's recommendations	1
5. Inquiry for additional diagnostic tests:		
	No/ Accessible tests	3
	Accessible tests with an investment of significant expenses (work, money)	2
	Inaccessible tests	1
6.Expert has propose:		
	One clinical program	3
	A few clinical programs	2
	Preconditions for formation of the program	1
7. A few distant experts take a part:		
	Yes	3
	No	1
8. Transportation after teleconsultation		
	Yes	1
	No	3

document's applicability to a given subject or query. For telemedicine I am offered the following formulation.

Relevance of teleconsultation: Conformity of the distant adviser's answer to information and medical needs of the attending physician (inquirer).

There are two kinds of an estimation of relevance (Rel): subjective and objective. In the clinical practice for value judgment we are use an approximate individual estimation on 3 mark scale: discrepancy of answers to questions - 1 point; incomplete conformity of answers to questions, an illegibility of formulations and recommendations - 2 points; full conformity of answers to questions, presence of the additional confirming information (articles, links, references, similar clinical cases etc) - 3 points. By the given scale it is possible to define quantity and relative density of high, average and low relevant answers in group of homogeneous teleconsultations (by pathology, by technical system etc).

For an objective estimation author had developed the questionnaire (see table). The questionnaire for definition of relevance includes 7 questions with several variants of answers. Each answer is estimated from 1 up to 3 points. The score within the limits of 17-21 points shows on high, 12-16 - average, 7-11 - low relevance of the lead teleconsultation. Also, there is an opportunity to define relevance for telemedical system (Rel_{sys}) for the some period of time:

$$Rel_{sys} = \frac{TK_{rel}}{TK},$$

TK_{rel} - quantity of teleconsultations with specific relevance (high and/or average), TK - total quantity of teleconsultations. Accordingly, in ideal situation this parameter aspires to 1.

Economic feasibility. Most often define the prime price (S_{tk}) and profitability (R_{tk}) of teleconsultations. Definition of one teleconsultation's cost can be spent proceeding according laws and instructions accepted in the given state (at the base of calculation of the cost price of medical service). For example, calculation of cost of simple medical service:

$$S=S1+S2=Z+H+M+I+O+P,$$

S1 - direct charges, S2 - indirect charges, Z - salary, H - taxes, M - charges for medicines, equipment etc, I - deterioration of materials, O - deterioration of equipment, P - miscellaneous costs.

Also, it is possible to use already developed methods. For example, the cost price of telemedical service (teleconsultation) by Kamaev et al, 2001:

$$S_{tk}=(S1+S2+S3) * (1+S)+A+D+C+G+SO+P,$$

S1- salary of the medical personnel; S2 - salary of the technician personnel; S3 - salary of the other personnel (administrative, auxiliary); S - deductions in social funds; A - amortization of the equipment; D - deterioration of equipment; C - cost of materials; G - general charges of establishment, SO - services of other organizations (providers etc); P- profit.

Profitability (R_{tk}) of telemedicine services of hospital, clinics etc is defined by the formula (where C – price of rendered services, S – prime cost of rendered services):

$$R_{tk} = \frac{C-S}{C}.$$

After calculation of S_{tk} and R_{tk} researcher can compare results with other servicies. For example, there is an opportunity to economically compare telemedical consultation and traditional consultation.

Quality Indicators

Quality indicators estimate for certain sample of teleconsultations. For example, lead in the certain period of time or by specific technology. There are five quality indicators: parameter of presence/absence of the expert's answer (A); parameter of average duration (T); average quantity of the experts' answers (Aq); timeliness of teleconsultations (Pt); quality of teleconsultations (Pq). First three indicators are most simple. The A-parameter can have two values: 0 - absence of the answer, 1 - presence of the answer. It is possible to define a parity of taken place and not taken place teleconsultations by A-parameter. The T-parameter estimate for sample of teleconsultations as an arithmetical mean (in numerator - the sum of durations of all teleconsultations, in denominator - quantity of teleconsultations):

$$\overline{T} = \frac{\sum_{i=1}^{n} T_i}{n}.$$

Figure 5. Algorithm for an estimation of teleconsultations' efficiency

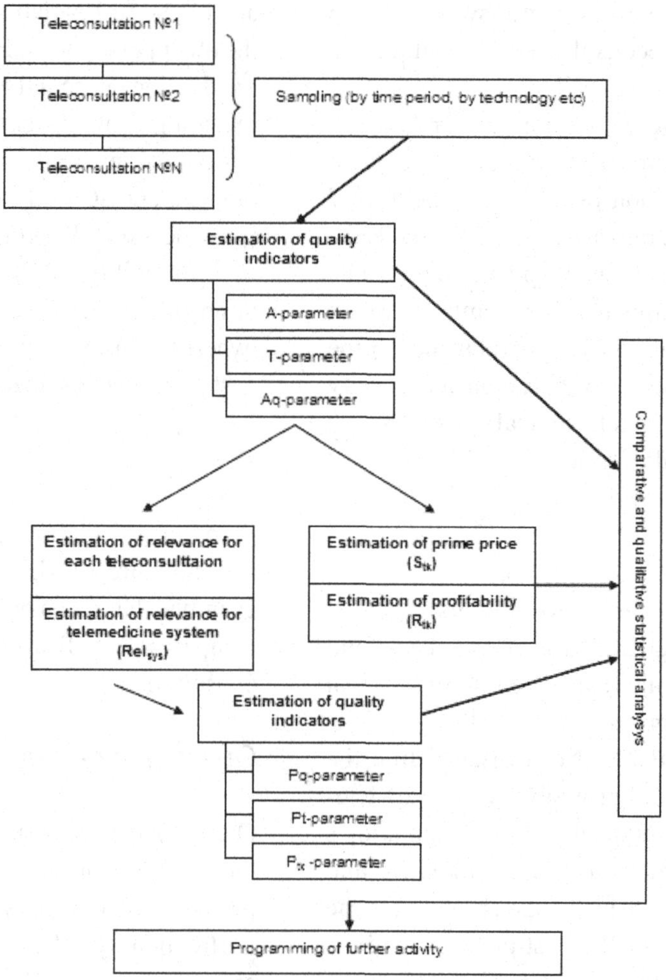

The Aq-parameter estimation, at the base of [14] (in numerator - quantity of answers (experts), in denominator - quantity of teleconsultations):

$$\overline{Aq} = \frac{\sum_{i=1}^{n} Aq_i}{n}.$$

Timeliness of teleconsultations (Pt) estimate on the basis of method by [4] (in numerator - quantity of duly received teleconsultations during certain time, in denominator - total quantity of teleconsultations for the same period of time):

$$Pt = \frac{m(t \le t_{cert})}{n_t}.$$

Quality of teleconsultations (Pq) also estimate on the basis of method by [4] (m - quantity of teleconsultations of admissible quality, n - total quantity of teleconsultations):

$$Pq = \frac{m}{n}.$$

It is possible to understand "quality of teleconsultation" as relevance or other certain estimation, for example, the quantity of teleconsultations with more than one answer so on. With help of two last criteria we can calculate probability of effective teleconsultation - (P_{tk}) (Gerasimov et al,2006):

$$P_{tk} = P_t * P_q,$$

In ideal situation this parameter aspires to 1. By P_{tk}- parameter researcher can estimate activity of telemedical system in general and, moreover, predict efficiency of teleconsultation after introduction of some technical, clinical, organizational, economical decision for telemedicine.

In Figure 5 you can see an algorithm for an estimation of teleconsultations' efficiency on the basis of the offered complex method.

Thus, there are three groups of parameters in complex method for investigation of efficiency (quality) of telemedicine consultations: relevance (Rel, Rel_{sys}), economic feasibility (compare of prime price (S_{tk}) and profitability (R_{tk})), quality indicators (A-parameter of answers, T-parameter of duration, Aq-parameter of answers' quantity, Pt-parameter of timeliness, Pq-parameter of quality, and also P_{tk} - probability of effective teleconsultation). In clinical practice it is better to use given method by special algorithm.

CONCLUSION

Thus, clinical teleconsultation is the process which include gathering of telemedicine work station, choice of telecommunication kind, participation of four parties (Inquirer, Adviser, Coordinator and Assistant - everyone of them has own special aims and functions), digitalisation of medical information, generation of telemedicine case record, information exchange, estimation of results and outcomes. Wide improvement of an effective telemedicine consultation systems in daily clinical practice open new ways for increasing of health care quality and capacity, "bring on" special care to rural and remote areas, makes clinical decisions easy and better.

REFERENCES

Aoki N, Dunn K, Johnson-Throop K. A., Turley J. P. (2003). Outcomes and methods in telemedicine evaluation. *Telemed J E Health, 9*(4),393-401.

Bashshur R. L., Sanders J. H., Shannon G. W., (1997). *Telemedicine: Theory and practice. springfield.* ILL. C.C. Thomas Publisher, Ltd.

Bergmo T. S. (1997). An economic analysis of teleconsultation in otorhinolaryngology. *J Telemed Telecare, 3*, 194–199.

Chan F. Y., Soong B., Lessing K., et al (2000). Clinical value of real-time tertiary fetal ultrasound consultation by telemedicine: preliminary evaluation. *Telemed J, 6*, 237–242.

Classic episodes in telemedicine. Treatment by telegraph (1917). *Excerpt from the obituary of John Joseph Holland (1876-1959).* JTT.1997;3:223.

Gerasimov B., Oxijuk A., Gulak N., (2006). Estimation of efficiency of the systems for support of decision-making. In *System of Support of Decision Making Theory and Practice.* Kiev, 25-7. (rus.)

Kamaev I., Levanov V., Sergeev D., (2001). *Telemedicine: Clinical, organisational, law, technological, economical aspects.* N. Novgorod: NGMA,. (rus.)

Lambrecht CJ. Telemedicine in trauma care: description of 100 trauma teleconsults. Telemed J 1997;3:265–268.

Nerlich M., Kretschmer R., (1998). The impact of telemedicine on health care management. In *Proceedings of the G 8 Global Health Care Applications Project (GHAP) Conference.* Regensburg, Germany, 21 November. Stud Health Technol Inform 1999; 64: 1-281

PalaninathaRaja M., Wadhwa S., Deshmukh S. G. (2006). Cost-benefit analysis on eHealthcare services. *Ukr. z. telemed.med.telemat, 1*(4), 53-64.

Rendina M. C., Downs S. M., Carasco N., Loonsk J., Bose C. L., (1998). Effect of telemedicine on health outcomes in 87 infants requiring neonatal intensive care. *Telemed J, 4*, 345–351.

Rosser J. C., Jr., Prosst R. L., Rodas E. B., Rosser L. E., Murayama M., Brem H., (2000). Evaluation of the effectiveness of portable low-bandwidth telemedical applications for postoperative followup: initial results. *J Am Coll Surg, 191*, 196–203.

Siden H. B., (1998). A qualitative approach to community and provider needs assessment in a telehealth project. *Telemed J, 4*, 225–235.

Vladzymyrskyy A., Chelnokov A., (2006). Relevance of telemedicine consultation. *Ukr. z.telemed.med.telemat, 1*(4), 99-100.

Vladzymyrskyy A. V. (2005). Four years' experience of teleconsultations in daily clinical practice. *JTT, 6*(11), 294-97.

Vladzymyrskyy A. V. (2003). Klynycheskoe teleconsultirovanie. *Rukovodstvo dlya Vrachei [Clinical Teleconsultation. Manual for Physicians]*. Sevastopol: OOO "Veber", 125 (rus.)

Vladzymyrskyy A. V. (2004). The Use of Teleconsultations in the Treatment of Patients with Multiple Trauma. *Europ J Trauma, 6*(30), 394-7.

KEY TERMS

Adviser: Expert or group of the experts considering the clinical case which was presented for the teleconsultation.

Assistant: Technical expert serving telemedical system.

Coordinator: Physician/nurse, expert in the field of computer technologies and telemedical procedures, which provides uninterrupted work on realization of telemedical procedures.

CT: Abbreviation of computer tomography.

Inquirer: Legal or physical person representing a clinical case for the teleconsultation. Most frequently inquirer is the "face-to-face" physician/nurse, also - patient or relatives (in case of self-reference for teleconsultation, "second opinion").

IP: Abbreviation of Internet Protocol.

ISDN: Abbreviation of Integrated Service Digital Network.

MRI: Abbreviation of magnetic resonance imaging.

MMS: Abbreviation of multimedia messaging system.

Relevance of Teleconsultation: Conformity of the distant adviser's answer to information and medical needs of the attending physician (inquirer).

Teleconsultation (Telemedicine, Remote Consultation): Remote discussion of the clinical case via special computer information and telecommunication system to get answers to precisely formulated questions for the help in clinical decisions.

Telemedicine Deontology: Is a professional etiquette and a complex of moral requirements for the persons practising a telemedicine, principles of behaviour for medical, technical and support personnel.

Telemedicine Work Station (TWS): Complex of the hardware and software (multitask workplace) with opportunities of digitalization, input, processing, transformation, conclusion, classification and archiving of the any kinds of the medical information and realization of telemedical procedures (teleconsultation).

TWS: Abbreviation of telemedicine work station.

Chapter XIX
Ubiquitous Healthcare:
Radio Frequency Identification (RFID) in Hospitals

Cheon-Pyo Lee
Carson-Newman College, USA

J. P. Shim
Mississippi State University, USA

ABSTRACT

Ubiquitous healthcare has become possible with rapid advances in information and communication technologies. Ubiquitous healthcare will bring about an increased accessibility to healthcare providers, more efficient tasks and processes, and a higher quality of healthcare services. radio frequency identification (RFID) is a key technology of ubiquitous healthcare and enables a fully automated solution for information delivery, thus reducing the potential for human error. This chapter provides an overview of ubiquitous healthcare and RFID applications. In this chapter, the background of ubiquitous computing and RFID technologies, current RFID applications in hospitals, and the future trends and privacy implications of RFID in hospitals are discussed.

INTRODUCTION

Advances in wireless networking, the Internet, and embedded systems move us toward ubiquitous computing. Ubiquitous computing refers to the creation and deployment of computing technology in such a way that it is embedded in our natural movements and interaction with our environments (Lyytinen and Yoo, 2002). Ubiquitous computing enhances computer use by making computers available throughout the physical environment, while making them effectively invisible to the user (Weiser, 1993).

With rapid advances in information and communication technologies, ubiquitous healthcare has become possible. Ubiquitous, or pervasive, healthcare refers to healthcare to anyone, anytime, and anywhere by removing location, time and other restraints while increasing both the coverage and quality of healthcare (Varshney, 2005). radio frequency identification (RFID) is a key technology of ubiquitous healthcare. RFID is a technology used to identify, track, and trace a person or an object without using a human to read and record data and enables the automated collection of important business information (Asif and Mandviwalla, 2005). In hospitals, RFID enables a fully automated solution for information delivery at the patient's bedside, thus reducing the potential for human error and increased efficiency (ITU, 2005).

The use of RFID technology in the healthcare market is on rise. A recent study reports that the global market for RFID tags and systems in the healthcare industry will increase steadily from \$90 million in 2006 to \$2.1billion by 2016 (Harrop and Das, 2006). The purpose of this chapter is to present an overview of ubiquitous healthcare and RFID in hospitals. Specifically, the chapter introduces the background of ubiquitous computing and RFID technologies, current RFID applications in the healthcare industry, the future trends and privacy implications of RFID, and the impact of RFID use on the healthcare industry.

HEALTHCARE INDUSTRY AND INFORMATION TECHNOLOGY

Healthcare is one of the world's largest industries. In the United States, for example, it accounts for 14 percent of GDP (Janz *et al.*, 2005). Healthcare is also arguably the most complex and regulated industry, regularly facing change brought on by federal, state, and local regulation, changing competitive landscapes, mergers and acquisitions, and the pressures of cost control (Finch, 1999). The healthcare industry historically has lagged behind other industries in the adoption of information and communication technologies partially due to healthcare managers and executives struggling to cope with environmental challenges in the healthcare industry (Menon *et al.*, 2000). Zukerman (2000) pointed out that it is the dynamic nature of the healthcare industry that leads organizations to struggle to survive in turbulent conditions.

While the healthcare industry historically has lagged behind other industries in the adoption of information and communication technologies, this is changing at a faster rate (Finch, 1999). Healthcare industry leaders and decision makers have begun to realize the supporting role of technology in their effort to maintain a focus on quality care while meeting the pressures from regulatory bodies, competition, and achieving business and performance goals.

The mobile workstation, which can be used for medical records, diagnostics, charting, pharmacy, admissions, and billing, is an example of recently adopted technologies in hospitals. With mobile workstations, physicians can write prescriptions at the point of care, from their offices or from home computers (Coonan, 2002). While inputting orders, physicians can be prompted about drug interactions, potential alternatives, formulary restrictions and patient limitations. As a result, generally illegible handwriting is not an issue and the electronic support systems at the bedside can deter errors.

UBIQUITOUS COMPUTING AND RFID

Rapidly progressing information and communication technologies have brought about increasingly connected computing devices which are so naturalized within the physical environment that users are not able to view the computers. The computing devices are embedded in the environment, track real-time information on current locations anywhere and anytime, and transmit and receive relevant data regarding the users and the context in which they are being used.

Ubiquitous computing places considerable requirements on both hardware and software development and support. Currently, numerous technologies including global positioning system (GPS), ultra-wideband (UWB), RFID, and cellular triangulation contribute to building ubiquitous computing. Among them, RFID is considered a key technology of the ubiquitous computing era (Römer *et al.*, 2004).

RFID technology has its origins in military applications during World War II, but its commercial applications did not begin to be realized until the early 1980s (AIM, 2001). The theory of RFID was first proposed in 1948 in a conference, and the first patent for RFID was filed in 1973 (Asif and Mandviwalla, 2005). However, technology and cost only recently became favorable for widespread adoption. The widespread adoption of RFID technology was also enhanced by mandates from large retailers and government organizations such as Wal-Mart and the U. S. Department of Defense. These organizations require all suppliers to implement this technology at the pallet level within the next few years (Asif and Mandviwalla, 2005).

The most familiar current RFID application is the automated toll-paying systems on highways (Asif and Mandviwalla, 2005). This system has reduced overhead for transport companies and facilitated travel for commuters (ITU, 2005). RFID applications have also been widely used in airport baggage handling, electronic payment, retail theft prevention, library systems, automotive manufacturing, parking, postal services, and homeland security (Smith and Konsynski, 2003). Most recently, RFID applications have been used to help to identify natural disaster victims. The US Disaster Mortuary Operational Response Team and health officials in Mississippi's Harrison County were implanting human cadavers with RFID chips in an effort to speed up the process of identifying victims and providing information to families (Kanellos 2005).

RFID technology has many benefits over the traditional bar coding that many firms have become accustomed to using. First, RFID technology is superior to barcode technology in that its user does not need to know where an object or person is and does not need to be close in order to collect the data (Smith and Konsynski, 2003). RFID tags can be read at a distance and do not require line-of-sight. Unlike barcode and magnetic strips mostly used inside store, RFID can help with the tracking of inventory inside and outside the facility. In addition, RFID technology has read/write capabilities to store and change data and an ability to read many tags simultaneously (Smith, 2005). Those features are expected to contribute to the improvement of the efficiency, accuracy, and security of both supply chain and inventory management through cost savings. RFID may also facilitate the improved use of warehouse and distribution center space. Goods will not need to be stored according to product type for manual location because RFID allows them to be stored in the most efficient manner based on size and shape (Jones *et al.*, 2005).

COMPONENTS OF RFID

RFID technology consists of three components – a tag, a reader, and a computer network (Fanberg, 2004). The key component of an RFID system is the tag itself. The tag contains a microchip with identification data and an antenna for transmitting its data. The readers use radio waves to read the tag, and the data then connects to some type of networked computer system or database in order to process the information.

RFID tags are essentially tiny computers. The most basic simply contain product identification information while the advanced tags include monitors that can be updated with information such as weight, temperature, and pressure. RFID systems are typically classified according to the functionality of their tag (Smith and Konsynski, 2003). For the most part, tags are either active or passive. As such, they are categorized according to the power source used by the tag.

Instead of a traditional barcode, electronic product codes (EPC) are stored in the RFID tag. Like the barcode, the EPC is a unique number that identifies a specific item in the supply chain and is composed of numbers that identify the manufacturer and product type. However, unlike the barcode, the EPC uses an extra set of digits for a serial number to identify unique items (Lai *et al.*, 2005). Therefore, while barcodes only distinguish among products, the EPC codes are unique to each unit and can provide more detailed information (Figure 1).

Figure 1. A 96 Bit electronic product code content

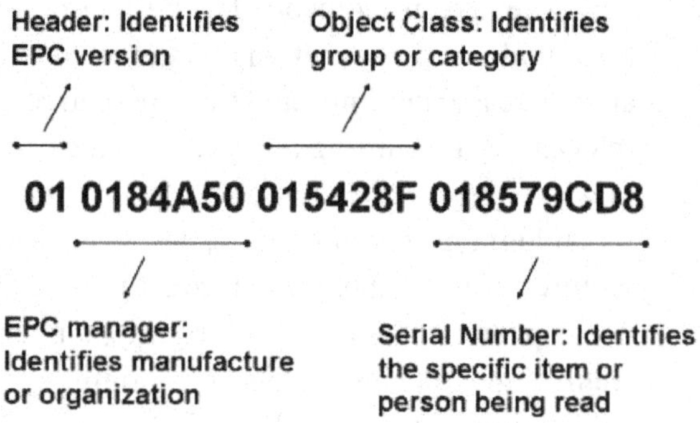

In a typical RFID system, RFID tags are attached to objects and send out EPC information when detecting a signal from the tag reader (Lai *et al.*, 2005). Tag readers, based on cellular technology, can scan products as needed so that a system can identify what products are located in a particular physical space. During reading, the signal is sent out continually by the active tag whereas in the passive tag, the reader sends a signal to the tag and listens (Asif and Mandviwalla, 2005). Regardless of whether this reader is a read only or read/write device, it is always referred to as a reader (ITU, 2005). Unlike barcode scanning, line of sight is not required and readers can deal with hundreds of tags at the same time (Smith and Konsynski, 2003).

The data collected by the RFID reader will be sent to backend databases via middleware to be utilized by enterprise systems. To distribute EPC codes quickly and efficiently, the network system, EPCglobal Network, which allows all parties in the supply chain to receive up-to-minute information about product movement, was designed using the Internet Protocol (IP) (Lai *et al.*, 2005). In this system, when any part of a supply chain needs a product or product movement information, a request for particular EPC information can be sent to the Object Name Service (ONS), which provides a global lookup service to translate an EPC into one or more Internet Uniform Reference Locations (URLs). Then, the URLs provide detailed information in a Product Markup Language (PML) format mainly based on eXtensive Markup Language (XML) (Angeles, 2005).

RFID AND THE HEALTHCARE INDUSTRY

In the healthcare industry, RFID can be used in various areas. First, the most practical area, and the one gaining the quickest acceptance among healthcare organizations, is to attach active RFID tags to expensive or vital supplies (ITU, 2005). The items can then be retrieved quickly when needed or monitored. There are almost 100,000 fatalities every year in the US that are a result of errors in dispensing medicine (Gazette, 2005). Therefore, a well monitored medical supplies and medicine is critical for the healthcare industry. According to Frost and Sullivan, the investments by pharmaceutical companies in RFID will reach $ 2.3 billion by 2011 (Barnes, 2006).

RFID tags can also be attached to the patient to track their location (Smith and Konsynski, 2003). Tracking the location of patients is particularly important in cases of long-term care, mentally challenged patients, and newborns (ITU, 2005). The ability to determine the location of a patient within a hospital can facilitate and expedite the delivery of healthcare. From a patient convenience and enhanced experience perspective, if hospitals used patient identification RFID tags, a nurse or other caregiver would not have to wake the patient up to verify their identity. As tags become more sophisticated, they could be used to monitor and transmit patient data (e.g., temperature, respiration, pulse) through wireless sensors that will interoperate within a broad network of generic readers (Smith and Konsynski, 2003). Other possible applications of RFID in the healthcare industry include tracking physicians within the hospital and cleaning of hospital beds. Table 1 summarizes the RFID applications in hospitals.

According a recent study, RFID and its related technologies in the hospital marketplace will reach $8.8 billion by 2010 (Sokol, 2005). The study reported that the market will be segmented into three general categories: RFID hardware and software integration ($1.3 billion), infrastructure support for RFID enablement ($2.7 billion) and hospital connectivity ($4.8 billion). Currently, less than 23 percent of RFID solutions implemented by hospitals are using passive RFID technology (Spyglass, 2006). Passive

RFID systems require a reader to be waved near a transponder with an RFID chip and have been used in healthcare to identify patients or drugs in medication administration. The study, however, found that many hospitals hope to use active RFID systems in the future.

OBSTACLES AND CHALLENGES FOR RFID ADOPTION IN HOSPITALS

The tremendous potential of RFID in hospitals is, however, being hindered by several obstacles including high cost, the lack of established standards, and privacy and security issues (ITU, 2005). Among them, the cost of tags is a major barrier to the adoption of RFID in hospitals. A study reported that 57 percent of healthcare professionals indicated that a major hurdle is lack of available

Table 1. RFID Applications in hospitals

RFID Applications	Examples
Tracking Medical Supplies and Medicine	• Holy Name Hospital in New Jersey is using an RFID asset tracking system which has enabled the staff to locate a piece of tagged equipment by using a PC. • St. Vincent's Hospital in Alabama is monitoring tagged surgical instruments for location and their maintenance schedule
Tracking Patient	• Bangkok hospital issues a RFID wristband to patients which is carrying the patient's name, age, gender, and dosage of any needed drug. • Jacobi Medical Center in New York traces the medical history of patients by reading information from the RFID radio wristbands.
Locating Medical Staffs	• Staff and patients at the Beth Israel Hospital in New York can be located using the tagged bracelets that they wear.
Other Applications	• Bielefeld municipal hospitals tested beds with integrated RFID chips in order to improve the deployment and cleaning of hospital beds.

funding, and 46 percent cited the cost of RFID tags and readers as a major barrier (BearingPoint, 2005). Although it has been projected that there will be a dramatic reduction in the price of the tags over the next few years, the current cost is still prohibitive for many routine applications (ITU, 2005). Currently, low-end tags sell for 7 to 10 cents each and readers cost between $1,000 and $3,000, depending on the features of the device (RFID, 2006).

The lack of established standards is also delaying the adoption of RFID technology (ITU, 2005; Lai *et al.*, 2005). There are currently no globally agreed upon standards, and there are literally dozens of manufacturers of tags and readers utilizing multiple frequencies and specifications (Twist, 2005). The lack of standards means that organizations will be forced to incur high costs to ensure compatibility with multiple readers and tags, and it is difficult for most firms to commit significant resources if they do not know whether their suppliers and customers will be using a compatible technology (Twist, 2005). A study reported that 60 percent of healthcare professionals said they have delayed some RFID activities while they wait for industry or government guidance on standards (BearingPoint, 2005).

In addition, the concern of privacy has become a major problem to those who adopt RFID in hospitals. Consumer advocacy groups (e.g., Consumers Against Supermarket Privacy Invasion and Numbering [CASPIAN]) have raised privacy issues about RFID technology (Shim *et al.*, 2006). The concerns revolve around consumer privacy and fears that if RFID technology is adopted, it could be used to allow hospitals to obtain information about patients and to track their movement without their knowledge (Jones *et al.*, 2005). Security has also become a major issue in implementing RFID since identification information on passive RFID tags can be easily stolen (Smith, 2005). Additionally, the extreme popularity of bar coding may be an obstacle in the way of RFID adoption since RFID would require significant financial investment and mind-set changes to those who have become accustomed to bar coding (Smith, 2005). Finally, it has been reported that many hospitals are concerned about the network infrastructure, scalability, integration capability and application availability of current RFID technology (Spyglass, 2006).

CONCLUSION

Ubiquitous healthcare will provide an increased accessibility to healthcare providers, more efficient tasks and processes, and a higher quality of healthcare services. As a key technology of ubiquitous healthcare, RFID enables a fully automated solution for information delivery in hospitals, thus reducing the potential for human error and increased efficiency. In spite of its tremendous global potential, RFID is still marginally adopted and in an early stage in hospitals. For widespread adoption of RFID in hospitals, it is imperative to find solutions to the current obstacles of RFID adoption including high cost, the lack of established standards, and privacy and security issues.

REFERENCES

AIM. (2001). *Shrouds of time: History of RFID.* Retrieved January 20, 2006, from http://www.aimglobal.org/technologies/rfid/resources/shrouds_of_time.pdf

Angeles, R. (2005). RFID technologies: Supply-chain applications and implementation issues. *Information Systems Management, 22*(1), 51-65.

Asif, Z., & Mandviwalla, M. (2005). Integrating the supply chain with RFID: A technical and business analysis. *Communications of the Association for Information Systems, 15*, 393-427.

Barnes, K. (2006). *RFID exploding into pharma industry.* Retrieved September 3, 2006, from http://www.in-pharmatechnologist.com/news/ng.asp?n=64786-gartner-frost-and-sullivan-rfid

BearingPoint. (2005). *Large healthcare organizations are embracing RFID.* Retrieved September 4, 2006, from http://www.nahit.org/cms/index.php?option=com_content&task=view&id=157&Itemid=148

Coonan, G. M. (2002). Making the most of mobility. *Health Management Technology, 23*(10), 32-36.

Finch, C. (1999). Mobile computing in healthcare. *Health Management Technology, 20*(3), 64-65.

Gazette. (2005). *RFID in the pharma supply chain.* Retrieved September 2, 2006, from http://www.rfidgazette.org/2005/11/rfid_in_the_pha.html

Harrop, P., & Das, R. (2006). *RFID in healthcare 2006-2016.* Cambridge, UK: IDTechEx.

Janz, B. D., Pitts, M. G., & Otondo, R. F. (2005). Information systems and health care II: Back to the future with RFID: Lessons learned - Some old, some new. *Communications of the Association for Information Systems, 15.*

ITU. (2005). *Ubiquitous network societies: The case of radio frequency identification.* Retrieved January 20, 2006, from http://www.itu.int/osg/spu/ni/ubiquitous/Papers/RFID%20background%20paper.pdf

Fanberg, H. (2004). The RFID revolution. *Marketing Health Services, 24*(3), 43-44.

Kanellos, M. (2005). *RFID tags used to track hurricane Katrina dead.* Retrieved September 2, 2006, from http://networks.silicon.com/lans/0,39024663,39152382,00.htm

Lai, F., Hutchinson, J., & Zhang, G. (2005). Radio frequency identification (RFID) in China: Opportunities and challenges. *International Journal of Retail & Distribution Management, 33*(11/12), 905-916.

Lyytinen, K., & Yoo, Y. (2002). Issues and challenges in ubiquitous computing. *Communications of the ACM, 45*(12), 63-65.

Menon, N. M., Lee, B., & Eldenburg, L. (2000). Productivity of information systems in the healthcare industry. *Information Systems Research, 11*(1), 83-92.

RFID. (2006). *The cost of RFID equipment.* Retrieved April 21, 2006, from http://www.rfidjournal.com/faq/20

Römer, K., Schoch, T., Mattern, F., & Dübendorfer, T. (2004). Smart identification frameworks for ubiquitous computing applications. *Wireless Networks, 10*(6), 689-700.

Shim, J. P., Varshney, U., & Dekleva, S. (2006). Wireless evolution 2006: Cellular TV, wearable computing, and RFID. *Communications of the Association for Information Systems, 18*, 497-518.

Smith, A. D. (2005). Exploring radio frequency identification technology and its impact on business systems. *Information Management & Computer Security, 13*(1), 16-28.

Smith, H., & Konsynski, B. (2003). Developments in practice X: Radio frequency identification (RFID) - An internet for physical objects. *Communications of the Association for Information Systems, 12*, 301-311.

Sokol, B. (2005). *RFID and emerging technologies market guide to healthcare.* Retrieved September 1, 2006, from http://www.rfidjournal.com/article/articleview/1534/1/1/

Spyglass. (2006). *Providers not passive about RFID.* Retrieved September 5, 2006, from http://healthdatamanagement.com/HDMSearchResultsDetails.cfm?articleId=12499

Twist, D. C. (2005). The impact of radio frequency identification on supply chain facilities. *Journal of Facilities Management, 3*(3), 226-239.

Varshney, U. (2005). Pervasive healthcare: Applications, challenges and wireless solutions. *Communications of the Association for Information Systems, 16*, 52-72.

Weiser, M. (1993). Some computer science issue in ubiquitous computing. *Communications of the ACM, 36*(7), 74-84.

Zuckerman, A. M. (2000). Creating a version for the twenty-first century healthcare organization. *Journal of Healthcare Management, 45*(5), 294-305.

KEY TERMS

Electronic Product Codes (EPC): A unique serial number that identifies an object or person. Currently, the 96-bit EPC is the most prevailing version and contains the detail information about the specific object or person being monitored.

Extensive Markup Language (XML): A general-purpose markup language, whose primary purpose is to facilitate the sharing of data across different information systems, particularly via the Internet.

Internet Protocol (IP): The method by which data is sent from one computer to another on the Internet. Each computer on the Internet has at least one IP address that uniquely identifies it from all other computers on the Internet.

Object Name Service (ONS): An automated networking service that points computers to sites on the World Wide Web.

Radio Frequency Identification (RFID): A technology used to identify, track, and trace a person or an object without using a human to read and record data.

Ubiquitous Healthcare: Healthcare to anyone, anytime, and anywhere by removing location, time and other restraints while increasing both the coverage and quality of healthcare.

Ultra-Wideband (UWB): A wireless communications technology that can transmit large amounts of digital data over a wide spectrum of frequency bands with very low power for a short distance.

Section V

Mobile Health Applications and New Home Care Telecare Systems

Chapter XX
Agile Patient Care with Distributed M-Health Applications

Rafael Capilla
Universidad Rey Juan Carlos, Spain

Alfonso del Río
Universidad Rey Juan Carlos, Spain

Miguel Ángel Valero
Universidad Politécnica de Madrid, Spain

José Antonio Sánchez
Universidad Politécnica de Madrid, Spain

ABSTRACT

This chapter deals with the conceptualization, design and implementation of an m-health solution to support ubiquitous, integrated and continuous health care in hospitals. As the life expectancy of population grows in modern societies, effective healthcare becomes more and more important as a key social priority. Medical technology and high quality, accessible and efficient healthcare is currently demanded by citizens. Existing technologies from the computer field are widely used to improve patient care but new challenges demand the use of new communication, hardware and software technologies as a way to provide the necessary quality, security and response time at the point of care need. In this scenario, mobile and distributed developments can clearly help to increase the quality of healthcare systems as well as reduce the time needed to react to emerging care demands. In this chapter we will discuss important issues related to m-health systems and we deeply describe a mobile application for hospital healthcare. This application offers a modern solution which makes more agile doctor and nurse rounds on behalf of an instant online access to patient records through wireless networks. We also provide a highly usable application that makes simple patient monitoring with handheld devices.

INTRODUCTION

The origins of health telematics and telemedicine did mainly focus on the benefits of communicating and making available medical information from a patient to a remote medical expert instead of having to displace the injured person to a health centre (Bashur, R., 1997). Thus, telemedicine aimed to support people at the point of care wherever, for different reasons, neither the health professional nor the patient could easily travel to meet each other face to face. In this context, multiple new scenario were imagined taking into advantage Information and Communication technologies (ICT) to provide care to people in isolated regions, emergency situations or environments where a difficulty exists to displace a patient who cannot receive on site medical attention. At a parallel pace, medical informatics started to devote significant efforts to deploy health information systems that ensure medical data availability "at the point of care". Both Hospital Information Systems (HIS) and Department Information Systems (DIS) aimed to provide health professionals with adequate tools that may integrate all the medical data required by health staff (medical doctors, nursery, administrative, health managers, etc.), to treat a patient (Winter A., 2003). Consequently, the concept of Electronic Health Record (EHR) raised and, with diverse levels of success at the market level, important standardization work have been active (CEN TC251, ISO215, HL7) making efforts to structure in a secure and efficient way the enormous amount of data that can be associated to a person's health history (Dolin R., 2006). However, the traditional view of Medical Informatics focused more on those situations where the health professionals are, for instance, present at their hospital or care centre office providing a consultation service rather than those scenarios that oblige them to be displacing in order to assist in-bed patients in the hospital or elderly and disabled people at home.

A solution for the challenge of mobile care support came from the concept of m-health proposed in the '90s to exploit the potentiality of mobile communications to assist care professionals or patients "in movement" (Istepanian R.S.H, 2004). The original scenarios of health telematics were changing and technologies were no longer expected to only provide medical information at a fixed computer or medical device where the specialist is supposed to be located, but to "bring" valuable information to the professional wherever he or she is located, in movement, whichever mobile or wireless network is available. Mobile networks were initially used to transmit data from mobile patients; furthermore, the m-health concept started to think about mobile professionals or wirelessly connected citizens who are displaced from a fixed location. A typical example from the first ideas was the utilization of emerging GSM systems to transmit biomedical signals, like an ECG or blood pressure, in emergency situations where an injured patient is moved from a mobile ambulance unit to the hospital (Pavlopoulos S., 1999). Most advanced research on m-health has mainly treated with the unobtrusive and ubiquitous integration of e-care or telemedicine services with remote health information systems through GPRS/UMTS, WLAN or WPAN technologies as well as provision of context aware health care ad-hoc support including Quality of Service features (Oliver N., 2006) (Wac K., 2007).

Innovative m-health solutions for health professionals rely on the possibilities to exploit the potential of next generation advanced mobile or wireless technologies (3G and above, WiFi/WiMax) together with the availability and affordability of usable and portable electronic devices such a PDA, smartphone, tablet PC or handheld that may provide health care professionals with a full EHR to support medical attention at the patient's point of care. It is unquestionably that successful e-health and m-health systems must be adapted to user's needs and capabilities. Whether the end user is a nurse or a patient, for example, the system will only be valuable if it provides in a usable and accessible way the health care information needed (Safran C., 2005). System utilization must provide useful, quick and effective information to users who, especially in medical scenarios, cannot afford delays or typical problems with computer tools that makes difficult or frustrating to receive the expected data. Most common communication networks must be considered by an m-health solution and the system should be supported by either available mobile communication technologies or private wireless networks ensuring additional security and performance requirements. In the past 10 years, the enormous advances in PDA capabilities, linked to cost reductions have brought that many health care professionals have familiarized with this kind of portable and easy devices. Initially, non-connected PDAs were used to facilitate professionals a daily agenda or local useful tools such as a vademecum or a small database to store patients′ records. These initial solutions faced a big inconvenient: they could not be connected and synchronization with medical information stored in a health care server was not possible. The increasing integration of WiFi and GPRS / UMTS capabilities into PDA or Smartphone devices has increased the number of potential mobile applications that can be applied to the health domain having always on mind safety and RF restrictions which might be compulsory in certain locations of health centers (DoH, 2007).

M-HEALTH RESEARCH OVERVIEW IN EUROPE

At present, the applicability of m-health has spread out in the economically developed countries were emerging mobile networks are having a broader penetration. Both in USA, Canada, Australia and European countries like Sweden, Norway, Spain, Great Britain or Greece, a range of mobile systems research and development (R&D) have been documented. For the purpose of this chapter, the focus is given on the European activity as the pace of European Commission Framework Programmes as representative of the evolution of m-health trends.

A significant boost to m-health R&D was given in European Commission V Framework Programme (1998-2002), where the IST Programme Key Action 1 (System and Services for the Citizen) defined a priority research line called Applications relating to Health. In particular, the cluster of projects called intelligent systems for the health professionals aimed at assisting health professionals to cope with major challenges, including enhancement of health services provision and continuous learning and training, through innovative, user-friendly, fast and reliable IST technologies and systems. The main research work of the projects, covered topics as new generations of computerized clinical systems, advanced interactive environments for remote and timely access of available best medical practice and patient's medical files from anywhere, collaborative healthcare provision, evidence-based medicine and systems supporting continuous education. The added value of the cluster was centered on interoperability, standardization, clinical validation, awareness and dissemination. Among the large number of projects regrouped in the cluster, two main thematic sub-clusters were identified and reached critical mass and visibility: Intelligent systems for minimally invasive diagnosis and treatment planning and intelligent systems for mobility of health professionals. The projects in this last sub-cluster aimed at enabling health professionals to access remotely the best available medical advice and consult patient medical files whether from the surgery room, the hospital, the patients' home or site of accident. The work was mainly based on the integration of advanced interfaces (voice recognition, natural language understanding, etc) and mobile multimedia workstations with embedded means of communication referred to as advance mobile and wireless systems for health.

In the Area of Mobile and Wireless Systems for Health, work in the domain of Medical Digital Assistants at EC V FP concerned with the implementation and validation of speech recognition technologies for specific clinical environments such as the WARD IN HAND project (Mobile workflow support and information distribution in hospitals via voice operated, wireless networked handheld devices) in addition to the use of natural language understanding systems in health care like MOBIDEV (mobile devices for healthcare applications). Other experiences focused on evidence based medicine and decision support tools (SMARTIE, smart medical applications repository of tools for informed expert decision), as well as mobile and wireless technologies to support intelligent collaborative environments (CHILDCARE, intelligent collaborative environment for out-of-hospital children healthcare and TELELOGOS, and next generation of methods and tools for team work based care in language and speech therapy). Special consideration was given to the market of Medical Digital Assistants and business models for making a success of these applications; the MEMO project (Accompanying Measure for medical mobile devices) was coordinating these activities. In the area of Portable and Wearable Health Monitoring, EPI-MEDICS (enhanced personal, intelligent and mobile system for early detection and interpretation of cardiological Syndromes); AMON (advanced care and alert portable telemedical monitor); LIFEBELT (intelligent wearable device for health monitoring during pregnancy); WEALTHY (wearable healthcare system); and MOBIHEALTH (mobile health care) were the most mentionable projects.

The EC VI Framework Programme (2003-2007) dealt with m-health solutions by defining areas of interest like the development of telemonitoring personal intelligent systems with embedded biosensors; interactive teleassistance systems for patients and citizens; decision supported systems; and intelligent environments for professionals. The outcome of the ALLADIN project (natural language based decision support in neurorehabilitation) was a personal digital assistant for neurorehabilitation activities with speech recognition, DICOEMS (diagnosis collaborative environment for medical relevant situations) developed for portable system to support remote management of medical emergencies. In addition, MYHEART (fighting cardio-vascular diseases by preventive lifestyle & early diagnosis) developed and tested personal intelligent systems to prevent and monitoring heart diseases. As in previous EC FP, the development of Personal Health Systems continue in the VII Framework Programme (FP) by focusing on wearable, implantable or portable health systems, as well as Point-of-Care diagnostic devices, enabling independent living for elderly people. In the VII FP it is proposed to develop Personal Health Systems focusing on non-invasive, multiparameter health monitoring; multianalytical screening and analysis; and disease management within the citizens' ordinary living environments.

M-HEALTH CHALLENGES, BENEFITS AND DRAWBACKS

In addition to future issues such us context aware services or "always best connected" solutions coming from 4G perspectives, the main challenges that currently rise for m-health refers to the secure and interoperable integration with health information. Current commercial tools do still offer proprietary and close solutions whose interoperability is hardly available. Therefore, ongoing developments like the work presented in this chapter opens the way for interconnectivity reducing dependency from ad hoc solutions and offering expected usability and organizational benefits.

The most important factors that have propelled the implantation of m-health in clinical care routine deal with quality of care, accessibility and efficiency issues. In particular, the time reduction to identify and react to a medical emergency is seeing as an important added value thanks to the enhanced access to data and medical information. Furthermore, improvements in care, perceived by patients, and care services are being identified linked to added value possibilities for specialized care and increases in medical productivity (Yu P., 2006). It is envisaged that the time reductions can be also obtained from digital information collection at the point of care as well as included processing mechanisms.

Also, one of the major drawbacks for m-health comes from the lack of relationship between devices and networks as well as standards for mobile devices. Each user may have a different operative environment (Windows Mobile, J2ME, and Symbian), different devices with distinct Graphical User Interface and different mobile network facilities (from GSM or GPRS to EDGE, UMTS, HDSPA or HSUPA), or wireless network technologies (WiFi, WiMax, Bluetooth, ZigBee, RFID). Certain highly cost hardware infrastructure, specifically for Body Area Network sensors or advanced PDA is still a problem, and m-health have to be extended to the users' community. Besides, health care industry and organizations are very practical and will not invest on m-health services unless sort time benefits may be demonstrated in clinical routine. From a HW point of view, devices autonomy (battery, weight) is still an issue to be solved as, for example, the daily and quick activity of health care staff should be supported independently of connectivity restrictions. From the software point of view, usability, accessibility and the complexity in the protocols stack are still problems to be solved in order to easily extend, develop and use services in the m-health world, including care professionals, patients, disabled people, relatives and informal careers.

AN M-HEALTH SYSTEM FOR REMOTE PATIENT CARE

On behalf of the wonders of wireless networks, there is an increasing popularity for developing and using mobile applications. Ubiquitous and pervasive computing (Hassmann U., Merk L., Nicklous, M.S., Stober, T., Korhonen P., Khan P. and Shelness N., 2003) exploit the advantages of handheld devices and provide efficient and modern solutions for users who demand mobility. The need of nurses and doctors to make more efficient patient care procedures has brought the development of a PDA application able to increase the response for those patients who demand a quick attention. This section addressed several issues related to the construction and usage of mobile applications for the health care domain and describes an m-health application developed at the University Rey Juan Carlos.

Hospitals and geriatric centers employ an increasing number of nurses that take care of patients using the classical "nursing rounds" protocol. Nurses' rounds are conducted regularly every 1 or 2 hours to decrease patients' use of call lights. As a result, an increasing level of safety and patient satisfaction is achieved. The usage of mobile devices like a PDA may improve hospital health care systems by making more agile nurse rounds and having a better control of the regular cares patients need. The agility that mobile devices can offer to doctors and nurses during the regular daily schedule, is achieved by exploiting on-line access to patients' records using handheld devices. Therefore, the importance for having available such key information for monitoring the evolution of patients (e.g.: elderly, critical cases) along the day, becomes a strong motivation to use specific handheld applications.

In this research we have developed GEMA, which is a PDA application aimed to support ubiquitous patient care. This application modernizes a very few similar products traditionally used by Spanish hospitals and enhances and extends some of the capabilities offered by other systems. The aforementioned application was mainly thought for clinical institutions, hospitals and geriatrics centers, in which most of the medical staff need to perform a precise and continuous control of elders and for those people with special cares. Therefore, the scheduling of nurse rounds during the patient visits can be optimized using mobile technologies because patient records are already available using the PDA application.

First, will we explain the main features of the functionality supported by GEMA. Second, we will outline the high level description of the system by detailing its software architecture and the main functional parts of the application. A connection to Web services is described for remotely accessing the corporate hospital database system. In addition, security issues such us authentication using an LDAP server will be discussed. Third, we will describe in detail the functionality offered by GEMA to support doctor and nurse rounds for monitoring patients with high availability to patient records to make more agile hospital rounds.

Functionality and Main Features of GEMA

Because hospitals are special organizations that frequently need an updated and on-line access to patients' records, doctors and nurses are the principal stakeholders and potential users of mobile applications that provide access to patients′ information , and make more agile the rounds for monitoring the status of their patients, in particular those who need special cares.

The main goal of GEMA is to provide mobility and agility for nurses and also doctors who want to have access to patients′ records using handheld devices. With GEMA, nurses and doctors will have an instant and on-line access to patient records during their rounds. Also, such information will be automatically updated to hospital server databases on behalf of the wireless connection.

As mentioned before, GEMA supports different stakeholders' roles for which each one may have different permission levels which have to be authenticated against and LDAP server. Patients' records have to be previously stored by the own hospital information system, and such databases could be exported to be used by GEMA. In other case, GEMA should be fully integrated with the HIS platform. In addition, GEMA was specifically designed to assist nurses during their rounds but also doctors can be key users of the system. The application can be tailored for each hospital or medical center that want to define their own medical protocols, constants registry, or patient evaluation levels. The main features of the system are summarized as follows:

- **Access to GEMA:** Only authorized hospital members may access to different information levels depending on the role assigned to each user type. Initially, three types of users (i.e.: nurse, doctor, auxiliary staff) are defined. Each type of user has different privileges for accessing relevant information from patient records. In addition, each specific user may browse which patients have been assigned daily by the schedule system. For each patient, nurses and doctors can browse the patient's record as well as know which current cares have to be performed, the specific medication needed, or the status of a particular diagnostic.
- **Patient monitoring and evaluation:** GEMA facilitates users to monitor each patient's status and check current medication. The aim of monitoring is to define the correct actions ensure that the patient's status evolves positively. Monitoring activities in GEMA includes the following tasks:
    - **Patient evaluation:** Nurses can fill evaluation sheets for each patient to

reflect the medical symptoms during the evaluation. These evaluation sheets have different evaluation criteria that can be defined by each particular hospital and they should be grouped into subgroups in order to facilitate the input data. For instance, a group of symptoms might be breathing difficulty, which can be associated to certain difficulty signs as well as implies an effort from the patient like: rapid breathing, apnea, and lung diseases among others.

  - **Insert comments on patient's evolution:** GEMA will allow the insertion during the rounds of new comments about the evolution of patients.
  - **Introduction of vital constants:** GEMA allows users the input of vital constants during monitoring. The allowed types and ranges of vital constants should be defined by each hospital, but most of them are common for all medical centers.
  - **Query the evolution of patient's constants:** The application also permits users to query the sequence of the constants of each patient. Such information can be displayed graphically to clearly show the evolution of the patient.
  - **Incidents:** All the issues happened during monitoring of enough relevance that cannot be registered using the options offered by GEMA can be registered as incidents in simple text form.
- **Maintenance:** The mobile application GEMA allow patient healthcare tasks basically consisting in the administration of medicines, as well as personalized programmed care plans defined for specific care agendas. The basic tasks defined for this functionality are the following.
  - **Care agenda:** Each patient should have a personalized healthcare agenda elaborated by the doctor and monitored by the nurse or any other specialized medical staff. This medical staff will administer each event and this will be registered in the care agenda of each patient. Initially, all the cares should be pre-programmed by the hospital before the rounds.
  - **Medical agenda: Each patient should** have an agenda for the medical prescriptions containing all the medicines and the amount of medicines each patient needs. After this, the agenda must be updated using the application.
  - **Incidents:** Similarly as for patient monitoring, every incident happened during patient maintenance tasks should be registered in the agenda. Incidents that might be produced by the administration of a specific care or medicament must be necessary registered in the system, in such a form that specifies the origin and the causes observed.
- **Common infrastructure:** The proposed applications include some features common to the entire application, and we highlight the following ones.
  - **Communication between clients:** The application permits an instant text message communication between PDA users by means of the facilities provided by the network infrastructure. A user name or code identifies who sent a message to another user.
  - **Legal issues:** All the communications and actions realized with GEMA should be registered according to specific country regulations. In the case of Spain, the LOPD ("Ley Orgánica de Protección de Datos") law, that develops the European recommendations given by the European Network and Information Security Agency (ENISA), should be taken into account to protect confidential information of patients.

- **Access to patient records:** Only authorized user with appropriated permissions can access patient records.
- **Home healthcare:** In special situations when needed, GEMA can be used for home healthcare in a transparent form by means of appropriate wireless radio protocols (e.g.: GPRS/UMTS).

All these features represent the core of the functionality of GEMA, were specified with 27 functional requirements, 4 non-functional requirements and 3 hardware requirements. Because the goal of this chapter is to show how a mobile healthcare applications works, and its benefits over the traditional healthcare, we have preferred to omit a detailed list of software requirements. Instead, we will focus on the description of the security issues and how HIS databases will be accessed. After this, we will explain the main parts of the software architecture we developed to support GEMA's features.

The GEMA's Architecture

GEMA is designed for use inside buildings with wireless technologies like WiFi, but GPRS/UMTS can be also employed for connecting to remote databases when needed. Traditionally, GPRS/UMTS radio networks are not longer used inside hospitals to avoid the potential impact of radio transmissions. Thus, the most effective connection to the remote databases for accessing patient record is offered using wireless networks. The physical architecture deployed for GEMA application is shown in Figure 1.

As shown in Figure 1, the mobile GEMA application installed on the PDAs may connect to the hospital or specific GEMA databases via GPRS/UMTS or by means of the private hospi-

Figure 1. Physical architecture of GEMA using PDA devices for remote access to patient records

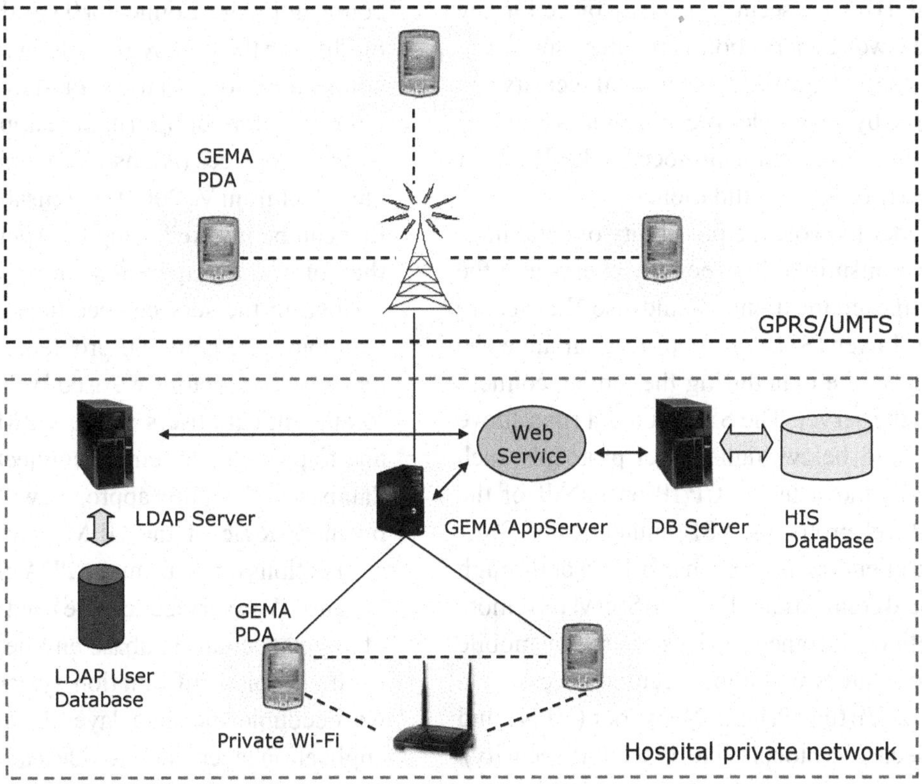

tal wireless network. The way in which GEMA mobile users access remotely the patient records is transparently to the wireless protocol selected. GPRS for those patients who need distance healthcare. Otherwise, inside the hospital the remote connection will be provided by the wireless infrastructure. In both cases, the connection will be established to an IP address for any authorized IP addresses valid range.

Securing Remote Connections

Information from patient records constitutes valuable and confidential information that must be legally protected and secured against unauthorized users. Therefore, authentication for hospital information system (HIS) becomes and important issue that should be carefully treated. In GEMA, the first thing we did for PDA users is to authenticate them to a secured users database, which consists on an LDAP Lightweight Directory Access Protocol) server that contains the list of authorized users (e.g.: doctors, nurses, etc.) of the hospital. Because security is a key piece for any HIS, password encryption is required for safety remote communications. Additional security can be offered by the wireless access points by means of wireless encryption protocols like WEP or WPA-PSK or MAC validation.

In order to avoid the possibility of data interception transmitted between the clients and the server, the connections should use the Secure Sockets Layer (SSL) protocol to guarantee the integrity of the data during the remote connections to the server. The SSL protocol runs above TCP/IP and below higher-level protocols such as HTTP, and it uses TCP/IP on behalf of the higher-level protocols. SSL authenticates SSL-enabled clients to an SSL-enabled server through encrypted connections. For GPRS/UMTS remote connections, intranet services offered by mobile phone operators will allow secured accesses on behalf of Virtual Private Networks (VPN) and using secure protocols like IPsec (IP security). IPsec is implemented by a set of cryptographic protocols for securing packet flows and for internet key exchange. IPsec can be used to create VPN for end-to-end communications between clients and the server. Integrity validation (ensuring traffic has not been modified along its path) and authenticating the peers (ensuring that traffic is from a trusted party) are facilities offered by IPsec. Using this scheme, home care patient records can be securely accessed from networks external to the hospital.

Web Services for Accessing HIS Databases

Many PDA applications that need to access information stored in databases employ specific connectors or drivers that have to be installed and configured for each PDA client. In many cases and depending on the target language or technology employed, compatibility problems between the language (e.g.: Java 1.1.8) and the PDA operating system may appear for a specific remote database connector (e.g.: Connector/J) or driver. Besides, modifying the PDA registry to indicate where the connector is located in the PDA directory may be a problem for configuring the application.

Web services (Alonso G., Casati, F., Kuno H. and Machiraju V., 2003) are reusable components that can be invoked using Internet protocols and they offer a transparent solution to the user described in the service specification. In order to overcome the potential problems using specific database connectors, we used Web services (WS) to authenticate users in the GEMA application and to provide the remote connection to GEMA databases. With this approach we can isolate the business logic of the GEMA system from the connections made from the PDA clients, and also because Web services can be used independently of any particular database engine of current use in the hospital information system. As a result we decouple the data layer from the business application layer, and provide a modern and scalable solution that can be integrated with different HIS, in a transparent way to the user. Another advantage of using Web services is the reuse of code for similar applications. Web services may facilitate maintenance tasks when new system requirements demand, for instance, a platform change. The compatibility of PDA users with other existing applications at the hospital requires that GEMA mobile application may allow different ways to authenticate users. The Web service provides adequate authentication support through specific connections to the LDAP server. In other environments, other authentication methods can be considered and be integrated appropriately with GEMA. Again, security for HIS databases is considered a key issue to deploy a Web server, where specific methods have to be included in order to protect critical data against embedded SQL sentences (SQL-InJection). In this way, the Web server will check the SQL sentences before its execution and will test that the arguments provided by the user do not contain such embedded SQL sentences. In other case, the service will block the user query.

General Use Case

In order to understand the main functionality of GEMA from a high level point of view, in this subsection we show one of the most interesting use cases (UCs) which describes the main activities carried out by the nurse subsystem. As shown in Figure 2, nurses can interact with patients assigned to a specific hospital unit. The nurse will monitor the status of each patient and will carry out the pre-programmed care plans including the administration of medicines. In addition, the role of the doctor stakeholder is to elaborate healthcare plans and is the unique authorized user to alter the diagnostic and the prescriptions of medicines. Therefore, specific profiles with individual grants are defined in GEMA in such a way that permissions are loaded when the users logons in the system. Depending of each particular hospital,

Figure 2. Use case for the nursing care subsystem

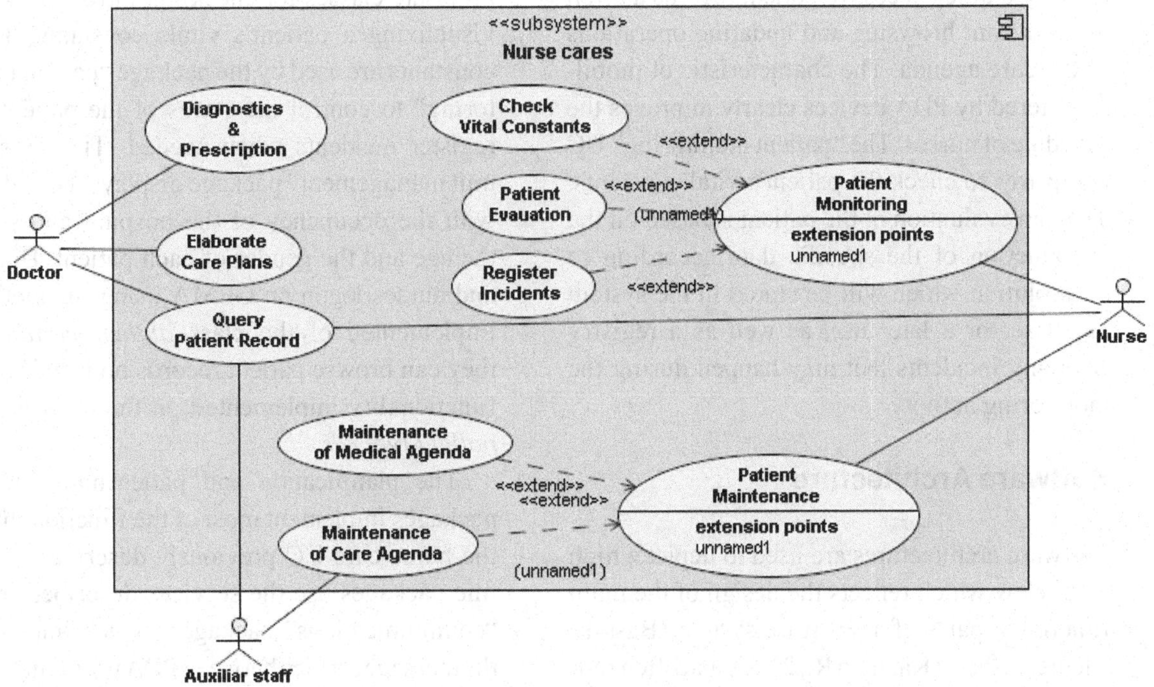

doctors may be involved in patient monitoring activities. In addition, auxiliary staff belongs to nurses with restricted tasks aimed to apply the cares defined in the care agenda.

More specifically, the "diagnostics and prescription" use case (UC) deals with the evaluation made by the doctor who, in consequence, prescribes the most appropriate medicaments to the patient. In tight relationship with this task, the medical agenda reflects each prescription. The "care plans" UC covers the realization of a specific care plan made by the doctor. This use case generates a set of tasks which are gathered in the care agenda. Each authorized hospital staff may have a care agenda for each individual patient. The whole set of care agendas form the care plan. Moreover, patient records can be accessed to browse some personal data of each patient and a brief summary of his/her disease. The maintenance of the care and medical agendas belong to the "patient maintenance" UC. The other important part of this subsystem focuses on patient monitoring activities, which result of extremely importance for controlling the status of the patient. GEMA makes patient monitoring more agile by a quick access to patient records as well as an instant browsing and updating operations of the care agenda. The characteristic of mobility offered by PDA devices clearly improves the schedule of nurses. The "patient monitoring" UC comprises to check the patient's vital constants. This, an evaluation of the patient is based on the introduction of the specific data according to its evolution which will be stored in the system database for a later use, as well as a registry with any incidents that may happen during the monitoring activity.

Software Architecture

Software architectures are used to depict a high level view which reflects the design of the main functional parts of a software system (Bass L, Clements P. and Kazman R., 2003), and often represented from different viewpoints (Clements P., Bachmann F., Bass L., Garlan D., Ivers J., Little R., Nord R. and Stafford J., 2002). In this chapter we describe the "structural view" of GEMA by means of a description of the most important packages and subsystems and including some classes. We have used UML 2.0 (Unified Modelling Language) to represent the high level architecture of GEMA and the main relationships between the packages and classes, such as Figure 3 shows.

The description of the architecture of Figure 3 is as follows. This two-layered architecture describes how GEMA is structured. A third layer under the middleware layer belonging to the hospital databases is not shown in the figure for practical reasons. The upper layer describes the overall functionally of the client application installed on the PDA. Part of this functionality has been detailed in the nurse use case described in the previous section. The architecture of Figure 3 shows the decomposition into subsystems (packages), each package containing appropriate classes that implement the functionality of GEMA and accordingly to the requirements.

The "vital constants" package defines appropriate classes for checking, introducing, and visualizing a patient's vitals constants. These constants are used by the package "patient monitoring" to control the status of the patient and register incidents when needed. The "hospital unit management" package displays the bed map with the occupancy of the hospital and shows the age and the gender of each patient. Doctors and nurses logon on GEMA using the methods implemented of the class *authentication* and they can browse patient records on behalf of the functionality implemented on the class *browse patient records*.

The "planification" and "patient maintenance" packages implement most of the functionality of the nurse care UC previously described. These fine packages use the services described in the "communications" packages, which implement the message service between PDA users and a spe-

Figure 3. Software architecture (structural view) of the GEMA application

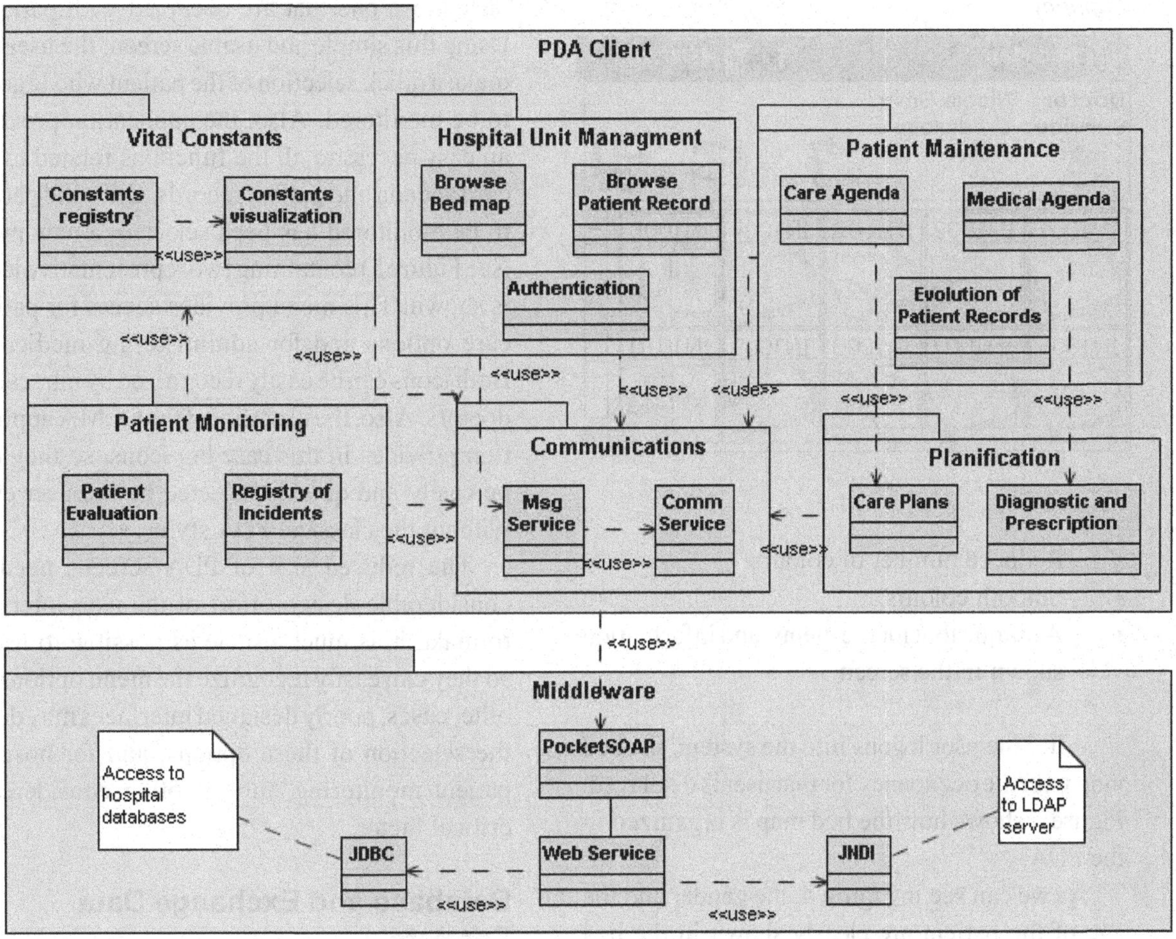

cific communication service which call the Web service by means of the "pocketSOAP" protocol for accessing remotely the hospital databases. The middleware layer mostly defines a class for the Web service for accessing such databases as well as the LDAP server for user authentication.

GEMA's User Interface

Because agility in nursing scheduling is a main concern to achieve, the organization of the menus has been designed according to the way nurses and doctors work. In addition, some of the menu options have big and representative icons in order to facilitate a quick identification by the user and a proper selection with the stylus of the PDA. The GEMA user interface has been designed according to the following characteristics:

- High usability level based on:
  - Structure of the menus according to the normal hospital procedures so that GEMA users can feel comfortable with GEMA operation mode.
  - No more than 3 menu levels.
  - Landscape mode to avoid the horizontal scroll as well as to ease the presentation of the information in the screen, such as the bed map.
- Screen resolution of at least 320x240.

Figure 4. Bed map with a partial view of the occupancy

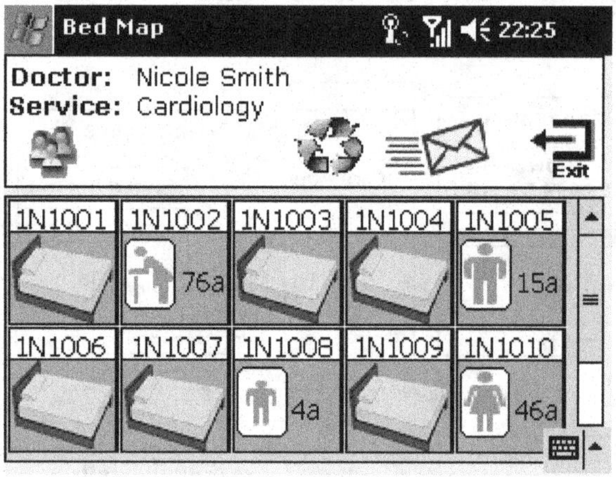

- Reduced number of colours.
- Smooth colours.
- A unique font for the menus and information shown in the screen.

After the user logons into the system, the bed map with the occupancy for that user is displayed. Figure 4 shows how the bed map is organized in the PDA.

As we can see in Figure 4, the gender and the age of the patient are clearly shown in the bed map. In addition, an icon in the left side of the screen allows the user to display all the beds or only those one that are occupied with patients. Using this simple and usable screen, the user can make a quick selection of the patient who is going to be monitored. Also, the application provides an easy access to all the functions related to the care agenda and patient records. Once the patient to be monitored has been selected, a new menu (see Figure 5) containing two representative icons is shown. This menu provides access for patient care options and for administering medicines. Both icons can be easily recognized by nurses and doctors. Also, the usability of the GEMA application provides in this case big icons, so they can be easily and quickly selected by the user even without the classical PDA stylus.

Figure 5. Contants input and graphics menu options

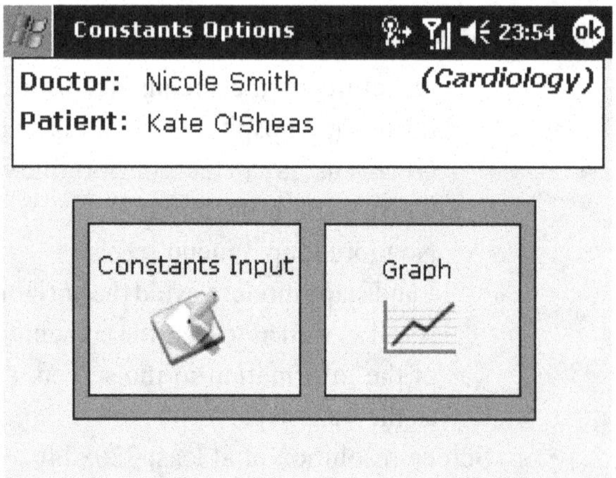

The reduced size of PDA screens needs a considerable design effort of the user interface to make it as much usable as possible to users, so they can easily recognize the menu options. In other cases, poorly designed interfaces may delay the selection of these options, and for hospital patient monitoring, time is often considered a critical factor.

Database and Exchange Data Formats

Because this first prototype of GEMA was implemented independently of any particular HIS, the database has not been fully integrated with any existing hospital server. In fact, GEMA was designed to be not only extensible to incorporate new features, but also opened to be integrated with existing platforms. The GEMA database system can be easily adapted or integrated with other database servers or existing data can be imported according to GEMA schema. Because many PDA installation and configuration problems with specific database connectors, we have developed a Web service that resolves the database connection by making it transparently to the user. In our case, a MySQL server is accessed from the Web service using a JDBC. The GEMA data model comprises 25 MySQL tables that store the information needed to implement the functionality described in the software architecture. In addition, the application is easily modifiable to change to a different database system like Oracle or Informix, which are frequently used in health care scenarios, without changing the functionality already implemented. In addition to the database model, the use of a Web service for database operations require the use of common data formats for all the operations with the data.

For instance, when we query the database, the problem turns out how to return a common structure that may include a different number of rows and cols as a result of a given query. To overcome this problem we decided to use the standard XML (eXtensible Markup Language) as an intermediate exchange data format, and the structure returned will dynamically compose the fields and the records obtained from the execution of SELECT sentence. Figure 6 shows an example of the common exchange data format using XML.

IMPLEMENTATION AND INTEGRATION

GEMA was implemented using PocketBuilder as the target language. In this section we will describe some relevant parts of the implementation and we will illustrate the problems encountered and the solutions provided. We prefer to explain the solutions already implemented describing the methods and the logical steps performed rather than showing a large number of source code sentences.

Web Service for Accessing HIS Databases

In order to avoid the potential problems that some PDA suffers when they directly use a specific database connector, we decide to implement a single Web services for managing the remote connections to databases server. Thus, the Web service (so-called GEMA_WS_DB), and implemented in Java, assumes the responsibility to interact with specific database connectors like JDBC for accessing MySQL tables. The GEMA_WS_DB

Figure 6. XML common format for exchanging information using a Web service for accessing hospital databases

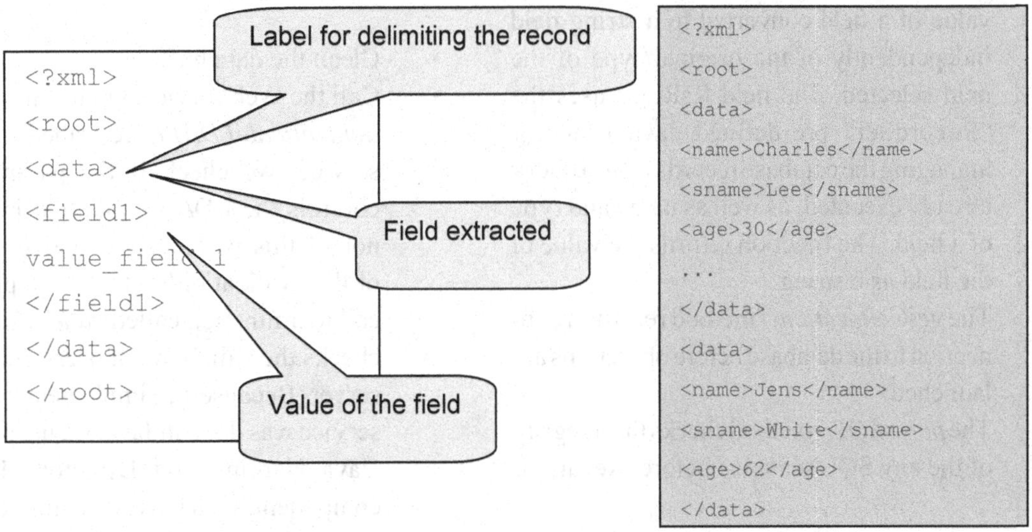

Figure 7. UML class describing the operations implemented in the GEMA_WS_DB Web service

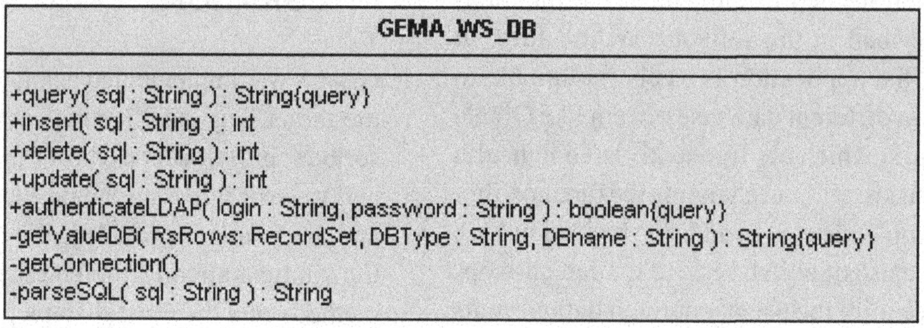

service is composed by a single class that access GEMA databases and provides user authentication through the LDAP server. Figure 7 shows the methods implemented in the class that describes the GEMA_WS_DB Web service, as Figure 7 shows.

GEMA_WS_DB
+query(sql : String) : String{query}
+insert(sql : String) : int
+delete(sql : String) : int
+update(sql : String) : int
+authenticateLDAP(login : String, password : String) : boolean{query}
-getValueDB(RsRows: RecordSet, DBType : String, DBname : String) : String{query}
-getConnection()
-parseSQL(sql : String) : String

The GEMA_WS_DB Web service defines five public methods; four of them, that is: *query(), insert(), delete(), and update()*) are used for accessing the hospital database, while the fifth one (*authenticateLDAP()*) implements the authentication process that validates users against the LDAP server. The remainder three methods are defined as private methods and the functionality of each of them is the following.

- The *getValueDB()* method returns the value of a field converted to a string field independently of the original type of the field selected. The field RsRows uses the "RecordSet" pre-defined Java type for managing the database records from a query already executed, as well as name and type of a field. The function returns the value of the field as a string.
- The *getConnection()* method returns a connection to the database before operations are launched.
- The *parseSQL()* method checks the integrity of the any SQL sentence before execution.

As an example, a typical scenario where a doctor wants to insert some specific data using GEMA, the application will create an instance of the GEMA_WS_DB service and build the call that invokes the insert() method in the service. Then, an internal process checks the integrity of the SQL sentence and stores it as an internal log file. This log file contains all the queries that have been executed due to security and legal reasons. After an SQL sentence is executed, the result is returned to the user if succeed. Otherwise, in case of failure and error is returned. Finally, the screen is refreshed with the information requested. Another example of Web service usage happens when users need to authenticated to the LDAP server. The service checks the user and password in the LDAP directory using the following process.

- Clean the data buffers
- Call the Web service. On behalf of method *authenticateLDAP()* described in the Web service, we check if the parameter that controls the LDAP validation is active or not. If this parameter is active, an object of the "validationLDAP" class produces a call to a function called *validation()* which checks the validation of users in the LDAP server. Because the implementation of the service was done in Java, we used the JNDI (Java Naming and Directory Interface) component, which uses a standardized API

for authenticating in different distributed directory systems like Microsoft Active Directory, Novell eDirectory, etc.

- Build the SQL sentence.
- Import the data from the buffer.
- Check if the user has been validated and if so, we select the profile for that specific user.
- The user is logged into the system, but a limited number of trials are permitted.

XML Data Exchange

As mentioned before, GEMA uses the XML format to display the data retrieved from the database. GEMA processes the data as XML files by exploiting the import facilities offered by PocketBuilder. The steps to do these tasks can be summarized in the following steps.

- Define the windows where the data will be presented.
- Invoke the query() method of the Web service.
- Import the data in XML format to the aforementioned window.
- The user access to the data to perform the desired operations.

One of the problems we encountered during the development of the first version of GEMA was the exchange of binary files. This is the case of, for instance, jpeg images containing the picture of the patient. If we are able to store these photos in the database we will need to implement a new function in the Web service able to return a BLOB (Binary Large Object) object. Nevertheless, we found an incompatibility problem with the BLOB field using the pocketSOAP protocol. This is due because the current implementation of the pocketSOAP component for pocketBuilder stores the data retrieved in string variables. During the communication between the service and the database, the pocketSOAP API realizes a conversion from BLOB to string but altering the content. Thus, the BLOB retrieved by the service cannot be properly interpreted and displayed. This problem doesn't appear if we use SOAP for transmitting the images from a PC or laptop. One alternative solution is to store the images locally in the PDA but this doesn't seem a realistic solution for the future. The second and most visible alternative is to change the transmission data protocol for accessing the images and replace pocketSOAP by FTP or HTTP. In other case, we should wait for an improved version of pocketSOAP for pocketBuilder. In this subsection we have discussed some key implementation issues of GEMA that we believe they could be useful for implementing similar applications, both in the same domain or in a different one. In next section we will provide an overview of the use of GEMA with appropriate screenshots guiding the habitual working schedule of nurse rounds.

AGILE NURSING ROUNDS WITH GEMA

In this section we will describe the operation practice using GEMA for m-health patient care. We will illustrate the logical steps of the activities usually performed by doctors and nurses to show how GEMA can help care assistance by making more agile the processes that most of them are often carried out manually. The instant on-line access to patient records during nurse rounds provides a powerful tool to get more agile care to patients, in particular to elderly or those who need special cares.

The first thing the user must do before using GEMA, is to log into the system with a user and a password, which are validated against the LDAP server using the Web service. Once the login information has been successfully, the application shows the user the profiles which are in current use for that user. GEMA users can select a specific role or clinic profile (i.e.: nurse, doctor, other staff)

Figure 8. Both screenshots constitute de main entrance to the GEMA system for user authentication and user profile selection

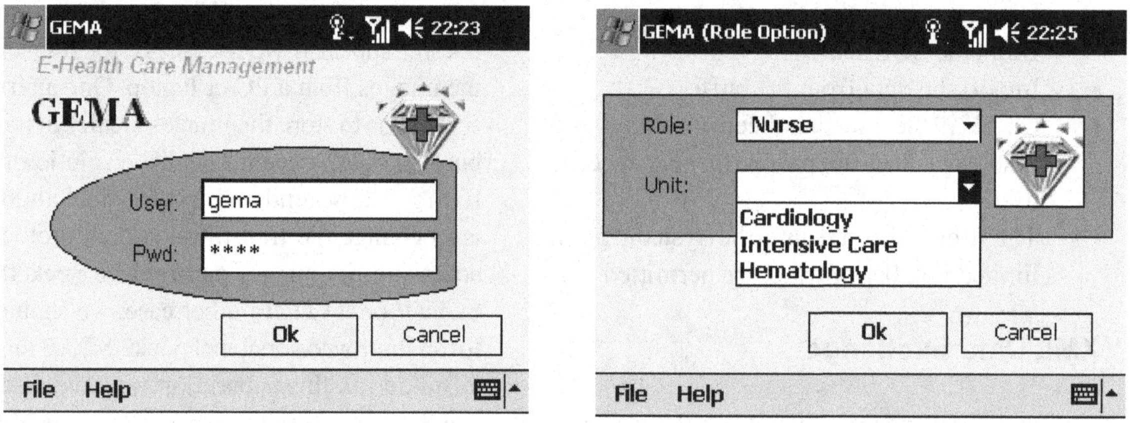

and a unit (e.g.: cardiology) for that profile. Figure 8 shows both screenshots used for authentication in the system and for selecting the profile and specific unit attached for that profile.

Once the user has selected his/her specific role and unit, the bed map of Figure 4 is displayed in the PDA showing the occupancy of the subset of patients assigned to that particular doctor or nurse. The top part of the screen of Figure 4 shows in the left side the type of user and the unit or service to which belongs. Also, three additional icons are defined to: update the data in the screen (the green recycle icon), show if user has incoming messages from other PDA user (an envelope turns its color to red), and the exit icon. The biggest area of Figure 4 is used exclusively to display the bed map. Each nurse and doctor can select one of the patients shown in the bed map to start the patient's medical history. After the selection of a particular patient, GEMA shows the user its entire functionality for mobile health care with on-line access to patient's records stored in the hospital information system or in a different database server. Figure 9 shows the main menu options with the processes supported by GEMA.

Using the functionality shown in Figure 9, a typical nurse round will start, for instance, checking the evolution of a patient that has just

Figure 9. GEMA main menu options for mobile health care

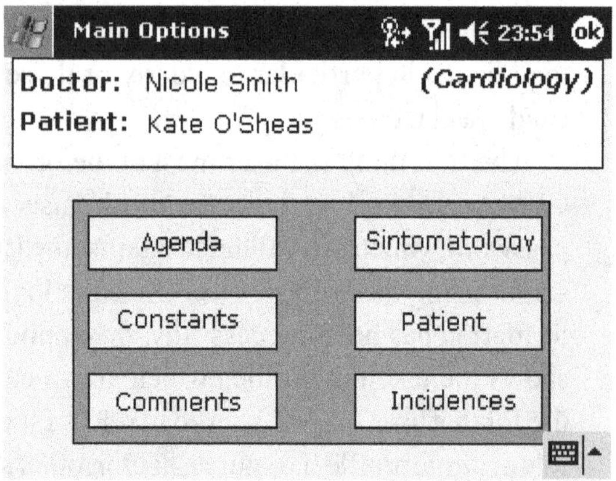

Figure 10. Symptomatology for a specific patient

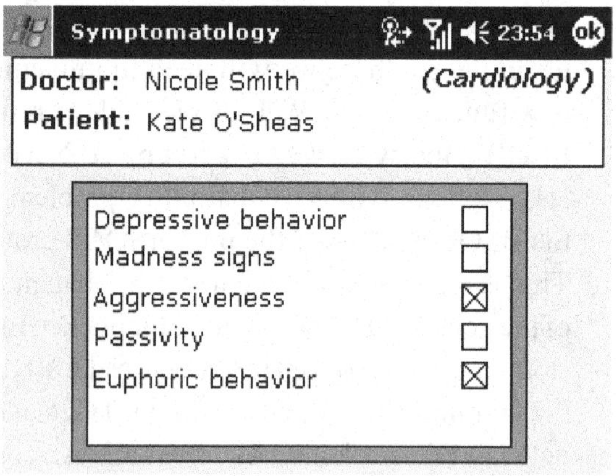

Figure 11. Histogram bar showing the diastolic tension constant evolution

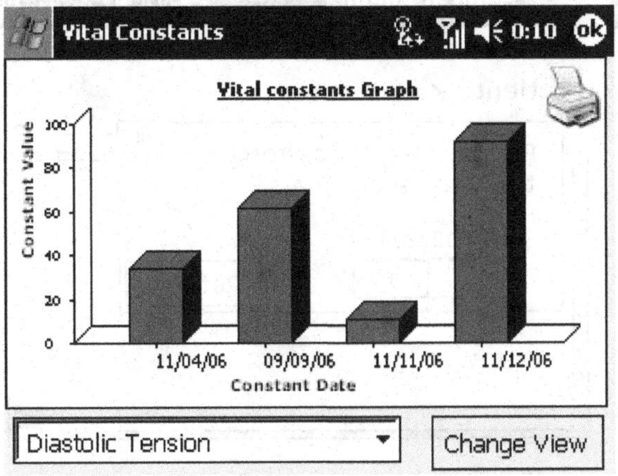

suffered a surgery operation. The nurse or doctor will start filling a symptomatology sheet using the **symptomatology** menu option. GEMA allows the user to select one symptom from a predefined list already store in the database servers and for that symptom the application displays more specific symptoms that can me marked according to the patient's status. Figure 10 shows an example of symptoms that have been checked during the round. The name of the patient and the nurse appear above the symptomatology features.

After the user has update the symptomatology of the patient, the **constants** option can be selected and a screen will appear to fill the appropriate constants for a patient who is being monitored. When all the constants have been recorded in the database, the user can check if every thing is right by a graphic dynamically built with the data already measured. A sample graphic displaying the constant for the diastolic tension is shown in Figure 11.

GEMA provides different visualization options for the graphics in the shape of histogram bars, pies, 3D view, solid line, etc, by only pressing the change view button and selecting the desired view (see Figure 12).

In addition, the graphics as well as some other data from other menu options can be remotely printed using, for instance, a bluetooth printer which should be previously configured for the GEMA application. Another key option for patient health care is the **medical agenda**, which stores the medicine doses that have to be administered to each patient. GEMA users can insert or new medicines or modify existing ones in the agenda for a specific date depending of the evolution of the patient. Therefore, the medical agenda is used by nurses to know each individualized patient care plan. Also, **comments** about the evolution of the patients can be added as a guide for the doctor to know if the medical agenda has to be changed or suppressed. Figure 13 shows a screenshot of the medical agenda.

Figure 12. Two different views of the same vital constant

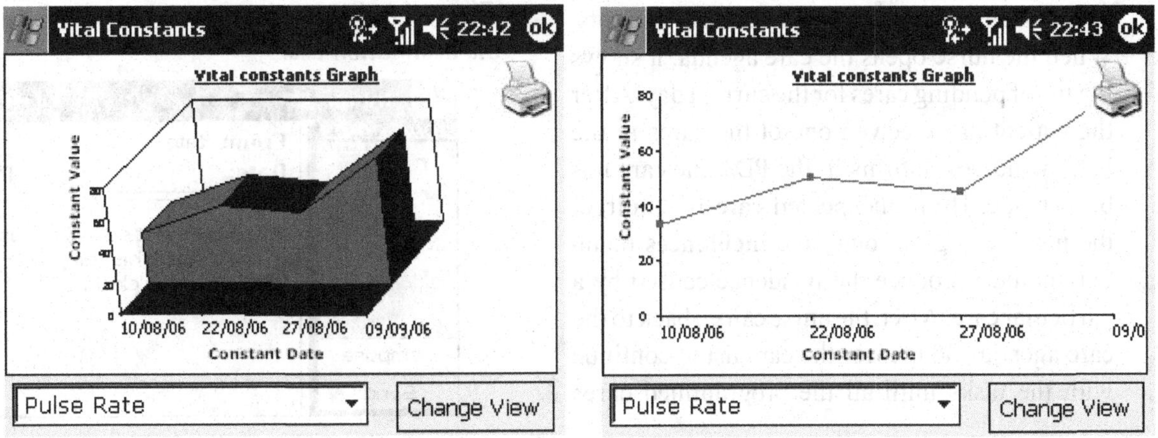

Figure 13. Perspective of the medical agenda with the insertion of a new care

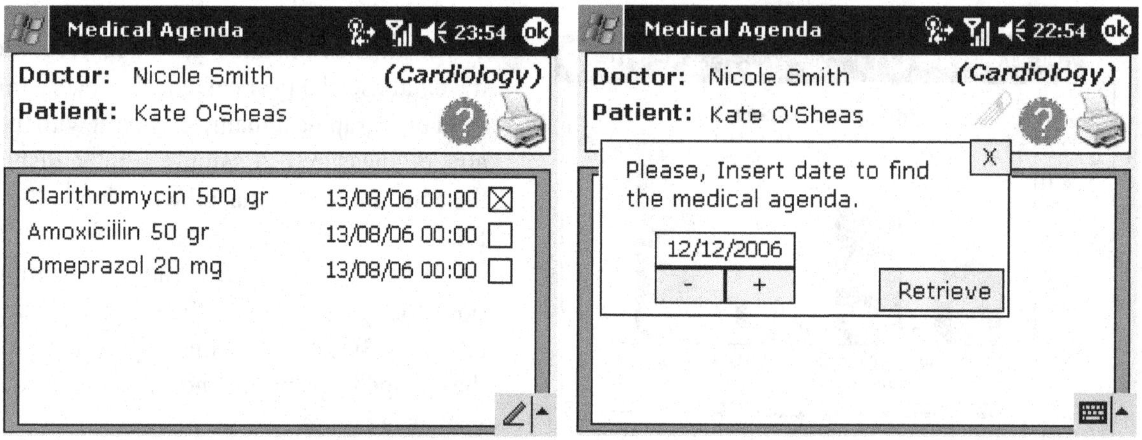

According to Figure 5, the mission of the **care agenda** is to define the set of specific care actions for each patient. Hospitals in which nurses, on average, take care of eight patients each have risk-adjusted mortality rates following common inpatient surgical procedures that are 31% higher than hospitals, in which nurses care for four patients each. Staffing hospitals uniformly at four versus eight patients per nurse would be expected to prevent 5 deaths per 1000 patients (Aiken L.H., Clarke S.P., Sloane D.M., Sochalski J. and Silber J.H., 2002). Therefore, there is a need for nurse staffing to receive more attention with regard to its potential to improve patient safety. The GEMA application eases this on behalf of the agility using PDA devices with on-line access to patient records and health care agendas for an effective surveillance of patients. When the nurse opens the care agenda, it shows the list of pending cares for the current day. After the patient has received one of the cares in the list, the nurse confirms in the PDA the care has been made. If an unexpected care is required, the nurse can go through the **incidences** menu option and introduce the incidence caused by a particular care. After, the nurse can go back to the care agenda and recover the care list to continue with the tasks until all the programmed cares have been applied and quickly move to the next patient. In order improve patient safety against unexpected situations, GEMA allows the user to send an instant message to another user like, as for instance, a doctor. The user will use the message icon to type a short message and selecting first the user where the message goes to. As the user receives the message, the icon message turns to red color indicating an incoming message. Figure 14 shows the message window.

This simple but effective communication systems between the handheld devices reduces the time needed to search for a particular doctor and contribute to patient's perception of doctor availability, as it enable best practices aimed to

Figure 14. An incoming message is displayed for the destination user

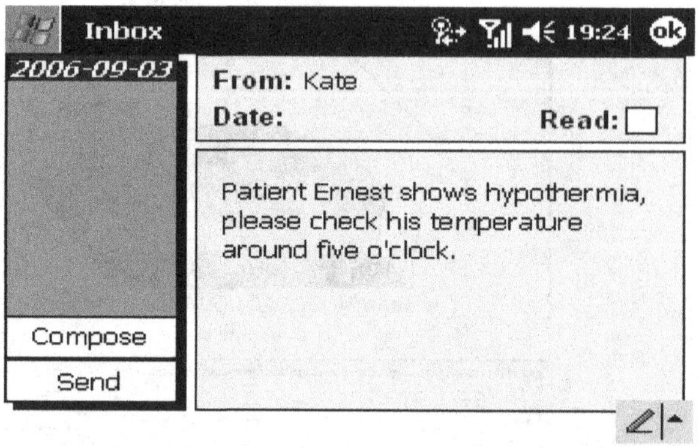

Figure 15. Abbreviated patient record information

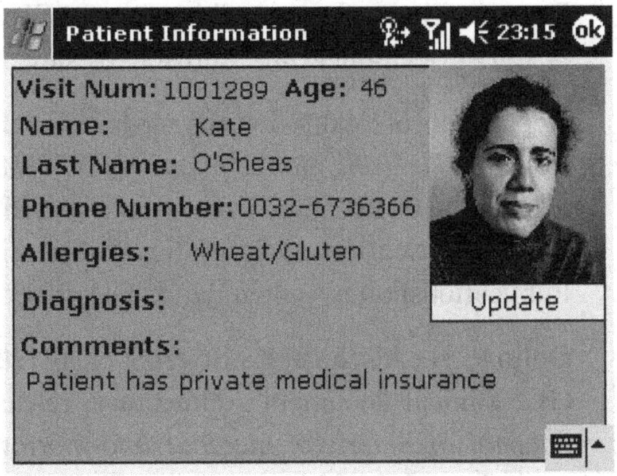

improve the communication of the hospital staff. To conclude, the goal of the **patient** option is to display a brief information of the patients records in order to clearly identify the basic history of the patient as well as his/her picture. This facility avoids that many times the doctor or nurse needs access to patient records and need to go to an authorized computer for this, which make take several minutes. With GEMA, basic patient information can be available in seconds without interrupting the nurse round. Figure 15 shows an example of basic patient record.

DISCUSSION

In this chapter we have addressed the importance of mobile application for hospital healthcare and we have stated this with the description of GEMA, a modern mobile application for m-health. The special requirements of hospital and similar medical centers requires the design and use of appropriate usable and accessible systems in order to cover the functionality demanded by patients, in particular elderly and disabled people, as well as those others with specific care needs.

At present, until being able to carry out a big scale hospital evaluation is too soon to extract results of the use of GEMA by doctors and nurses, and see how GEMA can make more agile nurse and doctor rounds. Is our aim to release GEMA as a commercial application, but at present we only have done three demos to hospital managers and computing chief directors. The feedback from these experiences was very positive but we will need more time to evaluate the benefits of using GEMA as an integrated application with any HIS platform.

From the more technical point of view, GEMA offers a usable and extensible solution for m-health which employs Web service technologies permit to connect with different databases and authentication servers what fosters real integration with existing HIS. Thus, the integration with other platforms should not be a problem and also to extend the functionality of GEMA allowing Web clients to connect to GEMA databases. Moreover, the use of open standards for data exchange like XML facilitate the description, storage, and exchange of patient records and other useful information between hospital databases. In addition, the modularity of the software architecture described in the chapter facilitates the extensibility of GEMA and fosters code reuse.

Finally, we have tested all the functionality described in GEMA both using a private wireless network and GPRS connections. We perceived that GPRS goes a little bit slower compared to Wi-Fi networks, but we believe UMTS or the more recent HSPDA protocol will provide more efficient ways of utilization. The advantage of using GPRS/UMTS protocols is that outside from the hospital, tele-medicine and tele-care can be improved by using m-health systems like GEMA.

CONCLUSION

This chapter has described a modern real-time m-health application and service with the capability of quick reaction and on-line data access in order to offer a proactive help to improve healthcare systems. As mean age is rapidly increasing in most societies, modern healthcare applications should be developed to provide a better, more accessible and quicker support to these citizens. The increasing interest in this kind of applications has brought the attention of researchers and developers and more applications like these are demanded. The satisfaction building GEMA can be mainly increased with its longer use in a real hospital environment to measure how patient care may become more and more effective.

One issue that needs to be analyzed in more detail is the proper integration with other HIS platforms and environments including the validation of use of appropriate standard data formats, like HL7 or CENTC251 among others, like XML to share medical information. More to the point, the use of Web services and other modern Internet technologies will facilitate the integration challenges that might appear in the future.

REFERENCES

Aiken L. H., Clarke S. P., Sloane D. M., Sochalski J. and Silber J. H. (2002). Hospital nurse staffing and patient mortality, nurse burnout, and job dissatisfaction. *JAMA*. Retrieved from http://www.webmm.ahrq.gov/perspective.aspx?perspectiveID=7

Alonso G., Casati, F., Kuno H. and Machiraju V. (2003). *Web services, concepts, architectures and applications*. Springer.

ANSI/IEEE Std. 1471-2000 (2000). *Recommended practice for architectural description of software intensive systems.*

Bashur R. (1997). *Telemedicine and the health care system in telemedicine, theory and practice*. Thomas, Charles C. (Ed.). Springfield, pp. 5-35.

Bass L., Clements P. and Kazman R. (2003). software architecture in practice, 2nd edition. *SEI series in software engineering.*Addison-Wesley.

Clements P., Bachmann F., Bass L., Garlan D., Ivers J., Little R., Nord R. and Stafford J. (2002). Documenting software architectures. *SEI series in software engineering.* Addison-Wesley.

Department of Health - Estates and Facilities Division (2007). *Using mobile phones in NHS hospitals*, (pp.5-10). Retrieved from http://www.dh.gov.uk/en/Publicationsandstatistics/Publications/PublicationsPolicyAndGuidance/DH_074396

Dolin R. H., Alschuler L., Boyer S. et. al. (2006). HL7 clinical document architecture, release 2. *Journal of American Medical Informatics Association, 13*, 30-39.

Hassmann U., Merk L., Nicklous, M.S., Stober, T., Korhonen P., Khan P. and Shelness N. (2003). *Pervasive computing: The mobile world.* Springer

Healy, J.C. (2004). Applications relating to health. fifth research and development framework programme 1998-2002. *Office for Official Publications of the European Communities.* Luxembourg, ISBN: 92-894-7432-7. Retrieved from http://ec.europa.eu/information_society/activities/health/docs/publications/fp5-ehealth-applications-relating-to-health.pdf

ICT for Health (2006). Resource book of eHealth projects. *Office for official publications of the European Communities.* Luxembourg. Retrieved from http://ec.europa.eu/information_society/activities/health/highlights/2006/index_en.htm

Istepanian R. S. H., Jovanov E. and Zhang Y. T. (2004). Guest editorial introduction to the special section on m-Health: Beyond seamless mobility and global wireless health-care connectivity, *IEEE Transactions on Information Technology in Biomedicine, 8*(4), 405- 414.

Oliver N. and Flores-Mangas F. (2006). Healthgear: A real-time wearable system for monitoring and analyzing physiological signals. In *Proceedings of Int. Conf. on Body Sensor Networks (BSN'06).* MIT, Boston. USA.

Pavlopoulos, S., Kyriacou, E., Berler, A., Dembeyiotis, S., and Koutsouris, D. (1999). A novel emergency telemedicine system based on wireless communication technology: AMBULANCE. *IEEE Transactions on Information Technology in Biomedicine, 2(*4), pp. 261-267.

Safran C., Pompilio-Weitzner, Emery, G. K. D. and Hampers L., (2005). *Collaborative approaches to e-Health: Valuable for users and non-users, connecting medical informatics and bio-informatics.* R. Engelbrecht, et al. (Eds). (pp. 879-884).

Wac K., Van Halteren A. Bults R. and Broens T. (2007). Context-aware QoS provisioning in an m-health service platform. *International Journal of Internet Protocol Technology, 2*(2), 102 – 108.

Winter A., Brigl B. and Wendt T. (2003). Modeling hospital information systems (Part 1), the revised three-layer graph-based meta-model 3LGM2. *Methods Inf. Med., 42*(5), 544—551.

Yu P., Wu M. X., Yu H. and Xiao G. C. (2006). The Challenges for the Adoption of M-Health. *IEEE International Conference on Service Operations and Logistics and Informatics (SOLI 2006).* Shanghai, China, pp. 181-186.

KEY TERMS

E-Health: Electronic Health. The term e-health encompasses all of the information and communication technologies (ICT) necessary to make the health system work (International Telecommunication Union – ITU, 2003)

Hospital Information System (HIS): Central medical information system in hospitals where health care related data (e.g.: personnel, patients and their medical history etc.) is stored.

Lightweight Directory Access Protocol (LDAP):. Is a software protocol for enabling anyone to locate organizations, individuals, and other resources such as files and devices in a network, whether on the public Internet or on a corporate intranet (SearchMobileComputing.com definitions).

M-Health (Mobile Health): It can be understood as mobile computing, medical sensor, and communications technologies for e-health (Istepanian R.S.H., Jovanov E. and Zhang Y.T., 2004).

Medical Informatics: The rapidly developing scientific field that deals with biomedical information, data, and knowledge - their storage, retrieval, and optimal use for problem solving and decision making.

Mobile Computing: Is a generic term describing your ability to use technology 'untethered', that is not physically connected, or in remote or mobile (non static) environments. The term is evolved in modern usage such that it requires that the mobile computing activity be connected wirelessly to and through the Internet or to and through a private network (Wikipedia).

Pervasive / Ubiquitous Computing Mobile Computing: Pervasive computing is the trend towards increasingly ubiquitous (another name for the movement is *ubiquitous computing*), connected computing devices in the environment, a trend being brought about by a convergence of advanced electronic - and particularly, wireless - technologies and the Internet (SearchNetworking.com).

Software Architecture: Architecture is defined as the fundamental organization of a system, embodied in its components, their relationships to each other and the environment, and the principles governing its design and evolution (ANSI/IEEE Std. 1471-2000, 2000).

Telemedicine: The use of medical information exchanged from one site to another via electronic communications for the health and education of the patient or healthcare provider and for the purpose of improving patient care. Telemedicine includes consultative, diagnostic, and treatment services (Websters's new world medical dictionary).

Web Service: A reusable component that can be registered, discovered, and invoked using standard internet protocols.

Chapter XXI
Mobile Health Applications and New Home Care Telecare Systems:
Critical Engineering Issues

Žilbert Tafa
University of Montenegro, Montenegro

ABSTRACT

This chapter describes the very actual issues on mobile health (M-H) and home care (H-C) telecare systems, reviewing state of the art as well as theoretical and practical engineering issues crucial for designing these applications. The purpose, advantages and overall information and communication technology (ICT) architectures of M-H and H-C telecare systems are firstly presented. There are several engineering fields involved in the design of modern M-H and H-C applications. Making the optimal application-specific choice in each engineering aspect and achieving the right balance between complementary coupled technological requests are of crucial meaning so the main critical engineering issues (weighted at sensing node's design and the wireless communications) are presented in details as well. Systematic theoretical review and accentuation of the design and realization problems given in this chapter can contribute in better understanding of crucial engineering issues and challenges on this topic as well as in giving the proper direction lines to approaching the practical realization of M-H and H-C telecare systems.

FROM DESKTOP TELEMEDICINE TO THE NEW WIRELESS SOLUTIONS

For more than 30 years, the achievements in IT, electronics, telecommunications and biomedical engineering have been used to facilitate the quality of health care delivery. This kind of approach has provided great benefits in improving the health of population generally, especially by assuring the timely diagnostics and therapeutic treating of patients. Taking the historical view of the technologies that have been used in classical telemedicine applications, one can notice that these applications mainly were designed for fixed-based infrastructure remote monitoring, professional teleconsultations and in providing medical help to remote patients treatment. These applications were concentrated on transferring biomedical and video signals, as well as the medical images and sounds, with the main aim of providing the remote health care service. But, the main drawbacks of the early health delivery systems are contained in the fact that they were not designed to provide the mobility, autonomy of measured subject and health care delivery integrated into patient's everyday life.

Current and emerging developments in microelectronics and wireless communications integrated with developments in pervasive and wearable technologies will have a radical impact on future health care delivery systems (Istepanian, Jovanov, and Zhang, 2004). The results of these developments make possible the realization of the wireless medical sensors with networking capability. Such medical sensor networks greatly enhance the ability of physicians to timely examine and treat complex biological systems at a distance and effectively reduce the infrastructure cost at hospital side and the travel expense at the patient side. The use of new wireless technologies in health delivery systems, offers many advantages, especially in continuous remote monitoring of patient vital signs. The most important improvements are achieved in earlier illness detection enabling timely medical intervention as well as in the treatment of chronic diseases . The integration of emerging wireless technologies in health delivery applications today is separated in two new engineering challenged disciplines – **mobile health** and **home care telecare** systems. Newer concepts represent M-H as a form of e-health evolution from traditional desktop telemedicine to wireless mobile configurations. M-H provides remote medical service delivery (especially the monitoring of biomedical signals) even while patient is in a move and regardless of geographical location of the patient. Home care systems, on the other hand, provide usually more functionality but these systems have the reduced range of mobility. In this case, the mobility range is usually limited to the level of the house, hospital or office. So, the main functional difference between M-H and H-C telecare systems is related to the mobility area. By using small-scale sensing and processing hardware attached to the patient's body or embedded into patient's everyday life ambience, both M-H and H-C systems make possible: more often or continuous inspection of patient's health condition generally, the monitoring of daily variable medical parameters (ECG, SpO2, blood pressure, glucose level, EEG etc.) which variations can point to specific medical conditions and illness etc. The advantages of using the modern m-health and home care applications can be summarized as follows:

- Medical treatment even when the patients are not situated in medical institution,
- Continuous, "real time" or store-and-forward insight into patient's health parameters
- Mobility and comfort of patients while medically treated
- Intelligent monitoring systems with the ability to generate alarms
- Multi-parameter and multi-user health care delivery

- Tele-consultations and flexibile access to expert opinion and advice at the point of care without delay
- Easy integration into greater telemedicine systems.

M-HEALTH AND HOME CARE APPLICATIONS

Applications related to the applying of wireless concept in medicine, usually have been realized for portable teletrauma systems (Chu & Gantz, 2004) and in systems designed for remote medical monitoring of mobile or "semi-mobile" patients (Lin et al, 2005, Anliker et al 2004, Fadlee et al 2005, Boquete, 2005). In the case of teletrauma systems, realized applications provide the transmission of medical parameters as: biomedical signals, images, video signals and voice assuring better understanding of the problem by medical professionals residing at remote location and, consequently, better assistance to the medical trauma team. On the other hand, systems designed for continuous remote monitoring of physiological parameters, usually are dedicated to the treatment of patients with chronicle disease as well as in case of post-hospital home care and also in cases when monitoring of some parameter's daily variability are of crucial meaning. Teletrauma and similar systems along with systems for remote continuous long term health monitoring are today known as M-H and H-C telecare systems, respectively. The first ones primarily aim to provide the ubiquitous health delivery while the second ones provide the home environment for patients while medically treated, which can be very impotant for the recovery process. Beside the main, medical advantages, the usage of these systems have economical meaning (especially when applied for longer patient-to-hospital distances) and social meaning too (in elderly population care). Health parameters which are often monitored using these systems are: ECG (electrocardiogram), HR (heart rate), SpO2 (arterial oxygen saturation), and blood pressure which are usually named as vital signs. But, signals as EEG (electroencephalograph), patient's physical activity, respiration, blood glucose etc. are also often included in these applications. Besides the basic meaning of these parameters, when monitored together, their inter-relational meaning can extend the range of the diseases that can be detected. For example, SpO2, heart beat, blood pressure, and respiration can form together an indicator of the oxygenation of the patient's brain in trauma care (Hailiang, 2006), or, when temperature and humidity sensors are used along with ECG sensor, the correlation between environment conditions with heart conditions can be derived. In all of these applications, the intention is to provide health care delivery not affecting significantly (or not affecting at all) the patient's everyday life and activities. For example, in home care applications, sensors can be embedded in

Figure 1. Example of a typical M-H application architecture

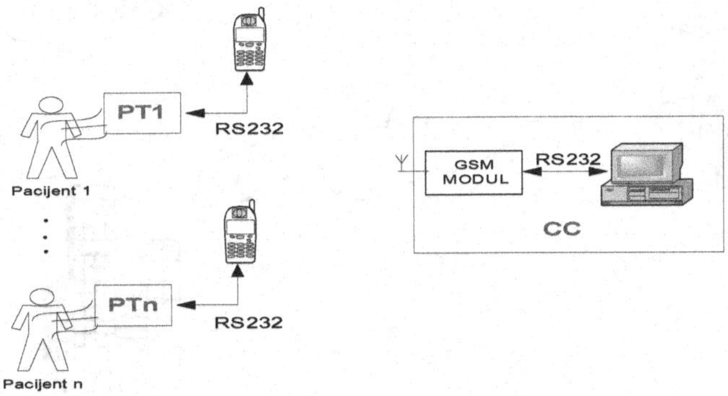

bed and wrapper (Seo, J.Choi, B.Choi, Jeong, and Park, 2005), chair and computer mouse (Kim, J., Park, J., Kim, Chee, Lim, and Park, K., 2007) and so on. On the other hand, the main benefit of using M-H monitoring system is contained in fact that the patient can be medically monitored while being in car, office, or generally, anywhere else in the area of M-H network coverage. The patient's data can be send using mobile phone (GSM, GPRS, 3G etc). An example of a step-by-step application developing process is given in (Boquete, 2005). Functional modules of the system are shown in Figure 1.

In this figure, PTn is abbreviation for the *patient terminal n* (which does the sensing and signal conditioning tasks and transfers data to the mobile phone thought RS232 interface), and CC is the abbreviation for the *control center* (which does the data storing and screening). The transmission here is done in "RS232 over GSM" manner. Typical H-C system organization is given in Figure 2 (Turner J. Kenneth, Gemma A., Campell and Feng Wang, 2007).

The main drawback of M-H system is the link capacity and the resource capacity fluctuation within the mobile environment while the main H-C system's limitation is contained in the mobility range. So, M-H and H-C systems overlap regarding the purpose – remote monitoring of human health parameters and remote health care delivery generally, but the mobility range and the wireless link capacity seems to make the main border on choosing between M-H and H-C systems in general.

ARCHITECTURAL ISSUES

The choice of the adequate technology for each sub module of the system for wireless remote medical monitoring and the way in which various technologies are implemented and integrated into these systems are still application-dependent. Some applications are designed for long term monitoring so they are limited to low power consumption technologies and design. Others are primarily constrained with the mobility range or link capacity, extended functionality etc. The view on typical M-H and H-C telecare system's position into a global Telemedicine system is shown in Figure 3.

It becomes obvious that there are 3 main architectural parts either in M-H and H-C systems:

- Hospital core information system (servers, core network, database organization etc.)
- Communication infrastructure (wired and wireless)

Figure 2. A typical H-C telecare system

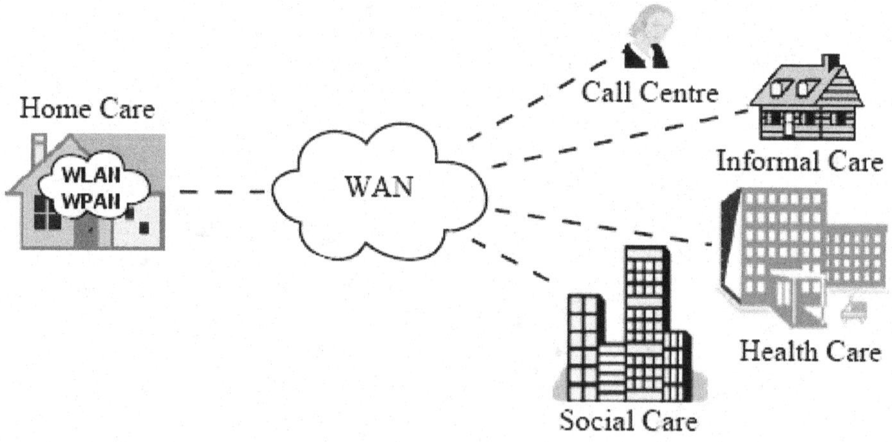

Figure 3. The view on the position of the M-H and H-C modules in telemedicine architecture

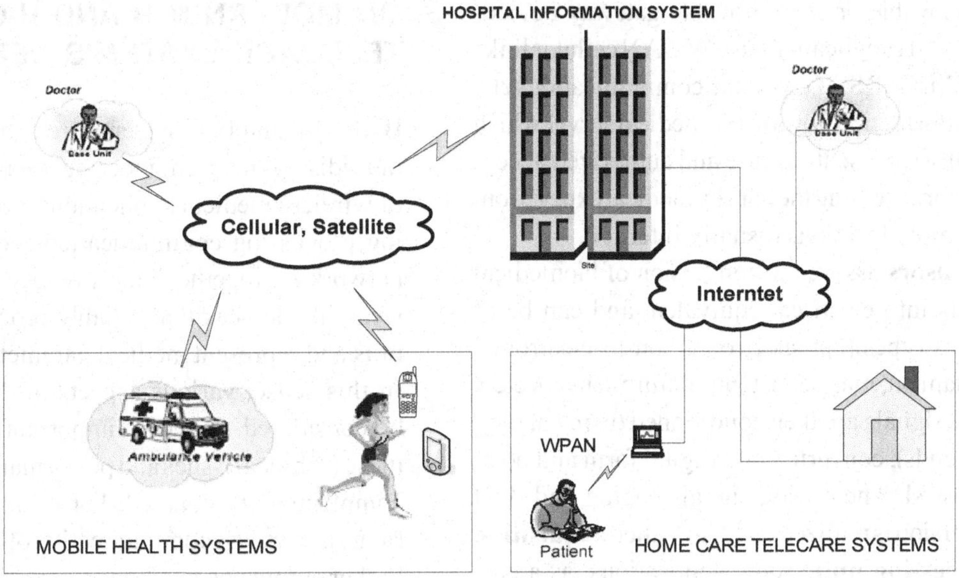

- Mobile subsystem (hardware and software modules)

Hospital core Information system is the framework where different kind of applications are attached to and integrated into. Modern Telemedicine networks support various kind of data flow. M-H and H-C systems are just a part of these networks. Modern telemedicine IT system enables the hardware and software for storing the biomedical, financial and social data. It enables the distributed connectivity, offering various levels of authorized access to the patient's data. Patient and medical professionals can access needed information through secured Telemedicine network (or Internet) links.

Communication infrastructure depends on various factors as: the location and the level of access, the type of transferred data, etc. It is based on standardized networking devices and technologies and does not basically differ from ordinary general purpose computer network infrastructure. In architectural sense, the differences are only noticeable at the level of the remote data upload, specific for M-H and H-C applications, and regarding the end-user networking devices.

A module specific to all wireless medical systems (as new M-H and H-C telecare systems are) is **mobile subsystem** or **personal server.** In case of H-C systems, mobile subsystem contains sensors (along with signal conditioning electronics), digital processing unit and the radio-device. In M-H systems, mobile subsystem contains the gateway device too, which is one additional difference in architectural sense between M-H and H-C systems. In modern wireless H-C applications data are sent through short range wireless links to the fixed wireless ADSL router or some other wireless / cable-based gateway device though Wireless wide area networking (WWAN) links are sometime used as well. Generally, sensing module, equiped with the wired or wireless interface, sends medical information to the gateway device. This module is attached to the monitored patient and is supposed to transmit medical data while the patient is on the move. M-H or H-C applications differ in the way the gateway device achieve the connection to the medical server. home care applications make WAN connections using fixed non-movable or semi-movable gateway devices while M-H applications use WWAN cellular links as GSM, GPRS, 3G, satellite communications etc. The information flows to the medical server which actually represents secure and authorized access point for accessing the data by medical expert from the remote locations (usually Internet).

Sensors assure the conversion of biomedical signals into electrical equivalent and can be of various types (optoelectronic, ion-to-electronic, mechanical, magnetic, temperature sensors etc.). These signals are then conditioned (using analog front ends), converted into digital form and post-processed. The analog signal shaping and A/D conversion is realized in the so-called **acquisition / processing unit**. Some applications, as a part of this unit or the gateway device functionality, provide the possibility for directly viewing the data and generating alarms. Signals are further transferred to the communication module which is used to communicate with gateway device. **Gateway device**, if designed for only transferring the data, can be of miniature dimensions. In case of M-H applications, it is usually mobile phone, PDA or Laptop PC. In these cases, for communication with gateway, the processing unit uses wired connections or some of WPAN technologies (usually Bluetooth or some other widely used technology). In some applications the processing unit and gateway device can be integrated in one, in form of PDA or laptop computer. These systems usually have extended functionality (but greater physical dimensions and weight too). For example, sensors can directly be connected to laptop computer (as it is often case in emergency care applications) and the laptop computer can act as a processing and gateway device, offering direct data screening, data storage capabilities and providing expert system as well.

CRITICAL ENGINEERING ISSUES ON MODERN M-H AND H-C TELECARE SYSTEM'S DESIGN

Both M-h and H-C systems are considered to be multidisciplinary engineering areas. The design of wireless medical applications integrates sensing, processing, communications, computing and networking together into a reduced volume for wearable devices that reliably processes, transmits and represent medical parameters and data. In this sense, various aspects of design should be considered. It is very important to point that these technical issues and performances are often complementary coupled. For example, a longer range in wireless communication often means the higher output power of the transmitter, which implies the higher power consumption which further shortens the battery life or enlarges the overall system costs and the implementation complexity. As it can be concluded, main engineering aspects that are specific to the M-H and H-C application's design, can be summarized in:

- Electronic, electrophysiological, and electromechanical design of sensor nodes - sensing
- Wireless communications and networking
- Software engineering

Sensing in M-H and H-C Applications

To monitor human health constantly without disturbing the user's normal daily activities, the wearable sensors and devices for physiological data collection should be designed to be compact, durable, accurate, small, and noninvasive, to have a fast response time, and provide disturbance rejection capability. It is not always easy to meet all these requirements because, beside the accuracy, electrical, processing/software, mechanical,

Figure 4. Block diagram of a typical sensing node

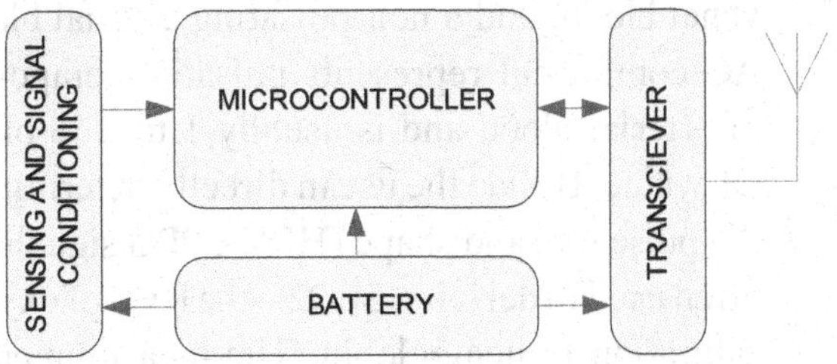

and practical aspects, communication aspect of these modules should be treated as well. Block diagram of typical sensing/acquisition unit is shown in Figure 4.

Because of the uniqueness of telemedical applications, non-invasive M-H and H-C measuring nodes should strictly follow some special limitations as in:

- Adequate sensing, signal shaping and digital signal processing capability, compared to the predefined medical standards
- Miniature physical dimensions
- Low power consumption
- Multi-functionality
- Resistance to various sources of noise (electrical, electromagnetic, chemical, mechanical, ambient noise etc.)
- Must be non-intrusive, acceptable for most patients, and have easy-to-use interface
- Must have the adequate wireless communication performances.

Medical signal recognition begins at **sensor's** end. Generally speaking, biomedical sensors are a subset of specialized sensors responsible for sensing physiological or biological measurands (Yeow, 2006). The biomedical measurands are used as indicators for clinical diagnosis or in therapeutic purposes. Most often, a biomedical sensor node is used as a diagnostic tool.

Many different kind of medical sensors are now available on the market, ranging from conventional sensors based on piezo-electrical materials for pressure measurements to infrared sensors for body temperature estimation and optoelectronic sensors monitoring SpO2, heart rate, HRV, and blood pressure.

In the sense of achieved measuring functionality, biomedical sensing is based on one of the three principles:

- Direct measuring of the electrical activities of organs (heart, brain, muscles, etc.) – bio potentials
- Measuring the influence of physiological processes on some external source of energy (light, ultrasound etc.)
- Injecting substances and detecting their flow by special detectors (as in case of the detection of injected radioisotopes by gamma cameras).

M-H and wireless H-C systems are typically dedicated to non invasively measuring of basic physiological signals (ECG, SPO2, heart rate, blood pressure, etc.). In some special cases, images and video signals are transmitted too (as, for example, in mobile emergency care diagnostic systems). So, It is very important for the designer to be aware of electrophysiological and other (electronics, mechanical) measurement aspects of sensor's node design.

ECG sensor's functionality is based on electrical activity of the heart. As a result of cell's depolarization and repolarization, ionic current is spread over human body. This current can be detected (and transformed into electronic current) using various types of sensors, so called electrodes. Very important issues when using these sensors are: good electrical contact with the body of the measured subject and mechanical stability, the number of used leads, and the position of the leads. The number and the position of the leads determine the range of measure sophistication – the number of the diseases that could be detected. Good electrical contact and mechanical stability directly influence the quality and accuracy of measurement. Bad contact means higher signal attenuation and noise while mechanical instability (vibrations and other mechanical movements) usually introduce so called artifact. An efficient low-noise transducer design can often reduce the need for extensive subsequent signal processing and still produce a better measurement (Semmlow, 2004).

Pulse rate, SPO2, HRV (heart rate variability), and blood pressure are usually derived from the measuring method called PPG (photoplethysmography). PPG is non-invasive method for the detection of cardiovascular pulse waves propagated around the human body based on the determination of optical properties of vascular tissue using light source and photo detector. It is also the mostly used sensing method to monitoring the physiological signals in M-H and H-C applications. There are two PPG approaches based on transmission or reflection of the light (**transmission mode** and **reflection mode**, respectively). Transmission mode is limited to areas such as finger, earlobe or toe, since the light emitter and receiver should be positioned on opposite side of tissue but should also be in close distance to each other. On the other side, reflective mode can be used virtually on any skin area, because the emitter and the receiver are positioned in parallel (and close) to each other. Experience in using PPG sensors in wearable sensor applications for wireless data transmission shows that the finger-base PPG may be most acceptable to users and provides excellent access to an arterial blood signal. PPG is based on the fact that, when directing the light on tissue, the light absorption (and consequently reflection) depends on the concentration of blood in vessels, which is generally given by Beer-Lambert law (Ward, 2001). Using this technique, usually pulsating current is measured and conditioned on the detector side and this pulsating current corresponds to pulse rate. PPG signal has two components: DC and AC component. DC component is relatively constant because it represents the absorption/reflection of the light by constant values as: skin, bones, venal blood, and a non-pulsating arterial blood. AC component represents pulsatile component of arterial blood and is usually 1 to 2 % of the DC value. Beside the use in directly determining the pulse rate and shape (HRV), PPG signals are often used in deriving SpO2 – the level of oxygen saturation in hemoglobin. The measurement is based on the fact that deoxyhemoglobin (Hb) is more absorbed by red (R) then infrared (IR) light and on the other hand oxygenated hemoglobin (HbO2) is more absorbed by IR than by R light. Saturation of hemoglobin is estimated by the following formula:

$$S_pO_2 = 110 - 25R \quad (1)$$

where

$$R = \frac{AC_{RED} / DC_{RED}}{AC_{IR} / DC_{IR}} \quad (2)$$

where alternated current (AC) and direct current (DC) components are firstly calculated.

SpO2 is a very important physiological parameter which gives information about respiration. On healthy subjects, the SpO2 values should be above 96 %. This parameter is often monitored during anesthesia but is also used in M-H and H-C applications alone or together with other parameter's monitoring.

Blood pressure is also one of the basic physiological parameters which are often monitored in typical M-H and H-C applications. There are few standard methods for blood pressure monitoring such as: invasive canola based monitoring (which is never used in M-H and home care systems), sphygmomanometer, oscilloscopic method, and lately some efforts are made in the direction of using pulse transit time (PTT) derived from PPG measuring sensors. Cuff-based method (oscilloscopic) is most popular for classical home but is also used in M-H and H-C applications (Anliker et al, 2004). The PTT based method measures the time distance between R or Q wave of the ECG and point of 50 % of the pulse magnitude. Consequently, ECG and PPG sensors should be used together in order to derive the PTT value, but since most of M-H and H-C applications already monitor ECG and PPG signals, the PTT calculation may extend the application functionality without any additional hardware. It should be noted that PTT based measurement of blood pressure is not well correlated to the absolute value of blood pressure at the given moment. PTT actually enables the prediction of the blood pressure variations for short time intervals.

As can be concluded, PPG method offers the creation of multifunctional non invasive sensor nodes and as such is very suitable for use in M-H and H-C applications. Signal sampling is often based on so called chopper mode – when sampling is triggered by some external source (microcontroller, oscillator etc.), making the module low power consumer. The main drawback of PPG sensing method is noise: **ambient light and artifact**. In order to reduce ambient noise, instead of usually used LED-PIN (light emitting diode – P type intrinsic N type) configuration, a LEDs in reverse bias mode are lately being used as photo detectors. This measuring process assures greater immunity to ambient noise since LED detector operates as band-pass filter. In order to face the artifact, many methods are being proposed. They are usually based on mechanical modeling of sensor node (Booho Yang, Harry H. Asada, S. Rhee, 1999) or on using accelerometer which enables the use of active noise cancellation algorithms based on adaptive filtering (Shaltis P., Wood L., Reisner A. & Asada H., 2005).

Along with transducers, **signal conditioning sub module** is the most important part in achieving the needed quality of the signal for further processing and transmission. Output signal from sensor can be in digital or analogue form. In order to achieve the needed quality of the signal (satisfying magnitude level and low noise influence), it is always necessary to make some further signal conditioning as amplifying, filtering etc. The tradeoff is usually made between the complexity (the size and the price) of **front-end** and the accuracy. For example when using higher filtering degree, higher quality of output signal can be achieved but this implies bulkiest hardware and some more power consumption as well as greater overall physical dimensions. When designing this part of the system, it is important to do some quantitative observations, comparing the achieved results to some professional widely used instrument. It is crucial to know the all technical (electrical) characteristics of measured physiological parameters, and the most important ones being: the signal magnitude and the frequency range. Depending on these parameters and the way the physiological signals are electrically represented (as current, voltage or frequency), proper amplifying and filtering should be realized. For example, when conditioning ECG signal, designer should keep in mind that the voltage derived from electrodes is in range of 1-5 mV and that the frequency band of ECG signal is between 0.02 Hz and 150 Hz (though 1 KHz limit is often used at hospital devices). Although ECG is specified to have a wider frequency band, when monitored using low cost, low power wearable devices, usually only the band from 0.02 Hz to 50 Hz is treated and this quality is very satisfying since the main energy concentration of ECG spectrum belongs to this band.

Summarizing, in biomedical measurements and consequently in M-H and H-C applications, unwanted signal variability has four different origins: physiological variability, environmental noise or interference, transducer artifact, and electronic noise.

As mentioned previously, one of the main limiting factor to be considered in wireless sensor node's design is **power consumption**. In M-H and H-C applications, mobile subsystem is battery supplied. Bearing in mind that these systems are dedicated for long term continuous monitoring, it is obvious that this parameter directly affects most of the system's performances. Duty cycle reduction in conjunction with the so-called power save modes of the MCU and RF transceiver, are often used in order to reduce the power consumption. For example, when using CC1000 transceiver supplied by idealized AA batteries, with duty cycle of 2%, the autonomous battery supply is expected to last up to about a year. But this power consumption reducing method can be used only where the real time monitoring is not a primary limiting factor. In the sense of power consumption, most important sub module is radio device. As it will be described further, many telecommunication and architectural aspects affect the overall power consumption (such as operating frequency, modulation technique, output power, etc). Actually, radio device usually consumes more than 70 % of overall power consumption of the sensing node. Processing units (microcontrollers) today are designed to be ultra low power devices. Their current consumption is expected to be in the range of 0,5 to few mA. Some other (but much lower) power consumption is expected from the rest of signal conditioning electronics (voltage regulators, etc.)

Processing unit enables A/D conversion, digital signal processing, and transmission of the signal to the communication module. In multifunctional applications where the data are needed to be screened from the sensing module directly, more powerful microcontrollers would be needed. Sometime this means some more external memory modules which, on the other hand, can enlarge the overall physical dimensions. Processing unit is not a critical part of the system because developments in today's microelectronic device's design offer very high performance products with: high processing speed, large memory space, low power consumption, high resolution, small physical dimensions, power saving modes, many I/O lines etc.

In the next section, special weight is given to the wireless communication's characteristics and performances since these communications make M-H and H-C applications differ from classical approaches in medical monitoring.

Wireless Communication Issues and the Emerging Wireless Technologies for M-H and H-C

Emerging wireless communications open new solution to health care delivery systems. The appliance of wireless communications in medical systems for remote monitoring such as M-health and home care telecare systems have the potential to transform the way health care is currently provided. Regarding the wireless communications, most important parameters that are considered when designing the M-H and H-C applications are:

- Range
- Data rate
- Resistance to the noise and disturbance
- Power consumption (of the radio-device)
- Physical dimensions (of the radio devices and antennas)
- Networking issues
- Security issues
- Easiness of implementation (the cost) and the ability to integrate smaller communication systems into larger systems (as larger networks or Internet) etc.

There is no actual wireless technology optimized on each of given parameters. These parameters depend on telecommunication aspects as well as the radio-technique architectures of used radio devices and usually are complementary coupled. In this sense, most important issues to be considered are:

- Operating frequency and the bandwidth
- Transmitter power, antenna gain, receiver sensitivity

- Modulation and multiplexing techniques
- Networking topology
- Higher networking protocols.

Although some wireless applications are based on using visible or near-visible optical spectrum, RF communications are mostly used (especially in wireless telemedicine systems). RF section of electromagnetic spectrum lies between the frequencies of 9 kHz and 300 GHz. The RF bands which are used for most wireless networking (including short range telemedicine modules) are the unlicensed ISM (instrument, scientific and medical) bands as: 314 MHz, 433 MHz, 868 MHz (for Europe), 915 MHz (for North America), 2,45 GHz and 5 GHz. Unlicensed in this sense means that the band is free for use and it is up to users to resolve any interference problems, while when dealing with licensed bands, the FCC and similar bodies have a role to play in resolving interference. The choice of **operating frequency** is directly correlated to some very important parameters as: range, power consumption of the radio device and (indirectly) the influence of electromagnetic noise and disturbance. Free space loss is the most important factor affecting the received signal strength. It depends on the signal frequency and transmission distance according to the formula:

$$Lfs = 20 \log (4\pi D \backslash \lambda) \qquad (3)$$

Where D is the transmitter to receiver distance in meters and λ is the wavelength of the radio signal in meters which can also be expressed as:

$$\lambda = c / f \qquad (4)$$

As can be noted from the given formulas (3) and (4), losses are larger when higher operating frequency is used. This is a very important conclusion, especially for the outdoor communications (as this calculation assumes the clear line-of sight between transmitting and receiving antennas). Lower frequencies better penetrate the walls but, in practical indoor situations, the differences in losses due to the difference between used frequencies are small compared to other environmental effects. The most important factor here is the material of the indoor construction and sometime the thickness of walls. Losses are in range from 2-4 dB for non tinted glass, wooden door, cinder block wall, or plaster to over 15 dB in case of metal and silvering (mirrors). Lower losses consequently imply typically lower energy consumption, so, generally, lower frequency transmissions mean lower consumption too. One drawback of using lower frequency is greater antenna length (l ~ λ\4). On the other hand, much higher operating frequencies (70 GHz) are sometime used as suitable for very short distances at the order of centimeters but they are not widely used in medical applications. When choosing the operating frequency, it is also important to choose the one which will not interfere with other networks at the same environment. This helps in preventing and minimizing the influence of the interference and noise.

Regarding the transmission frequency band, RF communications are often categorized as: **narrowband** and **wideband**. Data rate, as very important communication parameter, is directly correlated to the bandwidth: the greater the bandwidth, the higher capacity of the communication link. Narrowband devices generally have lower overall power consumption though some wideband systems can be highly effective in the sense of power consumption per transmitted bit (UWB). In order to avoid the interference and eavesdropping, today's technologies often use some of the Spread Spectrum (SS) techniques. Most important spread spectrum techniques are DSSS (direct sequence spread spectrum) as used by ZigBee networks, and FHSS (frequency hopping spread spectrum) as used by Bluetooth technology. It is important to note generaly that the choise in **operating frequency** and the **bandwidth** directly influence data rate and the range. Higher data rates require more spectrum. But, more spectrum can only be found higher in the frequency band. Using higher frequency band, on the other hand means greater propagation losses, which implies the lower propagation range.

Beside telecomunication aspects of the wireless links, some radio-technique characteristics are also very important as: **output transmitter power, antenna gain, and the receiver sensitivity**. Along with losses, these factors make so-called **link budget** - the balance of power plus gain required to compensate for losses in the link so that sufficient signal strength is available at the receiver to allow data decoding at an acceptable error rate (Webb, 2007).

Output transmitter power is one of the most important characteristics of the radio device because, along with other parameters, it often directly determines the range of RF communications. For the radio devices operating at ISM bands, some strict regulations exists regarding the output signal strength. For example, in Europe, at frequency of 2,4 GHz, oputput power is limited to maximum 100 mW.

Antenna shape and the directivity can have great impact on strength and the quality of transmittet signal and sometime can influence the link security too. Directive antennas are more effective but in M-H and H-C applications they can not be used because the factor of mobility. In implementation process, in order to avoid losses and reflection, it is important to match antenna impedance with the output impedance of the radio device. The higher directivity of the antenna, the lower possibility to eavesdropping the data.

Receiver's sensitivity is the lowest limit of the signal strength that can be detected by the receiver. Typical values for receiver's sensitivity of the low power WPAN devices (which are usually used in H-C and M-H applications and in wireless sensor systems generally) are < - 85 dBm.

The bit stream must be **modulated** in order to be sent by the radio waves. It can be modualated onto either a single or multiple carrier frequencies but also can be modified regarding the position or shape of the signal. Right choice on modulation technique has impact on some important communication parameters as:

- Spectral efficiency (achieving the desired data rate within the available spectral bandwidth),
- BER (Bit Error Rate) performance – achieving the required error rate given the particular factors of the degradation (interference, multipath fading etc.),
- Power efficiency – particulary important in mobile health applications,
- Implementation complexity – wich direcly influences the cost of the hardware though some aspects of the modulation can be implemented in software (not influencing the cost of implementation).

On these parameters some tecniques can be more or less efficient and usually the choise depends on the purpose and on which parameter is application more limited to. For example, constant envelope of modulated signal, practically means higher efficiency of the output power amplifier (even to 50 %) achieved by using nonlinear part of the transfer function in contrast to other types where efficiency can be up to 10 %, so in the sense of power efficiency, these techniques can be more appropriate where power consumption is the primary limitation factor.

For combining multiple analog message signals or digital data streams into one signal, **multiplexing techniques** are used. These techniques define the way multiple users access the common medium and can be of types as: TDMA (time division multiple access), FDMA (frequency division multiple access) or OFDMA (orthogonal FDMA), SDMA (space DMA) and CDMA (code DMA). The combination of two techniques is used as well. For example, GSM uses FDMA/TDMA with eight time slots available in each 200 KHz radio channel.

Networking topology is one of the first issues that are considered in the process of M-H and H-C application's design. At the beginning of the project, the designer usually determines some basic architectural parameters as: wireless coverage, number of sensing nodes, redundancy, extendibility, connectivity to higher level Telemedicine networks etc. All these aspects more or less depend on the choice of the networking topology. For example, when designing simple typical home care application for only one user (e.g. in continuous monitoring of ECG, SpO2, blood pressure etc.), a simple **point-to-point** link can be used without the need for wireless networking in the sense of dealing with greater number of nodes and considering medium sharing and addressing. When dealing with smaller size network (for ex. in ambulatory monitoring of few patients), usually the simple **star topology** can be appropriate. The main advantage of star topology is the simplicity. The drawbacks are: a simple central node (which, in case of error, can break down the whole network), relatively small range and bandwidth sharing. Central node can be: PC, PDA, WiMAX base station, Wi-Fi access point, Bluetooth master, ZigBee PAN coordinator, embedded Web server etc. Typical indoor range of wireless short-range star topology networks (as in Home/Office/Hospital Care low power communications) is 30 m. **Tree topology** (extended star) is very popular and mostly used one because of: extended range (usually using wired infrastructure partially), simplicity and more efficient in using the overall bandwidth. **Mesh topology** enables greater functionality of the network. The main advantages are the redundancy and roaming. The data routing function is distributed throughout the entire mesh rather than being under the control of one or more dedicated devices. These networks are also known as mobile ad hoc networks (MANET) in which nodes are mobile and communicate directly with adjacent nodes not needing any central controlling devices. Distributed control and continuous reconfiguration allows for rapid re-routing around overloaded, unreliable or broken paths, allowing mesh networks to be self-healing and very reliable (Rackley, 2007). It is clear that for the network to be really meshed and mobile, routing protocols should be implemented in each node. This implies the increased node's complexity, since more processing power should be implemented also affecting the overall power consumption of the nodes which can be a critical factor in most Telemedicine applications. Wireless mesh networks are rarely used in typical M-H and H-C applications, mostly because of their complexity. When ubiquitous monitoring is needed (as in mobile health applications), cellular networks are used.

Higher communication and networking protocols are important in achieving wider network functionality and more reliable data transfer as well as in accomplishing better efficiency in sending different types of data. Generally, there are five categories of medical data that can be transferred: biological signals, live scene images, administrative data (e.g., access control, device configuration signals, etc.), control commands for remote devices, and warning signals (Polley, 2006). Because the telemedicine applications use different interconnected networks, protocols as TCP (transmission control protocol) and UDP (user datagram protocol) are usually used. TCP is connection-oriented reliable protocol with flow control and congestion control mechanism, whereas UDP uses a simple datagram with no congestion control. TCP is more suitable for transferring data which require small portion of bandwidth and high reliability. Very imprtant issue here is setting the various priorities for various data types. As an example, ECG, PPG and other vital signs, should be sent via high priority TCP link. On the other hand, bandwidth-hungry images transfer quality will satisfy the purpose by using low priority UDP protocol, since congestion control mechanism of the TCP protocol with retransmitting (especially in a wireless environment) would cause extra delays.

In M-H and H-C systems, security issues have to be considered as well. This factor should be treated as the priority one, since medical data are very sensitive so the data integrity is very important. Different technologies offer different mechanisms in this sense. Higher protocols (as encryption algorithms and others) are usually integrated into a technology-specific protocol stack. For example, Bluetooth technology uses integrity check system SAFER+ and the 128 bit E0 encryption. Some extension in security issues can be achieved by appropriate software development at the application level.

Engineering aspects mentioned previously are very important in choosing adequate technology which would be optimal for a given purpose. Some of standardized technologies are often used. Knowing their technical characteristics, the designer should be able to make the choice of the appropriate one.

Generally, today's wireless communication systems can be categorized as (Webb, 2007):

1. **Mobile:**
   - 2G
   - 3G
   - WiMax
   - 4G
2. **Private mobile radio (PMR):**
   - Analogue
   - Digital
   - Mobile mesh
   - Emerging technologies including cognitive radio and software defined radio (SDR)
3. **Fixed wireless:**
   - Point-to-Point
   - Point-to-multipoint
   - Fixed mesh
4. **Short range:**
   - WLANs (802.11)
   - WPANs (Bluetooth, ZigBee, UWB)
   - RFID (Passive and Active devices) – WBAN.
5. Conventional analogue and digital broadcasting

Since applications designed for continuous monitoring of physiological parameters mostly use some of standardized cellular or short range (WLAN and WPAN) technologies, these technologies will be described in some more details.

As mentioned, M-H application's primarily advantage is the network coverage which enables ubiquitous mobile health care delivery. Consequently, these systems use cellular networks as 2G (and the extensions as GPRS, MMS, HSCSD, WAP, EDGE etc.), 3G, and (in future) 4G networks. Beside the coverage, the advantage of these networks is contained in the fact that they are very much present in cellular phones, so their integration into telemedicine systems is easy. 2G systems, through EDGE for GSM, can provide (in "ideal" occasions) the data rate of up to 300 kb/s. In typical practical use, data rates are much lower. On the other hand, 3G systems were designed against criteria of delivering 2 Mb/s but they practically can achieve data rates up to 400 kb/s which open a wide range of opportunities for use as: video calls, video streaming, real time monitoring (with very satisfying data rate and coverage) etc. As such, they are very appropriate for use in M-H systems when sending medical data in real time manner such as video signal, images and other measured medical parameters. The problem with 3G is that this technology is still not widely deployed. 4G technology, beside cellular character, is expected to integrate other short range technologies as: Bluetooth, ZigBee, UWB etc. Very high data rates are expected to be achieved, even up to 100 Mbps.

Indoor data and voice traffic transmission, however, converge to short range communications systems because these systems generally have some important advantages over cellular (and other long-range) networks when integrated into telemedicine applications as: lower price, higher data rate, networking capabilities (supporting ad-hoc networking), longer battery life, smaller device's dimensions etc. New home care telecare systems are supposed to assure the mobility in range of ambulance, hospital sector, office or house. So, there is no need for the only advantage which mobile cellular networks offer over short range communications – the outdoor coverage. That's why, in these systems, short range communications are mostly deployed. On the other hand, in typical M-H applications, short range communications (for communication of sensor node with the gateway device) are often used too. For example, cellular phone can communicate with sensor node using Bluetooth technology and, at the same time, can act as a gateway device transferring data to some medical server or directly to some other mobile phone using cellular networks.

Almost all **WLAN** networks are covered with IEEE standard 802.11. Most popular versions are: "a", "b", and "g". Greatest advantage of 802.11 is data rate which can theoretically go up to 54 Mbps. Technically, IEEE 802.11 use ISM frequency 2,4 GHz (versions "b" and "g") and 5 GHz (version "a"). Version "a" is under the lower influence on disturbance because a small number of technologies use this frequency, but, on the other hand, this shortens the range, which can be up to 7 times shorter compared to standards "b" and "g". For collision avoidance, CSMA/CA (Carrier Sense Multiple Access / Collision Avoidance) is used and, on physical layer, techniques as DSSS (at version "b") and OFDM (at versions "a" and "g") are used too. Indoor range is typically 50 m while outdoor links can be in rage of km using special antennas. Another sdvantage of IEEE 802.11 devices is very good Internet connectivity which makes this networks suitable for use as backbone (in conjunction to UWB or other short range technology). On the other hand, typical WLAN devices are not suitable for the integration into wearable medical nodes, primarily because of their power consumption and physical dimensions. WLAN technology can be very appropriate in ambulatory/hospital monitoring where sensor node can be wired to Laptop PC or PDA or can be wirelessly connected using some WPAN link, while the transmission to the medical server can be accomplished by WLAN link.

UWB technology uses very wide frequency band, between 3.1 GHz and 10.6 GHz. Because of the bandwidth, power limitations are regulated and very strict. UWB is designed for short range communications (typically 10-20 m) of very high data rates (few hundred Mbps). This technology is most suitable for PC connectivity and wireless connection of home devices (DVD players and plasma screens etc). UWB transmission has the lowest consumption per bit but overall power consumption is typically higher than at Bluetooth or ZigBee devices. This technology could be a good choice when transferring larger medical data loads at short distances as when transferring medical images and video signal.

Bluetooth was initially designed to serve as cable replacement technology for data communications between mobile phones. When new improved versions appeared, it became clear that Bluetooth will do much more than that. Today, Bluetooth devices, beside their initial purpose, are used in creating wireless sensor networks and especially in forming WPAN (Wireless Personal Area Networks) for mobile health and home care telecare applications. From the technical point of view, Bluetooth works at frequency range 2,402 – 2,480 GHz using FHSS, GFSK modulation and TDMA multiplexing. Bluetooth defines 3 power classes: class 1 (maximum output power of 20 dBm), class 2 (maximum output power of 4 dBm), and class 3 (maximum output power of 0 dBm). Networking architecture is of type master/slave and usually forms star topology called **piconet**. Bluetooth network can be extended into **scatternet** – set of two or more piconets. Main characteristics of Bluetooth technology can be summarized as:

- Data and voice transfer at typical distances 1-100 m

- Various networking topology supported
- Data rates can be up to 723 Kbps (versions 1.x) and up to 3 Mbps (version 2.0)
- Small current load (typically from few mA to 30 mA) and usage of power saving modes as *sniff, hold*, and *park*.
- Robustness
- Miniature radio devices (typically 20mm x 20mm or smaller)
- Great presence in mobile telephone devices.

These characteristics make Bluetooth technology a good choice when simple short range star topology is needed, with solid data rate and small power consumption. As such, Bluetooth is often found in M-H applications as a communication method between wearable sensor and mobile phone, PDA or Laptop. At home care applications, fixed cable based gateway can be used and the communication between gateway and sensor node can be done using Bluetooth links.

ZigBee is another WPAN technology which works at 3 frequency ranges: 2,4-2,4835 GHz (with 16 channels and maximum data rate of 250 Kbps), 902-928 MHz in North America (with 10 channels and maximum data rate of 40 Kbps), and 868-868,6 MHz (only one channel and maximum data rate of 20 Kbps). The first one uses OQSK (Offset Quadrature Shift Keying) modulation technique and the other two use BPSK (Binary Phase Shift Keying). ZigBee uses DSSS and, for collision avoidance, CSMA/CA. Performances of ZigBee technology can be summarized as:

- Ultra low power consumption
- Miniature radio devices
- Capability of creating large ad hoc networks
- Ranges 10-75 m

Because of the mentioned characteristics, especially power consumption, ZigBee technology tends to become optimal choice in wireless sensor networks where power consumption is most critical parameter, while the high data rates and advanced capabilities of Bluetooth are not needed. In Telemedical applications, ZigBee would be an optimal solution in long term continuous monitoring of some slow changing signals (i.e. PPG) or in the case of implants and signal acquisition from different parts of human body (forming wireless body area network).

Critical Issues on Software Design

As mentioned before, the design of systems for remote monitoring of medical data belongs to so-called middleware engineering which, beside some physiological and electrophysiological aspects, includes the knowledge on hardware design, communications, and the software design. Most of the hardware and device's communications should be supported by appropriate software modules. Software design in M-H and H-C systems is related to the microprocessor / sensor unit programming, network programming, and the user graphical user interface (GUI). Also, some software integration into a hospital core information system are needed as transferred data need to be correlated to other patient's data. Sensor units for continuous monitoring of biomedical signals as used in M-H and H-C systems contain programmable units such as microcontrollers or microprocessors with the extensions (memory modules, etc.). There are different software platforms on which the functionality of these units is based. For example, C programming is often used as very efficient with high speed processing capabilities. Some sensors are programmed using the operating system called TinyOS, which is currently the industrial standard for wireless sensor network operating system. TinyOS also provide well-defined set of API's for programming the Motes and some on-board data processing. It supports the execution of multiple threads and provides a variety of additional extensions like virtual machine and the database (TinyDB).

Typical software modules implemented into a microcontroller unit contain routines as: ports and timer's initialization, I/O initialization and communication routines, A/D routines, storage of digitized sampled data, interrupt routines, often CRC calculation routines etc. Beside this, some application-specific communication protocol is usually needed. For example, sensor initialization is usually made by the healthcare provider at the remote site. After that, the protocol might include some frames either for synchronization or for identification. To ensure the link security, some applications include special coding techniques. Into a software design, node control and administration often should be included in order to configure devices for various uses.

Generally, most important issues on remote health monitoring system software design can be summarized in following limitations:

- The ability for real time processing and (sometime) data compression
- User friendly GUI
- Security issues (authentication, authorization, encryption)
- Networking scalability and multi user platform
- Multi-functionality
- Database store and access for various types of patient's data as: medical, financial, insurance, etc.

The sensor node's software has to be able to efficiently capture and process data as well as to transmit them to the wireless radio device's interface. There are two ways of data processing storing and transferring at mobile subsystem's end: *real time* and *store and forward.* In order to achieve efficient and, for the purpose of the particular application, satisfying level of data processing and the transfer, it is very important to calculate and treat some parameters as: needed sampling period, duty cycle, etc. Depending on the fact if the data processing means buffering or not, some memory calculations sometimes are needed too. For example, if 4-Mb SRAM (static random access memory) is available and 10 min ECG signal buffering is needed, knowing the sampling rate (typical of 128 Hz or 250 Hz) and the resolution (typical 8-16 bit), leads to the calculations for the memory space. If the values are 14 bit resolution, 250 Hz sampling, and 10 minute recording of the ECG signal, then the amount of memory needed is *sampling rate x number of bits per sample x duration* = 250 x 14 x 10 x 60 = 2.1 Mb (Fadlee, 2005). This is about half of the SRAM capacity. Therefore there is a scope to alter the sampling rate, quantization level, and duration of the data according to the clinical need. It is also important to take into account the real transmission capacity of the system. For example, in order to transmit 2, 1 Mb of data through 32kb/s GPRS link, 66 seconds would be needed, so when programming the A/D conversion and buffering, it is important to make appropriate space between transmissions in order to avoid frame overlapping. In case when data are shown directly to user (as when using PDA or Laptop connection to the sensor node), the user friendly interface with easy and secure configurability should be designed. There is no practical limitation on which programming platform to use. The platform can be important mostly in the sense of portability.

At the core information system's end, software architecture is often comprised of a set of user-friendly software modules, which can receive data from the remote Telemedicine devices, transmit information back to it and store important data in local database. Authorized user (i.e. doctor) should be able to access patient's data either directly (while being logged on local hospital network), or through secured remote connection (i.e. using Virtual Private Network). These software modules should be flexible and integrated into the user-friendly GUI's functionality comprising together encircled software architecture for remote health care delivery.

CONCLUSION

M-H and H-C systems are new concepts that, beside classical integration of microelectronic design and computing in medical telecare application, include wireless communications as well. Biomedical signals are captured using sensors. They are further conditioned and processed using signal conditioning front-ends and the microprocessor unit, respectively. After digitally represented, medical data are sent to the medical server, partly or fully, using wireless communications. Medical server deals with remote connections, medical databases, networking etc. This approach assures continuous access to the patient's health parameters even when the patient is in move and usually regarding the geographical location. The benefits of this kind of health care delivery are shown in much aspects (medical, social, economical), but the essential one is facilitating the health condition of population which is already improved in countries and medical systems where these approaches are applied.

REFERENCES

Anliker, U., Ward, J.A., Lukowiez, P., Tröster, G., Dolveck, F., Baer, M., Keita, F., Schnecker, E., Catarsi, F., et.al. (2004, December). A wearable multiparameter medical monitoring and alert syste. *IEEE Transactions on Information Technology in Biomedicine, 8*(1), 415-425.

Booho Yang, Harry H. Asada, S. Rhee, (1999, October). Design of an Artifact-Resistive, Finger-Ring Plethysmographic Sensor. *MIT Home Automation and Healthcare Consortium*, Progress Report No.2-4.

Boquete,L., Bravo, I., Barea, R., Ascariz, J.M.R., and Martin, J.L.(2005, May). Practacal laboratory project in telemedicine: Supervision of electrocardiograms by mobile telephony. *IEEE Transactions on Education, 48*,(2).

Chu, Y. & Gantz, A. (2004, December). A mobile teletrauma system using 3G networks. *IEEE Transactions on Information Technology in Biomedicine, 8*,(4), 457-461.

Fadlee, M., Rasid, A., and Woodward, B. (March, 2005). Bluetooth Telemedicine Processor for Multichannel Biomedical Signal Transmission via Mobile Cellular Networks. *IEEE Transactions on Information Technology in Biomedicine, 9*(1), 35-43.

Hailiang Mei, Ing Widya, Aart van Halteren, Bayu Erfianto, (2006, December). A flexibile vital sign representation framework for mobile healthcare. I*nternational Conference on Pervasive Computing Technologies for Healthcare*. Innsbruck, Austria.

Istepanian, R.S.H., Jovanov, E., and Zhang, Y.T (2004, December). Guest editorial introduction to the special section on m-health: Beyond seamless mobility and global wireless health-care connectivity. *IEEE transactions on information technology in biomedicine, 8*(4), 405-413.

John L. Semmlow (2004). *Biosignals and biomedical image processing*. New York: Marcel Dekker.

John T. W. Yeow (2006). Biomedical sensors. *Wiley Encyclopedia of Biomedical Engineering*. University of Waterloo.

Kim, J., Park, J., Kim, K., Chee, Y., Lim,Y., and Park, K. (2007). Development of nonintrusive blood pressure estimation system for computer users. *Telemedicine and e-Health,* 13(1).

Lin, Y., Jan, I., Ko, P., Chen, Y., Wong, J., Jan, G. (2005, December). Wireless PDA based physiological monitoring system for patient transport. *IEEE Transactions on Information Technology in Biomedicine, 8*(4), 443-447.

Polley R. Liu, Max Q.-H. Meng, Peter X.Liu, Fanny F.L. Tong, M.Phil, and X.J. Chen, M.Phil, (2006). A telemedicine system for remote health and activity monitoring for the elderly. *Telemedicine and e-Health, 12(6).*

Seo, J., Choi, J., Choi, B., Jeong, D., and Park,K.(2005). The development of a nonintrusive home-based physiologic signal measurment system. *Telemedicine and e-Health, 11(4)*, 487-495.

Shaltis P., Wood L., Reisner A. & Asada H. (2005, September), Novel design for a wearable, rapidly deployable, wireless noninvasive triage sensor. *27th Annual International Conference of the IEEE/EMBS*. Shanghai, China.

Tomas Ward (2001), *The Photoplethysmograph as an instrument for physiological measurement.* Department of Electronic Engineering, NUI Maynooth.

Turner J. Kenneth, Gemma A., Campell and Feng Wang (2007, June). Policies for sensor networks and home care networks. In *Proceedings of 7th Int. Conf. on New Technologies for Distributed Systems*, pp. 237-284.

William Webb (2007). *Wireless communications: The future*. West Sussex, England: John Wiley & Sons Ltd. Key Words

KEY TERMS

Home Care: Home care is health care provided in the patient's home by healthcare professionals (often referred to as home health care or formal care; in the United States, it is known as skilled care) or by family and friends (also known as caregivers, primary caregiver, or voluntary caregivers who give informal care).

Mobile Health: M-health can be defined as emerging mobile communications and network technologies for healthcare. This emerging concept represents the evolution of e-health systems from traditional desktop telemedicine platforms to wireless and mobile configurations.

Physiological Signals: Physiological signals are acquired and processed to form psycho-physiological measures. These measures affect game play both through team understanding and altered game mechanics.

Sensor: A sensor is a device which measures a physical quantity and converts it into a signal which can be read by an observer or by an instrument. For accuracy, all sensors need to be calibrated against known standards. Sensors are used in everyday objects such as touch-sensitive elevator buttons and lamps which dim or brighten by touching the base. There are also innumerable applications for sensors of which most people are never aware. Applications include automobiles, machines, aerospace, medicine, industry, and robotics.

Telecare: Telecare is the term given to offering remote care of elderly and vulnerable people, providing care and reassurance needed to allow them to remain living in their own homes. Use of sensors allows the management of risk and as part of a package which can support people with dementia, people at risk of falling or at risk of violence and prevent hospital admission.

Vital Signs: Vital signs are measures of various physiological statistics often taken by health professionals in order to assess the most basic body functions. Vital signs are an essential part of a case presentation.

Wireless Communication: Is the transfer of *information* over a distance without the use of electrical conductors or "wires". The distances involved may be short (a few meters as in television remote control) or very long (thousands or even millions of kilometers for radio communications). When the context is clear the term is often simply shortened to "wireless". Wireless communications is generally considered to be a branch of telecommunications.

Section VI

Distributed Problem-Solving Environments and Medical Imaging

Chapter XXII
A New System for the Integration of Medical Imaging Processing Algorithms into a Web Environment

José Antonio Seoane Fernández
Artificial Neural Networks and Adaptative Systems Group, Spain & University of Corunna, Spain

Juan Luis Pérez Ordóñez
Center of Medical Informatics and Radiological Diagnosis, Spain & University of Corunna, Spain

Noha Veiguela Blanco
Artificial Neural Networks and Adaptative Systems Group, Spain & University of Corunna, Spain

Francisco Javier Novóa de Manuel
Center of Medical Informatics and Radiological Diagnosis, Spain & University of Corunna, Spain

Julián Dorado de la Calle
University of A Coruña, Spain

ABSTRACT

This chapter presents an architecture for the integration of various algorithms for digital image processing (DIP) into web-based information systems. The proposed environment provides the development of tools for intensive image processing and their integration into information systems by means of JAVA applets. The functionality of the system is shown through a set of tools for biomedical application. The main feature of this architecture is that it allows the application of various types of image processing, with different computational costs, through a web browser and in a transparent and user-friendly way.

INTRODUCTION

The rapid advance of the medical imaging field is revolutionizing medicine. Technologies such as computed axial tomography (CT Scan), magnetic resonance imaging (MRI), Helicoidal CT Scan, and the fusion of CT Scan and positron emission tomography (PET), all provide an effective map of the human anatomy in a non-invasive manner.

Clinical practice usually relies on computing techniques to simplify the diagnosis of the medical expert. Medical imaging is not restricted to the visualization of anatomical structures, it is also used for diagnosis, surgical planning, simulation, radiotherapy planning, etc. These applications enable the clinicians to virtually interact with the anatomical structures and as such achieve the knowledge that enhances their performances. All the aforementioned techniques belong to a discipline known as Digital Image Processing (DIP). Traditionally, the medical DIP applications were carried out in expensive work-stations provided by the CT or PET machine supplier. These kinds of applications have certain drawbacks, such as administration and maintenance, which make them unsuitable for some environments.

The current trend in software development is the creation of applications that can be integrated into a Web environment and enjoy advantages such as placement independence, centralized application maintenance, and the use of firewalls without changing the filter rules. Web applications have proliferated due to their rapid learning and easy use as well as their personalization capability that provides a user-friendly interface. This trend towards Web developments is also being introduced into the medical field, to the detriment of the traditional clinical applications. DIP-related applications have high computational costs and therefore hospitals have to invest heavily in computing equipment in order to provide the clinicians with powerful mainframes. At this point, it seems logical to differentiate between algorithms of low and high computational cost.

It should be borne in mind that, as DIP is not a recent discipline, there exist libraries that include different algorithms for digital image processing. Already implemented algorithms should therefore be reused in new developments.

State of the Art

There currently exists a wide range of applications that allow the digital processing of medical images by means of a Web browser. The following list represents applications with two common factors: the DIP is processed at the client and the implemented algorithms tend to have a low computational cost.

- RAIM Java is a DICOM (Digital Imaging and Communication in Medicine) image viewer for biomedical imaging that was developed by the Biomedical Digital Imaging Center of UDIAT-CD S.A. (http://www.cspt.es/webcsptcastella/udiat/default.htm). This viewer was developed with Java technology and can therefore be used in almost any computer and graphic operative system. Since the visual display was conceived as an applet, it has to be executed within a Web browser; this allows the images to be processed in various ways, such as change of visualization window (Window-Level), rotation, scale, etc.
- CHILI: Digital radiology (http://www.chili-radiology.com) is a set of software components oriented towards tele-radiology and PACS (Picture Archiving and Communication Systems). It is a product from CHILI GmbH (Germany) and was developed in cooperation with the German Cancer Research Center and the *Steinbeis Transferzentrum Medizinische Informatik* company. CHILI WEB is one of its products and is composed by the CHILI/Web Server with the CHILI/Web Client. The CHILI/Web Server first receives the images of the

modalities through the DICOM protocol and later stores them in a relational data base. The CHILI/WEB Server can work with an existing PACS. The CHILI/Web Client is a platform-independent program developed with Java.

- RemotEye (http://eng.neologica.it/prodotti/remoteye) is a DICOM display developed by NeoLogica.it. which allows the visualization of DICOM imaging though Internet and offers the possibility of performing certain types of digital image processing such as geometrical transformations, changes of brightness and contrast, etc. It can easily be integrated with the PACS.
- MagicWeb/ACOM.Web (http://www.medical.siemens.com) was developed by Siemens and provides the publication of images and reports for an entire welfare centre with the aim of allowing clinicians to consult from different places. One of its characteristics is the optimization of imaging visualization, since images can be seen with different brightness and contrast levels, augmentation, compression, cinema mode, filters, etc.

On the other hand, there also exists a series of applications that use intensive processing for the performance of different algorithms and rely on complex computing developments, since they can not be executed within a Web browser. The following list represents various developments with complex computational DIP requirements.

- A good option for the development of distributed applications is the CORBA interface for communication among remote objects. This technology allows not only the integration of various languages on different machines but also a total interconnection among all the applications. An example of the use of this technology is the Image Processing Tool (http://imageprocess.sourceforge.net), a distributed processing system based on open-source software that uses a client-server architecture. The main shortage of this software is that, inherently to the use of CORBA, two machines cannot communicate through the Internet due to possible intermediate firewalls.
- The IRMA (image retrieval in medical applications) (http://phobos.imib.rwth-aachen.de/irma/index_en.php) is a distributed system developed by the Computing Department of the University of Aachen (Germany). This system provides not only uniform access to different modalities of medical imaging but also the application of different types of distributed processing algorithms to the images. The proposed architecture has a client-server structure and involves a central database, a task planner, and several processing daemons. The planner distributes the processing load among the different processing daemons installed at processing stations, which provides a low cost and high performance system. The main disadvantage of such a system is the communication between the client and the server on TCP-IP through non-standard protocols, and the non-multiplatform nature of the client.
- The Diamond Eye (Burl et al, 1999) architecture was developed by NASA laboratories and created initially to recover images and use them for data-mining tasks. This architecture involves the use of a Web browser to gain access to images stored in a database through a Java Applet. The architecture enables the client to access and process the images independently from the platform. The data-mining operations with a high computational cost are performed in a network of workstations (NOW) of Sun UltraSparc II. The requirements of the client are handled to the server, which executes in parallel the algorithm at the processing network by means of message-passing libraries [9].

- Distributed architectures are a good alternative to the supercomputers in terms of processing power when executing high-cost computational tasks. Another architecture based on message passing is the proposal of Li, Veeravalli and Ko, (Li et al, 2003) that uses the PVM (Parallel Virtual Machine) library (http://www.csm.ornl.gov/pvm) to pass communication messages to and from the processors of various workstations. This approach is based on the division of the image into several parts in order to be distributed among the network nodes and processed afterwards; the approach of He, Wu, Liu and Zheng (He et al, 2003) explores the best way to distribute the data among the different processors.

Among all the aforementioned architectures, only he Diamond Eye developed by NASA achieves distributed processing using the Web browsers as front-end by means of Java applets. However, this system is very specific and does not allow the integration of different types of tools. A framework is therefore needed for the integration of heterogeneous tools into an information system that can support high computational costs through the Internet.

PROPOSED ARCHITECTURE

Considering the vast amount of existing medical imaging modalities and their respective processing needs, the proposed architecture had to be independent from both software and hardware and integrate several image processing algorithms. Our architecture provides access to the processing services through a Web interface. The present work proposes a framework for the development of tools that are able to provide a medical team with all the processing power required for high

Figure 1. Physical framework architecture

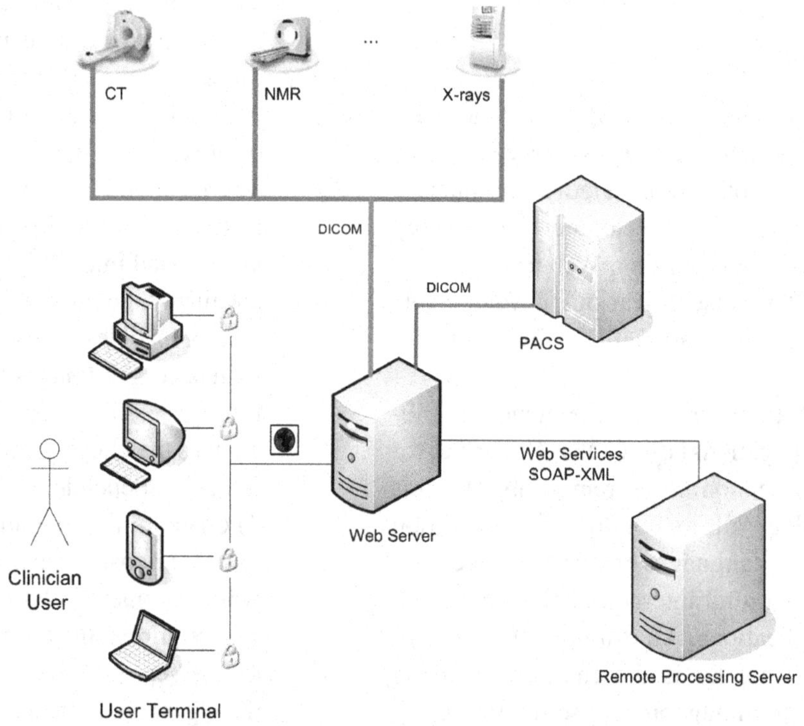

cost visualization, planning, and simulation tasks by means of a remote server. These tasks can be performed independently from a physical location, since only an Internet connection and browser are needed.

This section describes, from two different viewpoints, a solution for the integration of processing algorithms for biomedical digital imaging into Web systems. The first perspective is that of the physical placement of each element, whereas the second perspective focuses on the logical structure of the architecture.

Physical Framework Architecture

The main parts of the architecture are the following: the user terminal, the web server, and the remote processing server (Figure 1).

The user terminal is located at the Web browser and is integrated in an information system, whose data could be used for digital image processing operations. Once the user has selected the images that will be processed, the tools and the possible environments for digital processing are shown. An applet is executed when selecting a tool; this applet involves a display and a simple processing kernel and shows the images and processing options.

The Web Server is in charge of four fundamental tasks: it has to communicate with the kernel of the display for the transfer of images and other patient-associated data, it communicates the image information system for independently retrieving images and its associated information from various data sources, it performs the digital processing of the images with high computational requirements (remote processing), and it gives access to the different remote processing servers.

The use of remote processing servers offers the following advantages: the distribution of computational loads related to the digital processing, the integration of algorithms developed with different languages, the calculus transparency (how and where) for the developer thanks to Web access, and lastly, a higher processing capability. The architecture provides a uniform access through Web services and has a high scalability, which means that multiple queries can be received and processed at the cluster and that results can rapidly be returned by means of the distributed computation paradigm (Foster, 1999).

Logical Framework Architecture

The tools and components are defined so as to obtain a homogeneous and configurable interface.

Tools: A tool comprises the set of specific functions that are needed to work with a certain type of image, i.e for each possible environment for digital image processing. For instance, the functions for working with hemodynamics imaging are not the same than the ones used for oncology imaging; however, there might be common functions for both tools. Each tool has one or more components.

Components: Each component performs a specific function in the system, ranging from information management to digital image processing, with optional forms for the modification of processing parameters that are visualized at the applet. An example of a component is the function that changes the brightness and contrast of an image. The components have two different parts attending the place where they are executed: one of them inside the applet of the client's Web browser, and the other inside the application server, where it processes and manages the remote information. When building these two parts, interfaces must be defined for the good functioning of the parts.

Each component usually works with one or more DIP, such as for instance the segmentation of a hemodynamics image. Depending on the complexity of such algorithms, they will be located inside the applet, inside the application server or inside the remote processing server.

Local processing: If the processing algorithms have simple computational requirements, their execution is performed at the kernel of the client applet, located at the user terminal. This type of processing is known as local processing.

Application server processing: This second type of processing is especially indicated for algorithms of medium complexity, which will be executed by the application server. Each component is divided into two parts: the local part at the user browser and the remote part at the application server. The algorithm parameters are established at the local part of the component. When executing the processing, a request is sent to the application server through the tool, the kernel of the display, and the applet. After arriving to the servlet -where the component that has to be executed is identified- the remote component of the algorithm will be invoked to execute the algorithm and return the result.

Remote server processing: Finally, the remote processing servers are used for load distribution and to provide support to the algorithms that are developed with various programming languages. In this case, the remote part of the component -located at the application server- sends the request to the Web service, where the algorithm is executed. The result is sent back to the remote part and, from there, to the display. The different parts of the remote processing server can be observed in Figure 2.

A remote processing server model with three parts is built as follows: the first part, the web services proxy, collects the external processing web requests that come from the information system. These requests are sent to another server where the processing manager is located and where they are directed in accordance with both, the needed processing type and the original object that made the request to the web service. The third part is represented by the physical remote processing servers, which are able to perform one or more different intensive processing algorithms. The remote object manager instantiates a remote processing object on the subsequent server in charge

Figure 2. Remote processing server detail

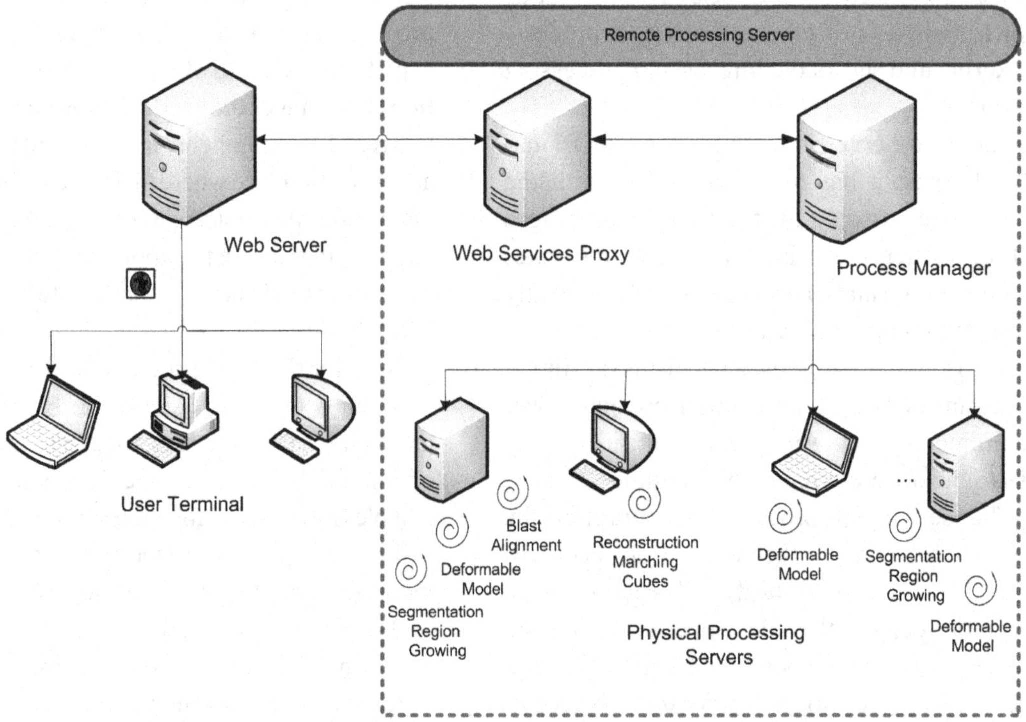

of executing the needed processing algorithm, keeping the result at the local memory of the machine where the algorithm is being executed, and returning that result when needed.

There are two reasons for dividing the remote processing server into three parts. Firstly, processing is usually quite costly and may collapse the reception, so we must separate the reception of the web server queries from the server that performs the intensive processing Secondly, the objects that are instantiated on the web server have no state, since every time a remote call is made from a web server, an object is instantiated; this object disappears as soon as it returns (web services behaviour). This fact reduces the functionality, because it does not allow the interaction with the remote object, but also acts as a call to a function that replies with a result. This architecture provides the web services with a virtual state that allows us to carry out several calls on the same object to assign parameters, modify them during the execution, and test the processing status.

The web services proxy implements only one processing method. The parameters of this method are an identifier of the object that invokes the web service, the operation type realised at the processing, and a list of parameters needed for performing that operation. This method invokes an operation from the remote object hosted at the processing manager that controls the processing objects. Distributing the processing manager among several machines provides a higher failure tolerance and a simpler maintenance, since each machine carries out only one function.

The object manager instantiates the processing objects that are needed to execute the processing algorithm required by the web services proxy; it also distributes the load among the different physical servers and it manages the security of the transactions. At the first call of an algorithm, the object manager instantiates a new object on one of the processing servers and then all the processing calls are directed towards that object.

Finally, the processing servers execute one or more processing algorithms. The remote object manager determines which physical processing server is more suitable for executing the new processing, according to the algorithms that every server has and the processor load at that moment.

IMPLEMENTATION

This section describes the technologies that were used to implement the architecture. The user terminal was developed with Java applets because of their multiplatform nature and also because it is a common solution for providing a web environment with processing capacities (Laird et al, 2003). In this part, where the local processing takes place, the algorithms must be developed with Java and with the option of using the advanced API for image processing of JAI (Java Advanced Imaging) (http://java.sun.com/products/java-media/jai).

The application server was developed with the J2EE platform, because it is portable, scalable, and safe, and because it uses open standards. The implementation that was used for J2EE is the Apache Tomcat 5.0.28. Since in this part the remote processing can be performed, we can integrate the developed processing algorithms that use either Java or C. Link libraries known as Java Native Interface (JNI) are used for algorithms developed with C.

The communication with the remote processing servers was established by means of web services, whose hardware and software are platform independent, which widens the range of implementation possibilities for the various remote processing servers. The algorithms developed with Java or C could be integrated using the same scheme for the web server. If the algorithm is developed with another language, or if the used technology is different, the algorithm's developing framework will only have to be supported by web services.

The validity of the remote processing system is proved by implementing two remote processing servers, one developed with Apache AXIS Java libraries, the other with a .NET Framework. In this case, the previously proposed remote processing server was implemented. An ideal processing scenario would imply three or more machines for the processing server: the first machine could have Internet Information Services (IIS), to collect the requests from the application server, or a stand-alone application that may require this type of processing by means of web services; the second machine would host the processing manager, and the remaining machines would house the specific processing servers. The technology used to intercommunicate the proxy with the object manager and the latter with the processing servers is .NET Remoting over TCP. In all these servers .NET framework must be installed. The use of .NET consists in integrating the developed algorithms by means of any .NET-supported language such as Visual Basic, C#, Visual C++, etc.

The standard network topology implies one or more J2EE application servers that respond to the requests of the client's applets. The remote processing server will need one or more machines with Internet Information Services (IIS) to serve the web services requests. These are the only machines that would have to be provided with an external connection. Security will be implemented by means of SSL certificates provided by the IIS (Seely, 2002), which warrant the Internet transaction security. On the one hand, the LAN network, which contains the IIS, has a machine provided with a *ProcessManager* for client control and the processing types of the system. The related data of previous versions will remain in a data base and as such allow several machines to provide this service. On the other hand, there exists a network of physical processing servers where every machine can execute one or more algorithms of intensive processing.

Integration into an Information System

The architecture was designed for to be easily integrated into an image information system. In this case, it was integrated into a biomedical imaging information system known as Web-SMIIS that is part of the SMIIS project (Pereira, 2003). The SMIIS is essentially a PACS for the retrieval of information from any modality that might support the DICOM standard, and the subsequent storage of that information into a data base for consultation. The SMIIS was developed by the Centre for Medical Informatics and Radiological Diagnosis (IMEDIR) of the University of A Coruña (Spain).

The integration between the two systems is focused on a point where the architecture has to obtain the images. This place depends on each information system. In the Web-SMIIS, the facade "*QueryFacadeDelegateFactory*" is the access to the SMIIS.

Also, this architecture could be integrated into any PACS DICOM thanks to a module that allows the extension of the system's functionality in order to achieve its compatibility with the DICOM standard and, more specifically, with the storage query/retrieve services.

RESULTS

This architecture was implemented in two Spanish hospitals, the *Complejo Hospitalario Universitario Juan Canalejo* and the *Instituto Médico Quirurgico San Rafael* in A Coruña. The first is the most important hospital of the city and a centre of reference for a geographic area of more than 500.000 people. The second is one of the most important private hospitals of A Coruña. The processing architecture is currently being validated by a group of 7 medical experts of the

Table 1. Hospital and validation data

	CHU Juan Canalejo	IMQ San Rafael
Beds	1.430	148
Total annual external consultations	672.295	44.310
Emergencies	179.101	7.949
Total annual admissions	44.814	4.605
Interventions	29.924	6.045
Implantation and Validation	Hemodynamics Service	Radiology Service
Service Volume	2.896 annual catheterisms	34.700 radiological tests
Validation team	7 persons	3 persons
Number of Tests	63 Validated studies	231 Validated studies

Hemodynamics Service of the Juan Canalejo Hospital, which carries out 3.000 catheterisms each year. The processing architecture is currently available in the radiology service of the San Rafael hospital.

Validation protocols are long and complex. The hemodynamics unit of the Juan Canalejo Hospital validated a total of 63 angiographs in groups of 2 to 3 members; the San Rafael Hospital validated 213 radiology studies (TC, MRI, medical ultrasonography, etc.) in groups of 3 members each.

We developed two tools for the semi-automatic analysis of angiographs in collaboration with the clinicians of the Hemodynamics Unit of Juan Canalejo in order to establish a score pattern for coronary stenosis. The first tool uses for segmentation tracking techniques (O'Brien and Ezquerra, 1994) (NEzquerra et al, 1998), the second tool uses morphological operators and techniques of region growth (Haris, 1999)(Kirbas, 2003). Figure 3a shows a screen capture of this tool.

This architecture was also used for tool development in the cooperative thematic research network INBIOMED (Pérez et al, 2005). With the collaboration of the Pharmacology Group from the University of Santiago de Compostela (Spain), a tool was developed for the analysis of protein and DNA electrophoresis gel (Figures 3b). It allows the application of low cost image preprocessing algorithms such as low-pass filtering, image-enhance filter, image rotation operator, etc., as well as the semiautomatic detection and analysis of the lanes and bands that contain this kind of image in order to obtain the protein weight represented by the relative position of the bands in each lane. Another tool that was developed by the INBIOMED network provides a fast and user-friendly cell count for immunohistochemical images using adaptative thresholding (Chow and Kaneko, 1972)(Chan et al, 1998) (figure 3c), applying not only low-cost image processing to the client side, but also algorithms with a high computational cost that are executed at a separate processing server that communicates with the system through Web services.

Finally, we developed a tool for the segmentation and subsequent reconstruction of three-dimensional medical image volumes. It uses algorithms with a high computational cost such as 3D region growth to segmentate the desired regions and marching cubes to reconstruct and visualize these regions in a Java applet on an internet browser. Both techniques are implemented in the remote processing server because of their high computational cost.

Table 2 shows the test results for the proposed architecture. Three high computational cost tests

Figure 3. (a) Stenosis detection tool (b) electrophoresis gel analysis tool (c) inmunohistochemical count tool

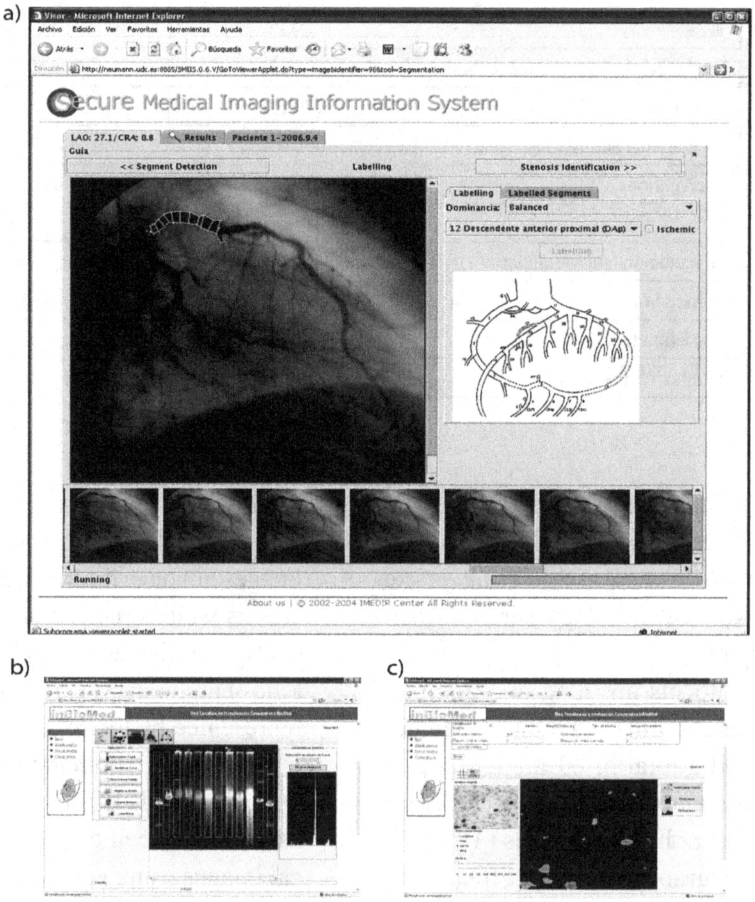

focused on development: cell counting in high resolution color images, segmentation of a skull in a CT set of 106 512x512 slices, using region growth, and reconstruction of this segmentation with marching cubes algorithms (Lorensen and Cline, 1987) (the processing time does not count image loading time). The tests were carried out according to three approaches: an applet, a stand-alone application, and the proposed architecture (10 processing units), with one, five, and twenty

Table 2. Test results

	Cell counting	Region growing	Marching cubes
Applet	40.8 s	(not enough memory)	(not enough memory)
Stand-alone application	12.6 s	19.3 s	5.6 s
Proposed architecture 1 request	15.3 s	22.1 s	6.8 s
Proposed architecture 5 request	22.1 s (4.4 s/req)	26.8 s (5.3 s/ req)	8.2 s (1.64 s/ req)
Proposed architecture 20 request	47.6 s (2.3 s/ req)	56.1 s (2.8 s/ req)	18.2 s (0.91 s/ req)

requests. A normal PC (Pentium IV 3GHz with 1GB RAM) was used in the one-machine test.

CONCLUSION

We propose a system that allows medical experts to analyze patient data through a web browser by integrating processing algorithms of biomedical imaging into web-based information systems.

The design is based on the use of both design and architectural patterns and provides the simple integration of this kind of architecture with information systems carried out under a "model-view-controller" paradigm such as SMIIS. Also, the design of new processing tools based on the "view-tool-component" model allows the developers of digital processing algorithms to easily integrate them and obtain new components and tools.

The remote processing server allows the incorporation of the architecture into new types of distributed systems, since it provides the developer with a façade that hides the placement, the functioning, and the situation of each specific remote processing server; it also provides a common interface and only one entry point for all the processing algorithms implemented in the system.

Another advantage of the remote processing server architecture is its communication with the application server by means of web services, because this implies remote processing through the Internet without any port redirection problems, firewalls, etc.; it also means that the application server may be located in a different place from the network of processing servers.

From the point of view of the user, we have achieved transparency with regard to the execution of the process. The clinician carries out data analysis and processing, regardless of whether the processing is simple and can be done at the local machine with the Web browser, or it is expensive and implies the joint work of several equipments.

ACKNOWLEDGMENT

This work was supported in part by the Spanish Ministry of Education and Science (Ref TIC2003-07593, TIN2006-13274), Ministry of the Treasury (PROLIT/SP1.E.194103), the INBIOMED network (Ref G03/160) financed by the Carlos III Health Institute (FIS-PI061524), and grants from the General Directorate of Research of the Xunta de Galicia (Ref. PGIDIT03-PXIC10504PN PGIDIT04-PXIC10503PN, PGIDIT04-PXIC10504PN). The work of Juan L. Pérez is supported by an FPI grant (Ref. BES-2006-13535) from the Spanish Ministry of Education and Science.

REFERENCES

Burl M.C., Fowlkes C., Roden J., Stecher A., Mukhtar S. (1999). Diamond Eye: A distributed architecture for image data mining. Presented in *SPIE Thirteenth International Symposium On Aerospace/Defense Sensing, Simulation and Controls.*

Chan F. H. Y., Lam F. K. and Hui Z. (1998), Adaptive thresholding by variational method. *IEEE Transaction on Image Processing. 7*(6), 468-473.

Chow C.K. and Kaneko R. (1972). Automatic boundary detection of the left ventricle from cineangiograms. *Comp. Biomed. Res. 5*, 443-452.

Ezquerra N., Capell S., Klein L. and Duijves P. (1998). Model-guided labelling of coronary structure. *IEEE Transactions on Medical Imaging, 17*(3), 429-441

Foster I. and Kesselman C. (1999). *The grid blueprint for a new computing infrastructure.* Morgan Kaufmann Publishers.

Haris K., Efstratiadis S., Maglaveras N., Pappas C., Goruassas H. and Loruidas G. (1999). Model-based morphological segmentation and labelling of coronary angiograms. *IEEE Transactions on Medical Imaging, 18*(10), 1003-1015

He X., Wu Q., Liu D. and Zheng L.H. (2003). A Distributed and Parallel Edge Detection Scheme within Spiral Architecture. In *Proceedings of Visualization, Imaging and Image Processing 393* (pp 303-311).

Kirbas C. and Queq F. (2003). *A review of vassel extraction techniques and algorithms*

Laird S.P., Wonng J.S.K., Schaller W.J. Ericksin B.J., de Groen P.C. (2003). Desing and implementation of an internet-based medical image viewing system. *The Journal of Systems and Software. Col. 66*, 167-181.

Li S. L., Veeravalli B., Ko C. (2003), Distributed image processing on a network of workstations. *International Journal of Computers and Applications, 25*, 2.

O'Brien J., Ezquerra N. (1994), Automated segmentation of coronary vessels in angiographic image sequences utilizing temporal, spatial and structural constraints. *Visualization in Biomedical Computing.*

Pereira J. (2003), Nuevo Enfoque en el desarrolo de un sistema de información de imágenes Médicas. *Una herramienta de apoyo a la toma de decisión clínica. Doctoral Thesis.* Universidade da Coruña.

Perez D., Crespo J., Anguita A., Pérez, J.L., Dorado J., Bueno G., Feliu V., Estruch A. and Heredia J. (2005). Biomedical Image Processing Integration Through INBIOMED: A Web Services-Based Platform. Lecture Notes in Bioinformatics. LNBI 3745 pp. 34-43.

Seely S. (2002), *Seguridad http y servicios web en ASP.NET.* Retrieved from http:// www.microsoft.com/spanish/msdn/articulos/archivo/111002/voices/httpsecurity.asp

KEY TERMS

Client-Server Architecture: The most fundamental distributed architecture. A client-server architecture is simply a client process that request services from a server process.

Common Object Request Broker Architecture (CORBA): Is a distributed object architecture defined by the Object Management Group. This architecture provides an interface that invokes other CORBA objects across a network.

Digital Imaging and Communication in Medicine (DICOM): A standard format and application protocol developed by the NEMA (National Electrical Manufacturers Association) to communicate systems over TCP. This protocol allows the integration of PACS, workstations, and TC, MNR, and other image scanners.

J2EE: Java 2 Enterprise Edition is a widely used platform for server programming in Java language, used to deploy distributed multi-tier Java software running in an application server. It is also known as Java EE in versions 1.5 and following.

Java Advanced Image (JAI): Is an image-processing toolbox, developed by Sun, that provides an object-oriented interface for the support of high-level programming models that allow images to be easily manipulated in Java applications.

Marching Cubes: A computer graphics algorithm for the extraction of a polygonal mesh of a set of volumetric data.

.Net Remoting: A distributed-object architecture by Microsoft to develop distributed applications over Microsoft platforms.

Network of Workstations (NoW): Is a computer network that connects several computer workstations with special software forming a cluster, to act as a distributed supercomputer on a building-wide scale.

Parallel Virtual Machine (PVM): Is a software package that allows a heterogeneous collection of computers hooked together by a network to be used as a single large parallel computer.

Picture Archive and Communication System (PACS): A storage system composed by different computers and networks dedicated to the storage and retrieval of medical images.

Platform-Independent: An application that can be run on many different server platforms, e.g. Java.

Region Growing: A segmentation technique based on the similarity of adjacent pixels. A region is started with a single pixel (seed pixel) and the adjacent pixels are added to the current region if they are similar to the region.

SSL: A secure socket layer is a secure protocol that provides secure communication over the internet based on cryptographic techniques. At present it is also known as TLS (Transport Layer Security)

Transmission Control Protocol/Internet protocol (TCP-IP): Is the basic family of network protocols for the Internet.

Web Services: Software system designed to support interoperable machine to machine interaction over web. It uses SOAP protocol and XML messages to receive request and offer responses.

Chapter XXIII
PACS Based on Open-Source Software Components

Daniel Welfer
Instituto de Informatica — Universidade Federal do Rio Grande do Sul, Brazil

Jacob Scharcanski
Instituto de Informatica — Universidade Federal do Rio Grande do Sul, Brazil

ABSTRACT

This chapter discusses the concept of open-source picture archiving and communication systems (i.e. PACS), which are low cost, and easy to re-configure and to customize for the specific user needs. Open-source PACS are based on relatively low cost computational resources, and are built by integrating open-source software components that implement basic services of a PACS. These services are described in this chapter, as well as how to integrate them. As an illustration, a PACS based on open-source software components for angiographic studies is discussed. Using the open-source approach, we expect to help diffusing the PACS technology by reducing its development and maintenance costs by using components easily available (e.g. desktop PCs).

INTRODUCTION

Nowadays, there is a growing tendency of integrating the technologies used in medical digital imaging for acquisition, storage, management, transmission, reception and visualization, and moving towards systems known as picture archiving and communication systems (i.e. PACS). These systems comprise software and hardware components, and often adopt the open DICOM standard for image representation, archiving and communication (Hludov, Meinel, Noelle & Warda, 1999). The DICOM standard was originally proposed to facilitate the interoperability between imaging equipments and health informatics systems. This standard also specifies services, such as archiving and retrieval of medical images, messaging syntax, and file formatting based on specific tags that represent objects (e.g. the 2D matrix pixels) (Bankman, 2000).

The digital images managed by PACS can be recovered locally or remotely, and such systems also can be considered as teleradiology tools (Engelmann, Schröter, Baur, Werner, Schwab, Müller & Meinzer, 1998). In the context of teleradiology, specifically, PACS provide mechanisms to facilitate the access to images and associated information, fastening the interpretation of medical studies. Known examples of such systems are the *eFilm Workstation* (Sachpazidis, Ohl, Polanczyk, Torres, Messina, Sales & Sakas, 2005; MERGE, 2007), the *Impax* family of products (Agfa, 2007), *Centricity Imaging PACS* (General Electric, 2007) and *Osirix* (Rosset, Spadola & Ratib, 2004). Nevertheless, the widespread utilization of these systems still is limited, mostly because of cost and technological issues. The patent protection of PACS software components imposes license costs and restricts the access to this technology to more affluent societies (Fogel, 2005), and is one of the most important issues preventing the widespread utilization of PACS. Coincidently, the most pressing needs to increase health care efficiency often are found in less affluent societies, especially in developing countries.

Recently, open-source software components to support the development of several PACS services became available. For example, nowadays there are available several open-source software components to implement DICOM services, such as image compression and transmission, storage, query, retrieval, and media management, among other services. Besides, the open-source software approach for constructing PACS allows to further develop and customize the system software components, while substantially reducing the development and maintenance costs, as compared to patent protected software.

The first Section of this chapter presents a survey of the PACS open-source software components currently available; next, a PACS model based on the integration of open-source software components is presented, and a test case illustrating the application of this PACS model to hemodynamics series management is discussed. Finally, we present some concluding remarks.

INTEGRATING OPEN-SOURCE SOFTWARE COMPONENTS TO BUILD A PACS

A PACS can be understood as integrated systems that provide the functionalities to facilitate medical image storage, management and communication, and these functionalities (i.e. services) are the system building blocks (i.e. the system components). These building blocks often are inter-dependent, and organized hierarchically, with some components providing the infra-structure to other components perform their functions. In this chapter, the term component is used as a binary, functionally self-contained software which interacts with its environment (i.e. the other components in a PACS) via a well-defined interface (Stal, 1999). This Section discusses the characteristics of the open-source components currently available, and the services they provide in the PACS environment.

Open-Source Components for PACS

Nowadays, most PACS rely on the DICOM standard for image representation and communication (Bankman, 2000). For this reason, we initially present a lower level component that performs DICOM decoding (i.e. the DICOM decoder), which provides the basic infra-structure for several other

PACS components. Basically, it is responsible for sequentially reading and decoding all the information in a DICOM file, and all bytes read (i.e. de-serialized) are converted to other formats, more useful to other PACS components. An important feature of the DICOM decoder is its ability to support different DICOM modalities. DICOM is a standard, but there are substantial differences in implementation among manufacturers, affecting the contents of DICOM files. For example, the CT DICOM modality requires the decoder to extract single images from a file. However, an XA modality requires the decoder to read multiple frames per file. The DICOM standard establishes the rules for decoding the files provided by these different modalities (NEMA, 2004). Besides decoding single images or multiframe sequences, the decoder must decode the textual information (i.e. technical annotations) in a DICOM file header, and to identify/access specific tags in the file header. For example, to make a DICOM file anonymous, some private DICOM tags must be removed, or modified, for confidentiality reasons, so the DICOM file can be published without exposing the patient or institutional information. The decoder is used to find and edit specific groups of tags, or specific tag elements, that represent the private data we want to protect. Nowadays, there are a few open-source DICOM decoders available (e.g. the DCMTK decoder). The DCMTK is a C-library designed to facilitate the development of DICOM-based applications (DCMTK, 2005), and it includes a DICOM decoder. Two others DICOM decoders freely available also should be mentioned, namely the decoders included in the libraries PixelMed Java toolkit and ImageJ DICOM plug in (Clunie, 2005; Rasband, 2006). All these open-source components will be explained in details in the next sections.

According to Isaac Bankman (Bankman, 2000), a PACS has three major sub-systems: acquisition, image archive and the viewer sub-system. The first one is responsible for the acquisition of medical digital images in compliance with the DICOM standard. These medical images (i.e. CT or XA modalities) are generated by equipments (made by different manufactures), and transmitted to a PACS. The PACS manages the images generated by these different modalities. The second sub-system is the viewer, which consists of software and hardware to display images for medical interpretation and diagnosis. More details of the viewer will be provided later. The third sub-system is the archive server, which stores and manages all DICOM images received by the acquisition sub-system. The archive server can be a computer with a database system and high storage capacity (i.e. hard disks, compact disks (CDs) or digital versatile disks (DVDs), or it can be based on other technologies like digital linear tapes (DLTs). The archive server usually does not store all the medical images, only manages the location where these images are stored in a local or remote file system (Bankman, 2000). The database tables contain demographic patient information that can be used later to retrieve the image studies from a local or remote file system using high level queries, like patient name, study date, study time, patient sex, pathology, and other attributes, or by their combination. Some of the available options in terms of open-source database system are MySQL and PostgreSQL (MySQL, 2006; PostgreSQL, 2007). Both are very popular relational databases in the open-source software community, and these database systems are installed by default in some free Linux distributions like SUSE 9.2 (http://www.novell.com/linux/).

These three sub-systems are connected to by communication network for data/image sharing purposes (Bankman, 2000). Thus, the network can be seen as a complementary low-level component because other components depend of its functionality. When an image is requested by a viewer, there is a handshaking process over the communication network, between the archive server and the viewer. This operation is known as query/retrieve, and the viewer is the Q/R SCU (query/retrieve service class user) element, and the archive server is the Q/R SCP (query/retrieve service class provider) element. The Q/S SCU (i.e. viewer) sends a query to the Q/R SCP (archive server), which sends back the requested image. This uses the client/server concept, where the SCU is the client and the SCP is the server. The same process occurs in the data exchange between the medical image modality (acquisition equipment) and the archive server. The image modality requests the storage of an image in the archive server. Thus, the modality is the client entity. The archive server accepts the request and receives the image files transmitted by the modality. After that, the process is finished. This is named as C-STORE DIMSE Service. This is a typical point-to-point communication between a server (archive) and client (modality), and it occurs under the TCP/IP protocol usually using sockets as a middleware. This unidirectional communication is not considered a drawback, besides TCP is a reliable protocol and assures that data stream will be received in the correct sequence in the receiver side, that is, in-order delivery of data packets from sender to receiver. The DCMTK and PixelMed toolkits provide this service implementation. An alternative to perform Q/R SCU and Q/R SCP and share DICOM files over a communication network, when clients and servers use different operating systems is SAMBA. The SAMBA tool makes it possible to set images to read-only mode in the archive server, guaranteeing their integrity (Eckstein, Brown & Kelly, 1999). Moreover, SAMBA is a default application of some open-source operating systems distributions, and its configuration is simple. In this way, no middleware is needed to transmit and receive DICOM (image) files. For example, to display an image on the viewer it is only necessary that this image files are accessible via SAMBA to the viewer. This approach makes the file reading process transparent, and the images appear to the viewer workstation as they were located in the local hard-disk. Besides, the systems interoperability is preserved, even across different hardware platforms and operating systems.

The PACS viewer subsystem consists of several components, and depends of the several other ones. It depends, for example, on the proper operation of all components of the archive server and on other PACS components. So, the database system, the DICOM decoder, the short and long-term storage, the network communication must all to be operational. Given these requirements are satisfied, other components can to be incorporated to the viewer (e.g. the image processing components).

Image processing open-source components also can be relevant in a PACS, since they help improving the image quality, and consequently the diagnosis quality (Bankman, 2000). Unfortunately, image processing algorithms tend to be time consuming, especially when several studies or frame sequences must be processed. Besides, no alterations must propagate to the stored images (i.e. the DICOM files should not be modified after their acquisition), so each time a study is viewed it may be processed at the viewer workstation. Histogram equalization, contrast adjustment, image scaling, rotation, image calibration and image negative are some popular algorithms. However, in some situations it may be convenient to save the processed image (e.g. to present it later as teaching example, etc.), or even to clip an image detail to substantiate an opinion (e.g. in a second opinion to confirm/disconfirm the diagnosis of a study). In order to not leave these needs unattended, some components must be included to save images, or yet frame sequences, in standard file formats supported by most Windows and/or Linux applications. These components export still images to common graphics files like jpeg (joint pictures expert group), tiff (tagged image file Format), or bmp (windows bitmap); or they export dynamic images to common file extensions like MPEG (moving picture experts group) and AVI (audio video interleave). The idea is to increase the portability of the image visualization process, since these common file formats are supported by many image and video tools. However, some of the graphic formats described previously implement lossy algorithms, that is, image coding algorithms that cause information loss in the converted image (i.e. are not bit preserving). The DICOM standard (part 5) defines lossy compression schemes, but defining adequate parameters for the adopted compression scheme is beyond the scope of the DICOM standard (NEMA, 2007). Therefore, the compression parameters must be selected judiciously, in a way that relevant details are preserved during the image compression process, and the reconstructed (uncompressed) image still can be useful from the clinical point of view. Furthermore, exporting an image to common graphic file formats does not imply in corrupting the original DICOM image file. A sound implementation police is to keep the original DICOM in raw or lossless data in the archive server, and to convert only an instance of this image. Using this approach it is possible to display images in devices with limited memory and/or low power, like smartphones or personal digital assistants (PDAs). For the purpose of image conversion, there are some open-source components and application programming interfaces (APIs). The C/C++ DCMTK toolkit contains resources to export a DICOM file to PPM/PGM (portable pixel map/portable gray map), PNG (portable network graphics), TIFF, BMP and JPEG. The C/C++ DCMTK toolkit also provides components that perform image processing operations like scaling, flipping, rotation and display of overlays. Besides, Java open-source DICOM toolkits like PixelMed or the ImageJ plug also offer resources to perform these operations. Also, the available Java imaging tools could be used, like the Image-I/O and the JAI (Java advanced imaging) APIs that perform several image operations (JAI, 2006; Image-I/O, 2006). These tools do not come with the Java development kit (JDK), but are available at Sun Microsystems Web site (http://java.sun.com/). These APIs provide high-level interfaces for image processing and to file format conversion.

A PACS MODEL BASED ON THE INTEGRATION OF OPEN-SOURCE SOFTWARE COMPONENTS

In this Section we discuss how to integrate the open-source software components described in the previous section, and assemble a DICOM-based PACS. Depending on the desired PACS functionalities, this integration requires some software development to customize and integrate the different components. For instance, for the DICOM viewer perform operations like accessing and viewing a DICOM file over a network, other components must be integrated and customized to operate within the context of a PACS (e.g. the DICOM decoder, the image processing toolbox, and the network communication interface). Therefore, larger systems can be assembled by integrating more components.

Figure 1. PACS architecture based on open-source component integration

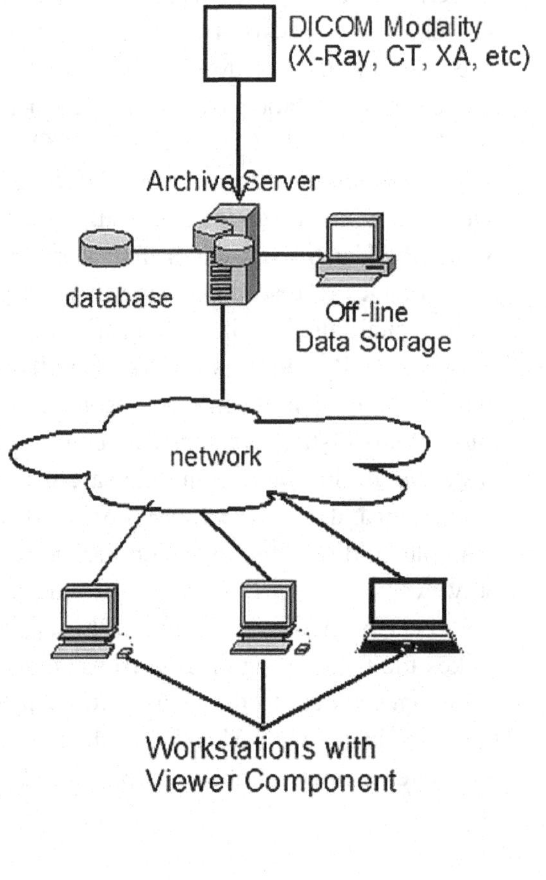

The PACS architecture presented in this Section has four main software components responsible for specific tasks, namely (1) the DICOM server; (2) the on-line manager; (3) the off-line manager; and (4) the DICOM viewer. The DICOM server and the online manager are installed in the DICOM archive server. The off-line manager is installed in a host computer, connected point-to-point with the archive server. The viewer is installed at the client workstations. Figure 1 illustrates the system architecture, including the software sub-systems and the host machines.

According to the architecture model depicted in Figure 1, the medical imaging equipments, namely the DICOM modalities, generate DICOM image files and transmit them to a DICOM node (archive server), using the network communication infra-structure. The DICOM modalities act as file sender systems, and often are integrated to the architecture based on TCP/IP connections and socket middleware. The files sent by these modalities to the archive server are handled by a file receiver. It shall be noted that this file receiver may be implemented in a language that is different of that used to develop the file sender, or run in a different platform. Next, we discuss some useful details to implement this architecture with open-source components.

Implementation Details

A popular open-source DICOM-compatible file receiver is the "storescp" class, available in the DCMTK toolkit. This component runs in the same hardware unit as the archive server, and it is the SCP entity that performs the storage service (see previous section). The DCMTK toolkit also has a file sender called "storescu", which is used to transmit the DICOM files, but usually the file sending service is embedded in a DICOM-compatible imaging modality (provided by the manufacturer) and does not need to be implemented. In the DCMTK "storescp" class default implementation, all DICOM files are received and stored in a common directory. This approach may be inconvenient because different medical image studies (even of different patients) are stored in the same directory, and as the number of studies in the directory grow becomes increasingly more difficult to handle and access individual studies of a given patient. Thus, we suggest a modification in this version of the file receiver, so that each image study is identified and stored in its own directory, and the image series of that specific study are stored in their own sub-directories (as opposed to storing all study series in the same directory). The archive server uses Linux as operating system, and the hardware architecture is IBM-PC based. The file receiver is now named DICOM server, and runs in the environment as the archive server (i.e., in the same hardware unit).

The MySQL database can be installed in the same machine where the archive server runs, and two tables could be used to manage the PACS information. The first table stores patient record information like name, study modality, and study time; this table also records some system information like the path to the directory where a given patient study is located (i.e. the internet address of the archive server, for example "192.168.123.123"), the file size of the patient study, and the information if a specific study is available in the archive server, or if it was transferred to long-term storage devices. If a study is now in a long-term storage device, this study can not to be retrieved automatically as if it was on-line. In this case, it is necessary to make a request for it, and these requests for studies stored off-line are handled using the second table. The second table contains information to retrieve older image studies, stored off-line (e.g. in media devices like DVD or CD). This table stores information about the off-line media like the media ID, and a field that controls if the study storage process was successfully finalized.

It is advisable to have a software component to update the information in the first table, named on-line manager. Like de DICOM server, the online manager runs on the same computer as the archive server. The on-line manager runs as a background application (i.e. like a daemon server, similar to the DICOM server), accessing all image study directories created by the file receiver (the DICOM server application), and generating the database indexes for each study automatically. The on-line manager uses the DICOM decoder to extract tag values from the image series to add these information in the first table.

The old studies are managed by the software component named off-line manager, running on a machine which has network access to the machine where the archive server runs. The off-line manager is constituted by two sub-systems: a) off-line recording sub-system that does the procedures to store old image studies in the long-term storage, and b) off-line retrieval sub-system that performs the procedures to retrieve the image files from the long-term storage and copy them to the archive server again. Both sub-systems can run simultaneously in the same computer where the archive server runs, but it is advisable to install them in a dedicated computer (for performance reasons).

The goal is to keep in the on-line storage (e.g. in the hard-disk of the archive server) only the files accessed most frequently, optimizing the utilization of this storage area, which has a higher cost compared to the long-term storage. If the choice for a long-term data storage is low cost media (like DVD or CD), it is necessary to add a DVD/CD reading/writing software tool - especially a software tool that allows reading/writing DVDs or CDs with command lines (so, it can be programmed). Among the different choices, we should mention the Nero Burning Rom (http://www.nero.com), and the K3b CD/DVD creator for Linux (http://www.k3b.org/). The Nero tool is an option for Windows-based systems, it is stable, but it is not open-source nor freeware. The K3b option runs on Linux, it is licensed under the GPL (General Public License), and has a graphic user interface so it is easier to use than Nero Burning ROM.

The off-line retrieval sub-system, which is part of the off-line manager, copies the DICOM images files stored off-line (in the long-term storage) to the on-line storage, in the archive server. We do not know of any open-source component to perform this task, so it must be developed for a specific PACS implementation. The tasks that must performed are: a) read a request for a study stored off-line and to restore it to on-line (the study location is the off-line records database table), b) copy the requested studies from de long-term storage to the on-line storage, and update the database system. Normally, this study remains on-line in the archive server by a few hours, and then we recommend automatically removing it from the on-line storage and update its location in the database system.

The network communication can to be based in any technology that uses the TCP/IP protocol, like Ethernet standards wireless or wireline cabling technology. If the communication link is fast, the image study transportation will be fast, consequently the image visualization will be speedy.

The DICOM viewer is another component of the PACS model illustrated in Figure 1. It should be as user friendly as possible, and make the actual process of accessing a study for display transparent to the clients; in other words, the viewer should occlude the details of how the images are retrieved and displayed, since the user does not need to know where the images are stored, or how they actually are accessed, copied and transmitted. Thus, the viewer must interact with the network communication infra-structure, the database system and the archive server in a way that is transparent to the user.

The next Section describes a test case implementation of the PACS model presented here.

Angiography: A Test Case

To illustrate the proposed open-source PACS model and clarify some of its implementation details, this Section presents a version of this model customized for the DICOM XA (X-ray Angiography) modality. The XA modality generates dynamic images, and the amount of information to be managed is quite large. Consequently, it provides a good benchmark for the proposed model. Figure 2 illustrates the structure of an XA DICOM study, organized in series, and series in frames.

Each frame in a series has two possible resolutions, 512x512 or 1024x1024 pixels, and each pixel in a frame can have 8 or 12 bpp (bits per pixel) depending on the type of angiographic study obtained (Bankman, 2000). So, 300 frame series can easily reach DICOM file sizes larger than 450 MB (1024x1024x12x300), which has a significant impact in terms of storage autonomy and network communication requirements. For example, a study with a file size of 800 MB, transmitted over a 10 Mbps Ethernet network link, would take 80 seconds to be received by a viewer application in a remote workstation, and an ISDN link with a rate of 1.92 Mbps would take 416 seconds (Guan, Kung & Larsen, 2001), imposing an undesirable delay to access the data. In fact, the delay for accessing data tends to be higher in the daily practice, because the communication link is simultaneously used by different applications, and the delay time to start displaying the frames of an XA series can be larger than the aforementioned. In our viewer implementation, we tried to minimize the delay to display a study by showing the image series progressively, i.e. the first frame of each study series is initially shown in a reduced resolution (thumbnail format). The user can access all image series clicking on the thumbnail images, and the selected series is displayed. In our implementation we use raw DICOM data, and more efficient data compression would reduce the network traffic and speedup displaying the image data. In fact, both approaches could be taken to optimize the image retrieval and visualization process.

The viewer was developed in Java, which by itself runs slower than applications in other programming language like C or C++, especially in image processing operations. For example, to perform a grayscale inversion of a complete XA sequence could take several seconds, therefore in our viewer, image processing algorithms are only applied to the frames selected by the user. Other possible ways of reducing the processing delays are to re-write the image processing algorithms in C or C++, and/or to use a computer with a faster processor and more memory.

The Java programming language was used to integrate all open-source components. It was chosen because of its portability and to make easier developing more sophisticated graphic user

Figure 2. The XA configuration

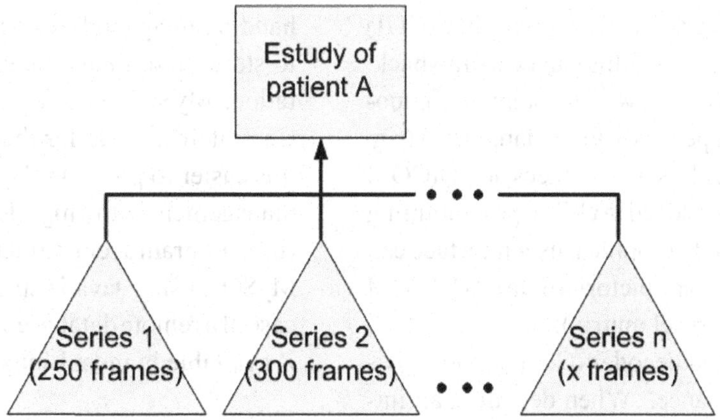

interfaces (e.g. such as those used in the off-line manager and in the viewer).

The viewer uses the SAMBA to access the images in the archive server, and it does not use the C-STORE DICOM service to retrieve the images, which is only used between the acquisition equipment and the archive server. We recommend using SAMBA to simplify the access to the images available in the archive server, since this tool provides a simple alternative to share the DICOM image files through the network. Therefore, in this case the DICOM network services are integrated with the viewer.

The SAMBA is a network file sharing component that was chosen because it is open-source, stable, easy to configure and manage. Besides, with SAMBA it is possible to protect the image files in the archive server by assigning read-only permissions to them. Also, we can control the access to the archive server in the case of having multiple instances of the viewer application trying to connect and copy image files from it.

The DICOM decoder used by the viewer was the ImageJ plug-in (Rasband, 2006). To justify its choice, we present features of DICOM decoders:

- The DCMTK decoder was implemented in ANSI C and C++. This decoder is fast, stable and efficient to use, however it is fairly complex to use with other applications that are not ANSI C based. For example, it is not straightforward to integrate this decoder with a graphical user interface (GUI) developed in Java. This can be a drawback, especially when we wish to integrate components developed in different languages (e.g. few graphical user interfaces for DICOM have been developed in C/C++ programming language, and a graphical user interface can be used to display pictorial data of a DICOM file, like the pixel matrix).
- The PixelMed decoder (Clunie, 2005), has low performance. When decoding an image sequence (in the case of a multiframe modality), the decoder reads and stores in a buffer the entire sequence, and not a specified number of frames only. This feature may be undesirable, especially when the DICOM series have many frames, and we wish to display a few frames while the other frames of the sequence are decoded in the background (i.e. waiting to decode the whole sequence may take a substantial amount of time, and could be frustrating to the user);
- The ImageJ DICOM plug in (Rasband, 2006) allows to read and display an image matrix in a graphical form quickly. In spite of supporting multiframe modalities, it does not support DICOM encapsulated types. Its code is easier to follow than in the case of the PixelMed DICOM decoder, and it is well commented. As in the case of the PixelMed decoder, all sequence frames must be read into a buffer before any frame can be accessed, however it is faster. Both DICOM decoders run on the IBM-PC platform, and can be extended to other platforms because of the Java portability features.

The on-line manager also was developed in Java, and it indexes image files in a database, so these files can be retrieved by queries programmed in the SQL language. The approach taken by Image Central Test Node (i.e. 'imagectn' of the DCMTK toolkit) provides an alternative way of handing image indexes, since it uses binary files to store these image indexes. In our implementation, MySQL was used instead of the Image Central Test Node for the following reasons: (a) it is easier to program the queries used in image management with a high-level language like SQL; (b) to program a remote (network) connection with MySQL using Java is straighforward (i.e. in the case of a remote database system); and (c) MySQL is available in most Linux distributions.

In our implementation, we chose to store older DICOM files on DVDs long-term medias. The off-line retrieval component is semi-automatic, because it depends on the user to operate the DVD media driver manually (i.e. to insert the DVD media containing the studies that must be retrieved and copied to the on-line storage). The off-line manager also was developed in Java, and the K3b CD/DVD creator was adopted. Methods for database connection and updating were implemented in this off-line manager too.

The implemented DICOM server (i.e. the file receiver) was a modified version of the "storescp" application, provided with the DCMTK toolkit. The modification introduced in this version of the file receiver was to have each image study stored in its own directory, identified by the study UID, so the image series of that study are stored in their own sub-directories under the study directory. Since it is a common practice to process XA series and measure some features showing in the frames (e.g. to evaluate the extension of a lesion), some common image processing algorithms are available in the viewer, like image gray level inversion, image calibration, movie control (i.e. stop and play an angiographic series like a movie), frame and video format conversion, besides some other processing tools like anonymization of a complete XA series. For that, we used the image processing tools of the Java Advanced Imaging (JAI) and the Image-I/O package, and some classes of ImageJ project. To reduce the computational cost, some of these algorithms only are executed on user selected frames. These algorithms can be executed when necessary, at any moment of the visualization process.

We should mention that Osirix is another open-source PACS, but developed for the MacOS X platform (Rosset, Spadola & Ratib, 2004). It also uses open-source software components like libraries for processing and image rendering, DICOM network communication, and other DICOM services. The programming language used to aggregate these components was the Objective-C with the help of object-oriented and cross-platform framework named Cocoa. Osirix is fairly complete and effective PACS for multiple modalities, but it has been designed specifically for the MacOS X platform. Our goal is to show how open-source components can to be used to develop an open-source DICOM-based PACS, which can also be cross-platform, easily customized and flexible in terms of resources.

CONCLUDING REMARKS

This chapter presented a review of PACS services and components currently available with the open standards and open-source software perspective. Besides, it presented a new PACS model based on open-source software components, which is less demanding (i.e. restrictive) in terms of computational resources than comparable systems (e.g. the network infrastructure is based on known TCP/IP, the computer hardware is based on the popular IBM-PC architecture, and the operating system is Linux-based). To illustrate implementation details, we discussed a version of this open-source PACS architecture customized for DICOM XA (x-ray angiography) modality. Thus, the proposed approach helps turning the PACS option for the automation of radiological image services more feasible, and contributes to increase the availability of patient information for E-Health applications

REFERENCES

Afga. (2007). Retrieved February 2007 from http://www.agfa.com/en/he/index.jsp

Bankman, I. N. (2000). *Handbook of medical imaging: Processing and analysis.* Academic Press.

Clunie, D. A. (2005). PixelMed Java DICOM toolkit. Retrieved October 2005 from http://www.pixelmed.com/, Accessed in

DCMTK. (2005). The DICOM Offis toolkit. Retrieved December 2005 from http://dicom.offis.de/

Eckstein, R., Brown, D. C., Kelly, P. (1999). *Using Samba, 1st Edition*. O'Reilly & Associates, Inc. .

Engelmann, U., Schröter, A., Baur, U., Werner, O., Schwab, M., Müller, H. and Meinzer, H.-P. (1998). A three-generation model for teleradiology. *IEEE Transactions on Information Technology in Biomedicine*, *2*(1), 20–25.

Fogel, K. (2005). *Producing open source software*. O'Reilly Media, Inc. ISBN: 0-596-00759-0

Guan, L.; Kung, S.Y.; Larsen, J. (2001). *Multimedia image and video processing*. New York: CRC Press.

General Electric. (2007). *General Electric Healthcare Company*. Retrieved February 2007 from http://www.gehealthcare.com/worldwide.html

Hludov, S., Meinel, C., Noelle, G. and Warda, F. (1999). Pacs for teleradiology. *12th IEEE Symposium on Computer-Based Medical Systems*.

Image-I/O. (2006). Java advanced imaging image-I/O tools 1.1. Retrieved October 2006 from http://java.sun.com/javase/6/docs/technotes/guides/imageio/index.html

JAI. (2006). Java advanced imaging 1.1.3. Retrieved September 2006 from http://java.sun.com/products/java-media/jai/

MySQL. (2006). Retrieved August 2006 from http://www.mysql.com/

MERGE. (2007). Retrieved February 2007 from https://www.merge-emed.com/index.asp

NEMA - National Electrical Manufacturers Association (2007). *Digital imaging and communications in medicine (DICOM) part 5: Data Structures and Encoding Publication* PS 3.5-2007, Rosslyn, VA .

NEMA - National Electrical Manufacturers Association (2004). *Digital imaging and communications in medicine (DICOM) part 2: Conformance* PS3.2-2004, Rosslyn, VA .

PostgreSQL. (2007). Retrieved May 2007 from http://www.postgresql.org/

Rasband, W.S., (2006) ImageJ, U. S. National Institutes of Health, Bethesda. Maryland, USA, http://rsb.info.nih.gov/ij/, 1997-2006.

Rosset, A. ; Spadola L. and Ratib O. (2004) OsiriX: An open-source software for navigating in multidimensional DICOM images. *Journal of Digital Imaging, 17*(3), 205-216.

Sachpazidis, I. A., Ohl, R., Polanczyk, C. A., Torres, M. S., Messina, L. A., Sales, A. and Sakas, G. (2005). Applying telemedicine to remote and rural underserved regions in Brazil using eMedical consulting tool. *IEEE Engineering in Medicine and Biology -27th Annual Conference*, Shanghai, China.

Stal, M.: OBJEKTspektrum (1999): Des Knaben Wunderhorn", Kommentare des Fachbeirats Komponenten-Forum. In *OBJEKTspektrum* 1/99, S. 18-20.

KEY TERMS

AEs: Acronym of application entities. Any PACS application is named AE (i.e. the service class user entity).

API: Acronym of application programming interface. It is a set of ready routines for use.

DIMSE: Acronym of DICOM message service element. It is a set of DICOM services performed between Application Entities.

IBM-PC: Personal computers appeared in the 1980s. Initially projected with open architecture and operational system. It continues in development and expansion however, much more complex.

JAI: Acronym of java advanced imaging. It is an API for image handle.

SCU: Acronym of service class user. It is an application entity that requests some service.

SCP: Acronym of service class provider. It is an application entity that offers a specific service.

Section VII
Medical Decision Support Systems

Chapter XXIV
Case Based Reasoning for Customizing Treatment Processes

Carolin Kaiser
University of Erlangen-Nuremberg, Germany

ABSTRACT

This chapter introduces a case based reasoning (CBR) system for customizing treatment processes. The CBR system enables the generating of inpatient and outpatient treatment processes and the supporting of e-services in heath care networks individually customized to the patients' needs. According to the CBR paradigm, which solves problems based on past experience, the proposed system uses old treatment processes of similar former patients and modifies them for new patients. In general, CBR is an established and well suited artificial intelligence method to support medical decision making. However, CBR systems capable of planning treatment processes by adapting old treatment processes to fit new patients are rare. The aim of this system is to increase the treatment quality of the patient by providing physicians with valuable treatment propositions and to contribute to the development of medical CBR Systems by introducing procedures enabling the generating of new treatment processes by modifying former treatment processes.

MOTIVATION

In the age of a growing flood of information on medical data and knowledge, medical decision support systems are becoming more and more important. Various artificial intelligence methods have been implemented in numerous systems to support the medical reasoning process. Among these methods case based reasoning (CBR) was established to support medical decision making. CBR (Amodt & Placa, 1994) solves problems by using past experiences and general knowledge. Past experiences are saved in form of cases in the case base. For solving a new arising problem the CBR system searches for similar problems and attempts to adapt their solutions to fit the new problem. CBR is particularly suited for helping find solutions to medical problems (Heinisch et al., 1998, p. 1) as it resembles the physicians' cognitive process of recalling former patients and reusing past experiences. Furthermore, the collection of patient records which represent a valuable knowledge resource can easily be integrated in a CBR system as a case base.

Medical CBR systems can be divided into different categories depending on their purpose-oriented properties and their functional properties. Purpose-oriented properties (Nilsson & Sollenborn, 2004, p. 179) describe the general aim which the system fulfills and allow the separation of medical CBR systems into diagnostic systems, classification systems, tutoring systems and planning systems. While diagnostic systems are intended to support the whole diagnostic process, classification systems focus on special diagnostic problems (e.g. image classification). Tutoring systems aim at teaching students medical knowledge based on patient records. Planning systems provide assistance by configuring medical processes (e.g. therapies) consisting of several steps. Considering the functional properties CBR systems can be classified into case-match-systems and case-adaptation-systems (Goos, 1996, p. 15). Case-match-systems only enable the retrievement of similar patient cases, whereas case-adaptation-systems also allow the adaptation of past cases to fit new patients. Most of the medical CBR systems developed in the last years are classification systems or diagnostic systems and they support case-matching only (Nilsson & Sollenborn 2004, p. 182). Moreover, the majority of these systems focus on inpatient treatment and specialize in one certain disease. Planning systems which realize the adaptation task, which support inpatient and outpatient treatment processes in health care networks and which implement disease independent algorithms are missing.

This chapter describes such a CBR system. The system proposes inpatient and outpatient treatment processes in health care networks based on the adaptation of treatment processes to new patients and can be applied to the treatment of various diseases. Besides the treatment steps to be fulfilled by the physicians, the generated propositions also contain e-services to satisfy the coordination and informational needs of the health care providers and the patients.

In order to clarify the functionality of this appraoch, all functions of the CBR systems are illustrated by example of heart failure treatment. Heart failure is a syndrome which is caused by cardiac disorder and which weakens the pumping capability of the heart supplying the tissue with blood and oxygen (Hoppe & Erdmann, 2004, p. 11). It is one of the most frequent and severest diseases of the industrialized countries with an approximate prevalence ranging from 0.3% to 2% and an estimated incidence of 0.1% to 0.5% (Cowie et al., 1997, p. 211). The medical treatment of the multitude of patients is important. However, in practice many patients do not obtain an adequate therapie compliant to actual guidelines (Hoppe & Erdmann, 2004, p. 15; Stödter, 2000, pp. 6, 18f). So the application of the Medical CBR system to the treatment of heart failure will hopefully contribute to the improvement of this situation.

CASE BASED REASONING FOR CUSTOMIZING TREATMENT PROCESSES

Introduction

CBR solves problems by using past experiences saved in form of cases in the case base. Each case

Figure 1. CBR-cycle

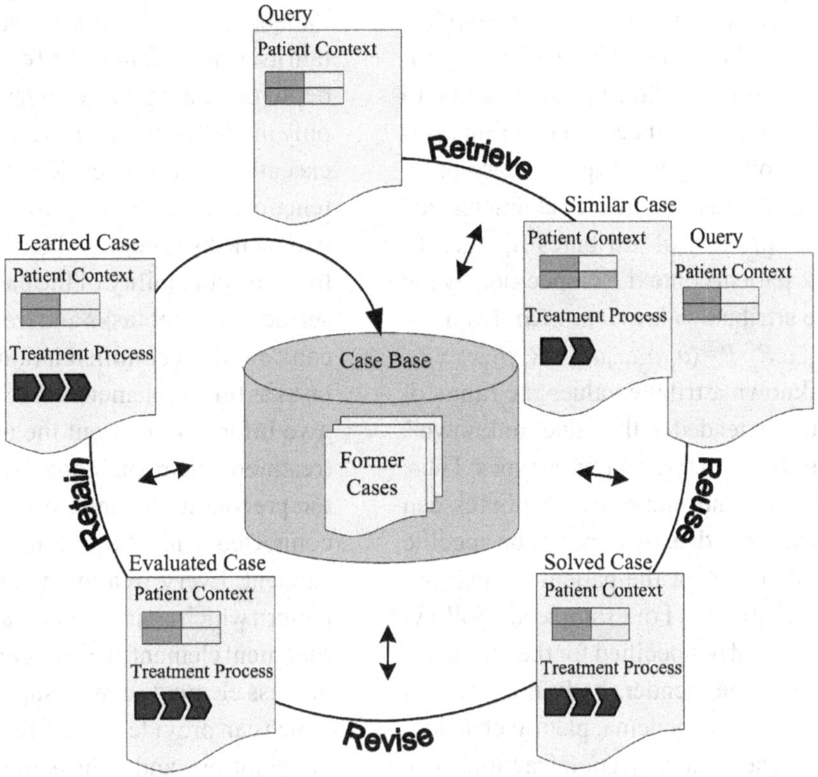

consists of a problem description (patient-context) and a solution (treatment process and its e-services). The functionality of a CBR system can be described by a cyclic phase model consisting of the retrieve phase, the reuse phase, the revise phase and the retain phase (Amodt & Placa, 1994, p. 47). Figure 1 illustrates the cyclic phase model. Given a new patient, the retrieve phase aims at searching for the treatment process and its e-services of the case base whose patient context is most similar to the new patient context. The retrieved treatment process and its e-services serve as a base for the treatment process and e-services of the new patient in the reuse phase. During the revise phase a new treatment process including its e-services is executed. Depending on the success of the treatment process and its e-services the retain phase decides on its inclusion in the case base. The development of a CBR system for the customization of treatment processes and e-services requires that an adequate representation of patient contexts, treatment processes and e-services is determined and that suited methods for similarity measurement, search, adaptation and maintenance are found.

Definition and Representation of Patient Contexts, Treatment Processes and E-Services

Each case consists of the patient context (problem) as well as its treatment process and e-services (solution). The patient context characterizes the patient and his disease pattern and contains information about his basis data, symptoms, findings, previous diseases, diagnoses and therapy relevant data. This information is represented by Attribute-Value-Vectors (Richter, 2003, p. 412), since they resemble the natural form of medical records and enable an efficient and effective similarity calculation. A further advantage of Attribute-Value-Vectors is the easy handling of incomplete information since many attribute values are unknown at the beginning of the treatment and will not become available until certain examinations are executed. Following this type of representation the general patient context is characterized by a certain number n of attributes $A_1,A_2,...,A_n$. One concrete patient context P is specified by the vector of the attribute values $a_1,a_2,...,a_n$ from the ranges $R_1,R_2,...,R_n$: $P=(a_1,a_2,...,a_n) \in R_1xR_2x...xR_n$. To allow unknown attribute values the range of each attribute is extended by the value "unknown". The attributes can be of three different types. Thus, nominal, ordered and numerical attributes can be used. Since every disease depends on specific factors, the attributes of the patient context are defined for each disease. For example, the following attributes could be specified for the treatment of heart failure: age, gender, body mass index, compliance, dispnoea, oedema, pleural effusion, blood pressure, heart rate, ejection fraction, type of heart failure, ventricle, NYHA class, etc.

The treatment process describes the treatment services and sub-services executed by the health care providers, the coordination tasks enabling communication and cooperation of the health care providers, the patient tasks concerning the patients' way of life as well as the supporting e-services. Treatment processes can consist of several treatment elements having different hierarchical and order-based relationships. In order to reflect this complex structure of treatment processes an object-oriented representation is chosen. In this type of representation all treatment process elements are characterized by classes. A concrete treatment process with its e-services contains a set of instances of these classes. The following section describes how treatment processes and e-services are defined in this project.

A treatment process consists of one or more treatment services which are provided by health care suppliers and it can contain several patient tasks which the patients have to fulfill. Each treatment service includes one or more sub services. Patient tasks and treatment sub services can contain itself as an element and enable any hierarchical depth of nesting. Order-related relationships are only modelled at service level. The exact order of execution of the sub services lies within the competence of the health care providers. The order of the patient tasks is neither fixed in the model but left to the responsibility of the patient. The treatment services, patient tasks and treatment sub services can contain recommendations and coordination tasks as further elements. While recommendations give information about the appropriateness of a treatment element, coordination tasks specify the preconditions and postconditions which are connected with the execution of the treatment element. Every treatment element is based on a pattern which contains general information on the treatment element. The execution of the treatment process elements can be supported by e-services which can provide several functionalities in form of operations and their parameters.

Before treatment processes with their e-services can be saved in the case base, the patterns of all treatment process elements have to be defined. Possible service patterns for heart failure can be the examination by the cardiologist or the practitioner. Exemplary sub service patterns are electrocardiogram or medication. Patient task patterns can be periodic measurement of heart rate or blood preasure. E-services supporting the treatment of heart failure can be electronic programs which organize the reimbursement of expenses or provide information on medicaments.

Figure 2 illustrates an exemplary patient with his treatment process. The attribute values characterise the patient as a 80-year old, overweight man who is suffering from a left-ventricular systolic heart failure in NYHA-Class II. In order to provide a clear illustration of the treatment process, Figure 2 only shows the types (e.g. Service) and the pattern names (e.g. examination by the cardiologist) of the treatment elements. The treatment process of the exemplary patient

Figure 2. Exemplary patient with his treatment process

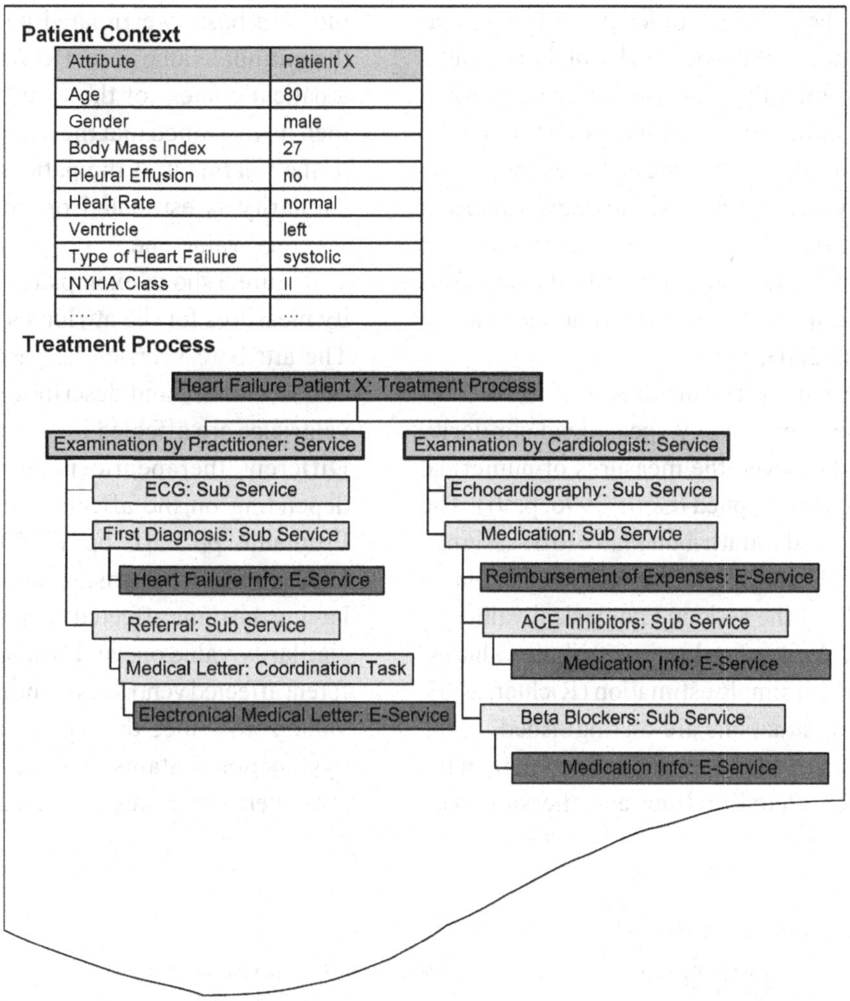

consists of an examination by the practitioner and by a cardiologist. During the examination the practitioner uses an electrocardiogram and refers the patient to the cardiologist with a first diagnosis of heart failure. The cardiologist confirms and concretizes the diagnosis by using an echocardiography and exhibits appropriate medicine. The treatment process is supported by the e-services Heart Failure Info and Medication Info which provide information, by the e-service Electronical Medical Letter which supports the communication between physicians, and by the e-service for the reimbursement of expenses.

Definition of Similar Patient Contexts

The retrieve phase aims at finding the treatment process and e-services of the patient in the case base, who is most similar to the given patient. For calculating the similarity of two patients local and global similarity measures are used. Similarity measures are two-digit functions on the problem space having a value range between zero (minimal similarity) and one (maximal similarity). While local similarity measures compute the similarity of two attribute values, global similarity measures assess the similarity of two patient contexts by aggregating the local similarities (Stahl, 2003, pp. 50ff). The definition of local similarity measures depends on the type of value of the attribute. For determining the local similarity of nominal attributes similarity tables (Goos, 1996, p. 90f) are used. Similarity tables are matrixes containing similarity values for each pair of query value and case value. In order to measure the similarity of numerical attributes several similarity functions such as linear and exponential functions can be used (Stahl, 2003, p. 54ff).

For the similarity calculation of ordinal attributes there are not any specialized similarity measures. However, the measures of numerical attributes can be applied (Goos, 1996, p. 91). The values of the ordinal attributes have to be assigned to numerical values. The similarity is calculated on the basis of the assigned numerical values.

The similarity of unknown attribute values is calculated by a simple estimation (Richter, 2003, p. 417). Two situations are distinguished. If the attribute value of the query is unknown, then the value is considered missing and the similarity between it and the value of the patient context of the case base is estimated pessimistically with the minimal value zero. However, if the value of a patient context of the case base is not known then it is assumed that the value had no relevance to the treatment of the patient. In this case, the similarity is estimated optimistically with the maximal value one.

Figure 3 shows exemplarily two local similarity measures for the attributes ventricle and age. The attribute ventricle is part of the diagnosis of heart failure and describes which of the heart ventricles are affected by a cardiac dysfunction. Different therapeutic methods are indicated depending on the affected ventricle (Hoppe & Erdmann, pp. 55ff, pp. 179ff). The exemplary local similarity measure assigns two patients having the same affected ventricle to the maximal similarity value one and two patients having different affected ventricles to the minimal similarity value zero. Since the therapy of a biventricular dysfunction contains some treatment steps which are either appropriate for a left or right ventricular

Figure 3. Similarity measurement

Local Similarity Table for Attribute Ventricle

Case/ Query	left	right	biven-tricular
left	1	0	0.25
right	0	1	0.25
biven-tricuar	0.25	0.25	1

Local Similarity Function for Attribute Age

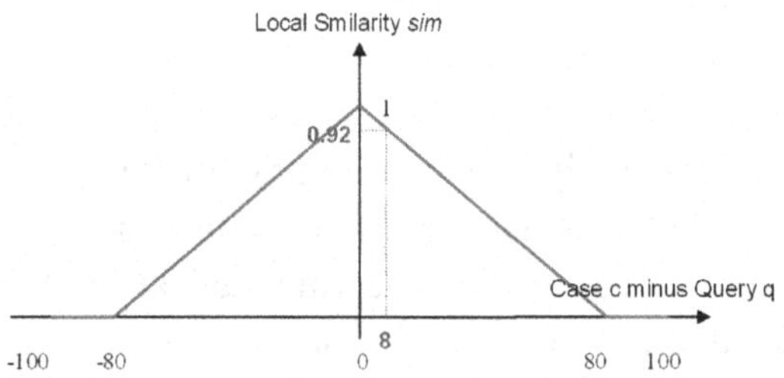

Global Similarity Measurement

Attribute	Query Patient Q	Patient of Case Base C	Local Similarity sim	Weight w	Global Similarity
Age	72	80	0,92	0.06	
Gender	male	male	1	0.07	
Body Mass Index	28	27	0.98	0.01	
Compliance	good	satisfying	0.2	0.03	$\sum w_i \cdot sim_i$
Pleural Effusion	yes	no	0	0.05	
Heart Rate	tachycardic	normal	0	0.04	
Ventricle	left	left	1	0.05	
NYHA Class	II	II	1	0,07	
...	...	...	...	...	

dysfunction, the local similarity value 0.25 is assigned to these cases.

The age influences the prognosis of heart failure and is an indicator for the general condition. Patients of different ages need different treatment steps. Therefore, a local similarity measure must be chosen, whereby the local similarity decreases with the increase in difference of age. Since many treatment steps are appropriate for young and old patients, a linear function is preferred to an exponential function. Figure 3 shows a possible similarity measure.

The global similarity of two patient contexts is calculated by a weighted average aggregation function. The weights resemble the relevance of the attribute and range between zero (low relevance) and one (high relevance). All weights have to be defined by a physician for each disease separately. Figure 3 demonstrates example weights for the attributes of heart failure. For instance, a high weight is assigned to the NYHA class since it serves as a measure for the severity of the symptoms and since most treatment steps are indicated in dependency of it.

The manual definition of similarity measures is very time-consuming and requires a great deal of explicit domain knowledge. Therefore a learning algorithm is implemented to ease the definition of the global similarity measure and to optimize the measure. The learning algorithm modifies the initial weights of the attributes as long as the global similarity measure enables retrievement of useful treatment processes. A gradient descent method (Stahl, 2003, pp. 105ff) is used for fulfilling the learning task. The gradient descent method requires input training data sets, which contain information from the user of the CBR system about the order of the usefulness of the proposed treatment processes for a given patient context. This information can be collected while using the system. The user must put all propositions of the system in order of their usefulness (Stahl, 2003, pp. 144f, pp. 140ff). An error function is defined by comparing the order of the proposed treatment processes preferred by the user with the order calculated by the similarity measure (Stahl, 2003, pp. 105ff). The gradient descent method aims at minimizing the error function by modifying the weights. The direction of the modification is determined by the gradient of the error function. The process of the modification is repeated until the error function converges to a minimum or a certain number of process iterations is reached.

Search of Similar Patient Contexts

The intention of the search algorithms used in the retrieve phase is to find those cases of the case base which are most similar to the query considering the defined similarity measure (Wess, 1995, p. 159). Searching the most similar cases can be realized by various strategies all requiring a compromise on quality, time and flexibility. For the search of similar patient contexts two alternative algorithms are provided: sequential search and knowledge-poor indexing using the extended k-d-tree (Wess, 95, pp. 209ff). Both algorithms guarantee finding the most similar patient contexts but differ in efficiency and flexibility. While the sequential search algorithm allows any ad-hoc-queries, the extended k-d-tree enables a quick standardized search.

The sequential search calculates the similarity of the query patient and all patients of the case base in sequential order using the defined similarity measures (Wess, 1995, pp. 163ff). The patients of the case base are put in order according to the degree of their similarity to the query patient.

The basic idea of the extended k-d-tree is to partition the case base into k dimensions using a tree (Wess, 1995, pp. 180f). The dimensions correspond to the attributes of the patient context (Goos 1996, pp. 69f).

The extended k-d-tree consists of a set of nodes and edges (Goos, 1996, pp. 69ff). While the root node represents all patients of the case base, the

Figure 4. Extended k-d-tree

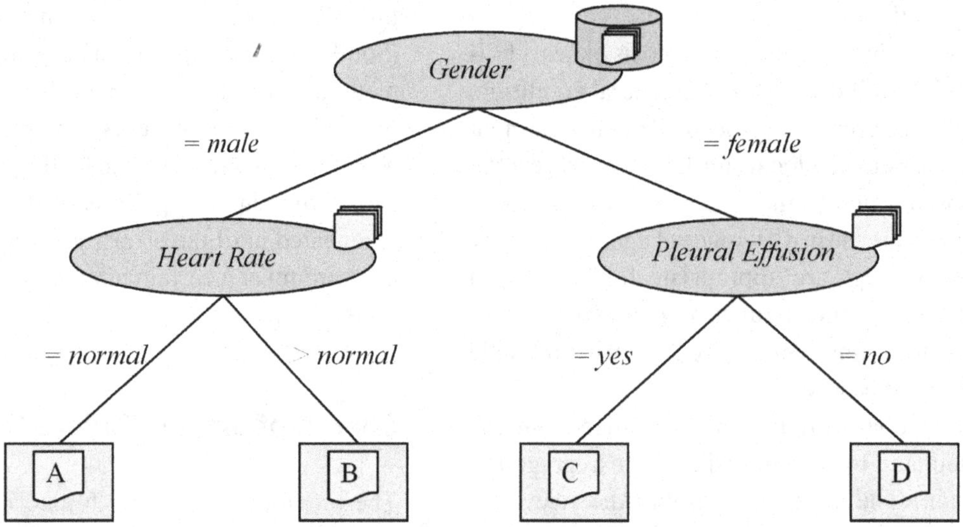

interior nodes describe a sub set of the case base. A small sub set of patients are saved in the leaf nodes. The root node and the interior nodes enable a partitioning of the set of cases which are represented by them. For this reason, each node has a discriminatory attribute and its outgoing edges are supplied with value conditions which specify the partition.

Figure 4 shows an extended k-d-tree which partitions the case base with the four patients A, B, C, D according to the attributes gender, heart rate and pleural effusion.

The tree can be generated automatically by a building procedure (Wess, 1995, pp. 198ff, pp. 182f, pp. 217ff). The building algorithm starts at the root node. There it determines the discriminatory attribute and partition value, which partition the case base best, using a selection method. Afterwards child nodes are created. The edges leading to the child nodes are labelled with conditions concerning the partition value (e.g. "= partition value"). Each child node inherits those patient cases, whose attribute values satisfy the edge labels. This procedure is executed recursively for all child nodes. The recursion stops and turns a node into a leaf node when the number of patient cases falls below a certain limit. These cases are saved in the leaf node.

The building procedure structures the tree in such a manner, that the similarity to the query patient has to be calculated only for a few patients of the case base in order to find the most similar patients (Goos 1996, p. 71). For this reason the selection method searches for the discriminatory attribute and partition value which divide the cases of a node in such a way that the cases in each child node are as similar as possible to each other and the cases of different child nodes are as dissimilar as possible. The mean value of the average similarities of the partitions can serve as selection criterion.

The search algorithm (Wess 1995, p. 188, pp. 234f) starts at the root node and follows the paths of the tree, whose edge conditions are fulfilled by the attribute values of the query patient, as long as a leaf node is reached. The cases contained in the leaf node are put in order of their similarities to the query. Since the algorithm does not aim at searching those patient cases which correspond to several attribute values of the query patient but those which are similar to all attribute values, the search is not over yet. In the next step, tests based on the discriminatory attributes and the partition values are executed which check if there are patients who are more similar to the query as the ones already found. In this case the search continues at the father node recursively.

Adaptation of Treatment Processes and E-Services

The adaptation taking place in the reuse phase aims at modifying the treatment process and its e-services of the retrieved patient to fit the new patient (Fuchs et al. 1999, p. 105).

The adaptation takes different turns depending on the goal of the query. Two goals can be differentiated: the generation of a new treatment process with e-services and the extension of an existing treatment process and its e-services. If the goal of the query is to generate a new treatment process with e-services then the old treatment process including its e-services is copied. If, however, the query aims at extending an existing treatment process and its e-services then the elements of the existing and the retrieved treatment process and its e-services are composed. Afterwards, a substitutional and structural adaptation as well as a consistency assurance are executed in order to adapt the copied or composed treatment process and its e-services to the new patient.

The compositional adaptation aims at building up a new treatment process and its e-services out of the existing treatment process and e-service elements of the query patient as well as of the similar patient of the case base. All completed and ongoing treatment process elements and e-service elements of the query patient are included in the new treatment process. Furthermore, treatment process and e-service elements of the similar patient are added. To guarantee a reasonable order of the treatment services, the retrieve-procedure only selects those cases, in which the service order corresponds to the order of the completed or ongoing services of the query patient. For example, take a query patient who has already consulted the practitioner and whose treatment process should be extended by the CBR-System: In the retrieve phase, only treatment processes starting with a practitioner service are considered during the similarity measuring. In order to build up the new treatment process for the query patient, the compositional adaptation includes the completed practitioner service and adds the services and its sub elements of the retrieved treatment process which follow the practitioner service.

The substitutional adaptation modifies the attribute values of the treatment elements and the e-service elements according to predefined rules. For example, the status is set to "planned" and the dates of the treatment services are uptated. Furthermore, the service providers are selected for each service according to the patient's preferences. Preferences can depend on former treatments, distance of the doctor's practice to the domicile of the patient and recommendations of other patients.

During the structural adaptation the structure of the treatment process and its e-services is modified. Depending on the mutality and differences in the attribute values of the query patient and the retrieved patient, components of the retrieved treatment process and its e-services are removed, new components are added or the order of the components is changed. The structural adaptation is realized by an additional CBR system, called ACBR system.

The cases of the ACBR system are generated with the aid of the case base of the main CBR system (Jarmulak et al., p. 1013). This procedure enables an adjustment of the adaptation cases of the ACBR system to the adaptation requirements of the main CBR systems. Each adaptation case consists of the adaptation conditions and the adaptation need (problem) as well as the adaptation actions (solution) (Wiratunga et al. 2002, pp. 426ff). The adaptation conditions describe the attributes of the patient context and the abstract treatment process, where the adaptation actions can be applied. The adaptation need indicates the differences between the attribute values of the query patient and the similar patient, which require the execution of the adaptation actions. The adaptation actions contain the modifications in which manner the treatment process has to be changed in order to adapt it to the new patient. Several types of actions can be differentiated: Add-Actions, Delete-Actions, Change-Order-Actions, Change-Structural-Relationship-Actions.

Figure 5 shows an exemplary adaptation case for heart failure. The adaptation conditions specify that the adaptation case is suited for elderly, female, overweight query patients who suffer from a left-ventricular systolic heart failure in NYHA-Class II. Furthermore, the planned treatment process of the query patient must include an examination by the practitioner and the cardiologist. According to the adaptation need the adaptation case is applicable to a query patient and a patient of the case base who differ in the attribute pleural effusion (fluid retention in the pleural cavity). Unlike the similar patient of the case base the query patient suffers from pleural effusion. In such a situation the adaptation case recommends a prescription of a diuretic in addition to the other medicaments of the similar patient in order to elevate the rate of fluid excretion.

Figure 5. Exemplary adaptation case

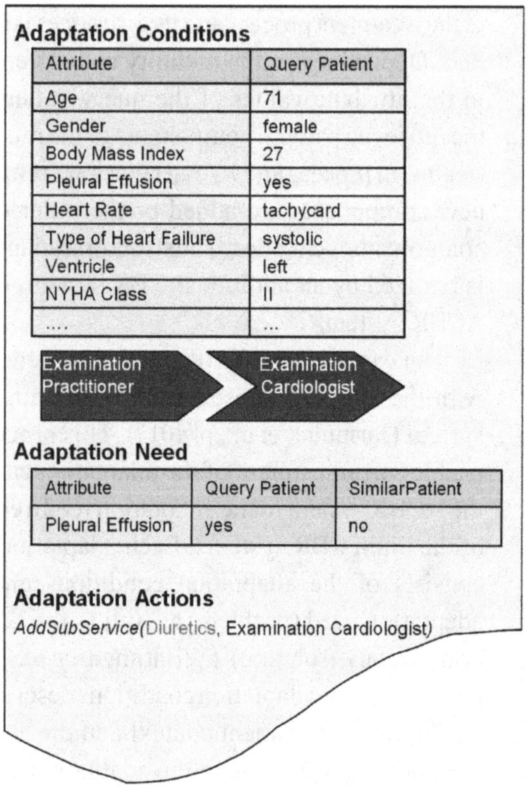

The structural adaptation searches the adaptation case, which contains the best adaptation actions for a given query patient and the similar patient of the case base. For this reason the main CBR system generates an adaptation query based on the query patient and the patient of the case base. The adaptation query is passed to the ACBR system which selects the case out of the adaptation case base being most similar to the adaptation query and returns it to the main CBR system. The main CBR system executes the adaptation actions of the adaptation case.

To assure the consistency of the adapted treatment process the last adaptation step executes local and global consistency testing methods. While the local consistency testing methods check for appropriateness of the treatment steps to the patient context, the global consistency testing methods deal with the interdependences of the treatment steps. Correction actions are executed if inconsistencies are detected. The consistency assurance is based on rules which are defined by domain experts. The rule antecedents ("if parts" of the rules) are tested and the rule consequences ("then parts" of the rules) are executed, if necessary.

For local consistency assurance, the rule antecedent consists of logically connected attribute value conditions of the patient context. The rule consequence can contain correction actions, which enable addition, deletion or replacement of the elements of the treatment process and the e-services. Local consistency rules can be used to specify contraindications. For example, the active ingredient digitalis is contraindicated for heart failure patients suffering from a bradycardic heart rate. This fact can be implemented by the following rule: If (heart rate = bradycardic) then DeleteSubService(digitalis).

The antecedents of global consistency assurance rules include treatment process elements. The rule consequences can contain actions calling for addition, deletion or replacement of the elements of the treatment process which are dependent on the element mentioned in the antecedent. For instance, a beta blockers therapy requires a periodic measurement of blood pressure and heart rate by the patient. This interdependency can be expressed by the following rule: If TreatmentProcessContains(beta blockers therapy) then AddPatientTask(measurement heart rate) and AddPatientTask(measurement blood preasure).

Execution of Treatment Processes and E-Services

The result of the adaptation is a proposal of a customized treatment process including e-services based on the collected treatment knowledge. During the revise phase, parts of the treatment process are executed. Besides proposing treatment processes and e-services this approach also has the aim of supporting the execution of the proposed e-services. The right e-services should be provided at the right time in the right place to satisfy the coordination and information needs of the health care suppliers and patients (Schicker et al., 2007, p. 724). Therefore the treatment process proposal is transformed into a XML-based representation and passed to the meta-orchestration engine for execution.

The meta-orchestration-engine (Schicker et al., 2007, p. 726) is based on the principle of web service based workflows and web service orchestration. Classic web service orchestration systems have little flexibility, are difficult to use and do not support individual orchestrations. By serving as a middleware the meta-orchestration-engine reduces these deficiencies. The process owner is able to modify the treatment process and its e-services proposed by the CBR system and to instantiate them. The technical configuration is executed at run time, e.g. the meta-orchestration engine activates the execution of the classic web service orchestration.

Maintenance of the CBR System

Changes in application environment and medical knowledge can reduce the quality of the result and efficiency of the CBR system (Wilson, 2001, p. 1). Therefore, maintenance which takes place in retain phase aims at preserving and correcting the knowledge of the CBR system to guarantee high quality and efficiency (Roth, 2002, p. 30). For customization of treatment processes and e-services the knowledge containers similarity knowledge and adaptation knowledge are automatically maintained by learning algorithms. The knowledge container vocabulary, which consists of the patient context attributes and the treatment process elements, is maintained manually by a domain expert.

The maintenance of the knowledge container case base is automatically executed in three maintenance steps, called retain step, review step and restore step (Roth, 2002, pp. 55ff). During the retain step intra-case quality-measures decide on inserting the treatment process with its e-services in the case base. Within the review step the treatment processes and e-services are checked for intra-case quality, inter-case quality and efficiency and deleted by the restore step, if necessary.

Intra-case quality-measures test the quality of a treatment process independently from other treatment processes (Reinartz et al. 2000, p. 253). Five different intra-case quality-measures are applied: solution success, local intra-case consistency, global intra-case consistency, up-to-dateness and completeness. The solution success measures the success of a treatment process and is judged by a physician according to the achieved improvement of the quality of life and the prolongation of the expectation of life (Stödter, 2000, p. 31). The local intra-case consistency evaluates to what degree the the treatment process is suited for the patient with respect to medical guidelines. Local consistency rules defined for adaptation can be used to determine the local intra case consistency. The global intra-case consistency checks each treatment process element if its dependent elements are contained in the treatment process. The calculation of the global intra-case consistency is based on the interdependency rules of the global consistency assurance of the adaptation phase. The up-to-dateness describes to what degree the treatment process elements are up-to-date. Its measurement takes into account the fraction of up-dated and out-dated treatment elements. The completeness evaluates to what degree the patient attributes are completely documented and is calculated with respect to the missing attribute values. All treatment processes whose mean value of all intra-case quality-measures falls below a ceratin quality limit are not inserted into the case base during the retain-phase and are deleted during the restore-phase.

In contrast to intra-case quality-measures, inter-case quality-measures determine the quality of a treatment process in relation to other treatment processes (Reinartz et al., 2000, p. 253). The inter-case consistency is used as inter-case quality-measure. A treatment process is judged as inter-case consistent with the case base if there are no other treatment processes in the case base which contain the same patient attribute values but different treatment steps. This measure allows the recognizing of alternative treatment processes. In the restore phase, the treatment process with the best intra-case quality is kept in the case base and all other treatment processes are deleted. As a result, the case base only contains the best treatment alternative for each combination of patient attribute values (Reinartz et al., 2000, p. 254).

In oder to increase efficiency, all redundant cases must be found and deleted exept for one. Therefore redundancy is taken as a measure for efficiency. Two treatment processes are considered redundant if they contain equal patient attribute values and treatment steps. During the restore phase, the case, which has the best intra-case quality, is left in the case base, while all its redundant cases are deleted.

CONCLUSION

The growing amount of medical information and knowledge requires the use of Medical Decision Support Systems. Among numerous artificial intelligence methods CBR is an especially recognized and established method for supporting medical decision making. Due to the lack of Medical CBR systems capable of planning and adaptation, a CBR system enabling the customization of treatment processes and e-services was developed. The aim of this system is to provide physicians in healthcare networks with valuable propositions of treatment processes and supporting e-services individually customized to the patients' needs in order to improve the quality of treatment. The concept is based on intelligent methods for selecting existing treatment processes and e-services as well as methods for adapting the found treatment processes and e-services. During the adaptation transformational procedures are applied. Compositional, substitutional and structural adaptation procedures as well as a consistency assurance are executed. The application of the CBR system is especially sensible in an environment where service-oriented architectures and possibilities for technical configuration of e-services exist. The installation and maintenance of the CBR system is time-consuming. This means that patient-context attributes, treatment process steps and e-services must be defined and maintained. Furthermore, the data must be adapted to the changes in environmental conditions and user requirements during the usage phase of the system. However, this task gives the opportunity of formalizing and expatiating on medical treatment knowledge. The proposed CBR system represents a base method for customizing treatment processes and supporting e-services and can be extended by further algorithms such as the prediction of unknown patient-context attributes.

REFERENCES

Aamodt, A., & Plaza, E. (1994). Case based reasoning: Foundational issues, methodological variations and system approaches. *AI Communications 7*(1), 39-59.

Cowie, M. R., & Mosterd, A., & Wood, D. A., & Deckers, J.W., & Poole-Wilson, P. A., & Sutton, G. C. (1997). The epidemiology of heart failure. *European Heart Journal, 18*, 208-255.

Fuchs, B., & Lieber, J., & Mille, A., & Napoli, A. (1999). Towards a unified theory of adaptation in case based reasoning. In Althoff, K.-D. et. al. (Eds.). *Case Based Reasoning Research and Development* (pp.104-117). Berlin: Springer.

Goos, K. (1996). *Fallbasiertes klassifizieren: Methoden, integration und evaluation.* Sankt Augustin: Infix Verlag.

Heinisch, R. H., & Weber, R., & Martins, A., & Barcia, R. M. (1998). Representing medical decision making strategies in a CBR system. In *Proceedings of the 6th German Workshop on Case based Reasoning - Foundations, Systems, and Applications*. Berlin.

Hoppe, U. C., & Erdmann, E. (2004). *Herzinsuffizienz – fortschritte in diagnostik und therapie*. München: Urban & Vogel Medien und Medizin Verlag.

Jarmulak, J., & Craw, S., & Rowe, R. (2001). Using case-based data to learn adaptation knowledge for design. In *Proceedings of the 17th IJCAI Conference*. Morgan Kaufmann, 1011-1016.

Nilsson, M., & Sollenborn, M. (2004). Advancements and trends in medical case-based reasoning: An overview of systems and system development. In *Proceedings of the FLAIRS Conference*, AAAI Press, 178-183.

Richter, M. M. (2003). Fallbasiertes Schließen. In Görz, G., & Rollinger, C.-R., & Schneeberger, J. (Eds.). *Handbuch der Künstlichen Intelligenz* (pp. 407-430), 4th ed. München: Oldenbourg Wissenschaftsverlag.

Reinartz, T., Iglezakis, I.; Roth-Berghofer, T. (2000). On quality measures for case base maintenance. In Blanzieri, E.; Portinale, L. (Eds.). *Advances in Case-Based Reasoning - Proceedings of the 5th European Workshop on Case-Based Reasoning.* Berlin: Springer Verlag, 247-259.

Roth-Berghofer, T. (2002). *Knowledge maintenance of case based reasoning systems - the SIAM methodology.* University of Kaiserslautern, Dissertation.

Schicker, G., & Kaiser, C., & Bodendorf, F. (2007). Individualiserung von Prozessen und E-Services mithilfe von Case based Reasoning. In Oberweis, S., & Weinhardt, C., & Gimpel, H., & Koschminder, A., & Pankratius, V., & Schnizler, B., *eOrganisation: Service-, prozess-, market-engineering* (pp.713-730). Karlsruhe: universitätsverlag karlsruhe.

Stahl, A. (2003). *Learning of knowledge-intensive similarity-measures in case based reasoning.* University Kaiserslautern, Dissertation.

Strödter, D. (2000). *Therapie der Herzinsuffizienz.* Bremen: UNI-MED Verlag.

Wess, S. (1995): *Fallbasiertes problemlösen in wissensbasierten systemen zur entscheidungsunterstützung und diagnostik.* Sankt Augustin: Infix Verlag.

Wilke, W., & Bergmann, R. (1998). Techniques and knowledge used for adaptation during case-based problem solving. In *Proceedings of the 12th International Conference On Industrial and Engineering Applications of Artificial Intelligence and Expert Systems, Lecture Notes in Computer Science* (pp. 497-506). Berlin: Springer Verlag.

Wilson, D. C. (2001): *Case-base maintenance: the husbandry of experience*. Indiana University, Dissertation.

Wiratunga, Ni., & Craw, S., & Rowe, R. (2002). Learning to adapt for case-based design. In *Proceedings of the 6th European Conference on Case Based Reasoning, Lecture Notes in Computer Science*, vol. 2416. Berlin: Springer Verlag, 421-435.

KEY TERMS

Attribute-Value-Vectors: Format to represent knowledge. It is often used to represent case knowledge in Case Based Reasoning (Richter, 2003, p. 412). The knowledge is characterised by a certain number n of attributes $A_1,A_2,...,A_n$. One concrete piece of knowledge P is specified by the vector of the attribute values $a_1,a_2,...,a_n$ from the ranges $R_1,R_2,...,R_n$: $P = (a_1,a_2,...,a_n) \in R_1xR_2x...xR_n$.

Case Based Reasoning: Method of Artificial Intelligence. It enables the solving of problems based on experience (Goos, 1996, S. 13). The experience is saved in the form of cases in a case base. Each case consists of two part: a decription of the problem and a description of its solution. In order to solve a new problem, Case Based Reasoning searches for the case of the case base which is most similar to the new problem and reuses its solution.

Extented K-D-Tree: Approach to save and retrieve knowledge in an efficient way. The basic idea is to partiton the knowledge base into k dimensions using a tree consisting of nodes and edges (Weß, 1995, pp. 180ff). While the leaf nodes of the tree save the knowledge, the inner nodes and the edges contain testing conditions, which direct the search of the knowledge. In Case Based Reasoning it can be used to save and search for cases efficiently.

Gradient Descent Method: Method for searching a local minimum of a function. In order to find a local minimum, the algorithm moves in the direction of the negative gradient (vector of the partial differentiations) of the function. In Case Based Reasoning it can be used to optimize the global similarity measure according to the preferences of the user (Stahl, 2003, pp. 105ff). For this purpose an error function must be defined by comparing the order of the cases preferred by the user and the order calculated by the global similarity measure. The gradient descent method searches the minimum of this error function.

Maintenance: Preservation and recoverage of the Case Based Reasoning System. The aim of the maintenance is to garantuee high quality and high efficiency of the Case Based Reasoning System throughout its whole life-cycle (Wilson, 2001, p. 1). The tasks of the maintenance are monitoring the status of the Case Based Reasoning System in order to recognize changes, which decrease the capability of the Case Based Reasoning System, and executing counteractive measures.

Medical Case Based Reasoning: Case based reasoning for supporting medical decision making. Medical Case Based Reasoning Systems can be applied to different medical purposes. They are often used in diagnosis and classification (Nilsson & Sollenborn 2004, p. 182). Further fields of application are tutoring and planning therapies.

Object-Oriented Representation: Format to represent knowledge. In comparision to Attribute-Value-Vectors it provides better posibilities of representing structural knowledge. In this type of representation knowledge is characterised by classes. A concrete piece of knowledge is composed of a set of instances of these classes.

Similarity Measures: Two-digit, real-valued function on the problem space: *Sim*: $PxP \rightarrow [0;1]$. The value range of similarity measures is restricted to the interval between zero and one, whereas the value zero represents minimal similarity and the value one symbolizes maximal similarity. Similarity measures enable the calculation of similarity between the problem of the query and the problem of the case of the case base (Stahl 2003, S. 47).

Structural Adaptation: Adaptation approach of Case Based Reasoning. It allows adapting the structure of the solution of a case from the case base in order to fit the problem of the query. Depending on the differences of the problem of the query and the problem of the similar case from the case base, components of the solution of the similar case are removed and reordered or new components are added (Wilke & Bergmann 1998, p. 500).

Section VIII
Virtual Environments in Healthcare

Chapter XXV
A Holistic Perspective of Security in Health Related Virtual Communities

I. Apostolakis
National School of Public Health, Greece

A. Chryssanthou
Greek Data Protection Agency, Greece

I. Varlamis
University of Peloponnese, Greece

ABSTRACT

A significant issue in health related applications is protecting a patient's profile data from unauthorized access. In the case of telemedicine systems a patient's medical profile and other medical information is transferred over the network from the examination lab to the doctor's office in order for the doctor to be able to perform a diagnosis. The medical information transferred across the network should be encrypted, secured and protected until it reaches its final destination. Patients' medical profiles should be accessible by their doctors in order to support diagnosis and care, but must also be protected from other patients, medical companies and others who are not certified by the patient to access his medical data. A very important element of virtual communities is trust. Trust should be built upon the same specifications for secure data transfer and leveled access with medical information. Furthermore, trust requires a strict policy based mechanism, which defines roles, access rights and limitation among community members, as well as a flexible identification mechanism, which allows anonymity of patients, while in the same time guarantees the truthfulness of doctors' identity and expertise.

INTRODUCTION

The Web offers access to many databases that contain medical information, and has significantly changed the way patients seek medical help. According to recent surveys, 50% of patients access medical information via the internet before visiting their doctor and this information affects their choice of treatment (Ferguson, 2002). The assistant role of virtual communities for patients who search for medical help and advice is undeniable. Researchers, practitioners, medical industry and patients jointly contribute their findings, products and experiences, to the community's knowledge base. The information transferred inside a health related virtual community and the stockpiled knowledge must be carefully protected from unauthorized use and validated in order to be qualitative and useful.

The issues of security, which traditionally applies to telecommunication applications, and confidentiality, which applies to healthcare applications, smoothly converge towards trust, which is the basis and apex of communities (Mezgar, 2005). This chapter examines various aspects of a health related virtual community always under the prism of information security and user protection. We provide several paradigms where patient information may be at risk and others where the integrity of the exchanged information can be questionable due to security faults.

The following section provides an introduction to the main community concepts and defines the structure of a typical health related virtual community. The critical features of communities (aim, limits, roles, services) are examined in the scope of a health related community. The third section deals with health information in general and with the security issues, which might arise when using medical services from distance. In the third section, we argue for the need to protect medical data on access, in transit and in storage, we summarize the possible security risks and state the need for an integrated security management system. The last section, uses an fictitious example in order to demonstrate the use of security policies, which can be help virtual communities to protect knowledge and information sharing and guarantee integrity.

Our objective in writing this chapter is:

- To enlighten the public in the security and integrity issues inside community,
- To raise the level of security awareness: a) of IT professionals, who develop, maintain or contribute to health related communities, b) of patients that reveal their privacy to a "virtual doctor" and make use of medical advices shared by other community members,
- To propose a set of technologies, which can under circumstances ensure that patients and doctors benefit from using community services without the fear of being a pray for phishers, spammers, hackers and crackers,
- To define the steps for building a trustful health related virtual community.

HEALTH RELATED VIRTUAL COMMUNITIES

This section provides a short introduction to the role of virtual communities in healthcare giving emphasis to the community structure and presenting the critical features of a healthcare community (aim, limits, roles, services). The section concludes with issues such as confidentiality and integrity of the community services and content.

In the process of psychological and medical support of patients with special needs three different types of participants can be distinguished: care providers, care givers and patients (Varlamis & Apostolakis 2007): *Care providers* are healthcare professionals, doctors and nurses, who treat and support patients as part of their work. The group is extended with researchers and scientists that convey their expertise on diseases and potential medical treatments. *Care givers* are those people who help a patient as friends or family of the patient. The group is extended with people who help voluntarily or otherwise deal with a specific disease, such as cancer. *Patients* are the "receivers" of the support. Care providers should be constantly informed on the scientific and industrial advances, on new products, treatments and devices. Researchers and scientists should disseminate their findings and guide industry and practitioners in favour of patients. Care givers should exchange information and useful hints concerning patients' care and support. Patients' needs vary over time, in the course of their disease experience: they want information in the first phase, when they learn about their disease and treatment alternatives; later, they are more interested in compassion and request emotional support (Varlamis & Apostolakis 2006). The BCANS community site (http://bca.ns.ca/) is a perfect example of patients and medical staff working in harmony by the means of a virtual medical community to fight the monster as they call it, namely breast cancer. They are performing that in a status quo of:

- Deep trust, where users share trusting interpersonal relationships built on liking and mutual appreciation between people that have to work together on a mutual goal

Or:

- Thick trust, where users trust each other based on personal experience or up-to-date info about a person's trustworthiness

Or:

- Swift (scatter) trust, where users trust each other based on some background of shared social network (Patricia Radin, 2006)

Tasks and Roles

One of the most important tasks in a virtual community is the coordination of discussion groups, which is handled by the group moderators (Moon, 2005). An important task which contributes to the building of trust inside the community is the administration of user profiles. The profile moderators check members' credentials and guarantee the truthfulness of their profile. This is possible through mini self-biographies. New users, who are "lurking" in the community's forums, need to feel comfortable enough, in order to participate in the community by talking about their problems, offering compassion or participating in group activities. Administrators protect the community from fraud and guide new members to the appropriate discussion and support groups based on their individual profiles. They guarantee the patients identity, distinguish care givers from medical professionals and in the same time protect patients' privacy by assigning them a virtual identity. In order to guarantee the quality of information provided to the community members, an additional moderator role is necessary: the content moderator, who is made responsible for reviewing and filtering all published material and acts as a liaison between information providers (experts, doctors, etc) and consumers (patients).

The aim of restricting access to the community only to members, is to build a status quo of thick trust among members and to protect them from outsiders (i.e. spammers, who advertise products, or ***phishers***, who gather and exploit personal data of members).

The different roles and tasks carried by each type of community's users are displayed in Figure 1. In the same figure the two valuable community sources; the Knowledge and Profile base offer multilevel access to members according to their role. Only registered community members are able to communicate and collaborate.

Figure 1. Community roles and responsibilities

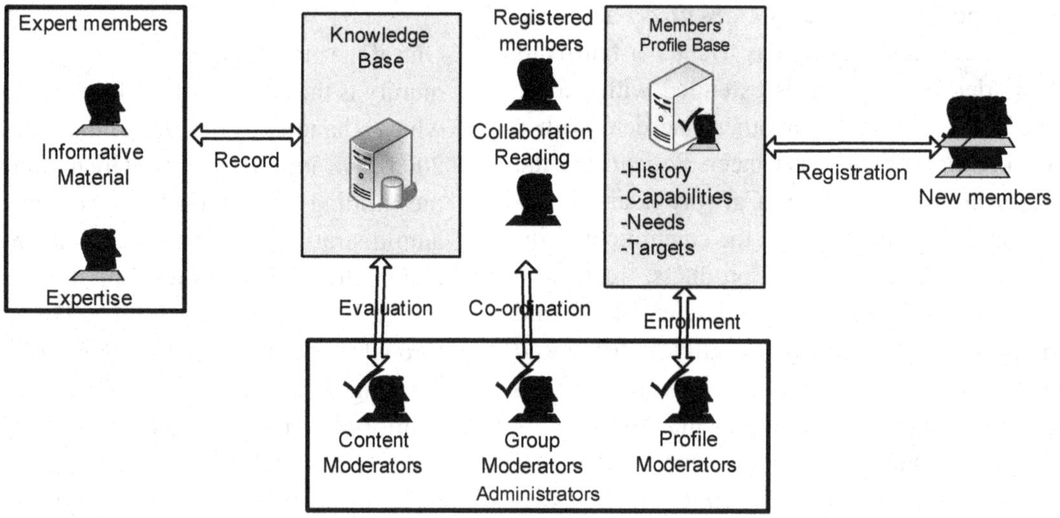

We consider health related virtual communities as a large-scale distributed system, which offers services and allows transfer and storage of data. An important issue for the designers of a community is the building of trust among members. This requires that the administrators are aware of the complete profile of a member, whilst all other members have partial access. The protection of members' *anonymity* (Tygar, 1998) is crucial in a community of support and can be attained through the virtual identity of members. Virtual identity is always bound to the same user and stands for the static profile, thus allowing doctors to keep a history of their patients, while at the same time, preserves personal data of patients.

Secure use of Services

The services provided to the members of a supportive community must be carefully designed in order to be as useful to patients as possible. Extra care should be taken to guarantee accessibility of content and services and to avoid member exclusion. A patient joins a virtual community in order to obtain medical advice and care by doctors or support by fellow people, or co-patients. It is crucial for the patient to be able to access the community's services and content 24 hours a day 7 days a week. Consequently, computer security measures, such as the ones that will be analyzed later in this chapter, are necessary to ensure constant availability of the virtual community. Furthermore, appropriate access control mechanisms need to be in place to allow authorized users, namely the members of the virtual community, to enter the community site and benefit from its services, while blocking any unauthorized individuals from being able to enter the site with malicious intent. Access controls, such as security tokens, will be discussed further in this chapter. Data stored in the medical community's site should be regularly backed up offsite, so that they can be recovered safely in case of a disastrous incident.

The most widely used service is the distribution of ***informative content*** (i.e. medical documents, surveys, medical advices, news etc.). Content should be easily located and retrieved from patients. This subsumes that content should be available in various formats, so that it can be accessible to people with disabilities (deaf, blind etc). In order to facilitate new users, content can be forwarded to patients via e-mail through the appropriate mailing lists. For frequent users, content can also be published through a Web portal. It should be organized into meaningful categories and a search service should allow retrieval of the appropriate information.

Information dissemination through the Web Site of the virtual community or by means of mailing lists requires security measures to be taken in order to ensure the safe transfer of medical data. In the first case (Web Site transmission) cryptographic protocols, such as ***SSL (secure socket layer)***, can be used by a member to communicate with the community site. Provided that the users use an e-token to enter the site, as suggested later in the chapter, the encryption process is handled entirely by the token, which requests from the server to "speak" a common cryptographic algorithm during their communication. Therefore, the patients need simply to enter a password for the e-token to communicate securely. The ***E-token USB device*** encrypts the whole communication between the end-user (member of the virtual community) to the virtual community's Web server with a 256-bit security key.

An alternative could be the use of Virtual Private Network technology as an access control measure. A ***virtual private network*** (VPN) is a private data network that makes use of the public telecommunication infrastructure, maintaining privacy through the use of a tunneling protocol and security procedures. Since the users of the virtual community enter the community site by means of an encrypted tunnel any conducted communication is private therefore secure.

In the case of ***e-mail communication, public-key cryptography*** should be used to ensure that mail communication can be read only by the intended recipient. In public key cryptography both communicating parties have a pair of keys, a public and private key. If a fictitious character named Bob wants to send a message to a person named Alice by using public-key algorithms, he just has to obtain Alice's public key and encrypt his message with it. After encrypting the message the only person capable of decrypting the message is the one holding the private key, thus only Alice can decrypt the encrypted message and read it.

Interaction between community members is increased with online and offline discussions (Rada, 2005). ***Discussions*** can be asynchronous (by posting questions and answers) or synchronous (in a discussion ***forum*** or in private chat-rooms). The aim of discussions is bi-fold: to support patients and their families and to allow experts to exchange knowledge. Debates are more meaningful, when their topics are predefined and organized. The discussions in the community forums should be moderated by expert users that filter informa-

Figure 2. Secure Communication by means of an e-token usb device.

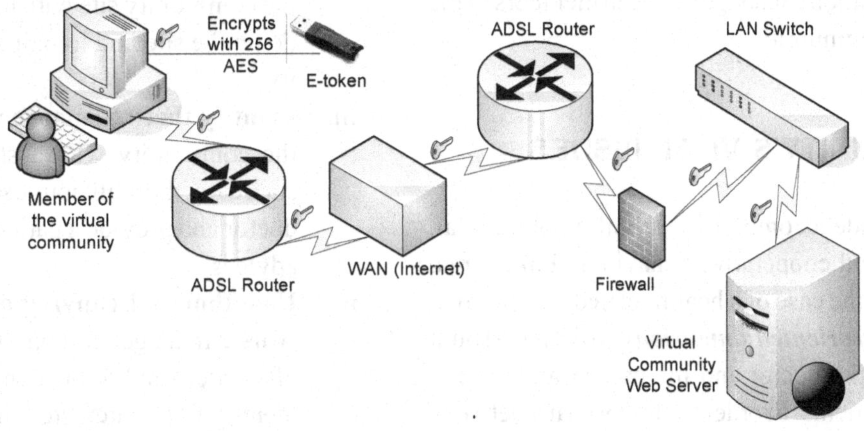

tion when requested, facilitate members or consult members about the forum rules. The presence of professionals (doctors, nurses etc) in a forum adds to its value and increases participation.

Additional services allow members to provide information about themselves to the community and build their profile. The part of the ***user profile***, which is provided by the user himself, is his static profile and remains unchanged. Both patient and doctors should be able to update their member profile so that the community knows their current interest or expertise. Another part of the profile, which evolves all the time, is the dynamic profile which encompasses all actions of a member inside the community. In order to increase member interaction with the community and exploit the expertise of members, moderator roles could be assigned to frequent members, who will be requested to submit their feedback on the community operations.

Finally, in an autonomous community members should be able to make their own, ***self-supportive groups*** inside the community. Members of a group should be able to set-up or attend chat sessions on topics of interest, to participate in point-in-time surveys or straw polls on a topic to allow communities to gather consensus and determine community activity, to start new communities related to specific problems and steer the content according to their collective needs. The security measures mentioned above (encryption, tokens) apply naturally to all types of information exchange between members of the virtual community.

COMMUNITY'S VITAL ISSUES

Trust inside a community is built upon regular, honest, and cooperative behaviour (Fukuyama, 1995). In the case of a health related community, the ***person oriented dimension*** of trust is first built between the doctor and his patient and second among patients. In order to support trust between doctor and patients, the doctor's identity should be valid and accessible to the patient and on the other side, the patient's profile should be made available to the doctor.

The other two dimensions of trust, as stated by (Fogg & Tseng, 1999), more specifically the ***trust in the object*** (such as computers, networks, and software) and ***process*** (such as tele-healthcare, or tele-consultation) can be met but more slowly. Although, many technological issues have been solved, the building of trust towards networks, security mechanisms and other technology issues is difficult. The build of trust towards the process can be facilitated with the definition and implementation of access policies to the medical information and services. A presentation of the approaches that capitalize on the building of trust in a health related virtual community follows.

Threats for the Virtual Medical Community

Threats that might damage the virtual community and cause the circulation in public of important medical data are among others:

i. **Unauthorized access:** A malicious user manages to infiltrate the community site and gains access to all these data that the community needs to protect.
ii. **DOS (denial of service) attacks:** Malicious users use a number of computers to flood the community site with messages and take down the site and impair service availability.
iii. **Identity theft:** Someone manages to enter the community with a stolen identity. In such case, the malicious user might pose as a doctor and provide a patient with erroneous advices.
iv. **Unauthorized copying of medical data:** A user manages to copy the medical data of a patient and sell it along with a patient's identity to an interested third party.

v. **Eavesdropping:** A malicious user is spying information exchanged between community members and collects useful information.

The above mentioned threats could come from internal users (patients, the doctors and the moderators) as well as from external ones (McClure et al, 2003), such as:

i ***Hackers:*** Skilled programmers, who attack information systems, aiming to achieve absolute knowledge of information technology
ii ***Crackers:*** Skilled programmers, who attack information systems, aiming at personal gain either in financial or information level (information is power for the one who holds it)
iii **Script-kiddies:** Good programmers, who employ hack tools in order to find exploits in the community platform and bring it down.

The potentiality of these threats depends on various factors:

i Main elements of the community infrastructure
ii Technical Vulnerabilities of the community systems
iii Handling of security issues by the members of the community
iv Value of the community's information for people outside looking in, such as crackers.

Securing the use of Health Services

All members of a community -patients, their families, doctors, nurses and students of medicine- make use of the community services for their own reasons. Patients, for example, access the community in order to get the results of a medical examination or to obtain some medical advice, doctors in order to edit a patient's data or perform a diagnosis etc. Tele-medicine and tele-advice are two important services of health related communities, which both require the transfer of medical data.

Transfer of Medical data (examination results, medical information, medical advice etc.) obeys to the laws of CIA, where CIA stands for ***Confidentiality, Integrity*** and ***Availability***. Medical data is confidential, must be accurate and available during all times and is protected by Data Protection Laws. A process must be applied upon design and on launch and operation of the virtual community, which will guarantee that care providers, care givers and patients discuss in a secure manner. No user is eavesdropping, no one is collecting data (medical condition, mail address, financial data) for ***phishing*** or spamming purposes. This process must follow international standards such as BS7799 and ISO 27001, which define the lifecycle of an Information Security Management System.

A framework that has already been used in other medical information systems is the Octave Risk Management Framework. The framework consists of an organizational, a technology and a strategy and plan development phase. According to the framework a risk assessment identifies critical assets and potential threats in the first phase. In the second phase, key components and technical vulnerabilities are identified. In the final phase mitigation plans and a protection strategy are designed.. The goal is to build a security "stronghold" of information, where medical data and confidential discussions remain private, is not altered in any way and is constantly available.

Securing Medical Data

In this section, we argue for the need to protect medical data on access, in transit and in storage. Technologies such as Web sign-on, cryptographic algorithms, patch management suites and usage agreements are deemed necessary, so that all users, can use the community services securely (Chryssanthou & Kastania, 2006), (Chryssanthou, 2006).

Web sign-on can be used by members of a virtual community upon login on the virtual community site. By using this technology users can identify themselves correctly and communicate with each other by means of a cryptographic algorithm. ***Web sign-on*** is performed usually by using an ***e-token*** usb device which can be provided to the user upon registration. This e-token can store passwords in an encrypted state and when used encrypts the user's communications with algorithms such as AES. ***Cryptographic*** algorithms ensure confidentiality of communication. Any eavesdropper will "hear" cryptographic gilberish. Depending on the quality of the used algorithm the potential eavesdropper might never get any useful data from "hearing" a user's conversation.

Computer systems are vulnerable to problems of the operating system and have several security holes. Most of these vulnerabilities are discovered also by members of the hacking community. Manufacturers update their software, in order to keep up with the "bad" hackers and ensure that their customer's data remain secure, but unfortunately they cannot avoid zero-day exploits. Zero-day exploits are exploits that are deployed on the net before a manufacturer has the time to provide a fix for a particular vulnerability. To tackle with zero-day exploits a further security component such as an ***intrusion prevention system*** is needed. This type of system will be able to block any suspicious traffic based on the characteristics of the received data.

The members of a virtual community discuss about sensitive medical issues, handle medical data and might disclose very sensitive private information, which would prove to be a goldmine in the hands of a skilful hacker, a spammer or a phisher. Thus, the members of the virtual community do not just need to feel protected against potential threats, they also need to be aware that even in a case of a breach the appropriate measures are in place, which will ensure that the potential perpetrator is found, before their data turn into a valuable asset for the highest bidder in the pharmaceutical community. The logs, which are maintained by an intrusion prevention system, will certainly play an important role in finding a potential perpetrator. A well justified and designed procedure that will guide the moderators in performing a ***forensic analysis*** of a potential incident, while recovering through a backup plan in the minimum amount of time, will be another important aspect of these measures. Forensic analysis (Chryssanthou & Apostolakis, 2006) is the procedure, during which the appropriate personnel, either internal or external, images hard disks, collects network traffic logs, system logs, hashes the evidentiary data, so that it can be used in a court of law. This vast amount of data is collected and analyzed by using special tools (i.e. Encase from Guidance Software and The Forensic Toolkit by AccessData, Helix and F.I.R.E).

It might also prove useful to set up a honeypot to draw back the perpetrator in order to trace him back to his location, collect data on the type of his illegal activity or just collect data that will help reveal the perpetrator's true identity. In computer terminology, a honeypot is defined a trap, which seems to contain information that would be of value to attackers, and which is set to detect or deflect attempts at unauthorized use of information systems.

Backup systems are also necessary so that the systems can return to a previous known state without the users losing their data and with the minimum cost in availability. A medical site should remain offline the least amount of time, because time is of great importance in all medical cases.

Usage agreements are not a technological security measure, but still play an important role in a network security infrastructure, especially in a Web community. They are written based on the results of the risk management process and according to the data protection laws governing medical data. Users have to know how the virtual community operates, what its purpose is, what is allowed and what prohibited and which legal consequences might arise on violation of the usage agreement.

Building Trust Inside the Community

In this section we focus on the necessary security policies, which can be implemented in health virtual communities in order to protect community members from improper use of services, deception and other possible hazards inside the community. This section crosses the technical barriers of information security and data privacy and presents a holistic perspective of security inside a community. This perspective examines people, processes, strategies and community culture.

A fundamental requirement for a successful community is to build trust among the community members and consequently enforce members' confidence to the community mechanisms. A community is trusted when it implements a security policy mechanism. The first action of community designers is to define the appropriate policies, to describe the roles inside the community, the access rights and restrictions for each role etc. The design of the community should follow the security guidelines: provision should be made for user roles and credentials and an access control mechanism should be implemented over information and services. This would be made possible by using access policy models. A prototype access policy for a medical community is the Cassandra trust management system for electronic health records (Becker & Sewell, 2005). Cassandra is a role-based access system (RBAC) expressed on a language based on Datalog with constraints. Access control is based on the member's role in the community. Furthermore, the data owner can define the sensitivity of his data, the people able to access it and the access rights, by which each allowed user can access his data.

For example, a treating physician can access a patient's entire medical file, while a receptionist can only view and alter (with the patient's authorization) his general data. Credentials can be distributed by registration authorities or by patients. For example, suppose that a patient needs to undergo a surgical operation. The patient grants the treating doctor access to his medical doctor to access his data in order to perform the surgery. The doctor can now give access to his data to the other members of the medical team so that they can assist during surgery. The roles assigned to the members of the surgical team (Register-team-episode) are valid only for a period of time (during surgery and for treatment. Upon recovery of the patient the roles are revoked. In a virtual medical community a similar semantic role-based policy has to be applied. The general roles (patient, doctor, advisor, etc) can be assigned by the moderators. Patients then can define which doctors can access their private data or which members can take part in a private held conversation. This access policy will be enforced by each user upon entering the site of the virtual community. On first registration, the users will have general access rights based on their type of user (doctor, patient, etc).

The access policy is supplementary to the access control mechanisms mentioned earlier. An access control policy will be implemented technically, explained to the user on registration and will be available as a written and electronic document so that the users have no excuse for violating other user's rights or the policy in general and the community is protected against users' misbehavior. This written document will explain everything, from login procedures, password quality, privacy rights to user roles and credentials.

In a health related community, the problem of trust is multifold: patients should be confident that their doctor (or medical consultant in general) is capable to support them, they should be sure that the communication with their doctor is sheltered from unauthorized access and that their doctor is discreet with their problem. The patients have to be certain beyond any reasonable doubt that they are talking to a doctor and not an impostor and that their conversation with a doctor is held in private (protected by doctor – patient confidentiality). In several cases, it is desirable for patients to hide their identity even from the doctor, thus allowing them to express their problems or worries more sincerely. On the other side, doctors share their expertise with the patients, and request access to patients' health profile in order to provide better diagnosis and support.

Inside a virtual community, patients and doctors are hidden behind their virtual identities. A user is anonymous without obtaining the right not to be liable for any disrespect or violation of the community's regulations. A difference between health related communities and other community applications is that the history of visits as well as the role of a member inside the community is of importance to other members. For example, patients, who engage on a discussion with a doctor, want to be absolutely certain that their interlocutor is a real doctor. Furthermore, they need to be aware of his/hers field of expertise. Similarly, doctors need to access the complete patient's profile and medical history before making their diagnosis. Doctors will be allowed to access the complete patient's profile only after obtaining the patient's consent by the means of a role assignment (for example treating physician role) through a properly formed semantic policy.

It is clear from the above that the virtual identities of all community members should remain unchanged throughout their "virtual life" in order to allow the creation of dynamic profiles and facilitate doctors' work. Parts of the real identity of doctors (i.e. their expertise) should accompany the virtual identity, in order that the users of the virtual community build a thick trust relationship. Enhancing the doctor's avatar with a short bio of his medical accomplishments will certainly convince the patients to open up about their problems, trust the doctor and obtain helpful medical advices.

User's Responsibility of Security

All the security technologies, which were analyzed and proposed earlier in this chapter, focused on protecting and encrypting communications on the one side and controlling access to the main infrastructure on the other. However, a basic factor has been left aside: end users. Kevin Mitnick used to say that there is no cure for human stupidity. The strongest security mechanisms are of no use when a naïve user shares his/her password with an unknown person. Users need to be security aware, not give their passwords or their keys to anyone and should not just hang on the security measures handed to them by the community. A fully updated antivirus product on their own personal computer can protect them from ***keyloggers***, namely programs that will try to log their keystrokes, ***trojans***, programs that do not perform just as intended, ***spyware*** and of course viruses. What's the point of building a secure channel if the one end of the connecting line is not secure? Both ends of a communication line need and must be secure in order for any security mechanisms to have a real effect.

Figure 3. The Information Security Management cycle

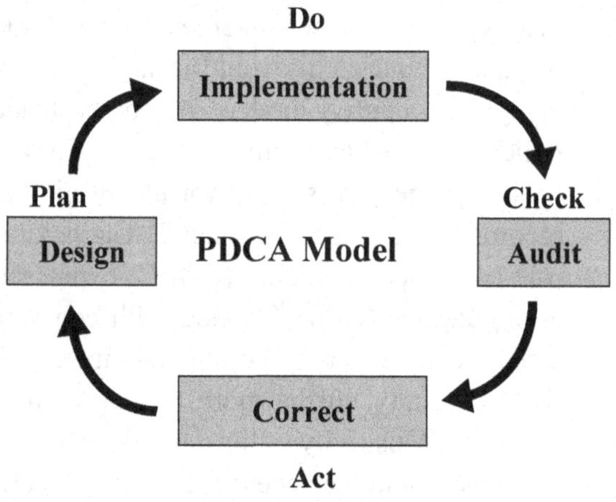

Combining the Strengths of BS7799 and ISO 27001

As a conclusion, in order to achieve international security standards during designing and implementing the community, an Information Security Management System has to be designed. The international standards in the computer security area are the BS 7799 (BSI, 2005) and the ISO 27001(IEC, 2005) (IEC_2, 2005). Both standards define the right way to implement an effective Information Security Management System. Building such a system is a result of a continuous cycle of procedures, which repeats itself as the needs of an organization change, the legal regulations change and security regulations evolve, while their "opponents", the tools, that the perpetrators of e-crime use, become more and more sophisticated. This cycle consists of 4 stages, namely: *Plan, Do, Check* and *Act* as depicted in Figure 3.

An Information Security Management System, in essence, is a "live" part of an organization, which has to be designed correctly (based on various parameters), implemented based on technologies, that are selected during the design phase and checked for its effectiveness. This check will result in identifying possible changes, which are necessary, in order for the system to improve or to adapt to new circumstances, such as a new stricter computer law act. If such a system is surpassed by technological developments then it stops being effective and the organization, which uses it, is in immediate danger of computer security breaches.

A VIRTUAL MEDICAL COMMUNITY SCENARIO

In order to achieve our objective a fictitious health related virtual community will be used as a paradigm. This community must be evaluated from a security perspective by the means of globally accepted security standards such as BS7799 and ISO27001. The community structure, the appropriate trust building mechanisms and policies will be discussed in the following.

If we abstract the interaction between a doctor and a patient inside a virtual community to a transaction between two people in which one requests assistance and the other offers it we can easier discover the critical security issues. In the following we describe a community comprising patients of a group therapy program and the affiliated doctors and this is our exemplar case study.

Both patients and doctors access the community Web server using their browsers. Patient's real identity must remain hidden to all community members, and only the community administrators should be able to access it. This type of anonymity is crucial for a group therapy community to attract potential members.

In order to support this partial anonymity we need a flexible patient profile, which contains both identity and medical information, and which has access control policies.

When patients and doctors log into the community, they apply the appropriate credentials and get a virtual id, which remains constant throughout their virtual life. This virtual identity offers anonymity while in the same time guarantees atomicity. Patients are identified as patients and their virtual profile is enhanced each time they join the community: the group therapy sessions in which they participate are recorded in their dynamic profile (history) and the same holds for their activities. This information is available for doctors who monitor patients' behavior. Doctors are identified in a similar way and their field of expertise appears in their publicly available profile. The identification of doctors and patients increases the confidence of patients to the community experts (psychologists, pathologists etc) and makes them more positive in participating to virtual group meetings or private sessions. The virtual identity conceals the real identity from unauthorized view and increases patients' openness in discussions.

Upon identification, patients gain access to their own space in the community server. There, they are able to update their personal and medical profile information. Patient's medical profile is valuable for the doctor but is of no use to the other patients and as such it must remain out of their access. The patient must be able to define which user groups or specific users should have access to their profile information (e.g. my doctor, my friends, user X etc) and to which specific part of it (i.e. medical information, personal information etc)

After updating her profile, the patient is able to contact a doctor and discuss her problem. The patient grants access to the medical profile to the doctor at any time. The doctor uploads a diagnosis and consultation and grants access to the patient (or to an accredited member of his family). No other doctor is able to access this medical profile unless the patient gives a grant option to the doctor. Similarly, the diagnosis is accessible to the patient only. The same holds with any examination results.

Define Sensitive Data

The first important asset of a medical community, whether virtual or not, is medical data. Medical data is twofold. It consists of the identity of the patient and its medical file. Having one without the other or being able to identify the other is useless for financial purposes. Having both provides a repository of information, which can be of value to patients, doctors, insurance, pharmaceutical companies and medical organizations. This type of data is sensitive and protected by international computer laws such as the EU 95/46/EC directive (EU, 1995) and national laws such as law no 2472 for the protection of an individual against unlawful processing of personal data (Greek Data Protection Authority, 1997). Medical data abide to the laws of CIA and need to be protected so that cases like the one of Privacy Rights Clearinghouse (PRC) v. Albertsons, where a chain of pharmacies was collecting data about their customers, which were used for illegal marketing of pharmaceutical products, are not repeated. (PrivacyRights.org, 2004) Such a case is clearly illegal in the EU, as this chain of pharmacies violated contract laws, connected medical files without authorized permission, violated the confidentiality of medical data and engaged in illegal marketing. Consequently, a virtual community must remain a virtual community; ***medical data*** must be protected ***in whatever form they are uploaded*** in the community, ***medical conversations*** must remain confidential and ***virtual identities*** must never by any means be identified with a patient's or a doctor's real identity. Medical data, medical conversations and virtual identities are the most important information assets of a virtual medical community, assets which must be identified by the designer of the ISMS in the design phase while performing risk analysis.

Defining Hazards

The first phase of the risk analysis was to identify the most important information assets, which need to be always protected. The second phase would be to identify what these assets need to be protected from and the potentiality of those threats. The hazards for the healthcare community comprise unauthorized access to data and services, attacks, data and credentials stealing, eavesdropping and have been detailed in the previous. The biggest threat for a healthcare community is eavesdropping because it is difficult to be detected and refers to sensitive personal data. DOS attacks are less likely in a healthcare virtual community. Other threats can be minimized by choosing and implementing appropriate security and identification mechanisms.

Choosing the Technologies

First of all, the community must be shielded against unauthorised copying. For this reason, a written policy will be sent to the users and must be agreed on during registration. This written policy will define security procedures, emphasize on the sensitivity of the exchanged data, and inform the users of the legal consequences of unauthorized copying or publishing of community's data as well as the consequences of damaging in any way the community's infrastructure. This written policy must be supplemented by an actual technically implemented policy which will assign specific rights to the users on first entry.

The access policy will be role-based and will follow the semantics model proposed earlier, in order to allow patients to assign different rights to their treating doctor than other doctors, who simply will need to see a portion of the data to provide them with an advice. Simultaneously, a doctor will be able to add hidden comments about a patient's medical condition without the patient knowing about it. Access to the repository of real identity information will be restricted only to the administrators group, will be allowed only when at least two administrators agree and any access will be audited. Auditing, of course, will be enabled for all access to sensitive data.

A second measure is to ensure that no one is eavesdropping. In order to achieve that all communications will be encrypted. Encryption is bi-fold: first, the Web server has to speak a cryptographic "language" such as SSL and second, the user's browser has to speak the same "language". The encryption algorithm has to be as strong as possible. Upon verification of a user's data and completion of the registration procedure, a Web sign-on e-token will be given to the user. The token will have a strong password and will comprise the community password. The only way to enter the community will be by using this token, which will encrypt the user's traffic. In this way, the possibility of identity theft and unauthorized access will be also reduced, as a malicious user would have to obtain a valid e-token in order to enter the community's site.

A third measure is to protect both ends of the communication. Users must install an antivirus in order to ensure that they are virus free and Trojan free. The infrastructure of the community must also be protected by a fully updated antivirus system and up-to date patched against technical vulnerabilities by means of a patch management suite. Furthermore an Intrusion Prevention System has to be in place with constantly updated signatures, in order to deal with hack attempts and DOS attacks.

The final step is to define a backup and recovery procedure. The community's data have to be backed up regularly so that the community can recover from a security breach or another form of damage. Backups should be kept in remote sites, while a recovery procedure has to be in place that will help regain functionality in the minimum amount of time in all possible scenarios.

These proposed solutions should be enough to protect a fictitious medical community against most important types of attacks. It hangs on the moderators and the support team to maintain security and achieve it. Security is a constant battle. Technologies change and attacks evolve, so measures must constantly be improved, while users must be always security aware.

CONCLUSION

This chapter presented a holistic approach in securing transaction inside a health related virtual community and building trust among members and trust to the community mechanisms. The major requirements of this approach are: technical solutions that secure transfer of medical information (such as encryption etc), identification mechanisms that guarantee atomicity and allow anonymity per case and security policies, which grant access to medical information only to the appropriate community members. The necessary technology infrastructure exists, however it must be adapted to the specific community needs.

REFERENCES

Becker, Moritz, Y., Sewell, Peter (2005). Cassandra: Flexible trust management applied to electronic health records. Published as *Technical Report UCAM-CL-TR 648*. University of Cambridge, Computer Laboratory, (pp 214).

British Standards Institution, BSI (2005). Information technology. Security techniques. Information security management systems. Requirements. British Standard / ISO/IEC / 18-Oct-2005/ ISBN: 0580467813.

Chryssanthou, Anargiros (2006). Security of information systems in health environments. *6th National Conference on Public Health & Medical Services*. Athens.

Chryssanthou, Anargiros & Apostolakis, Ioannis (2006). Network forensics: Problems and solutions. In *Proceedings of the 2nd National Conference with International Participation, Electronic Democracy*. Athens, ACCI.

Chryssanthou, Anargiros & Kastania, Anastasia (2006). Quality & Security in medical information systems. *Health Review, Tome 17, Issue 100*, pages 42-45.

Chryssanthou, Anargiros (2006). Gathering of digital evidence in a computer network : Problems & possible solutions. School of officers in research and informatics. *Informational leaflet in informatics & technology, issue 28*, May 2006.

The European parliament and the council of the European Union. (1995). *Directive 95/46/EC of the European Parliament and of the Council of 24 October 1995 on the protection of individuals with regard to the processing of personal data and on the free movement of such data*. Luxembourg. (Directive 95/46/EC).

Ferguson, Tom (2002). "From patients to end-users". *British Medical Journal, 324*, 555-556.

Fogg, B.J. & Tseng, Hsiang (1999). The elements of computer credibility. In *Proceedings of CHI'99*. Pittsburgh, PA.

Fukuyama, Francis (1995). *Trust—the social virtues and the creation of prosperity*. New York: The Free Press.

Greek Data Protection authority. (1997). *Individuals protection against the processing of personal sensitive data*. (Law 2472/1997).

International Electrotechnical Commission, IEC (2005). *Information technology - Security techniques - code of practice for information security management*. ISO/IEC/ 17799/ 01-Jun-2005.

International Electrotechnical Commission, IEC_2 (2005). *Information technology – security techniques – information security management systems – requirements*. ISO/IEC FDIS 27001:2005.

McClure, Stuart, Scambray, Joel & Kurtz, George (2003). *Hacking exposed, network security secrets and solutions*. McGraw Hill Osborn, (pp 408 -412).

Mezgar, Ivan (2005). Building trust in virtual communities. In Dasgupta, Subhasish (Ed.), *Encyclopedia of Virtual Communities and Technologies*. George Washington University, USA.

Moon, Jane (2005). Discussing health issues on the Internet. In Dasgupta, Subhasish (Ed.), *Encyclopedia of Virtual Communities and Technologies*. George Washington University, USA.

Rada, Roy (2005). Cancer patient-patient online discussion groups. In Dasgupta, Subhasish (Ed.), *Encyclopedia of Virtual Communities and Technologies*. George Washington University, USA.

Radin, Patricia (2006). To me, it's my life: Medical communication, trust, and activism in cyberspace. *Social science and Medicine, 62*, 591-601.

Tygar, Doug (1998 August 24-27). "Atomicity versus anonymity: Distributed transactions for electronic commerce. In *Proceedings of 24 International Conference on Very Large Databases (VLDB)*. New York City

Varlamis, Iraklis & Apostolakis, Ioannis (2007 February 18-20). Self supportive Web communities in the service of patients. In *Proceedings of IADIS International Conference on Web Based Communities* 2007. Salamanca, Spain.

Varlamis, Iraklis & Apostolakis, Ioannis (2006). Use of virtual communities for the welfare of groups with particular needs. In *Proceedings of the 4th ICICTH International Conference on Information Communication Technologies in Health.*

KEY TERMS

Confidentiality, Integrity and Availability: Medical data is confidential, must be accurate and available during all times and is protected by Data Protection Laws.

Eavesdropping: A malicious user is spying information exchanged between community members and collects useful information.

Healthcare Virtual Communities: Virtual communities comprising members from the healthcare domain. Members join the community in order to discuss health related subject, give or receive medical advice and support etc.

Intrusion Prevention System: A system which is able to block any suspicious traffic based on the characteristics of the received data and guarantees authorized access to the community information and services

Sensitive Personal Data: Data referring to a person, which cannot be revealed to anybody. In a health related virtual community, such data may refer to a person's health situation, nutritional restrictions, history of examinations and surgeries etc.

Trust: The most important factor for a long-living community. Trust can be deep, thick and swift depending on the strength of relation between community members.

Unauthorized Access: A malicious user manages to infiltrate the community site and gains access to all these data that the community needs to protect.

Chapter XXVI
Virtual Learning Environments in Health

Stamatia Ilioudi
University of Piraeus, Greece

Christina Ilioudi
University of Piraeus, Greece

Konstantinos Siassiakos
University of Piraeus, Greece

ABSTRACT

This chapter aims to present various virtual learning environments for medical purposes in the world. More than ever, medical students and healthcare professionals are faced to with floods of data of which the relevant information has to be selected and applied. The internet and the new media are a fertile ground to meet these requirements. More and more physicians unravel e-learning as new tool and as attractive adjunct to the traditional face-to-face teaching in medicine. This chapter describes the most important benefits for all parties of the simulation and learning environments in health sciences.

INTRODUCTION

Traditional training for health care providers follows a methodology of observation and repetition allowing the trainee to learn from those cases and situations presented within the short period of time a clinician attends school.

Simulation is a training and feedback technique in which learners practice tasks and processes under realistic settings and circumstances using tools and models, such as virtual reality, and utilizing feedback from observers, such as professors, peers, actor-patients, and video cameras.

Medical simulation improves patient safety, an a priori fact. Simulation technologies have a proven record in improving safety through decreased errors during technically challenging procedures, such as surgery and other interventions. Technical errors are reduced by improved training with a focus on error identification.

In addition to clinical skill development, simulation or training-based medical training provides realistic training in communication, leadership and team interaction and observation providing the student with the opportunity to repeat the materials until the student has mastered the information.

Distance education has emerged due to increased technological advances and the increased demands and responsibilities of learners. Historically, distance education was known as correspondence education, but is currently being replaced by a more electronic media (Schlais and Davis, 2001). Distance education programs primarily take place when facilitator and learner is separated by physical distance and therefore use different types of technology to deliver the subject content (Picciano, 2001). This makes learning interesting for both the facilitator and learner as the learners are given more responsibility as self-leaders to take initiative for the pace of their learning. As well, it allows the learners to think critically, preventing the facilitator to force them to learn. There is a focus on the needs of the learners as well as the requirements of the course. The needs of the learners involve their values and beliefs, as well as their available time. Assessing these needs will influence the development of curriculum and enrollment choices made by the learners.

As adult learners, health care staff will likely be involved in formalized forms of education throughout their lives that tends to be self-directed, independent and problem-based (Tight, 2002). A common model used for adult learning is an andragogical model which is based on the assumptions that adults need to know why they are learning something, that they have a self-concept of being responsible for their own lives, their experiences are a valuable resource, adults are ready to learn those things they need to know, adult learners are more motivated to learn as they bring their experiences to a relevant learning environment, and they are motivated by internal factors such as job satisfaction and self-efficacy (Knowles, 1984).

In the health care context, there is no question that the diffusion of Virtual Learning Environments (VLEs) has profoundly changed education and practice. Medical training on "real" patients is no longer acceptable (Gallagher & Cates, 2004) and there is an increasing demand for simulation-based medical education. Continuing advances in Virtual Reality (VR) technology and computer-based Simulations Devices, available at increasingly lowcost have opened new frontiers in teaching since the end of the 20th century.

Disparities in medical information and education are a major determinant of health practice inequities in developing communities. The recent diffusion of the internet is facilitating the creation and circulation of "new" VLEs in the health-care field, that overcome traditional boundaries of "space", "time", and "place". Yet, online learning environments bring along huge opportunities for learning and knowledge exchange among multiple users in remote areas of the world, but also new barriers.

The validity of the new internet mediated learning environments has still to be tested, especially for what concerns their ability to: (1) overcome "traditional boundaries" characterizing the learning experience and consequently change medical education and profession and (2) help educate patients and "health seekers".

DEFINITION OF A VIRTUAL LEARNING ENVIRONMENT

A virtual learning environment (VLE) is a set of teaching and learning tools designed to enhance a student's learning experience by including computers and the Internet in the learning process. The principal components of a VLE package include curriculum mapping (breaking curriculum into sections that can be assigned and assessed), student tracking, online support for both teacher and student, electronic communication (e-mail, threaded discussions, chat, Web publishing), and Internet links to outside curriculum resources. In general, VLE users are assigned either a teacher ID or a student ID. The teacher sees what a students sees, but the teacher has additional user rights to create or modify curriculum content and track student performance. There are a number of commercial VLE software packages available, including Blackboard, WebCT, Lotus LearningSpace, and COSE.

The terms virtual learning environment (VLE) and managed learning environment (MLE) are often interchanged.

VIRTUAL LEARNING ENVIRONMENTS IN HEALTH

One of the problems with e-learning is that medical students have to learn on their own without any interaction with teachers and other students. Interpersonal contact cannot be omitted by building virtual environment, because it is a crucial factor in training future physicians. That is why, only a blended learning model should be taken into the account, while discussing implementation of e-learning in graduate medical education. The term "blended learning" refers to the situation that combines a mix of on-line and face-to-face training. This approach allows using the best of e-learning (interactive multimedia presentations, online video transmission and simulations) together with important aspects of traditional training (gaining clinical experience by students).

Health professionals will need to develop the skills to use this technology in their clinical practice. Evidence suggests that consumers now have access to large amounts of unfiltered material via the Internet. Not only does this impact on the professional boundaries with consumers (Timmons, 2001), but adds further responsibility to the practitioner's role. Drucker (1994) argues that in the future anyone who wishes to be considered educated will be someone who has embraced the notion of lifelong learning. Nurses in the United Kingdom (UK) have a requirement to undertake educational activities to support their practice as part of the registration system. The ability to use a computer and effectively find and use the wealth of information that it enables access to, is a very useful tool in maintaining this lifelong commitment to education. information and technology (IT) skills being needed is becoming a universal truth for nurses and doctors working in many countries.

The National Health Service (NHS) was slow to develop IT as a strategic asset in the delivery of healthcare. However, national strategies have been developed since 1998 to address this situation. 'Information for Health' defined the strategic NHS approach when an information strategy was launched to improve use of information technology and provide staff with modern tools to improve treatment and care. It aims to improve management and delivery of services by provision of good quality data; support staff through effective electronic communications and support delivery of services designed around patients to be quicker, more convenient and seamless.

Online group discussions can potentially result in learning and change in practice because this active process allows integration of tacit and explicit knowledge. This has been increasingly recognised with the development of online networks or "communities", such as on the National Electronic Library for Health (NeLH), NHS University, and BMJ Learning websites. The potential of online networks for healthcare professionals will be realised only if barriers to online interaction can understood and overcome.

In 2003/4 the Information Management Research Institute, Northumbria University, conducted a research project to identify the barriers to e-learning for healthcare professionals and medical students. The project also established possible ways to overcome these barriers. The main barriers are: requirement for change; costs; poorly designed packages; inadequate technology; lack of skills; need for a component of face-to-face teaching; time intensive nature of e-learning; computer anxiety. A range of solutions can solve these barriers. The main solutions are: standardization; strategies; funding; integration of e-learning into the curriculum; blended teaching; user friendly packages; access to technology; skills training; support; employers paying e-learning costs; dedicated work time for e-learning.

Web 2.0 technologies such as wikis, podcasts and blogs could be quite effective tools in e-learning for health professionals in patients. The very interactivity of the technology could prove a boon for professional and patient education, providing that any changes and collaboration is effectively monitored, say researchers from the faculties of Education and Health and Social Work at the University of Plymouth. Interactivity with other students and learners could be beneficial for those unable to socialise in a normal learning environment. Active learning and feedback could also help to increase learning and retention.

A virtual learning environment (VLE) refers to the components in which learners and tutors participate in 'online' interactions of various kinds, including online learning. However, not all interactions have to be online since a Virtual Learning Environment can act as a focus for students' learning activities. Virtual Learning Environment software is currently being used across most UK health institutions to support a variety of different types of learning: for example, collaborative and co-operative, blended and distance learning. A virtual learning environment for medical purposes:

- Is web-based and accessible to both medical students and professors through a web browser on any computer connected to the Internet anywhere, any time;
- Organizes medical students into virtual classes, with individual, secure, logins;
- Comprises a range of integrated online tools that aims to support collaborative and co-operative student learning;
- Provides a focus for medical student learning activities;
- May support on-campus delivery (typically referred to as blended learning) or off-campus delivery (distance learning);
- Has a wide range of benefits for professors including improving the learning experience (through using the collaborative, communication and assessment tools) and assisting in course management and administration;
- Has the flexibility to support a range of learning scenarios but needs careful and thoughtful course design to ensure that the virtual learning environment is used to its fullest.

The Virtual Campus Rhineland-Palatinate (VCRP) is jointly held by the universities of applied sciences of Rhineland-Palatinate (http://www.vcrp.de). The VCRP (Efferth, 2002). does not comprehend itself as an independent university which claims substitution towards other universities. On the contrary, it aims to provide support for the implementation of new media into the universities. The VCRP pursues two directions of e-learning: (1) The support of teaching activities of universities is a main task and (2) the extension of teaching activities in the fields of continuing education. A further field of activities is the involvement of segments outside teaching activities in the fields of academic and students' self-administration.

A board of experts located at the Regional University Computing Center in Kaiserslautern is responsible for the maintenance of the technical platform of the VCRP. In the course of a public private partnership, Sun Microsystems sponsored a redundant server system to store and distribute net-based teaching contents of all universities of Rhineland-Palatinate. The locations of the universities are interconnected by an ATM-based net (rlp-net). A wireless local area network (W-LAN) is under construction. In 2002, the learning environment "WebCT" has been established at the VCRP to test this learning platform for providing learning contents and for performing administrative tasks with the aim to implement e-learning in existing syllabi and to create new study programs (Efferth, 2002).

Among other disciplines, the VCRP has a large number of medical online learning topics. The VCRP medical data base comprises more than 600 links to educational web pages out of 28 different medical areas. The students find virtual lectures and seminars, scripts, image collections, tutorials, animations and simulations, movie clips, search engines, virtual libraries, discussion platforms etc.

BENEFITS OF SIMULATION AND LEARNING ENVIRONMENTS IN HEALTH

Distance education using multimedia resources is a solution that will allow health care staff to enroll in continuing education sessions without adding stress to their current personal and work demands. It will allow them to participate in environments within their work setting. These types of learning environments can be successfully suited to meet the needs of adult health care learners using principles from the andragogical model and constructivist strategies together with their identified learning needs.

Simulation is an effective, efficient way to learn skills and teamwork behaviors. It is a way to provide consistency in training; objectivity in feedback and assessment; transparent, credible credentialing; a real-world evaluation of technologies and techniques under stressful conditions; and experience delivering services for the entire health care organization.

Simulation-based medical training provides better-trained health care providers, reduces medical errors, saves money, and improves the quality of patient care overall – all good reasons for using medical simulation.

Simulation can improve and provide:

- Safety;
- Efficiency in high-cost clinical settings;
- Optimal conditions for learning (learner-centered at the pace of individual);
- Objective and immediate feedback;
- Integration of multiple skills;
- Utility as an assessment tool; and
- Test-bed for research.

The e- learning and simulation-based medical training benefits all of us, as follows:

- Patients benefit from improved health outcomes and reduced errors and deaths.
- Patients with rare or unusual conditions benefit from better-trained providers.
- Patients and clinicians benefit by increasing the number of procedures and type of complex, risky procedures addressed and experienced during training.
- Consumers, patients, and families benefit from reduced health care costs and enhanced quality.
- Taxpayers benefit from tax dollars spent on equipment that can be tailored to different skill levels.
- Businesses benefit from the creation of high-tech jobs.
- Businesses benefit from greater worker productivity due to better health care.
- Physicians, nurses, and health professionals benefit from having better skills

- Society, health care systems, and physicians benefit from lower malpractice rates through demonstrated clinical competence.
- Health care organizations benefit from reduced adverse events.
- Insurers benefit from defending fewer malpractice claims.
- Students benefit from a flexible training curriculum that is tailored to their pace, learning comprehension, and schedule. Students have the opportunity to practice, make mistakes, and improve their skills and knowledge on the simulated patient without consequence to the patient.

CONCLUSION

Distance education using multimedia resources is a solution that will allow health care staff to enroll in continuing education sessions without adding stress to their current personal and work demands. It will allow them to participate in environments within their work setting. The aforementioned types of learning environments can be successfully suited to meet the needs of adult health care learners using principles from the andragogical model and constructivist strategies together with their identified learning needs. Change may be met with resistance when required to develop a competency plan, so simple and flexible solutions involving multimedia resources should be available to alert health care staff that continuing education will be relevant to their experiences and more importantly it will benefit their personal and professional growth.

REFERENCES

Badenoch D., Tomlin A. (2004). How electronic communication is changing health care: Usability is main barrier to effective electronic communication systems. *BMJ 2004, 328*, 1564-1566.

Coldwell, J., Wells, J. (2003). Students' perspective of online learning', In G. Davies & E. Stacey (Eds.), *Quality education @ a distance*. Norwell, MA: Kluwer Academic Publishers Group, (pp. 101-108).

Dawson, S. L., Kaufman, J. A. (1998). The Imperative for Medical Simulation. In *Proceedings of the IEEE,* 86/3, pp. 479-483.

Drucker, P. (1994) The age of social transformation. *The Atlantic Monthly*, (Nov), pp. 53–80.

Efferth, T. (2002). E-learning in medicine at the virtual campus rhineland-palatinate. In *Proceedings of the 7th International Conference on the Medical Aspects of Telemedicine.* Regensburg, Germany.

Giardina, M. (1992). Interactivity and intelligent advisory strategies in a multimedia learning environment: Human factors, design issues and technical considerations. In M. Giardina (Ed.), *Interactive multimedia learning environments,* New York: Springer -Verlag, (pp. 48-66).

Glowniak, J. V. (1995). Medical resources on the Internet. *Ann Intern Med., 123*, 123-31.

Harrington, J. J. (1993). *IEEE P1157 MEDIX: A standard for open systems medical data interchange.* Institute of Electrical and Electronic Engineers, New York City, NY

Ilioudi, S., Lazakidou, A. (2007). Principles and effects of electronic communication systems between healthcare providers and managed care organizations. *International Journal of Electronic Healthcare*, ISSN (Online): 1741-8461, ISSN (Print): 1741-8453, Vol. 3, Nr. 4, pp. 468-478.

Jadar, A. R., Delamothe, T. (2004). What next for electronic communication and health care? *BMJ 2004, 328,* 1143-1144.

Katz, S. and Moyer, C. (2004). The emerging role of online communication between patients and their providers. *Journal of General Internal Medicine*, *19*(9), 978–983.

Knowles, M. (1984). *The adult learner: A neglected species*. Houston, TX: Gulf Publishing Company.

Lazakidou-Kafetzi, G., Lazakidou, A., Siassiakos, K. (2008). Computer supported collaborative work systems and communication services in health. *International Journal of Healthcare Technology and Management, Special Issue: Learning Environments in Health Sciences*, ISSN (Online): 1741-5144, ISSN (Print): 1368-2156, Vol. 9, Nr. 2, 2008.

Lowery, Julie C. (1998). 'Introduction to simulation in health care. In *Proceedings of the Winter Simulation Conference*, J. M. Charnes, D. M. Morrice, D.T. Brunner, and J. J. Swain, (Eds.). IEEE, Piscataway. New Jersey, (pp. 78-83).

Lehner, F. and Nosekabel, H. (2002). The role of mobile devices in e-learning -first experience with a e-learning environment. In M. Milrad, H. U. Hoppe and Kinshuk (Eds.). *IEEE International Workshop on Wireless and Mobile Technologies in Education*, Los Alamitos, USA, (pp. 103-106).

Madiope, M. (2004). Web-based instruction for critical care nursing science: Lessons learned. In *Proceedings of the World Conference on E-Learning in Corporate, Government, Healthcare, & Higher Education 2004, 1*, (pp. 814-818).

O'Toole, R. V., Playter, R. R., Krummel, T. M., Blank, W. C., Cornelius, N. H., Roberts, W. R., Bell, W. J., Raibert, M. (1999). Measuring and developing suturing technique with a virtual reality surgical simulator. *Journal of the American College of Surgeons*, 189/1, 114-127.

Picciano, A.G. (2001). *Distance learning: Making connections across virtual space and time*. Columbus, Ohio: Merrill Prentice Hall.

Rhodes, R. S., Biesten, T. W., Ritchie Jr., W. P., Malangoni, M. A. (2003). Continuing medical education activity and american board of surgery examination performance. *Journal of the American College of Surgeons*, 196/4, pp. 604-609.

Siassiakos, K., Ilioudi, S., Lazakidou, A. (2008). Simulation and learning environments in health care. *International Journal of Healthcare Technology and Management*, ISSN (Online): 1741-5144, ISSN (Print): 1368-2156, Vol. 9, Nr. 2, 2008.

Schlais, D., & Davis, R. (2001). 'Distance learning through educational networks: The global view experience. In J. Stephenson (Ed.), *Teaching & learning online: Pedagogies for new technologies*. Sterling, VA: Stylus Publishing Inc., (pp. 112-126).

Tight, M. (2002). *'Key concepts in adult education and training*. New York: RoutledgeFalmer.

Timmons, S. (2001). Use of Internet by patients: Not a threat but an opportunity?', *Nurse Education Today, 21*(2), 104–109.

Youngblood, P., Parvati, D. (2005). A framework for evaluating new learning technologies in medicine. *AMIA Annu Symp Proc. 2005*, (pp. 1163).

KEY TERMS

Collaborative Virtual Environments (CVEs): CVEs are used to construct a virtual world where users can interact with one another and the environment in which they preside in order to perform, for example, a training exercise.

Distributed Collaboration: VR has been employed to allow geographically distributed people to do more than simply hear and see each other. For instance, VR technology is being used to develop highly interactive shared virtual environments, graphically orientated, for local and distance training and learning.

Simulation: A simulation is an imitation of some real thing, state of affairs, or process. The act of simulating something generally entails representing certain key characteristics or behaviours of a selected physical or abstract system.

Virtual Learning Environment: A VLE refers to the components in which learners and tutors participate in 'online' interactions of various kinds, including online learning.

Chapter XXVII
Multimedia Distance Learning Solutions for Surgery

Jelena Vucetic
Alpha Mission, Inc., USA

ABSTRACT

In the last decade, advances in medicine, telemedicine, computer technologies, information systems, Web applications, robotics and telecommunications have enabled creation of new solutions for training and continued education in various medical disciplines. This chapter presents most recent developments and future trends in distance learning for surgeons, focusing on the following goals: a) Building a comprehensive, world-wide, virtual knowledge base for various disciplines of surgery and telesurgery, including text documents, videos, case studies, expert surgeons' opinions, and relevant references; b) Building a virtual knowledge base for rare medical cases, conditions and recommended procedures; c) Interactive multimedia simulators for hands-on training in all surgical disciplines; d) Building a worldwide surgical community, which will accelerate the accumulation and sharing of the latest surgical breakthroughs and technological advances throughout the world. Above all these goals, the most important goal is to improve patient health and convenience, and reduce risks of mortality and complications.

INTRODUCTION

According to the U.S. Bureau of Labor and Statistics (http://stats.bls.gov/oco/ocos074.htm), employment of physicians and surgeons will increase annually 10% - 20% through the year 2012 because of the expansion of the health care industry. The growing and aging population will drive overall growth in the demand for medical services. Therefore, the demand for surgeons is expected to be favorable, although highly sensitive to changes in consumer preferences, healthcare reimbursement policies, and legislation. Reports of shortages in some surgical disciplines or geographic areas should attract new entrants (surgeons), encouraging schools to expand their programs and hospitals to expand available residency slots. On the other side, new entrants may be discouraged by demand for the long-term commitment and high expenses of surgical education and training. To become a surgeon, it takes 4 years of undergraduate school, 4 years of medical school, and 3 to 8 years of internship and residency.

Surgical training requires close supervision and evaluation. Technical competence of surgical learners is evaluated by the mentor and has always been subjective (Otta, 2005). Typically, qualitative rather than quantitative evaluations are performed in traditional surgical training.

Based on the most recent trends in surgery, distance learning represents a very attractive medium for training of new as well as continuing medical education (CME) for seasoned surgeons in:

- **Traditional Surgical Procedures:** Traditional surgery typically involves 20 to 80 cm long incisions into a patient's body in order to examine or treat a certain organ or tissue (Otta, 2005).
- **Laparoscopy Procedures:** Laparoscopy (minimal invasive surgery) is a relatively new surgical technique that enables major abdominal procedures with only four to five 1 cm long incisions into the patient's abdomen. The surgeon passes the video imaging scopes and surgical instruments into the abdominal cavity and completes the procedure while monitoring the operation on a display. The advantages of laparoscopy include: a) less postoperative pain, b) earlier patient's recovery and hospital discharge, c) reduced costs, d) earlier return to work or normal activity, and e) fewer complications (Otta, 2005).
- **Robotic Telesurgery:** In 2001, the first telesurgical operation (called the "Lindbergh Operation") was performed at a distance of 4,000 miles by a surgeon in New York, USA on a patient in Strasbourg, France. Using a satellite link to control remotely a surgical robot, the surgeon successfully removed the patient's gallbladder. This first telesurgery operation has demonstrated an enormous potential to expand the availability of surgical expertise to patients worldwide. On the other side, it has also clearly indicated that telesurgical technology needed to be improved with respect to tactile feedback, instrumentation, telecommunication speed and availability (Eadie, L. H., Seifalian, A.M., Davidson, B.R, 2003). In addition, new challenges in telesurgery have been discovered in the domains of education, liability, legislation, health insurance, and costs.

Laparoscopy and robotic telesurgery require skills that are very different from the skills required in traditional surgical procedures. Surgeons accustomed to using the sense of touch have to learn to perform surgery using a video monitor instead of direct vision, how to compensate for reduced depth perception, and how to distinguish nearly identical-looking objects.

INFORMATION TECHNOLOGY IN SURGICAL EDUCATION

Information technology has become a critical component of initial and continuing medical education (CME) as well as daily surgeons' practice. According to a survey done by American College of Physicians (2004), approximately 20% of physicians use computers for education. 41% of them prefer electronic formats (primarily, the Internet), 32% non-electronic, and 27% rated

Table 1.

Year	1998	1999	2000	2001	2002	2003
Physicians	37,879	79,556	181,922	230,055	329,110	577,903

them the same. Electronic educational formats are preferred among physicians younger than 40.

Although live meetings and courses still dominate CME, online education continues to grow in popularity. Traditional face-to-face courses and conferences accounted for 76% of the CME activities presented by the American Surgical Association (ACCME) accredited providers in 2003, which is a decrease from 82% in 2002. Internet CME accounted for 12.5% in 2003, an increase of 92% since 2002. Table 1 presents the number of physicians who have participated in Internet-based CME since 1998.

Online learning has changed medical education. The Internet has become an important force in how surgeons acquire knowledge, hands-on experience, and deliver care. A shift to increased use of online learning points to new demands for learners and providers. *Practice-based learning and improvement (PBLI)* has become increasingly important for surgery, and education providers need to introduce online tools for hands-on training and development of practical surgical skills into their programs.

The key steps in developing an effective surgical education Web site are (Cook and Dupras, 2004):

- Perform a needs analysis and specify goals and objectives;
- Determine technical resources and requirements;
- Evaluate and use preexisting technologies;
- Secure commitment from all stakeholders;
- Identify and address potential barriers to implementation;
- Develop the course content and design the Web site combining multimedia, simulation, hyperlinks, and online communication;
- Encourage active learning (self-assessment, reflection, self–directed learning, problem-based learning, learner interaction, and feedback);
- Evaluate learners and courses;
- Pilot the Web site before full implementation;
- Monitor and maintain the Web site by resolving technical problems, and regularly updating content.

DISTANCE LEARNING SOLUTIONS FOR SURGEONS

Effective surgery education in a distance learning environment combines: 1) Virtual-reality simulators that represent real-time, step-by-step execution of various surgical procedures; 2) Broadband distance learning infrastructure that enables remote access to the learning environment.

VIRTUAL-REALITY SIMULATORS

According to the relatively recent research conducted by Yale University and Queen's University Belfast (2002), surgeons who trained on computer simulators (on the Procedicus (r) MIST system) performed the operation 29% faster and made seven times fewer errors. This research has also shown that all the participating surgeons, the beginners and even those with more than seven years experience, demonstrated a "significantly improved" performance with the added experience of training on the virtual reality simulator. The conclusion of this research was that surgical simulators could be used both for initial training of new surgeons, and in CME programs for experienced surgeons, similar to the use of flight simulators for new and experienced airline pilots (to develop and/or maintain their flying skills).

Virtual-reality surgical simulators provide numerous advantages over the traditional surgical education, as follows:

- No risk or inconvenience (pain, injury, side effects, etc.) to the patient, because no patient is involved in simulation.
- Simulation can be repeated unlimited number of times, any time and anywhere. The marginal increase of education costs with the increased simulation (training) time is negligible, as compared to the costs of the equivalent increase of the equivalent, traditional surgical training time.
- The overhead (in terms of time and resources) is minimal, since the learner does not need to wait for the operating room, for specific patients, specimens or instruments. In addition, the learner does not need to waste any time on the preparation procedures that are unavoidable in a real operating room environment.
- In simulation, the learner can gain experience in treating very rare and complex cases, while in traditional surgical education it may not be possible at all due to the low probability that such cases will be available at that time.
- Simulation environment is very similar to laparoscopy procedures, which provides the learner with hands-on experience in monitoring the operation on the screen, and controlling the manipulation of each surgical instrument that is positioned within the patient's body.
- Simulation-based surgical education programs may provide more uniform curricula, while at the same time the learners will gain hands-on experience with a very broad scope of medical cases and procedures.

Using virtual-reality simulation in surgical education, the following objectives can be achieved:

- **Accurate examination of specified medical cases/pathologies:** The learner's performance should be evaluated based on the accuracy of the diagnosis for the examined case, the preciseness of the learner's dexterity with instruments and the timeliness of the examination. Any "tissue damage" (in the simulated surgical environment) or other wrong or imprecise instrument manipulation should reduce the overall performance score.
- **Mastery of the specified surgical techniques or procedures:** The learner's performance should be evaluated using a checklist that includes all steps in the specified surgical technique or procedure, and the "weighted" scores associated with each step. A weight should be assigned to each step according to the importance of the step for the overall technique or procedure.
- **Automated, virtual-reality feedback to the learner:** Similar to traditional tests, where a learner can see the correct test results upon his/her taking the test, the learner using a virtual-reality simulator should be able to review how well he/she has performed the specified task (examination, technique or procedure), and what elements have been done incorrectly or not done at all. The simulator should also provide a review of the correct way to perform the specified task, and notify the learner whether he/she has completed the procedure in a timely manner.
- **Progress report:** The learner should be able to review his/her progress report for each

simulation attempt, with a comparison to previous attempts, as well as with comparison to other learners in the program. Based on these progress reports, a comprehensive learner history log is created and updated automatically with each simulation attempt. This log should contain the number of successful attempts of specific surgical tasks, the number of hours spent in simulation training, and the most recent training date and time.

A virtual-reality surgical simulation system integrates:

- A high-resolution 3D graphics computer with a real-time visual simulation program (combining complex modeling systems and algorithms) – The learner can select different surgical procedures that he/she wants to practice from a remote location, while the simulator "leads" the learner through various scenarios that may occur during a surgery based on the decisions and actions that the learner makes throughout the process.
- Input peripherals to control the simulation – Similar to the corresponding real operating room scenario, the learner at a remote location uses specific surgical instruments and virtual-reality devices that serve as input peripherals to control the simulated surgical procedure.
- Output peripherals to display the outcomes of the simulation (based on advanced, high-resolution 3D computer graphics technologies) – Like in the corresponding real operating room scenario, the learner at a remote location monitors on the display the appearance and reactions of the simulated "patient's" body or a specific organ to the decisions and actions that the learner makes during the simulated surgical procedure.

Modeling Systems and Algorithms

A critical component of surgical simulators is the surgeon's perception of the patient on the operating table. In general, surgical simulators should include:

- Three-dimensional (3D) models of all human organs, displayed in the size and shape that corresponds to a specified patient's body measures;
- A 3D model of the overall human body, displayed in the size and shape that corresponds to a specified patient's body measures;
- Algorithms and programs that enable different presentations of human organs (from different angles, from inside or outside, with a different level of detail, etc.);
- Algorithms and programs that model the real-life reactions of organs to the interventions by various surgical instruments

Real-time, elastically deformable virtual organs and soft tissue [4, 6] represent a basis for haptic (tactile) surgical simulators. Although many techniques have been proposed for deformable object animation (Suzy, 1997), so far only few have provided the performance necessary for real-time applications. For example, still in research is an eye simulator (Webster, 2002), which runs on a Windows XP workstation with a 1.0 GHz Pentium processor (or higher) and an OpenGL graphics accelerator (e.g. Nvidia Geforce). The simulator reads the learner's motions with instruments on the simulated "eye" model, modifies the shape and the reactions of the model accordingly, sends the updated graphical presentation of the eye to the display, and at the same time collects various metrics (learner's name, updated number of simulation attempts, time spent on the specified surgical procedure, instrument movements, tissue tears, and severe tear errors).

Surgical Instruments and Virtual-Reality Devices

In order to control the simulation, surgical instruments and motion-tracking "virtual gloves" (5DT DataGlove) are used as an input system by surgeons in training (Haluck, 2002). This system records laparoscopic motions of the surgeon for learning and evaluation of his/her surgical skills.

Computer Graphics Technologies

Surgical simulators rely heavily on realistic 3D imagery representing the patient's organ or tissue being "treated" in virtual reality by the learner. Most recent surgical simulators (Webster, 2005) were developed using MUopenGL toolkit (an object-oriented applications programming interface that calls OpenGL graphics library), running on a dual Pentium processor workstation with an Nvidia OpenGL graphics accelerator and Windows XP operating system.

BROADBAND DISTANCE LEARNING INFRASTRUCTURE

For successful implementation of surgical distance-learning programs, several critical requirements need to be fulfilled:

- **Broadband Internet access to all learners:** The majority of applications require interactive, multimedia content to be transferred between each learner and the university's distance learning servers. The minimum data rate should be 384 Kbps.
- **University local area network (LAN):** A 100BASE-T Ethernet is recommended assuming combined voice, text, graphics and video data transfer among a large number of workstations. This LAN would ensure net data rates of up to 10 MBps
- **Large database systems:** In general, multimedia applications demand very large (order of several GBytes) memory space. In simulation-based surgical education, the resolution of the graphical content needs to be relatively high (640 x 480 x 24-bit, or at least 320 x 240 x 24-bit) in order to ensure the accuracy of the surgical training.

Figure 1 (Vucetic, 2005) represents a distance learning infrastructure for surgical education that includes a Distance Learning (DL) University and numerous remote learners. Learners are connected with DL University via broadband Internet links.

The following functional units are located in the DL University:

Figure 1. Distance learning infrastructure for surgical education

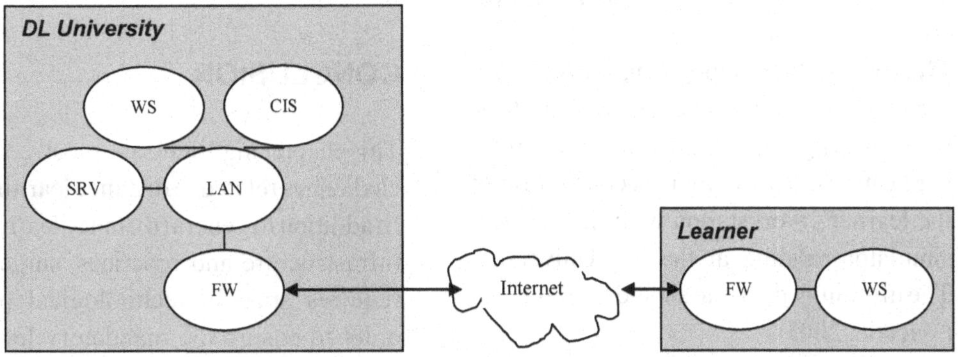

- **Central information system (CIS):** The information system that is used by the university for storage of various categories of records related to learners, employees, etc.
- **Local area network (LAN):** Combined voice, text, graphics and video transfers may vary from 1 MB to 100 MB. In a large DL University configuration, a 100BASE-T Ethernet is recommended to ensure net data rates of up to 10 MBps.
- **Servers/Firewall (SRV/FW):** Supporting the high-speed network infrastructure, Internet, Intranet, email hosting, file sharing, Web services, information security, load balancing, clustering, CIS interface and applications, messaging/groupware, high-performance applications (surgical simulators), extensive I/O, and a high memory throughput.
- **Workstations (WS):** General-purpose computers, such as a 3.60GHz 1MB L3 Cache Intel Pentium 4, with Windows XP or Vista Pro operating system.

The following functional units should be located at the learner's side:

- **Workstation (WS):** The WS integrates virtual-reality peripheral devices that collect the learner's hands' manipulation information, with a general-purpose computer (e.g. a 2.13 GHz Intel Pentium M 770 PC, with Windows XP or Vista Pro operating system).
- **Firewall (FW):** Supporting information security, the client side of web applications, workgroup email and workgroup applications. It also provides connection of the learner's workstation with the surgical simulator residing at the DL University. The minimum data rate should be 384 Kbps (Vucetic, 2005).

VIRTUAL SURGICAL UNIVERSITIES

In the last decade, numerous schools of medicine have introduced surgical tutorials, tests and case studies in an electronic form, either on the Internet or on CDs. However, only in the last couple of years have some surgical education programs started to use virtual-reality simulation of various surgical procedures.

One of the leaders in online laparoscopy training is WebSurg (http://www.websurg.com/), a virtual surgical university accessible from anywhere in the world through the Internet. The WebSurg project was launched at the European Institute of TeleSurgery (EITS) in Strasbourg, France, in collaboration with University of Virginia. The goal of this project is to provide online training in laparoscopic surgery worldwide, including diagnosis, standards of pre- and post-operative patient care, and practical surgical procedures.

Millersville and Penn State Universities have teamed up to develop a software suite for training and testing of surgical skills using a virtual reality surgical simulator with a sensitive touch (haptic) feedback and realistic 3D imagery.

University of California has also developed a virtual surgical simulator for training perceptual motor skills, spatial skills, and critical steps of surgical procedures, with the goal to eliminate laparoscopy-caused injuries that presently occur at a relatively high rate (2.2%) if procedures are performed by inexperienced laparoscopic surgeons.

CONCLUSION

This chapter highlights the most recent trends and challenges related to distance learning of surgery. In addition to general distance learning concepts, infrastructure and practices, surgery education requires specific technological provisions in order to ensure the mandatory level of quality. These provisions include: a) a broadband Internet access; b) a diverse set of simulators for various surgical disciplines (e.g. abdominal, endocrine, aortoiliac, urological surgery); c) high-resolution, 3D workstations with large memory space and high processing power; d) virtual-reality input peripherals; e) a comprehensive feedback and skills evaluation system.

So far, virtual reality surgical simulators have not been widely used in schools of medicine, but it is only a matter of time when they will be adopted as effective practical training tools for surgeons. After using these simulators in training, surgeons will be more efficient, accurate and thorough when operating on real patients. In addition, they will make less mistakes and injuries to the patients, and the overall examination time will be shorter.

Future trends in the area of distance learning programs for surgery include:

- Integration of individual, specialized research projects into a comprehensive, world-wide, virtual knowledge base for various areas of surgery and telesurgery, consisting of virtual-reality simulators, text documents, videos, case studies, expert surgeons' opinions, and relevant references. For example, a learner may decide to attend an online course in Emergency Surgery, where a suite of online, virtual-reality simulators will be available to practice the following procedures: peritonitis, appendectomy, small bowel obstruction and perforated ulcer.
- Building a comprehensive virtual knowledge base for rare medical cases collected around the world, along with recommended surgical procedures – Among major advantages of simulators in general is their ability to generate rare scenarios and cases of the simulated phenomenon or process. Likewise, surgical simulators will enable learners to practice unlimited number of times certain rare procedures and scenarios that they may never have a chance to do in traditional training, in a real operating room.
- Further technological advances in the area of virtual-reality simulators for hands-on training in all surgical fields – Current technological efforts are focused on increase in the processing power, increase in memory space and efficient access to critical data, improvement in algorithms for 3D manipulation, deformable object modeling and evaluation of surgical procedures performed on the simulator.
- Building a worldwide surgical community, which will accelerate the accumulation and sharing of the latest surgical breakthroughs and technological advances throughout the world.

REFERENCES

Accreditation Council for Continuing Medical Education (2003). *ACCME annual report data.* Retrieved from: http://www.accme.org

American College of Physicians Research Center (2004). *Member survey: Report of findings.* October 2004.

Cook, D.A., Dupras, D.M.. (2004). A practical guide to developing effective Web-based learning. *Journal of General Internal Medicine,19*, 698-707. Retrieved from: http://www.blackwell-synergy.com

Eadie, L. H., Seifalian, A.M., Davidson, B.R., (2003). Telemedicine in surgery. *British Journal of Surgery Society Ltd, 90*(6), 647-658.

Haluck, R. et al., (2002). Reliability and validity of endotower, a virtual reality trainer for angled endoscope navigation. In J.D. Westwood et al. (Eds.), *Medicine meets virtual reality.* IOS Press

Otta, D. et al. (2005). *Virtual reality in surgical education, division of surgical oncology.* University of Missouri. Retrieved from http://www.vmasc.odu.edu

Payandeh, et al. (2004). *On defining metrics for assessing laparoscopic surgical skills in a virtual training environment.* Simon Fraser University

Revolutionary Research on Virtual Surgery (2002). *Innovations Report, Forum for Science, Industry and Business.*

Suzy, A., (1997). A survey of deformable modeling in computer graphics. *MERL Technical Report* TR-97-19, November 1997

Vucetic, J. (2005). *Technological and business challenges and solutions for a successful emergency telemedicine venture*, IPSI-2005. MIT, Cambridge, MA

Webster, R. et al., (2005). Millersville University's research in haptic and surgical simulation. *A Joint Research Project in Surgical Simulation with the Penn State University College of Medicine.* Millersville University

Webster, R., Haluck, R., Mohler, B., Ravenscroft, B., Crouthamel, E., Frack, T., Terlecki, S., Sheaffer, J., (2002). Elastically deformable 3D organs for haptic surgical simulators. In *Proceedings of the Medicine Meets Virtual Reality Conference, MMVR '2002.* Newport Beach, CA, IOS Press, (pp 570-572).

KEY TERMS

Broadband Internet: A high data transmission rate Internet access, which ensures at least 200 kbit/s in one direction according to the FCC standard.

Haptic Simulators: Simulators in which the interface to the user is applied through touch, motion or vibration. Haptic feedback is the reactive force applied by the interface in response to the user's active, tactile force or pressure.

Laparoscopy (Minimal Invasive Surgery): A relatively new surgical technique that enables major abdominal procedures with only four to five 1 cm long incisions into the patient's abdomen. The surgeon passes the video imaging scopes and surgical instruments into the abdominal cavity, and completes the procedure while monitoring the operation on a display.

Practice-Based Learning and Improvement (PBLI): An educational approach in which a physician monitors, analyzes and improves his or her own practice behaviors, as well as keep up with advances in relevant medical disciplines. For monitoring and analysis, physicians typically use logs, critical incident journals, and charts. Physicians continue to learn and advance their practical skills and behaviors through recognition of their earlier mistakes, additional exercises of the particular skills that need improvement, and seeking feedback about performance.

Telemedicine: Delivery of clinical medical services at a distance using advanced telecommunications, robotic and computer technology and their applications.

Telesurgery: Surgical procedures carried out at a distance using advanced telecommunications, robotic and computer technology and their applications.

Virtual Reality: A technology that enables the user to interact with a computer-simulated environment implemented in the form of visual, haptic, sensory, and audio experiences.

Chapter XXVIII
Collaborative Virtual Environments and Multimedia Communication Technologies in Healthcare

Maria Andréia F. Rodrigues
Universidade de Fortaleza, Brazil

Raimir Holanda Filho
Universidade de Fortaleza, Brazil

ABSTRACT

This chapter shows how recent computing technologies such as collaborative virtual environments, high speed networks and mobile devices can be used for training and learning in healthcare providing an environment with security and quality of service. A number of studies have been conducted so far in these research areas. However, the development of integrated care has proven to be a difficult task. Therefore, we aim also to discuss the promising directions of the current work and growing importance on these subjects. This includes comparative analysis of the most relevant computer systems and applications developed so far that integrate modern computing technologies and health care. We believe this work is considered to be primarily for the benefit of those who are working in the field of computer science and health care, as well academic community, practitioners, and those involved in the development, implementation and study of integrated care using new computing technologies.

INTRODUCTION

In this chapter, we investigate how recent computing technologies such as collaborative virtual environments (CVEs), high speed networks and mobile devices can be used for training and learning in healthcare providing an environment with security and quality of service (QoS).

In our view, there is a considerable gap between the promises that the new computing technologies hold, and the expectations that they cause in the medical area, particularly, in the simulation and training of surgical procedures. The evidences indicate that these expectations should be fulfilled in the next few years. This partnership will require the improvement of several computational technologies (storage devices, high-speed networks, distributed systems for mobile environments, etc), as well as changes in the background of health professionals before their routine adoption. New areas of interdisciplinary research can emerge, such as multimedia surgical support, interventional radiology, and even less invasive surgical procedures. The development of system architectures utilizing new computing technologies that support interactive computer graphics and CVEs is another growing necessity. Examples are computer systems developed to support virtual training and learning, which are becoming more and more realistic (Blezek et al., 2000; Hosseini & Geordanas, 2001; Dev et al., 2002; Gunn et al., 2005a; DiMaio & Salcudean, 2005; Lee et al., 2006; Rodrigues et al., 2007). Some of these systems are used to construct a virtual world where users (trainer and trainees) can interact with one another and the environment in which they preside when performing training exercises.

Nowadays, geographically distributed computing technologies can be interconnected to create an integrated computing environment. Healthcare professionals in different places can collaborate using this environment. Collaborative virtual environments involve several participants working in a network, using a shared virtual environment to analyze the same object from different points of view, and in which the action of any participant is viewed by all others sharing the environment. In order to make communications more realistic the environment must supply voice, video and data multimedia applications. This will favor comprehension of the actual intent of each participant, thus improving the collaborative environment.

Networked computers and corresponding applications facilitate collaboration activities through a constellation of various tools (such as shared spaces, whiteboards, etc) having appropriate approaches to collaboration and social interactions. A World Wide Web tem proporcionado uma plataforma comum para que pessoas em qualquer parte do mundo possam interagir. Com o incremento do uso de dispositivos móveis, abre-se um vasto campo para novas pesquisas especialmente nas áreas de redes sem fio e colaboração distribuída. O aumento da disponibilidade de facilidades de comunicação tem provocado uma mudança no conceito de utilização de inúmeras aplicações, uma vez que dispositivos móveis possuem um comportamento diferente e oferecem possibilidades de interação diferentes, dependendo do contexto em que a aplicação está sendo usada. Para analisar estes diferentes cenários, muito esforço tem sido direcionado em pesquisas para mitigar possíveis ataques e para prover padrões mínimos de qualidade de serviço.

The World Wide Web has provided a collective platform where people in any part of the globe can interact. The increasing number of mobile devices in use has opened a vast field for new research, especially in the areas of wireless networks and distributed collaboration. The increase in availability of communications facilities has brought about changes in the concept of use of many applications, considering that mobile devices have a different behavior and offer different possibilities of interaction, depending on the context in which the application is being used. In order to analyze these different settings, a lot of effort has been directed to researches in mitigating possible attacks, and providing minimum standards of QoS.

Our discussion will also focus on recent wireless network technologies (Sharma & Nakamura, 2004) and mobility facilities (Pesch et al., 2007) that are highly recommended for the development of CVEs. One of the benefits of wireless data communication is the possibility of exchanging real-time messages among patients and medical staff. Wireless handhelds are becoming simple, direct and efficient communication paths with great potential for facilitating the access and flow of information. These new computing technologies are also important to be taken into account to provide better working conditions in the health area.

Finally, as consequence of the use of patient data, further attention is important to provide a secure network environment, specifically in the cases where wireless connections are used. In this scenario, authentication, authorization and cryptography procedures (Stallings, 2005) are mandatory to mitigate unauthorized users to get access to information, and to hinder data capture in promiscuous mode. Another relevant topic is to supply a network environment with minimum QoS guarantees for voice and video traffic (Ash, 2006). In this case, some network parameters such as delay and jitter are very important to assure QoS. Moreover, the traffic of huge image files should also be controlled in order not to affect real-time traffic classes.

Hence, the key to achieving all these requirements on current technology is to pay more attention to applications that aim at assisting in bridging the gap between theoretical workers in the medical field and those scientists involved in handling and simulating true life problems. In so doing, the former should be able to better identify the objective towards which future developments should be directed, and the latter will be provided with an insight of the possibilities and limitations of existing theoretical work. Our utmost interest is then to investigate the extent to which present computer technologies can contribute to training and learning in healthcare.

CVES IN HEALTHCARE

Although no attempt was made to be comprehensive, we have investigated the CVEs developed so far for training and learning in healthcare.

Many researchers have reported that Virtual Reality (VR) technology has proved to be an invaluable approach in Computer Graphics to represent real life problems within an interactive three-dimensional representation of an environment. Based upon these grounds, we can consider that VR technology is increasingly becoming an important component for simulation in surgical training, although it brings with it educational issues and practical implications. Further, qualitative findings reported in the literature, present that simulators can provide safe, realistic learning environments for repeated practice, underpinned by feedback and objective metrics of performance (Kneebone, 2003).

Some researchers have concentrated on the development of CVEs that have proved beneficial when groups or individuals need to share visual (graphics) or textual information. The most representative simulation-oriented learning environments support interaction, collaboration, and active learning. In general, the topics of training and learning are anatomy and basic surgical manipulations which involve a visual-haptic-audio experience. According to Dev et al. (2002), "while books, lectures, and multimedia are important routes to learning, the acts of touching, feeling, and cutting are believed to be essential in the training of surgeons". Therefore, simulated environments that deliver this experience with simultaneous viewing of the virtual world by all users are expected to form the next generation of technology-enhanced training and learning environments.

In some CVEs, haptic feedback devices are also used to improve the perceived virtual presence in these environments. In fact, they have been useful in building realistic computer based training systems in which users interact with virtual objects. In these systems, Web-based technology can be used to set the model parameters and run the simulation on a remote machine, while visualizing results on a low cost local machine. A library of objects, such as patients and medical devices, can then be created, and used to provide the component parts for a variety of virtual environments (VEs) that may be shared, simulated, analyzed, touched, and visualized by the virtual world of trainee and instructor.

In the last few years, implementation of shared virtual environments has been particularly active. As a result, distributed, multi-user simulations have been implemented, which generally allow the interactions of users with the virtual scenario by clicking on objects to carry out functions to reproduce typical tasks and conditions commonly available in a physical training environment (e.g., a surgical) or educational environment (e.g., a classroom). These actions can be shared and transmitted through the Internet to other participants to have the impression of being involved in a training exercise. One example is the work presented in (Gunn et al., 2005b).

Essentially, the main focus in implementing shared VEs that use haptic devices is to reduce delay in processing force information. Actually, touch is central in expertise in surgery. During surgery procedures, the surgeon should have the feeling in his hands of directly holding the medical instruments interacting with the patient. In addition, the integration of VR technologies and experiences with VR-based approaches for clinical assessment, treatment and rehabilitation offers powerful options that could revolutionize standard practices in these fields (Rose et al., 2005; Rizzo et al., 2006). There is a series of studies involving haptic devices which can display virtual textures, which are useful to perceive objects (tactile sensing). The haptic devices have potential for simulating real world objects and helping in the navigation of VEs, mainly for simulating minimally invasive procedures (to operate remotely and interactively) and assisting people with disabilities. The great importance of minimally invasive surgery resides in the fact that it has revolutionized many surgical procedures over the last few decades (Basdogan et al., 2004). One of the most important aspects of surgical simulation is to provide the user with estimated reaction forces that arise from surgical instrument and soft tissue interactions.

The advantages of using VR in the medical area through simulations (that could replace the process of building physical mock-ups of functional environments needed for human performance testing, training, and learning) have already been recognized by many research groups. These joint efforts point to a promising future for CVEs. As the field of VR matures, our expectations are indeed that CVEs can deliver substantial benefits to the healthcare area.

MOBILITY

CVEs in healthcare increase the needs for privacy of data. This is tightly linked to security. If data about patients are to be processed, the level of security should match the sensibility of the data with personal information (e.g. address, phone number etc.) calling for lower security, and secret information (like names, exams, test results, etc) requiring highest security and more access restrictions. Enhanced privacy and security furthermore result in added trust in the system. This should in turn increase usage and acceptance, whereas low security will almost certainly have detrimental effects.

Hence, the system needs to be secure. The necessity and the level of security depend on the data processed. Patient images and other medical content could be secured in a way that only authorized users (health staff) have access to them. This might be desirable from a medical point of view when the documents should not be widely distributed, for example, because they contain confidential information.

Recently, security concerns have been emphasized due to mobility issues, and due to access through wireless networks. Introduction of these new technologies have associated greater difficulties to these kinds of communications, demanding mechanisms, for example, to prevent attacks.

In order to provide mobility, wireless network technologies have expanded rapidly in the past few years, becoming accessible to the ordinary user, which may revolutionize the computing and learning environments. This concept affords the emergence of numerous possibilities, like the development of real-time, distributed collaborative applications in mobile devices.

The concept of mobility in CVEs is not entirely new. For example, a system was proposed in Satchel (Lamming et al., 2000) to provide access to any document, at any time from anywhere. Although this is not a Mobile-CVE, it requires sharing of resources from anywhere at any time. The scenario proposed in Satchel involved a worker outside his workplace, who needed remote access to documents, but couldn't do so effectively due to the high transmission times provoked by mobility. Satchel's scenario (Lamming et al., 2000) demonstrates the importance of resource (e.g. documents) sharing during the mobile process, and that it is even more important to diffuse the collaboration of not only resources, but also of information in the more ample sense of the word (such as chats, messages, etc.).

The new "computing anywhere, at any time" paradigm is generating a movement towards mobile services. In this case the concepts of e-commerce are being extended to m-commerce, and e-learning now includes m-learning. With mobility, advantages in the quality of education, and improved results in learning are both expected. M-learning is, therefore, the next step in the evolution of e-learning.

The need for mobile users to use mobile devices for collaborative purposes does not arise from the fact that they are mobile, but from the implication of mobility, that is, they do not have access to conventional means of collaboration through their desktop computers. As mobile devices and access networks become more adequate and trustworthy, people feel increasingly attracted to use collaborative computing on several types of platforms. These changes have brought about a transition from the traditional model of computing to an ubiquitous one, which enables the entire environment to be available to the user from wherever it may be required.

The use of mobile devices is also justified in emergency situations, where a worker (or team of workers) must be located to establish collaboration, but is presently outside the normal work environment, and therefore unable to access his (their) desktop computers. Therefore, it is necessary to evaluate the impact of transferring the use of a desktop computer to a mobile device, mainly in the issues related to QoS (quality of service) and security. Now we present some situations in the medical field where mobile devices can be employed: requests for a second opinion, remote attendance of surgical procedures, and the transmission of warnings concerning the state of patients.

New computing technologies have provided some tools to overcome some limitations, creating virtual environments that can bring people closer together. A fairly common procedure, nowadays, is the concept of a "second opinion". This procedure has progressed from the use of asynchronous communications (e-mails) to synchronous communications, by means of instant messages to relay information. More recently, this communication has progressed even further with the development of CVEs that allow healthcare workers to interact in real time with audio, video and data transfer based on Web standard interfaces. All of these concepts may obviously be available also in PDA (Personal Digital Assistant) type mobile devices, and the collaborators can be located anywhere, at any time. This has been made possible through the creation of an access infrastructure based on wireless networks. It was recently established that part of the resistance of healthcare professionals to working in remote areas originates from the feeling of isolation and not being able to share diagnoses.

In the case of transmission of patient data warnings, the idea is not limited to the use of Short Message Services (SMS) provided by cellular phone networks, but also the transmission of a warning followed by the relay of information that can be monitored at a given moment, allowing a physician to evaluate the gravity of the warning and issue procedures adequate for each case.

QUALITY OF SERVICE AND STABILITY

Present Internet network architecture was designed to relay information using a Best Effort service model, with no guarantees concerning QoS (quality of service) requirements. In the event of a congestion packets are discarded and there is a certain downgrade in the transmission rate, which does not guarantee that the application will be executed effectively. These problems result from the increase of traffic over the Internet, and the type of information carried over the network.

QoS is defined as a set of techniques used to provide differentiated treatments to the flow of data, according to the application. The requirements for each flow can be characterized by four main parameters: Delay – the time necessary for a packet to travel through he network, measured from the moment of transmission to the moment of arrival; Jitter - is the variation in delay, and is defined by consecutive pairs of packets (if D_i is the delay of the i_{th} packet, then the jitter of the pair of packets is defined as $D_i - D_{(i-1)}$); Reliability - is associated to the packet loss rate, which is the relation between the number of packets lost and the number transmitted, measured at the receiving end (this loss occurs when the router buffer is overloaded and no longer allows storage of packets); Bandwidth – represents the speed of the environment, in other words, the maximum transmission rate available at a given moment for communication between two knots of the network (Ash, 2006).

In a multimedia environment different types of traffic (viedo, voice, data, etc.) compete for the use of the same resources. Therefore it is important to understand the network requirements needed to provide satisfactory QoS performance. The introduction of QoS management mechanisms is necessary, as a measure to guarantee that applications sensitive to delay, jitter and packet loss are not affected.

Furthermore, to guarantee the continuous use of a mobile system, stability must be a premise. Stability, in the technical sense, means that the services must be carried out obeying parameters of speed and availability. This is a fundamental point when the link to the mobile device has low speed. Instability, in this case, such as connection losses and application interruptions, will cause loss of user data. If the system is functioning devoid of interesting information, users will lose interest in the system. Lastly, stability is also connected to maintenance. Programming errors may never be fully solved, thus the need for someone who is responsible for receiving bug reports and suggestions that should be incorporated to the system, in order to guarantee good acceptance.

MOBILE LEARNING

The premise of Mobile-education is based on the idea by Pascoe et al. (2000): "Using While Moving", which is basically what users need from a mobile computer system. Mobile-education affords distributed collaboration over wireless devices to generate learning opportunities. This is, therefore, a new approach that uses a virtual wireless community to facilitate learning activities through collaboration in a distributed environment. Mobile-Education is significantly different from traditional learning systems. In this new model collaborative activities are based on virtual communities, and offer a wide range of collaboration opportunities, such as synchronous and asynchronous peer-to-peer interactivity, allowing data visualization. All of this interaction will be possible from handheld devices.

MAIN CHALLENGES

Some challenges facing the CVEs and Multimedia Communication Technologies are briefly outlined in this section.

High performance computing and networking technology promise to offer great potential to link many medical centers and universities to each other. An interesting point to note regarding this fact, is that virtual anatomical models of the human body will be able then to be shared and used systematically, for various surgical simulation and learning applications through the Web. As a result, we believe that these applications will be able to generate immersive and highly adaptable VEs that will allow individual participants or teams to train and learn simultaneously. However, we need also to take into account the fact that CVEs are typically associated with high-performance computers and specialized input/output haptic devices, with high costs involved, which make operating them on a large scale still prohibitively expensive. Also, related to this issue is the problem of ensuring that each participant sharing an entity in the CVE has a consistent view of the environment. The consequences of differing state can be detrimental to the application as each user's perception of the interaction being performed would differ, thus, leading to a breakdown in the collaboration (Glencross & Chalmers, 2005).

Other important issues in typical CVEs are the most complex types of interactions possible, which are collisions (detection and response) and touch. Collisions are often the bottleneck of simulation applications in terms of calculation time, directly related to the geometric complexity of the VE, and sometimes involves a huge number of geometrical tests for determining which elements are colliding (Ericson, 2005). Colliding virtual bodies can be deformable or rigid. During their movements, a point located anywhere in space (centre of rotation) is associated with the surfaces. Rotational and translational velocities around that point define the instantaneous motion. These velocities are integrated forward in time to define the motion of the surfaces. It is appropriate to certify always during the collisions whether the surfaces are still both physically continuous and topologically contiguous. From a rendering point of view, for graphical display of VEs that support interactions between objects, such as collisions, one of the most important considerations is maintaining suitably high frame rates to guarantee the quality of the simulation.

In some CVEs, participants may change attributes of entities (with complex behavior), which have physical characteristics allowing them to deform or flow (Glencross & Chalmers, 2005). This type of interaction impacts upon the values provided to the algorithms used to compute the state and/or the geometric structure of the entities. Haptic feedback is one of the important stimuli that can be used to provide richer response for physical interaction with VEs by touch. However, simply adding haptic feedback to CVEs does not lead to usable medical applications. It is also essential to consider how to combine suitable force models to support correct perception of surface details (e.g, textures), entity-entity collisions, and motion during interactions.

As medical devices are becoming increasingly networked, ensuring the same level of existing health safety become crucial (Lee et al., 2006), especially considering that interactions in VEs still suffer from problems of accuracy. In addition, networked virtual reality (NVR) services with integrated multimedia components (and perceived "real-time" interactivity) impose certain QoS requirements at the user/application level as well on the underlying network (Skorin-Kapov et al., 2004).

IP technology, in its original conception, does not offer any type of guarantee of QoS. Also, in order for an IP network to support voice services with strict delay and jitter requirements, it is necessary to implement some functionalities to this protocol. The IETF (Internet Engineering Task Force) standardized two specific architectures to supply QoS in the IP environment: IntServ – Integrated Services, and DiffServ – Differentiated Services. The big challenge, however, consists of implementing an infrastructure capable of supporting these architectures.

Further, as devices become increasingly smaller in physical terms, but larger in software terms, they bring capabilities that are sufficient to provide the basis for mobile use. Equipped with small health applications these PDAs can be given out to a number of health agents, thus providing a higher coverage by giving many agents access to a computing device. Therefore, as mobility in collaboration is emerging as a research topic in itself, it is imperative that researchers in this field explore new methods of interaction and novel applications (Perry et al., 2001).

The type of device which can be used for a service is basically unrestricted as long as it is wireless. However, wireless does not mean that a constant connection to a server or network is required. A PDA that holds notes which were transmitted during synchronization using a personal computer is a mobile device just as is a mobile phone with a Wireless Application Protocol (WAP) browser, or a PDA with a Wireless Local Area Network (WLAN) connection.

The need for privacy and confidentiality is giving rise to increased expectations about data storage and transmission security, as data on demand emerges as a viable concept in healthcare. Regarding security, it is important to emphasize that unrestricted admittance is only possible with a valid user identity, which is controlled by the system. Adequate security is ensured by encrypting all data at 128 bit. For mobile admittance the user has to enter an identifier. When the infrastructure supports Wireless Identification Module (WIM), additional security can be established by unambiguously identifying a user.

ACKNOWLEDGMENT

The research was partly supported by The National Council for Scientific and Technological Development of Brazil (CNPq) under grant No. 303046/2006-6.

CONCLUSION AND FUTURE WORK

The medical field has been one of the most appealing areas for computer graphics and VR research. Further, we believe that CVEs can provide novice physicians, residents and students with a natural training and learning environment that may increase understanding of the anatomic relationships of the human body and improve healthcare, minimizing the risks to patients, thereby their ultimate safety. The advantage is that the novice, for example, will be introduced to uncommon conditions that would only arise rarely in clinical practice.

We also observe that while a range of VR medical applications do contain simulation and rich behavior to varying degrees, it is still very hard to quantify the realism of the computer models, since the human body is a system of complex interactions between organs and tissues. These interactions are particularly intricate in the case of soft tissues (very little information is currently known regarding their deformable behavior). In addition, there are ethical problems involved and the need of volunteers. Last, but not least, there is still the fact that collecting medical data takes time.

Beyond these issues are also the psychological and sociological barriers to implementation that any new technology should overcome. Crossing these barriers among professionals in Education, Training, Healthcare Delivery, Engineering, and Computer Science will require an integrated and collaborative approach. Actually, over the past few years, a movement characterized by increased collaboration among these professionals has started to take shape.

QoS makes it possible to offer better guarantees and security for Internet applications, once the traffic of advanced applications (such as voice, videoconference, etc.) is being given greater priority, while users of traditional applications continue to use the Best Effort approach.

Finally, we hope that CVEs and recent computer technologies can contribute not only to the advance and improvement of healthcare delivery, but also to do it more safely.

REFERENCES

Ash, G. (2006). *Traffic engineering and QoS optimization of integrated voice & data networks.* Morgan Kaufmann Series in Networking.

Basdogan, C., De, S., Kim., J., Munivandi, M., & Srinivasan, M.A. (2004). Haptics in minimally invasive surgical simulation and training. *IEEE Computer Graphics and Applications (special issue on Haptic Rendering – Beyond Visual Computing), 24*(2), 56-64.

Blezek, D.J., Robb, R.A., & Martin, D.P. (2000). Virtual reality simulation of regional anesthesia for training of residentes. *Presented at the 33rd Hawaii International Conference on System Sciences,* (pp. 1-8). IEEE CS Press.

Burdea, G. (1999). Haptic feedback for virtual reality. *Presented at the Virtual Reality and Prototyping Workshop,* (pp. 87-96).

Dev, P., Montgomery, K., Senger, S., Heinrichs, W.L., Srivastana, S., & Waldron, K. (2002). Simulated medical learning environment on the Internet. *Journal of the American Medical Informatics Association, 9*(5).

DiMaio, S.P., & Salcudean, S.E. (2005). Interactive simulation of needle insertion models. *IEEE Transactions on Biomedical Engineering,52*(7), 1167–1179. IEEE CS Press.

Ericson, C. (2005). *Real time collision detection.* Morgan Kaufmann. Elsevier.

Glencross, M. & Chalmers, A. (2005). High fidelity collaborative virtual environments. *Presented at the 4th International Conference on Virtual Reality, Computer Graphics, Visualization and Interaction in Africa (tutorial notes).* AFRIGRAPH.

Gunn, C., Hutchins, M., & Adcock, M. (2005b). Combating latency in haptic collaborative virtual environments. *Presence: Teleoperators and Virtual Environments, 14*(3), 313-328.

Gunn, C., Hutchins, M., Stevenson, D., Adcock, M., & Youngblood, P. (2005a). Using collaborative haptics in remote surgical training. *Presented at the Eurohaptics Conference and Symposium on Haptic Interfaces for Virtual Environment and Teleoperator Systems,* (pp. 481-482).

Hosseini, M., & Georganas, N.D. (2001). Collaborative virtual environments for training. *In the ACM Multimedia.* Ottawa, ON, Canada.

Kneebone, R. (2003). *Med Educ, 3,* 267-77.

Lamming, M., Eldridge, M., Flynn, M., Jones, C., & Pendleburry, D. (2000). Satchel: providing access to any document, any time, anywhere. *ACM Transactions on Computer-Human Interaction,* 7(3), 322-352.

Lee, I., Pappas, G.J., Cleaveland, R., Hatcliff, J., Krog. B.H., Lee, P., et al. (2006). High-confidence medical device software and systems. *Computer (special issue on Clinical Software Engineering)* , *39*(4), 33-38. IEEE CS Press.

Pascoe, J., Ryan, N., & Morse, D. (2000). Using while moving: HCI issues in fieldwork environments. ACM Transactions on Computer-Human Interaction, vol. 7, 3, pp. 417-437.

Perry, M., O'Hara, K., Sellen, A., Brown, B., & Harper, R. (2001). Dealing with mobility: understanding access anytime, anywhere. *ACM Transactions TOCHI, 8*(4).

Pesch, D., Irvine, J. & Klepal, M. (2007). *Mobile communication systems and networks.* John Wiley & Sons.

Rizzo, A.A., Klimchuk, D., Mitura, R., Bowerly, T., Buckwalter, Parsons, TD & Yeh, S.C. (2006). A virtual reality scenario for all seasons: the virtual classroom. *CNS Spectrums, 11*(1), 35-44.

Rodrigues, M.A.F., Silva, W.B., Barbosa-Neto, M.E., Gillies, D.F., Ribeiro, I.M.M.P. (2007). An interactive simulation system for training and treatment planning in orthodontics (article in press, doi: 10.1016/j.cag.2007.04.010). *Computers & Graphics*, Elsevier.

Rose, F.D., Brooks, B.M. & Rizzo, A.A. (2005). Virtual reality in brain damage rehabilitation: a review. *CyberPsychology & Behavior, 8*(3), 241-262.

Skorin-Kapov, L., Vilendečić, D., Mikić, D. (2004). Experimental performance evaluation of networked virtual reality services. *Presented at the IEEE MELECON*, (pp. 661-664). IEEE CS Press.

Sharma, C., & Nakamura, Y. (2004). *Wireless data services: Technologies, business models and global markets.* Cambridge University Press.

Stallings, W. (2005). *Cryptography and network security.* Prentice Hall.

KEY TERMS

Collaborative Virtual Environments (CVEs): CVEs are used to construct a virtual world where users can interact with one another and the environment in which they preside in order to perform, for example, a training exercise.

Distributed Collaboration: VR has been employed to allow geographically distributed people to do more than simply hear and see each other. For instance, VR technology is being used to develop highly interactive shared virtual environments, graphically orientated, for local and distance training and learning.

Haptics: It refers to technology which interfaces the user via the sense of touch by applying forces, vibrations and/or motions to the user.

Haptic Feedback: A crucial sensorial modality in VR applications. Haptics means both *force feedback* (simulating object hardness, weight, inertia, etc) and *tactile feedback* (simulating surface contact geometry, smoothness, slippage, and temperature) (Burdea, 1999).

Mobility: It is the ability of mobile devices to move or change the position.

Quality of Service (QoS): QoS refers to control mechanisms that can provide different priority to different users or data flows, or guarantee a certain level of performance to a data flow in accordance with requests from the application program.

Security: It is the practice of protecting and preserving private resources and information on the network from unauthorized modification or destruction.

Virtual Reality (VR): VR entails the use of advanced technologies, including computers and multimedia peripherals, to produce "virtual" environments that users perceive as comparable to real world objects. It offers great potential as a technology for computer-based training and simulation. It may be delivered to the user via a variety of input/output devices such as screen monitors, head-mounted displays, data gloves, etc.

Virtual Environments (VEs): VEs can be used to simulate aspects of the real world which are not physically available to the users of the application.

Wireless: Communication or transfer of information over a distance without the use of wires. It is generally used for mobile devices.

Chapter XXIX
Transforming a Pediatrics Lecture Series to Online Instruction

Tiffany A. Koszalka
Syracuse University, USA

Bradley Olson
SUNY Upstate Medical University, USA

ABSTRACT

A major issue facing medical education training programs across the USA is the recent advent of universal mandatory duty hour limitations and the time pressure it places on formal face-to-face educational sessions. In response to these mandates and associated issues many medical education programs are exploring the use of online instruction to address issues of accessibility. This chapter describes the instructional development process followed to transform a classroom-based pediatrics residency lecture series into an on-demand, video-enhanced, online instructional environment. An overview of the learning principles and instructional sciences that guided the design process is provided. The phases of the designed solution are then described in the context of enhancing the lecture series as it was transformed into online instruction. Implementation logistics are described followed by an overview of the benefits, barriers, and initial project outcomes. Plans for future enhancements and research projects are also discussed.

INTRODUCTION

Designing good instruction is predicated on understanding learning. Effective learning is predicated on accurately defining learning outcomes and providing instructional environments that support the achievement of learning outcomes. Both are essential to successful online instruction (Koszalka, 2007, p. 2).

Principles of learning and the instructional sciences were used to enhance the overall strength of the pediatrics residency curriculum at SUNY Upstate Medical University in Syracuse, New York. In response to the recent advent of universal mandatory duty hour limitations and the time pressure it places on formal face-to-face educational sessions, the entire residency curriculum, consisting of a year-long classroom-based lecture series, was transformed into a blended video-based online format supported by application-based classroom experiences. The online lectures component was not a straight conversion where lectures were simply videotaped and offered to the residents through a distance education program, rather the demand for change was used as an opportunity to re-evaluate the design of the lecture series and apply sound learning and instructional design principles to enhance the overall residency instructional process.

Application of learning principles. Learning at its foundation is about change, change in human condition based on experiences. Principles of social learning theories posit that learning is a construction of knowledge based on an individual's observations of, and interactions with, information and people around them. Learning can occur both at surface and deep levels depending on how individuals interact with new information.

Surface learning suggests storage and remembrance of information, facts, concepts, principles, and procedures. It often results in recalling basic information and demonstrating new procedures and behaviors, for example. Deep learning, or critical thinking, suggests activation of higher order thinking. Outcomes of this type of learning include constructing knowledge to evaluate, apply, diagnose, problem solve, debate, critique, and other activities that require successfully addressing complex and ill-structured problems, such as those encountered by medical professionals.

The construction or learning of knowledge at these different levels is supported through different types of interactions (instruction) with content and people that accommodate individual preferences and learning styles of the learner (Akdemir & Koszalka, In-press; Akdemir & Koszalka, 2005; Kidney, G., & Puckett, 2003). Thus, instruction is thought to be richest and most effective in facilitating deep learning when:

- Learners are *engaged* in solving real-life problems;
- Existing knowledge is *activated* as a foundation to new knowledge;
- New knowledge is *demonstrated* to the learner;
- When new knowledge is *applied* by the learner;
- When new knowledge is *integrated* into the learner's world (Merrill, 2000).

Application of instructional sciences and design processes. The instructional sciences inform how activities can be designed to prompt and facilitate required levels of learning that meet expected outcomes. To design instruction and learning experiences that apply learning principles successfully an instructional system design (ISD) process can be undertaken. The process includes: (A) analyzing the gap in knowledge (what does the learner know and what should they learn), (D) designing an instructional and learning solution, (D) developing the solution based on the design, (I) implementing and testing the solution, and (E) evaluating the results (Dick, Carey, & Carey, 2005; Smith & Ragan, 2005). An ADDIE approach, guided by principles of learning and instruction, is especially important when designing instruction for online applications, as the perceived separation of learner and facilitator can be distracting to the learner or fail to provide information and social learning interactions required by the learner.

Distance education of the past was designed to stand on its own as correspondence courses in which learners received an instructional packet and submitted assignments at their own pace. There was little or no social interaction with peers or an instructor. Distance education today however mostly refers to technology-delivered instruction and learning activities that are designed to provide informational and instructional elements as well as social learning elements to actively engage learners with content, peers, and the instructor through digital technologies (Grabowski & Small, 1997). The major benefit is posited to be providing instruction to those who have limitations of time or travel (Hawkridge, 1999; Stock-McIssac, 1999).

Incorporating these interaction elements however, comes at a price. Learners in distance education seem to have a wide range of technology skills and content application knowledge (Lamb & Smith, 2000). Thus, addressing the needs of such a wide variety of learners can be a challenge. Designing for such a diverse audience often means incorporating multiple and rich representations of the same information (e.g., lecture, readings, learning aides) and providing learners with multiple ways to interact with content and demonstrate their learning (e.g., discussion boards, online assessment, reflective journaling). Thus, it is critical when converting from classroom-based instruction to online delivery that instructional materials and learning activities be well integrated and aligned with expected learning outcomes, e.g., surface recall or knowledge application in problem solving.

THE PROBLEM WITH THE CURRENT RESIDENCY CLASSROOM-BASED CURRICULUM AT SUNY UPSTATE

Prompted in part by a recent citation for poor resident attendance at the pediatric core conference (classroom lecture) series a curriculum reform effort was undertaken at SUNY Upstate Medical University. As part of this reform an analysis of the formal didactic educational program was undertaken. This analysis revealed that as a result of significant clinical responsibilities the 36 pediatric residents could only attend approximately 30-40% of the offered lectures. This attendance situation has recently been made worse across the country in medical education with the introduction of mandatory work hour limitations that restrict residents' ability to attend standard face-to-face lectures series (Higgins, 2006). The curriculum analysis that was undertaken also revealed that the offered lecture series did not cover the necessary scope of content as outlined by the American Board of Pediatrics (ABP). As a result of these findings it was decided by Upstate's Pediatrics departmental administration to take advantage of distance education technologies to provide greater access for the residents to 'attend' the lectures and address the above noted challenges. Specifically, there were three gaps the institution has tried to overcome from the traditional formal didactic component of the pediatric residency program:

- Lack of overarching design in the core curriculum to cover a defined scope of content.
- Poor conference attendance due to mandatory duty hour limitations making lectures increasingly inaccessible.
- Lacked meaningful learning objectives and measures of knowledge acquisition in core lecture curriculum.

The previous core face-to-face lecture curriculum consisted of a 50-minutes didactic conference series offered 3 days per week. At the end of the academic year the same series was repeated with the assumption that any missed lectures would be attended the next year by the resident as needed. The 120+ annual lectures in this face to face lecture series were organized and presented monthly according to the identified clinical domains. See Table 1. It is important to note that missing from this list of face-to-face lecture topics are the domains of Dermatology, Genetics, Orthopedics and Pharmacology. Because Upstate has limited

Table 1. Pediatrics residency curriculum listing clinical domains

Clinical domain	*New Domains	Topics covered in clinical domain
Adolescent Med.		Adolescent History; Adolescent Physical Exam; Eating Disorders; Depression
Cardiology		
Developmental Peds.		Patterns of Development & Disability; Spinal Dysraphism; Disorders of Communication & the Autistic Spectrum Disorders; Disorders of Language, Learning & Cognition; Diagnosis and Treatment of ADHD; Cerebral Palsy; Parent Partners in Health Education: Introduction; Parent Partners in Health Education: Communication; Parent Partners in Health Education: Educational Advocacy
Dermatology	X	Principles of Atopic Dermatitis; Acne; Newborn Skin
Emergency Med.		
Endocrinology		Type 1 Diabetes; Type 2 Diabetes; Diabetic Ketoacidosis (DKA); Hyperthyroidism; Acquired Hypothyroidism; Congenital Hypothyroidism; Short Stature; Delayed Puberty; Precocious Puberty
Gastroenterology		Vomiting; Diarrheal Disorders; Gastroesophageal Reflux Disease (GERD); Jaundice (Part 1); Jaundice (Part 2); Gastrointestinal Bleeding; Malabsorption; Abdominal Mass; Refeeding Syndrome; Celiac Disease
Genetics	X	Prenatal Diagnosis; Newborn Screening & Metabolic Emergencies; Chromosomal Abnormalities; Teratogens; Malformations & Deformations; Common Genetic Syndromes
Hematology/Oncology		CBC Interpretation; Coagulation Disorders; Neoplastic Disorders; Pediatric Transfusion (Indications & Complications)
Infectious Disease		Public Health: Prevention of Infectious Diseases; Laboratory Diagnosis of Infectious Diseases: Bacteriology; Laboratory Diagnosis of Infectious Diseases: Virology; Infectious Gastroenteritis; Antiviral Therapy; Antibiotic Treatment of Common Respiratory Tract Infections; Pertussis; Tickborne Diseases; Enterovirus Infections; Respiratory Viral Infections
Intensive Care Med.		
Neonatology		Term Newborn - Part 1 (The Basics); Neonatal Resuscitation; Apnea, SIDS, and Sleep Position; Management of Jaundice; Hematologic Problems of the Newborn; Respiratory Disorders of the Newborn; Neonatal Abstinence & Fetal Alcohol Syndrome
Nephrology		Hematuria and Glomerulonephritis; Congenital & Inherited Disorders of the Urinary Tract; Proteinuria & Nephrotic Syndrome; Normal and Abnormal Renal Function; Urinary Tract Infection in Children; Hypertension
Neurology		
Outpatient Peds		Immunizations; Infant and Child Nutrition; Monitoring Growth and Development; Disorders of the Eye; Childhood Obesity; Child Abuse
Orthopedics	X	Infections of the Bones & Joints; Disorders of the Hip 2: Perthes and SCFE
Pharmacology	X	Developmental Pharmacology & Pharmacokinetics; Clinical Implications of Pharmacokinetics
Pulmonology		Hypnosis; Cystic Fibrosis - Diagnosis & Pathophysiology; Cystic Fibrosis - Treatment; Bronchopulmonary Dysplasia; The Wheezing Infant; Allergy & Related Disorders; Urticaria, Angioedema, Anaphylaxis & Food Allergies; Asthma (etiology, epidemiology & natural history); Asthma (diagnosis); Asthma (outpatient treatment); Chronic Cough; Breathing Disorders of Sleep; Spirometry, Chest X-ray & Blood Gas Analysis
Rheumatology		

**Expertise not previously available at Upstate to conduct classroom sessions in these domains* access to content experts in these fields robust face-to-face lectures in these content domains could not be delivered. However, with the development of the online curriculum content experts could be recruited to cover these domains so that our online curriculum covers a proper and expected scope of content.

The pediatrics faculty consists of 50 physicians all of who are content experts, but who have varying degrees of expertise in instructional design and no formal training in instructional concepts or designing online instruction. The lectures that they provided were of a similar quality typical of most academic medical institution. The lectures however consistently lacked educational objectives and rarely had measures of knowledge acquisition by which achievement can be assessed.

THE PROPOSED PEDIATRIC ONLINE CORE CURRICULUM

In order to address the issues of accessibility and lack of content scope it was decided by the department's education committee to develop an online core curriculum that covers the full scope of content outlined by the American Board of Pediatrics Blueprint Document (ABP 2006). The ABP outlines the content that is tested by the national board certifying examination.

The Associate Program Director for Resident Education at Upstate took the lead in developing the pediatric online core curriculum. This core curriculum now consists of approximately 130 learning units divided into 20 basic clinical domains. Figure 1 provides a view of the online table of contents of the clinical domains (menu on the left) that residents see once logged into the course. Refer to table 1 for a complete listing of the clinical domains and topics covered within each.

This online pediatric core curriculum is offered through a commonly used Course Management System (CMS) called Blackboard. Within each domain folder are the basic learning units that comprise the core content of that knowledge domain (figure 2). For example in the Genetic domain topics on prenatal diagnosis, new born screening and metabolic emergencies, chromosomal abnormalities, etc. are accessible. Within each of the topics is access to lectures, supporting slides, reading materials, and short self-assessment quizzes.

By clicking on one of the learning topic folders (e.g., Prenatal Diagnosis) inside the clinical domain (Genetics) the basic architecture of each learning unit is revealed. This structure has been

Figure 1. Main menu of pediatric core curriculum at Upstate Medical University

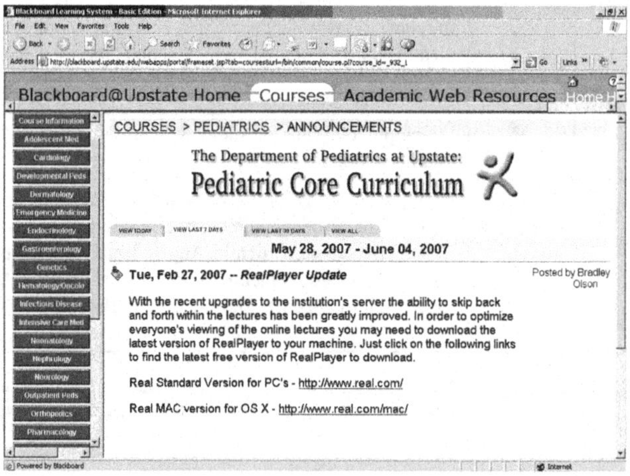

Figure 2. Learning unit architecture and navigation

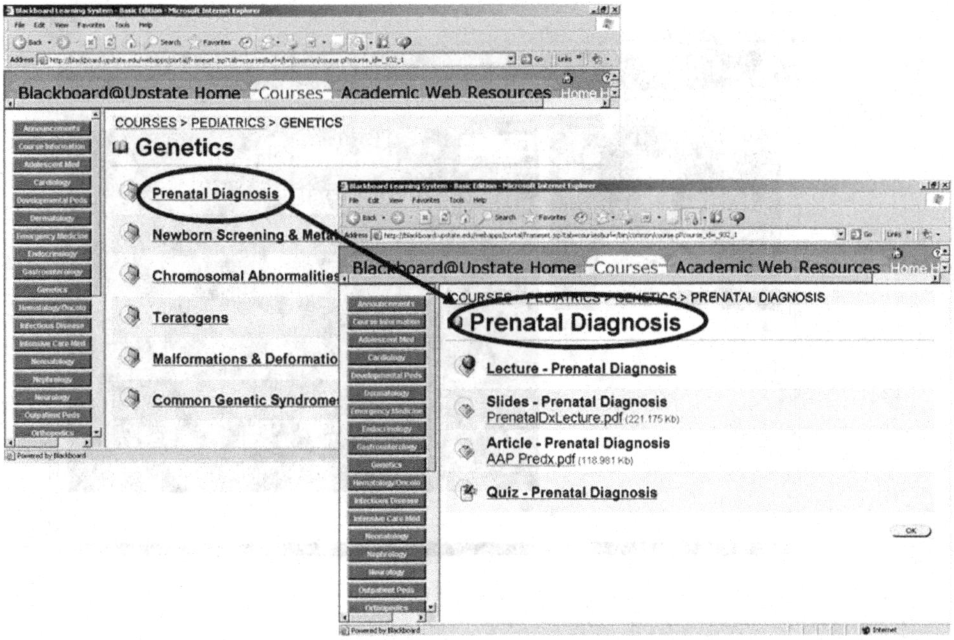

kept intentionally simple and consistent across domains to avoid interface complexity (Grunwald 2006). In designing online learning environments it is desirable to keep the basic architecture simple so that learners will quickly learn to navigate their way around the site without wasting time and effort learning complex linking and technology strategies. This way the learner dedicates a majority of his or her cognitive efforts towards learning the content rather than navigating a complex interface. A common mistake often found in the design of online learning environments is to use features of the technology simply because they are available (Gilbert & Moore, 1998; Kidney & Puckett, 2003; Koszalka & Ganesan, 2004). Non-purposive - not explicitly related to a specified learning outcome - use of technical features can inhibit learning (Kersley, 1997; Koszalka & Ganesan, 2004). Thus a consistent and easy to follow technical infrastructure is recommended.

The basic architecture of each learning unit in the pediatric core curriculum consists of four components: a video lecture that highlights the essential points of the learning unit, a printable copy of the lecture slides, a review article that serves as a summary document of the essential material, and a quiz that assesses the learners' acquisition of the content material. The video lecture is integrated with synchronized PowerPoint slides to effectively present of the topic content. See figure 3. This component mimics face-to-face lecture with the exception that learners have the advantage of being able to start and stop a video lecture at any time. They can also skip forward and backward within a lecture to review points that they recall from a previous viewing, supplemental reading or quizzing materials, or from outside experiences. As mentioned previously the learners may also download the PowerPoint presentations and review them without the video.

The overall design of the online core curriculum provides the residents with flexibility to review required content domains and topics when they have time and access. To help them develop deeper understanding of the content the lectures and presentation notes are supplemented with

Figure 3. Sample video and synchronized PowerPoint topic lecture

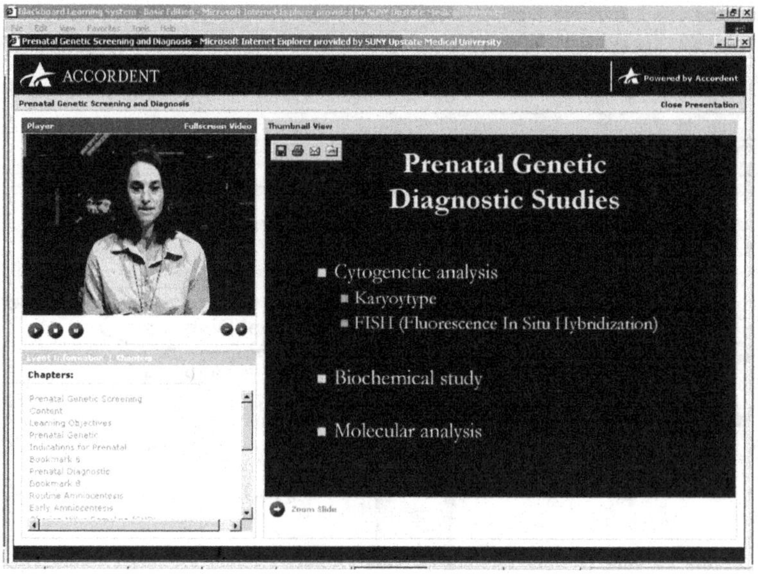

learning objectives, focused reading materials, and self-check quizzes. Although provided as a self-paced, anytime-anywhere accessible format, the delivery of the content online has also provided opportunities for the university to revise the format of classroom sessions.

The in class session are now more focused on case-based discussions that engage the residents in applying information from the online lectures and activities. Thus, residents are now engaged in surface and deep learning activities during all aspects of the new curriculum with a focus on discussion, application, and case-based social learning activities during classroom sessions.

IMPLEMENTATION: PROCESS, BENEFITS, CHALLENGES, AND INITIAL RESULTS

The pediatric online core curriculum is the result of a two-year educational reform effort that employed learning theory and the ADDIE model of Instructional development. This model involved the analysis, design, development, implementation, and evaluation of an instructional solution to Upstate's pediatrics residency education program challenges of non-attendance in lecture series, gaps in presented content domains, and weak/non-existent learning assessment approaches. This stepwise systems-based approach for designing and implementing instructional solutions involved analyzing instructional problems followed by designing solution that address identified learning and instructional problems. Once the solution was designed instructional materials were developed and the instruction was implemented and tested. Through out this process both the instructional product and the process were evaluated to verify that the product addressed the problem originally identified and learners were able to achieve expected outcomes. The following is a description of each of the phases conducted during the development of Upstate's pediatric online residency core curriculum.

Analysis Phase. The initial step in the curriculum reform efforts involved analysis of the curriculum content, learners, and environmental factors to define the instructional problem and scope of this project. As in any system, the educational systems is made up of multiple stakeholders (e.g., administrators, educators and learners) who may have differing opinions of the problem and different ideas of problem causes and what the next steps should be in reforming the current system. Lacking a common understanding of the problem will make it difficult, if not impossible to reach consensus on possible solutions. Thus, the analysis phase is critical in identifying gaps in knowledge and skills, describing the key problems (gap between current knowledge and expected knowledge), articulating causes of the gaps, and suggesting potential instructional and learning solutions.

The steps to perform a gap analysis primarily involve collecting a variety of data from key of stakeholders and the instructional and practice environments. Questions that are addressed to stakeholders should be designed to elicit information from their perspective on current practices, ideal practices, problems (gaps) faced by the educational organization, potential causes of identified problems, and potential solutions. The data collection methods that Upstate used included the following:

- External review of our educational program by a nationally recognized pediatric educator and leader.
- Telephone interviews of 10 former pediatric residents (5 in practice/5 in fellowship) concerning their perceived strengths and weaknesses after having completed training at our institution.
- Survey of all department chairs about their perceived educational needs within their departments.
- Analysis of an external governing agency's review of our educational program.
- Focus group discussions with current residents, faculty and the education committee about each group's perceptions of the strengths and weaknesses of the educational program.

The results of this data collection method were analyzed in order to clearly define the gaps faced by the educational program from the perspective of the various stakeholders. These gaps were then synthesized into 3 statements that were easily communicated and agreed upon by the entire faculty. The gaps that the Upstate pediatric residency program faced were as follows:

- The face-to-face core lecture series did not cover the full scope of content defined by the American Board of Pediatrics blue print document.
- Lecture attendance was poor (<30-40%) partially because of resident commitments to service obligations and mandatory duty hour limitations.
- There were no clearly defined learning objectives for each of the lectures in the core series and consequently no measure of whether our learners had achieved those objectives.

Once these gaps were clearly defined it was a relatively straightforward process to gain the acceptance of the faculty on an online curriculum that accomplished the following three goals.

- Create a designed curriculum that covers a defined scope (i.e. the *American Board of Pediatrics* blue print document).
- Create a lecture series that is accessible to the residents when and where they need it.
- Develop learning objectives for the core lecture series that covers the scope described above and provides learners with ways to check that they have achieved the objectives.

This proposal was presented to the faculty during a 3-hour workshop dedicated, in large part, to launching the online curriculum. The response of the faculty was overwhelmingly positive to this project proposal as they were able to easily see the gaps and follow the rational for a proposed solution that would be helpful in closing identified gaps.

Design Phase. The chief step in the design phase is to devise an instructional plan that specifically addresses the gaps outlined in the analysis phase. At Upstate the online curriculum was designed to address the 3 gaps in access, content, and learning assessment outlined above. In response to the gap in the content scope of the face-to-face curriculum the ABP blueprint document was used to define the scope for the new online core lecture curriculum. The ABP document, revised every 3 years, keeps up with the advances in medical knowledge and outlines the material that is covered by the annual certification examination, thus is useful in preparing instruction that readies residents for this exam.

A major decision during curriculum design for delivery with any type of media is to define the scope of the curriculum. Critical to these decisions is defining the boundaries of the core content knowledge that is required within a content domain. This is only possible in consultation with individuals who have sufficient domain expertise to make appropriate decisions as to what novices do and do not need to master within the specific domain. If the choices of what to study are left entirely to the novice scholarly research suggests that their learning will be less efficient and they will develop feelings of being overwhelmed by the volume of the material to cover (Leff, 2006). Thus the ABP was helpful in defining content updates to the lecture series.

Thus, Upstate's approach was to rely on an external source (ABP blueprint document) to define the boundaries of the overall curriculum. The project instructional designer partitioned the ABP document and distributed it to the various pediatric divisions with expertise to serve as the outline for the material that they were responsible for covering in the revised curriculum. This approach aborted any discussions/arguments that may have occurred between various stakeholders in regards to content ownership and facilitated the ultimate timely development of the curriculum material.

In order to address the accessibility gap the solution was to develop the new core curriculum for an online environment. By doing so the material would be accessible to learners anytime and anywhere. It is this accessibility that our learners cited as one of the most appealing aspects about the revised pediatric curriculum.

Finally, in addressing the 3rd gap, lack of learning objectives or measures of achievement, Upstate required each of the faculty to include specific learning objectives in their video presentation and 4-5 multiple choice questions that related specifically to those learning objectives and presented content. Each learning unit was designed with the same architecture of video lecture, followed by core reading material, and ending with self-test of knowledge acquisition in the form of an online quiz. By requiring the faculty to develop these basic components for each learning unit the development of a more uniform core curriculum focused on the most important aspects of the key curricular topics was fostered.

Development Phase. The chief task of the development phase was to build the instructional materials that were designed in the previous phase. During development of the online curriculum there were two main tasks to achieve. First the 50 faculty members in the department of pediatrics were introduced to models and sample templates of curricular materials in the new instructional medium, BlackBoard. In order to accomplish this, prototype lectures were first prototyped and piloted tested with pediatric residents. Once the pilot series was developed and implemented residents were surveyed to determine their satisfaction with online pilot curriculum, which was overwhelmingly positive. This pilot study provided important feedback that was used to enhance the prototype prior to sharing with the faculty.

Figure 4. Portion of the core curriculum revision project gantt chart

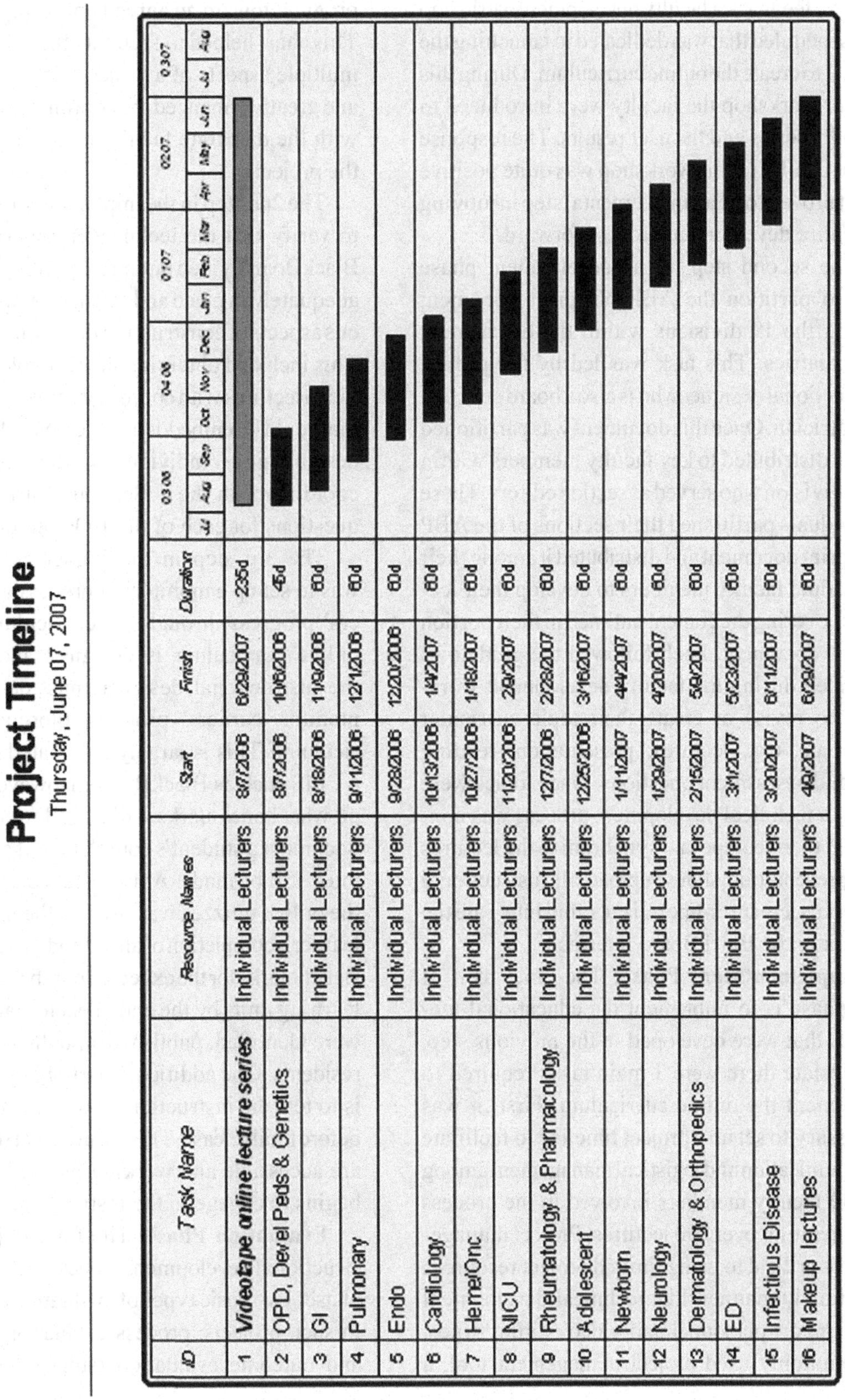

After testing the pilot series and obtaining positive feedback a faculty development workshop was scheduled that was dedicated to launching the project to create the online curriculum. During this 3-hour workshop the faculty were introduced to the pilot series and the user results. The response of the faculty to this workshop was quite positive and it proved to be an instrumental step in moving the entire development process forward.

The second step to the development phase was to partition the ABP blueprint document among the 19 divisions within the department of pediatrics. This task was led by the project instructional designer who is also a board certified pediatrician. Once this document was partitioned it was distributed to key faculty members within each division who served as section editors. These individuals partitioned their sections of the ABP blueprint document and distributed it among their individual faculty members to develop their lectures covering the content outlined in their portion of this document. Each followed the guidelines provided during the faculty development workshop to revise or create their topic curricular materials, e.g., lectures, presentation, reading list, and assessment questions. Once topics were ready a technical development process was conducted to videotape and synchronize the lectures and presentation slides, upload all instructional materials, create online quizzes, and integrate the topic into the BlackBoard interface.

Implementation Phase. The chief step of this phase is to implement the educational materials that were developed in the previous step. At Upstate there were 3 main tasks required to implement the online curriculum. First, it was necessary to set up a project timeline to facilitate communication and logistical management among the 50 faculty members involved in the process of generating over 100 lectures. Project management is critical to using limited project resources in a timely manner, like technical development and support personnel and video editing suites. A commonly used project management tool, a Gantt chart (see Figure 4.), was developed to show progress toward an agreed upon project timeline. This chart helped to facilitate the coordination of multiple aspects of a project within the timeline and greatly enhanced the communication process with the disparate faculty members involved in the project.

The 2nd step in the implementation phase was to verify that the technical infrastructure (e.g., BlackBoard, video taping and editing suites,) was adequately in place and set up to support the various aspects of constructing the online curriculum. This included obtaining the technology to create video lectures with coordinated PowerPoint slides that could be embedded in the CMS. It also meant designating an individual to serve as the central coordinator in the collection of articles & quiz questions for each of the 100+ lectures.

The 3rd step in the implementation phase was to set up a monitoring process for the learners' progress through the curriculum. Once an online curriculum is designed and developed the instructional designer must decide how to monitor learners' progress thorough the curriculum. This is largely automated when using a CMS such as BlackBoard. However, decisions on what benchmarks will be followed in order to document a student's completion of a curriculum must still be made. At Upstate the completion of the online quizzes was used as the marker of the learner's completion of an individual learning unit. Benchmarks for the expected number of completed learning units by the end of each year of training were identified, published, and distributed to the residents. One additional part of implementation is to test the instructional program and material before final release. This assures that the materials are accessible and working before the audience begins to engage in the instruction.

Evaluation Phase. The final step of the instructional development process is the evaluation phase. Two basic types of evaluation are common in such projects: process evaluation (formative) and outcome evaluation (summative). Process evaluation asks the questions, "is the project progressing according to plan and what enhancements need to be made before final release?" Outcome evaluation asks the question, "did the instruction address the gaps it was intended to at the outset?"

Process evaluation measures for this project included completion of the total number of lectures which have been placed into the CMS. Commitments were obtained from each of the divisions on the number of lectures that would be provided to cover their respective domains as outlined in the ABP blueprint document. As the curriculum has continued to be constructed over the past year it has been a simple matter of checking off each of the lectures from a master list once they have been completed and uploaded to the online course management system. At the time of this writing 90 of the final 130 lectures are complete and available to our learners through Blackboard.

One other measure examined as part of the formative evaluation was the results of a learner satisfaction survey. The two main areas of interest were (i) information on overall user satisfaction with the online curriculum and (ii) suggestions that the users had for improving the curriculum. The level of satisfaction questions resulted in >90% of the survey respondents rating the pilot curriculum as outstanding or very good. Several minor suggestions for improvements were provided based on the two following open-ended questions:

- Please describe any technical difficulties that you experienced with the pilot phase of the online lecture series.
- Please suggest any changes to the online lecture series that you would like us to make.

Suggestions in response to these survey questions as well as direct personal feedback from participating residents were used to enhance the final version of the curriculum. Continued data collection of satisfaction with the online curriculum will be solicited and analyzed to continually upgrade the online curriculum throughout its life.

The final (summative) outcome measures were designed to gauge whether the online curriculum effectively addressed the gaps that it was designed to address. We queried:

- Comparison of the scope of the final curriculum to the ABP blueprint document (verifying the final curriculum covers the full scope of content as outlined by ABP)
- The overall use rates of the online curriculum by the residents to verify that we have adequately addressed the issue of accessibility.
- Review of uploaded curricular materials to verify that each learning unit has a statement of the objectives followed by a measurement of the achievement of those objectives

The preliminary results of the review of the scope of the online curriculum compared to the ABP blueprint document reveal that of the nearly 90 lectures that have been developed to date, approximately 20% are entirely new lectures on material that was not previously covered in our face-to-face curriculum. This is a significant improvement over what our program was previously providing. When the curriculum is complete a final analysis will be performed to see if there are any significant gaps in the scope of content of the online curriculum compared to the ABP blueprint document.

The utilization rate that was expected of the residents and provided to them as a benchmark was a 50% completion by the end of the first year of the online curriculum. Our project team has been actively recording and posting the online lectures for the past 8 months so 90% of the curriculum was accessible. The overall use rate of the curriculum by the residents has been 40%. It is fully anticipated that the final use rate, after completing the first year of development, will meet the 50% threshold for the curriculum.

Finally, the online curriculum was reviewed to verify that each learning unit has learning objectives and accompanying measures of achievement. Nearly 100% of the posted curriculum complies with these criteria. Effective communications of requirements, sample templates, and review processes are credited with the nearly perfect compliance.

Thus, following a systematic process of instructional development, ADDIE, with accompanying project management checks and balances, professional development for faculty that provided rational for and clear steps toward curriculum re-form, technical support, and department buy-in led to the successful development of an enhanced pediatrics online curriculum. The learning and instructional design principles provided a framework that guided the construction of robust and effective instruction that seem to be well accepted by residents, the learners. Certainly enhancements will be necessary in the future as content revisions are suggested and new technologies emerge. There is also a greater need now to develop a better understanding of what affects this new delivery mechanisms is having on resident learning and practice in the long-term and the relationships between online learning and board scores.

PLANS FOR THE FUTURE: ENHANCEMENTS, RESEARCH, CONCLUSIONS

In moving forward with this project it will be important to measure the future achievement of the learners exposed to this new curriculum on norm referenced examinations like the American Board of Pediatrics' certification examination. The 3 and 5 year running averages will be followed to see how the new online curriculum effectives the performance of the pediatric residents on exams. Other interesting future areas of investigation may be to examine the barriers and affordances that promote and interfere with the use of online curriculum by pediatric residents or the use of new technologies to make the learning engagement more portable and on-demand with new technologies like smartphones. This will be particularly important to examine, as it appears that E-learning and the use of new portable technologies will continue to grow in medical education. The needs of users will need to be clearly understood in order to avoid developing curricula that are ineffective and under utilized.

Following established instructional design processes and considering learning principles becomes even more important as education shifts away from face-to-face modes. This work for the Upstate Medical University pediatrics residency program was deemed successful based on it approach to transforming its classroom lecture series to online instruction using instructional design principles and process.

REFERENCES

Akdemir, O., & Koszalka, T. (in-press). Investigating the relationships among instructional strategies and learning styles in online environments. *Computers and Education.*

Akdemir, O., & Koszalka, T. (Oct 2005). Expository and discovery learning compared: Their effects on learning outcomes of online students. Presented at *Association of Educational Communication and Technology 2005 annual conference*. Orlando, FL.

The American Board of Pediatrics (2007). Retrieved May 1, from https://www.abp.org/ABPWebSite/

Dick, W., Carey, L., & Carey, J. (2005). *The systematic design of instruction- sixth edition.* Boston, MA: Allyn and Bacon.

Gilbert, L., & Moore, D. (1998). Buidling interactivity in Web courses: Tools for social and instructional interaction. *Educational Technology, 38*, 29-35.

Grabowski, B., & Small, R. (1997). Information, instruction, and learning: A hypermedia perspective. *Performance and Improvement Quarterly, 10*(1). 156-166.

Grunwald, T., & Crosbie-Massay, C. (2006). Guidelines for cognitively efficient multimedia learning tools: Educational strategies, cognitive load and interface design. *Academic Medicine, 81*, 213-223.

Hawkridge, D. (1999) Distance learning: International Comparisons. *Performance Improvement Quarterly, 12*(2) 9-20.

Higgins, R., Cavendish, S., & Gregory, R. (2006). Class half-empty? Pre-registration house officer attendance at weekly teaching sessions: Implications for delivering the new Foundation Programme curriculum. *Medical Education, 40*, 877-883.

Kearsley, G. (1997). A guide to online education. Retrieved November 1, 2003, from http://gwis.circ.gwu.edu/~etl/online.html.

Kidney, G., & Puckett, E. (2003). Rediscovering the first principles through online learning. *Quarterly Review of Distance Education, 4*, 203-212.

Koszalka, T. (May 2007). The nuts & bolts of creating an online curriculum: A primer in: principles for designing effective online instruction. Presented at the *2007 Pediatric Medicine Conference*. Toronto CA.

Koszalka, T. (2001). Designing synchronous distance education: A demonstration project. *Quarterly Review of Distance Education. 2*(4), 333-346.

Koszalka, T. & Bianco M. (2001). Reflecting on the instructional design of distance education for teachers: Learnings from the instructors. *Quarterly Review of Distance Education. 1*(2), 59-70.

Koszalka, T. & Ganesan, R. (2004). Designing Online Courses: A taxonomy to guide strategic use of features available in course management systems (CMS) in distance education. *Distance Education, 25*(2), 243-256.

Lamb, A., & Smith, J. (2000). Ten facts of life for distance learning courses. *TechTrends, 44*(1), 12-15.

Leff B., & Harper G. M. (2006). The reading habits of medicine clerks at one medical school: Frequency, usefulness and difficulties. *Academic Medicine, 81*, 489-494.

Merrill, M.D. (2000). *First principles of instruction*. Retrieved December 5, 2007, from http://www.id2.usu.edu/Papers/5FirstPrinciples.PDF.

Merrill, M. (1997). Instructional strategies that teach. *CBT Solutions,* 1-11.

Oliver, R. (1999). Exploring strategies for online teaching and learning. *Distance Education,* 20, 240-250.

Olson, B., Koszalka, T., & Touhey, M., (May 2007). The nuts & bolts of creating an online curriculum. Presented at the *2007 Pediatric Medicine Conference*, Toronto CA.

Simonson, M., Smaldino, S., Albright, M., & Zvacek, S. (2003). *Teaching and learning at a distance.* Upper Saddle River, NJ: Merrill Prentice Hall.

Smith, P., & Raga, T. (2005). *Instructional design-third edition.* Hoboken, NJ: John Wiley & Sons, Inc.

Stock-McIssac, M. (1999). Distance learning: The U.S. version. *Performance Improvement Quarterly, 12*(2), 21-35.

Wittrock, M. (1990). Generative processes of comprehension. *Educational Psychologist, 27,* 531-41.

KEY TERMS

American Board of Pediatrics (ABP): The governing agency that certifies pediatric practitioners within the United States of America. The certification process involves passing a norm-referenced examination upon completion of pediatric residency training.

American Board of Pediatrics Blueprint Document: This is a 212-page document that outlines the core content of the *American Board of Pediatrics* certification exam that is taken upon completion of pediatric residency training.

Core Curriculum: The core curriculum is the agreed upon scope of material that defines the significant knowledge that is contained within a domain like pediatrics. It encompasses what would be reasonably expected for a practicing pediatrician to know.

Course Management System (CMS): A packaged program that is used for creating, delivering, and managing online instruction. Often course management systems include menu and template based tools to help developers easily build content, communication, testing, and other types of screens that support teaching and learning. These systems often also include management functions that support assignment grading, monitoring learner access, and completing course evaluations. Examples of popular CMS include BlackBoard, WebCT, and ANGEL.

E-Learning: Also referred to as online learning, it is the use of internet technologies to deliver a broad array of educational materials.

Instructional Design: Phase with the instructional systems design process where instruction in planned that is designed to close and instructional gap based on learning theory and instructional design theory.

Instructional Development: Phase with the instructional systems design process where instructional materials and processes are built based on a blue print developed during a design phase.

Instructional Systems Design: Systematic process for designing and developing instruction. Generally includes analysis, design, development, implementation, and evaluation phases.

Interface Complexity: A term that describes the degree of complexity that a user encounters when engaged with a digital medium like a website. With increasing complexity of the interface of a webpage, for example, the user required to dedicate cognitive energy to learning the intricacies of the interface as opposed to the content that is contained within the website.

Chapter XXX
Quality and Reliability Aspects in Telehealth Systems

Anastasia Kastania
Athens University of Economics and Business, Greece

Stelios Zimeras
University of the Aegean, Greece

ABSTRACT

In this chapter the authors investigate telehealth quality and reliability assurance. Various models and standards can be applied to assess software quality and reliability in telehealth platforms and there are also general principles for total quality management which can be adopted. There are also models to assess the quality of the system and the quality of care which are also presented. The approach based on user satisfaction, considers the expectation measurement as information which is not inextricably linked to quality. A different approach is the one based on expectations as well as on disconfirmation of user expectations. The underlying structural model is based on a modified SERVQUAL approach that consists of five dimensions (Tangibles, Reliability, Responsiveness, Assurance and Empathy) which have been consistently ranked by customers to be most important for service quality across all industries. The model can thus be used for evaluation of healthcare services and for planning improvements on services. All these aspects for telehealth systems design are discussed to formulate epistemic criteria for evaluation purposes.

INTRODUCTION

In this chapter the authors investigate measures and models for telehealth quality and reliability assurance. Telehealth is defined as "the exchange of health information and the provision of health care services through electronic information and communications technology, where participants are separated by geographic, time, social and cultural barriers" (Hebert, M., 2001). There are two basic components to quality: quality assurance and quality control (Whitney, C.W., Lind, B.K. and Wahl, P.W., 1998). The following quality evaluation issues should be considered in telehealth design and evaluation: system, software, care, patient satisfaction and management.

Very different measures are necessary for measuring the effectiveness of an information system. Related to the information systems effectiveness the dimensions of information systems success have been defined (DeLone, W. H. and McLean E. R., 2002). Other researchers (Cameron, K.S. and Whetten, D.A., 1983) have proposed a useful framework for selecting appropriate measures for future information systems research focused on organizational performance. In the scientific literature it is also proposed (Seddon, P.B., Staples, S., Patnayakuni, R. and Bowtell, M., 1999) that the diversity of information systems effectiveness measures is to be encouraged. Guidelines for standardisation of quality assurance in clinical trials are also described (Knatterud, G.L., Rockhold, F.W., George, S.L., Barton, F.B., Davis, C.E., Fairweather, W.R., Honohan, T., Mowery, R. and O'Neil, R., 1998).

The transcedental aspect of product quality (Ward, W.A. and Venkataraman, B., 1999) is identified with the sense of perfection that each person has. Because of this subjectivity, the methods and the models for the improvement of quality are necessary. With regard to the user view, a product is of quality if it satisfies the user. From the product view quality depends from its acquired characteristics and can be appraised from the presence or absence of certain attributes/characteristics. The manufacturer view is focused to the fulfillment of the required specifications and determines quality as a function. The value based view determines the quality as the means that offer the required services in financially accessible and acceptable cost. Empiric methods are also described to model the factors of software quality (Thomas, W. and Cerino, D. A., 1995). These are separated in functional characteristics (reliability), in programming characteristics (development cost and duration) and in maintenance characteristics. The method they propose (Thomas, W. and Cerino, D. A., 1995) is set from qualitative indicators for the evaluation of quality from the first stages.

Quality of care is a fundamental issue worldwide. There are many different approaches to monitoring the quality of services provided by an individual telehealthcare system, but one of the most valuable is obtaining feedback and opinions from users of the services. One of the main methodological problems in modern literature deals with the interpretation and the comprehension of the role of "expectation" in systems. "Expectation" represents a complex and dynamic concept (Harvey, J., 1998), defined within the framework of two prevailing trends. The approach based on user satisfaction, considers the expectation measurement as information which is not directly linked to quality. With respect to this there are a variety of tools for assessing the quality of a service but one of the most popular is SERVQUAL, an instrument designed by Parasuraman, and colleagues (Parasuraman, A., Berry, L.L., Zeithaml, V.A., 1988). This consists of a set of five dimensions which have been consistently ranked by customers to be most important for service quality, regardless of service industry. According to the general definition, expectations relate to the user's "predictions" for the services, whereas, on the basis of the second, expectations refer to the user's evaluation regarding the level of the services the provider needs to offer. The user's expectations of the quality of the healthcare services provided derive from a combination of characteristics and factors (Lewis, B.R and Mitchell, V.W., 1990) (Liljander, V. and Strandvik, T., 1994) (Rose, R., Uli, J., Abdul, M. and Ng, K., 2004) which are summarized as follows: (i) previous experiences the user has gathered from the service. (ii) third party suggestions (physicians, relatives, friends and other involved parties). (iii) factors relating to communication (direct & indirect) between the user and the service. (iv) factors relating to the Public or non -Public status of services: (iv.a) personal needs within the framework of the user value system, demographic – social- economic characteristics of the users etc. (iv.b) users perceive the healthcare system mainly through the institutional role of competent public services and the local administration. Lastly, measurement of the levels of user expectations allows the investigation of causes for quality problems in the organization.

ISO and standards facilitate the development of a quality management system, which serves as a basis for continuous process improvement and ensures consistency in processes (Hysell, D., 1999).

Worldwide, systems to measure service quality have been developed which have subsequently been modified according to the particular case and adopted by major organizations. With reference to the nature and structure of the service provided, the public sector is conducting user-satisfaction measurement research in competitive environments in order to develop prior principal and support services with the aim of improving the relationship between the providers and the user. User satisfaction and/or service quality (SERVQUAL) constitute essential components of healthcare (Donabedian, A., 1988). Users determine the strategy for quality management in healthcare services (Hasin, M.A.A., Seeluangsawat, R., Shareef, M.A., 2001). Methodological issues concerning service quality measurements have been discussed in the international literature (Lin, B. and Kelly, E., 1995) for many years and have been the subject of topical studies throughout the world (Ovretveit, J., 2000). Significant efforts have been made to develop user satisfaction models (Grigoroudis, E. and Siskos, Y., 2002) (Athanasopoulos, A., Gounaris, Sp. and Stathakopoulos, Vl., 2001) as well as to assess user satisfaction in healthcare services (Angelopoulou, P., Kangis, P., Babis, G., 1998) (Merkouris, A., Yfantopoulos, J., Lanara, V., Lemonidou, C., 1999) (Moumtzoglou, A., Dafogianni, C., Karra, V., Michailidou, D., Lazarou, P. and Bartsocas, C., 2000). The fact is that "user satisfaction" and/or "service quality" are complex phenomena involving intricate operations such as the measurement of quality in healthcare services, currently under examination, their perceived "value", and the social image of the organization.

DEFINITION OF QUALITY IN HEALTHCARE

Satisfaction with service quality depends on a large number of dimensions - both tangible and intangible attributes of the product-service offer. It is necessary to explain the importance of adopting common semantics when developing health geo-information services that span administrative boundaries and carry geographical information for the evaluation of the healthcare sectors. With reference to the nature and structure of the service provided, the public sector is conducting user-satisfaction measurement research in competitive environments in order to develop prior principal and support services with the aim of improving the relationship between the provider and the user. The final objective lies in increasing the market share of the organization. This observation also refers to the close relation between quality management and the marketing policy. With regard to healthcare services, a range of actions within the framework of a "special Marketing" can be introduced, which apart from taking into account the user satisfaction measurement will also aim at meeting user expectations. Quality measurement objectives in the Public Sector differ from the ones in the Private Sector as illustrated by the following statements (Robinson, St., 1999) (Teas, R.K., 1993): (i) Questions regarding service pricing rarely arise, whereas data concerning the user's perceived "value" of the service provided are taken into consideration. (ii) Often questions asked refer to the Public dimension of the Healthcare System, which must function in keeping with the concept of public interest, safeguarding its basic principles such as equal treatment, protection and safety, totality as well as accessibility to health services. (iii) The "user expectations" parameter assumes major importance for user "acceptance" of the services provided and also for the final "value" (Parasuraman, A., Berry, L.L. and Zeithaml, V.A., 1991) attributed to the public system of healthcare services. The trilogy for quality management (Juran, J.M., 1988), is consisting of Quality Planning, Quality Control and Quality Improvement. Quality planning involves identification of customers and their needs, and development of products to satisfy customer needs, and processes to produce those product attributes. Quality control involves evaluation of the gap between actual and targeted quality performances and the actions to fill the gap. Quality improvement deals with development of infrastructure, identification of improvement goals, establishment of project teams and allocation of resources to implement quality improvement projects.

The approach based on user satisfaction, considers the expectation measurement as information which is not inextricably linked to quality. Satisfaction is a cognitive state *(it follows the implementation of the service)* and derives from service quality. Moreover, it offers additional information such as meeting the needs *(expressed and implied),* perceived performance, perceived value of services and assessment of the benefit deriving from services. Therefore, according to this approach, quality determines the level of user satisfaction following a comprehensive assessment of the service provided. Similar approaches are the "service performance" (SERVPERF) which defines quality as equal to the user's performance perception of the service (*Service Quality = perceived performance*) and the approach of Teas (Teas, R.K., 1993), which presents a weighted SERVPERF model: *Service Quality = perceived importance × perceived performance.* A different approach is the one based on expectations as well as on disconfirmation of user expectations. In this case, the established model is the SERVQUAL "Service Quality" model (Parasuraman, A., Zeithaml, V., Berry, L.L., 1985). Moreover, within this approach Service Quality (SQ) is measured by comparing Perceptions "P" with Expectations "E" and is defined as the difference between perceptions and expectations (SQ=P - E). Regardless of the numerous distinct views voiced within the framework of this specific approach, (Liljander, V. and Strandvik, T., 1997) it is agreed that the user perceives "high" quality when perceived performance exceeds his or her expectations. Another broadly known methodology relating to the expectation disconfirmation approach lies in the expectation disconfirmation model (Oliver, R.L., 1996). The expectation concept is gradually incorporated into scientific approaches to Total Quality Management (Perkins, W.St., 1993) (Donaldson, W.G., 1995).

SERVICE QUALITY IN HEALTHCARE

Service quality is relating to meets customers satisfaction needs, leading to the investigation of preserved service quality in order to understand customers. Preserved quality is the difference between customers' expectation and their perceptions of the actual service received. Customer satisfaction is an individual emotional response to the evaluation of an object (or a service) (Parasuraman, A., Zeithaml, V., Berry, L.L., 1985).

It is difficult to measure service quality due to fewer tangible cues available when customers purchase services (Parasuraman, A., Zeithaml, V., Berry, L.L., 1985), fewer search properties but higher in experience and credence properties (Parasuraman, A., Zeithaml, V., Berry, L.L., 1985), as compared to services. There are a number of different definitions as to what is meant by service quality. One that is commonly used defines service quality as the extent to which a service meets customers' needs or expectations. Service quality can thus be defined as the difference between customer expectations of service and perceived service. If expectations are greater than performance, then perceived quality is less than satisfactory and hence customer dissatisfaction occurs.

Although the SERVQUAL model has raised debates about dimensionality, the need to measure expectations, the reliability and validity of difference-score formulation, and the interpretation of expectations, it have been the predominant method used to measure consumers' perceptions of service quality. It represents a multiitem scale that can be used for measuring expectations and perceptions of service quality- as perceived among consumers. The SERVQUAL model, a 22-item scale has five generic dimensions or factors and is stated as follows: (1) Tangibles, (2) Reliability, (3) Responsiveness, (4) Assurance, (5) Empathy (Figure 1). When referring to surveys related to healthcare institutions the dimensions of service quality can be adjusted as follows:

1. **Reliability:** Ability to perform the service dependably and accurately
2. **Tangibles:** Appearance of physical facilities and provision of appropriate equipment
3. **Responsiveness**: Willingness to help customers
4. **Assurance:** The knowledge of employees and their ability to inspire trust and confidence.
5. **Empathy:** The caring individualized attention the firm provides to its customers.

It is important to note that without adequate information on both the quality of services expected and perceptions of services received then feedback from customer surveys can be highly misleading from both a policy and an operational perspective. To improve quality services to these customers we must first of all understand their

Figure 1. SERVQUAL's five dimensions

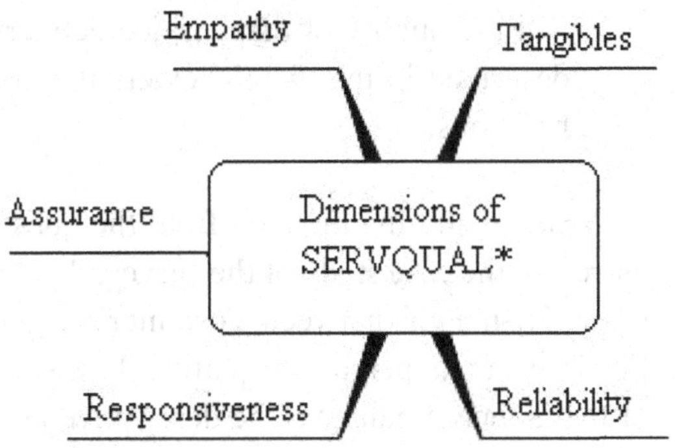

needs. In order to understand their needs, we must in turn understand the quality attributes embraced by the customers. People perceive quality differently.

When analyzing the data gathered most of the surveys are based on the '**gap theory**', that is, the difference between clients' expectations about performance of a service and their assessment of the actual performance of service. For example 'gap theory' in healthcare context has been used to develop a number of questions in order to compare what customers 'look for' (expect) and what they 'experience' from doctors, equipments, healthcare services e.t.c.

It is important to note, that the SERVQUAL is designed to investigate the aforementioned gap; nevertheless it is important to recognize the existence of four other gaps:

- **The understanding gap:** The difference between what consumers expect of a service and what management perceives consumers to expect.
- **The design gap:** The difference between the management perceives and consumers expect and the quality specifications set for service delivery.
- **The delivery gap:** The difference between the quality specifications set for service delivery and the actual quality of that service delivery.

- **The communications gap:** The difference between the actual quality of service delivery and the quality of that service delivery as described in the 'firm's' external communications.

When gathering the data from the questionnaires, in the case study of the survey, there may be a 'mismatch' between customer's expectations and their perceived quality. The analysis of the gathered data may be descriptive as well as inferential. A researcher assessed the scale's reliability by calculating the *Cronbach alpha*; for analyzing the service quality, the mean and the standard deviation scores for each of the items were calculated for the perception level (P) and the expectation levels (E). The mean perception scores were compared to the mean expectation scores for the various customer requirements and the design characteristics, so as to identify the Gap scores (P-E=Gap). The underlying dimensionality was tested through an exploratory factor analysis conducted on each of the correlation matrices of the perception, expectation, and Gap scores. The QDF matrix was framed with rows representing 'customer requirements'-'what'- and the columns representing the 'design characteristics'-'how'. Customers were asked the level of importance they assigned to the different customer requirements. They were also asked to give their perception of the relationship between items of each row and the items of each column. Thereafter the *QDF* matrix was used, wherein the respondent was required to specify the relationship between the customer requirements and design characteristics. Finally, the quality function deployment technique along with correlation analysis was used to identify the minimum set of design elements (synonymous to the quality components) able to cover the customer requirements.

Current literature on SERVQUAL applications in healthcare services describes variations of the initial model according to the following: (Robledo, M.A., 2001)

- The first category of the SERVQUAL model variations deals with the definition of different dimensions and/or service characteristics in order to measure quality (Brady, M.K., Cronin, J.J., Brand, R.R., 2002) (Conway, T., Willcocks, St., 1997) (Hwang, Li-Jen J., Eves, A., Desombre, T., 2003). In this specific field, it is hard to be original and consequently, similar characteristics are presented in dissimilar forms.
- The second category of SERVQUAL refers to the introduction or the non-introduction of different weight in the dimensions and/or characteristics. This way, models with similar or different weights are produced. The Overall Service Quality (OSQ) is estimated by the main value of the five dimensions. The weights employed in SERVQUAL models arise either by introducing a third section of questions for the estimation of weight by the users themselves or by the personnel in the organization through preliminary empirical studies *(structured survey or interview)* or through a combination of the aforementioned.
- The last category of the SERVQUAL model variations relates to the measurement scales employed. The Likert measurement scales may be identical or distinct per measurement section (perceptions, expectations and/or importance). The choice of scale is made on the basis of the respondents' understanding, the required level of sensitivity and the impact on the internal reliability of the questionnaire. The latest approaches to service quality (Rose, R. Ch., Uli, J., Abdul, M., Ng, K.L., 2004) (Butler, T., Kendra, J., Grimley, R., Taylor, B., 1996) (Kandampully, J., 1997) (Sohail, M.S., 2003) (Zimeras S., Lambrinoudakis C., Fournaridis G., Fournaridis I, 2005) involve a uniform high sensitivity Likert scale.

Figure 2. Likert scale

☹ 😐 ☺

0 1 2 3 4 5 6 7 8 9 10

(very low level) *(neutral)* *(very high level)*

In the SERVQUAL model gaps between user service perceptions and expectations are known as GAP 5. Gaps arise either when the service falls short of the user's expectations or when the service fails to meet the user's needs. Numerous surveys conducted in health services have provided information about GAP 5 (Butler, T., Kendra, J., Grimley, R., Taylor, B., 1996) (Kandampully, J., 1997) (Sohail, M.S., 2003). The *"Gap Zone"* is divided into positive (expectations exceed to a great extent user perceptions), intermediate (discrepancy observed between expectations and perceptions is not striking) and negative (expectations fall short of user perceptions). The extent of each of these zones allows the categorization of the GAP 5 SERVQUAL score gaps. The intermediate zone is of utmost importance because it relates to healthcare services that are generally considered tolerable (neither satisfying nor dissatisfying) by users and this is called Zone of Tolerance.

DATA ANALYSIS PROCEDURES

Some researchers, in order to test whether the initial conceptual framework was optimal, they use two types of factor analyses, namely exploratory factor analysis (EFA) and confirmatory factor analysis (CFA), followed by reliability analysis and qualitative analysis. Confirmatory factor analysis is first performed to evaluate the validity of the original SERVQUAL conceptual framework. Exploratory factor analysis is then performed for determining the number and structure of the dimensions that are underlying the data. Then the resulted dimensions from the exploratory factor analysis are then confirmed again by using the confirmatory factor analysis and reliability analysis. The derived dimensions and items are then compared with the findings of qualitative analysis for its validity and usefulness.

The use of statistical methodologies comprising multivariate analysis techniques (Mardia, K.V., Kent, J.I., Bibby, M., 1979) may elucidate the variables of overriding importance for the complex problems under investigation and depict correlations. Multivariate statistics provide the ability to analyze complex sets of data. Multivariate statistics are provided for analysis where there are many independent and possible dependent variables, which are correlated to each other to varying degrees. The method of principal components allows the replacement of the plethora of interrelated variables by groups of factors (hypothetical sections) exhibiting similar behavior to the major statistical variables. Principal components analysis (PCA) was applied to a single set of variables to discover which sets of variables form coherent subsets that are relatively independent of one another (Zimeras, S., Kostagiolas P. and Lambrinoudakis C., 2007).

Also cluster analysis could be considered in cases we investigate the effectiveness of the characteristics into spatial regions. Using this technique, we could justify which regions are important so we could direct our analysis to these areas. Cluster analysis is a technique used to classify objects into relatively homogeneous groups called clusters. Objects in each cluster tend to be similar to each other and dissimilar with objects in the other clusters (Malhotra N.K. and Birks H. 2003). A very useful graph in displaying clustering results is the dendrogram. The dendrogram is read from left to right. It shows where the clusters are joined together as well as the distance at which the clusters are jointed. It is very useful to decide the appropriate number of clusters.

In recent years, there has been an unprecedented demand for measures of quality in the healthcare industry. It is therefore crucial to develop effective tools for monitoring the quality of the medical services offered. Furthermore, in order to ensure the reliability of the results it is necessary to have a large number of patients, and in some cases medical personnel, participating in the evaluation process. With respect to healthcare, information services and the internet provides a unique platform that enables the creation of important information systems that can be accessed from anywhere and any time. The goal is to establish a consistent level of e-support to healthcare professional learners of Total Quality Management concepts, quality methods and tools.

Brainstorming, fishbone diagram, flowchart, run sheet, Pareto analysis, control chart and histogram are some of the tools that can help to zero in on quality problems. Quality function deployment helps to concentrate on customer needs while developing new services. For example *brainstorming* is a systematic approach to generate ideas from a group. A brainstorming group consists of individuals who can help to develop ideas relevant to a problem to be solved. Each individual suggests ideas (or directions) without regard to their validity. After all ideas are collected, they are critically reviewed. Brainstorming is a method to identify problems, develop ideas and improve creativity. Also *fishbone diagram* is a graphical approach to represent "cause and effect". The effect is desired outcome and causes are the spines. In practice most applications will have more branches where there will be a single outcome that we wish to improve or eliminate. A well drawn fishbone diagram can help to detect effects of quality quickly so that an alternative action can be taken. An alternative would be a tree diagram, which is much easier to follow. Finally a *control chart* essentially presents the expected range of variations in a stable process. A process is stable when all the data points fall within the prescribed control limits. Control chart is an excellent technique to monitor a process which is subject to variations. The control chart is a graphical representation of hypothesis testing. All these tools could be used for different purposes, considering the needs of the individual groups (doctors, technicians, administrative department, etc.)

CONSIDERATIONS FOR THE STRATEGIC EVALUATION OF TELEHEALTH SYSTEMS

The following aspects should be studied, criticized and adopted or adapted (Figure 3).

Figure 3. Telehealth evaluation aspects

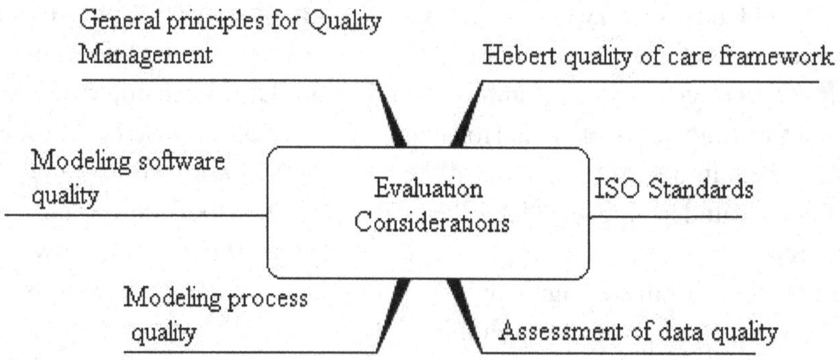

The Hebert Quality of Care Framework In Telehealth Applications

The Hebert Quality of Care framework (Hebert, M., 2001) contains inquiring questions related with the Quality of Care. For patients, providers and organizations the structure, the process and the outcomes are studied.

With regard to the *structure*, the individuals that participate in studies for the evaluation of quality of Information Systems in Health usually are individuals that have the study problem and after they are informed on this, they accept or not to participate. During the selection of these individuals we want not to be connected as relatives, to belong in a wide age-related spectrum, be from different regions and suffer from the same illness. Each one of them can participate for various personal reasons. Nevertheless they exist probably also other reasons. Somebody with a chronic/serious disease needs intensive medical follow-up and probably the intervention of an expert. Persons that live in borders and inaccessible areas are those with the bigger need and who will profit more from the program. Usually these patients have minimal alternative solutions for provision of care. The health care providers are selected on the basis of criteria that are determined by each research framework. They should be the more suitable and most capable for the particular place. They participate in the studies in order to contribute in the growth of their company, for projection, research and mainly in order to provide the better possible services of health in the patients. Alternative solutions for the providers exist but usually they choose the most lucrative for the interest of the company. Good provision of services ensures satisfied customers and consequently good quality. To provide services using a Health Information System their training is necessary. The organizations that use these technologies can be public or private health care providers. Various types of technology have been adopted. Computational systems, medical instruments, robotics, high performance computing and communications, videoconferencing contribute in the implementation of Telemedicine services.

With regard to the *process* the relation patient-doctor using telehealth is not anymore direct but indirect. The patient may not have personal contact with his doctor but he is provided the same medical care from distance. To achieve this a medical patient record should exist. Health care providers feel "comfortably" offering care with the use of electronic means, because they can offer more, time is saved from them and better service of patients exists. Nevertheless they are certain questions which influence the benefit of care with the use of telemedicine/telehealth technologies. Specialized personnel is needed and specialized patients to have knowledge of computers and be capable to handle the new technology. Via this technology the organizations want to achieve prevention, clinical care, even social support.

As far as the *outcomes* are concerned patient satisfaction is one of the desirable results. It becomes perceptible from the comments of patient on the program of care, but also from the perceptible improvement of his/her health. The outcomes that are important from the patient side are mainly the patient requirements satisfaction from the program. If the patient is satisfied and the program is characterized by ease of use then its success is ensured. The customer indications give useful information, empiric elements and indications for the needs, expectations and wishes, essential elements for the determination of objectives for customer satisfaction. From the health information systems and the interventions related to telehealth all patients can benefit from but mainly these with chronic diseases, these in some critical stage of health, and those that live far from health care centers. The organizations apply/adapt the technology depending on their needs and with that they want to use. The organizations change the initial way of technology use after certain comments from the patients, the providers or other colleagues in the organization. Success for a program is to achieve its initial aim, while at the same time increases its quality. The recording of these incidents becomes with many different ways. Usually via evaluation questionnaires or a Process Failure Mode Effects Analysis.

ISO Standards

According to the International Standards Organization, the ISO standards define the requirements for products of advanced technology, services, mechanisms, materials and systems, for evaluations of good conformity and for administrative and organizational applications. The most known existing models for quality certification are the Maturity Model in USA and the ISO standards that are recognized on International level (Saiedian, H. and McClanahan, L., 1995). A product to be imported in the European Union should be ISO- compatible. (Rada, R., 1996)

- **ISO 9000:** The International Standards Organization has developed a series of ISO standards for quality certification. Up to the 70's existed various models for the determination of quality. In November 1992, the countries of the European Union agreed to use ISO 9000 as the national model of quality (Dadoun, G., 1992)

ISO 9000 refers to quality management. This means that "an organization is supposed to satisfy the requirements of the customer for quality and the applicable regulating requirements, while at the same time it aims at continuous improvement of efforts".

ISO is divided in the parts 9001, 9002 and 9003. ISO 9001 refers in activities as planning, growth, production, installation and maintenance, ISO 9002 is applied in the production and installation and ISO 9003 covers the final control and trial (Dadoun, G., 1992). In the year 2000, the series 9001, 9002 and 9003 were included in ISO 9001:2000. This is the only standard in the ISO 9000 family that is certified by an external agency.

- ISO 9004: 2000: It extends the advantages of ISO 9001:2000 in all the interested teams (e.g. employees, employers, owners, providers and society). The 8 principles for quality management that are formulated in ISO 9000:2000 & ISO 9004:2000 are:
  - **Principle 1:** Focus in the customer
  - **Principle 2:** Leadership
  - **Principle 3:** Collaboration of individuals
  - **Principle 4:** Process based approach
  - **Principle 5:** Systemic approach in the Administration
  - **Principle 6:** Continuous improvement
  - **Principle 7:** Realistic approach in decision-making
  - **Principle 8:** Mutually beneficial relations of suppliers

These principles form the basis for requirements for ISO 9004:2000.

ISO 9000:2000 and ISO 9004:2000 have been designed as a single pair of standards, for easier use and flexibility. Starting from 9001:2000 a first level of performance can be reached. Applying then ISO 9004:2000 a more efficient system of quality management can be achieved.

ISO 9004-4 refers to the Administration of Quality and in the elements of Quality Systems. The 4th part provides governing directives for the Administration, so that Continuous Quality Improvement is applied in an organization.

- **ISO 15504 or SPICE:** Additional to ISO 9001. It offers confidence in the quality management of the suppliers and a framework that determines if the candidate suppliers are suitable. It also helps the evaluation process.

- **ISO 9126:** It is a extensive model for the sector of Medical Informatics. ISO 9126 provides a framework for the estimation of software quality. According to this the six characteristics of software quality are: Functionality, Reliability, Usability, Performance, Maintainability, and Portability.
- **ISO 15504 in comparison with ISO 9001:** ISO standards ensure the continuous improvement of quality; the user knows that he has to deal with regularly qualitatively products and services (Hysell, D., 1999). They provide better perception of quality, better recording of processes and control of operations. Due to the permanently increasing need for qualitative products and services, more companies record the processes, their tactics of operation and their organizational duties (Schuler, K., 1996).

The need for certifications of safety or interoperability helped in the growth of Information Technology Standards of safety (Ferris, J.M., 1994). These are developed under accreditations of the International Standards Organization and depending on the specifications that follow they can be characterized as international, national or even local.

ISO 9000 was developed for industrial operations (Averill, E., 1994). For software operations it was needed an extension that was given with the creation ISO 9000-3. ISO 9000 is important because (Rada, R., 1996) it provides directives with regard to the way that an enterprise will improve the quality and promotion of her products. The conformity of an organization with the ISO 9000 can be checked from the organization, or from the one in which are addressed the products or the services provided by this organization, or from a third independent organization that is specialized clearly in such certifications. For an organization to be certified, both its documentation and its human potential should follow the specifications of quality. Despite the fact that ISO 9000 began for constructional companies and organizations, it is also extended also in the health sector, where the certification of quality is very important. The certificates provided by certain third persons, are more prone in errors due to the involvement of the human factor (Ungureanu, V., 2001).

Assessment of Data Quality

A model has been proposed for data quality measurement from the user viewpoint. (Cappiello, C., Francalanci, C., Pernici, B., 2004). According to this, the users are separated in age-groups, where each age-group is constituted by users with common characteristics. The age-group of user selector determines which dimensions of data quality will be delivered with the information that the user has asked. The service sends the demand in the selector and depending on the characteristics of age-group of user, the department of evaluation sends in the end the data in the user with the results from quality evaluation. If the information is of low quality, that is to say if the requirements of user are not satisfied, an alert message is presented.

MedCritic system and the QUIL (Quality Indicator Language) are another way of quality evaluation (Advani, A., Shahar, Y., Musen, M. A., 2002). QUIL allows the determination quality indicators and the modeling of the medical directives so that the determination of quality from the side of patient is easier.

Another way of quality measurement from the user viewpoint is the protection of his/her personal data. A model exists (Kam, L.E. and Chismar, W.G., 2003) which combines the discretion in the collection of data from the patients, with the sensitivity of content and the qualitative feedback. A secure platform has been proposed (Taylor, K.L., O'Keefe, C.M., Colton, J., Baxter, R., Sparks, R., Srinivasan, U., Cameron, M.A., and Lefort, L. A., 2004), for personal data named Health Research Data Network (HRDN).

The collection of medical histories should have evident definitions of data, settled guidelines and specialized personnel for this purpose (Arts, D. G. T., de Keizer, N. and Scheffer, G. J., 2002). The guarantee of data quality depends from the prevention, the localization and the actions that will follow (Knatterud, G.L., Rockhold, F.W., George, S.L., Barton, F.B., Davis, C.E., Fairweather, W.R., Honohan, T., Mowery, R. and O'Neil, R., 1998).

Modelling Process Quality

A quality model for information technology systems has been proposed (Marchetti, C., Pernici, B., and Plebani, P.A., 2004) that separates evidently the planning of services, from the network and the devices. The quality as conceived by the user in such a system mainly depends from the quality of the media that are used for the provision of services (network, devices) and less from the quality the services it provides. The supplier of services and the user of services sign a contract agreement for the quality of services. This contract describes the offered quality level with regard to the quality of data, the safety and the availability. It is supported (Nejmeh, B. A., 1995) that the best methods of evaluation of progress of processes are: SEI (Software Engineering Institute) CMM (Capability Maturity Model), ISO9000, Tick-IT, SPICE (Software Process Improvement and Capability dEtermination) and the Malcolm Baldrige National Quality Award.

Modelling Software Quality

- McCall's Quality Model (McCall, J., Richards, P., and Walters, G., 1977): It describes the quality as relation between the factors, the criteria and metrics of quality (Ward, W.A. and Venkataraman, B., 1999).

Quality measurement is performed in the following steps:

1. Identification of all factors that can influence software quality
2. Recognition of criteria for each factor.
3. Definition of metrics for each criterion and determination of relation between metric and all the criteria that are reported in each factor
4. Assessment of metrics
5. Correlation of metrics with a line of directives that should follows each team of software development
6. Development of recommendations for metrics collection

- ISO 9126 (see aforementioned description)
- Dromey model (Dromey, R. G., 1995) is based on the following steps for the development of software quality models. In the first step, we define the attributes of high quality. Then we determine analytically the various parts of a product, and for each part we categorize the most important properties of quality. Afterwards we propose connections between the quality-carrying properties and the quality attributes. We repeat the aforementioned steps using a process of assessment and perfection.

General Principles for Quality Management

The fact that a lot of models exist for the improvement of quality can mean two things: either it is very difficult to model right the quality or it is impossible (Saturno P.J., 1999). The right collection, verification and interpretation of data is one of the most usual problems for the cost of data quality (Keogh W., Atkins M.H., Dalrymple J.F., 2000). Further research is needed in order to clarify the long-lasting dimensions of telemedicine and the derived results in the expenses of health (Roine, R., Ohinmaa, A., Hailey, D., 2001).

According to the Centre for Human services, any measure that improves the quality can be considered as Quality Assurance (QA). Usually it is constituted from a QA tool, a QA approach and a QA program. Teams from a variety of health care organizations have reported the successful usage of methods like team work, flow charts, data collection and graphic analysis of data (Plsek P.E., 1999).

Statistical Process Control (SPC) and various other examples of practical applications of control charts have been used in health care (Benneyan J.C., Lloyd R. C., Plsek P. E., 2003). Almost all these models have the same steps: "planning-monitoring –improvement".

To achieve quality at low cost is essential the adoption and use of methods as the Continuous Quality Improvement (CQI) or the Total Quality Management (TQM) (Shortell, S.M., Bennett, C. L., and Buck, G. R., 1998). CQI it is the continuous improvement of processes performed to offer a service that corresponds in the needs and expectations of customers.

There are quality concepts and criteria to record quality. The engineers and managers are responsible for the quality during the process of the construction of a product. Quality metrics check how much the product corresponds in the requirements of the customer. ISO and other standards have as basic condition the installation, maintenance and control of recorded remaining processes.

The challenge is in the planning of models that keep pace with good medical practice (Abston, C. K., Pryor, A.T., Haug, P.J., Anderson J.L., 1997). The implementation guidelines should include rules for when we begin and / or we avoid interventions in health care.

There are also data mining challenges (Kastania, A.N., 2004) in the design of telehealth platforms that should be taken into account during the telehealth quality and reliability evaluation process. Especially those related with intelligent decision systems participation in the evaluation process of telemedicine models for primary care (Kastania, A.N., 2004).

CONCLUSION

Herein, we have investigated aspects related to quality and reliability assurance in telehealth. We have defined quality and service quality in healthcare combined with data analysis strategies based on SERVQUAL as a tool for reliability assurance. Finally we have presented a set of considerations for the strategic evaluation of quality in telehealth systems.

REFERENCES

Abston, C. K., Pryor, A.T., Haug, P.J., Anderson J.L. (1997). Introducing practice guidelines from a hospital database. Presented at the *Proc/AMIA Annu Fall Symp (1997)*, (pp. 168–172).

Advani, A., Shahar, Y., Musen, M. A., Medical Quality Assessment by Scoring Adherence to Guideline Intentions (2002). *Journal of the American Medical Informatics Association, 9*(6), S92-S97.

Angelopoulou, P., Kangis, P., Babis, G. (1998). Private and public medicine: A comparison of quality perceptions. *Int. Journal of Health Care Quality Assurance,11*(1), 14-20.

Arts, D. G. T., de Keizer, N. and Scheffer, G. J. (2002). Defining and improving data quality in medical registries: A literature review, case study, and generic framework. *J Am Med Inform Assoc, 9*(6), 600-611.

Athanasopoulos, A., Gounaris, Sp., Stathakopoulos, V. (2001). Behavioural responses to customer satisfaction: An empirical Study. *European Journal of Marketing,35*,(5/6), 687-707.

Averill, E. (1994). Reference models and standards. *StandardView*, 2(2), 96-109.

Benneyan J.C., Lloyd R. C., Plsek P. E. (2003). Statistical process control as a tool for research and healthcare improvement, *Qual Saf Health Care, 12*, 458-464.

Brady, M.K., Cronin, J.J., Brand, R.R. (2002). Performance-only measurement of service quality: A replication and extension. *Journal of Business Research, 55*, 17– 31.

Butler, T., Kendra, J., Grimley, R., Taylor, B. (1996). Can we measure the effectiveness of our organizations. *International Journal of Health Care Quality Assurance, 9*(5), 37-38.

Cameron, K.S. and Whetten, D.A. (1983). Some Conclusions about Organisational Effectiveness. In K.S. Cameron and D.A. Whetten, (Eds.). *Organisational Effectiveness: A Comparison of Multiple Models*. New York: Academic Press, (pp. 261-277).

Cappiello, C., Francalanci, C., Pernici, B. (2004). Data quality assessment from the user's perspective, Information Quality in Informational Systems. In *Proceedings of the 2004 international workshop on Information quality in information systems*. Paris, France, (pp.68 – 73), ISBN:1-58113-902-0.

Conway, T., Willcocks, S. (1997). The role of expectations in the perception of health care quality: developing a conceptual model. *International Journal of Health Care Quality Assurance, , 10*(3), 131–140.

Dadoun, G. (1992). ISO 9000 a requirement for doing business. IBM Centre for Advanced Studies Conference. In *Proceedings of the 1992 conference of the Centre for Advanced Studies on Collaborative research*. Toronto, Ontario, Canada, SESSION: Software engineering environment, vol.1, (pp. 433-437).

DeLone, W. H. and McLean E. R. (2002). Information success revisited. *Presented at Hawaii International Conference on System Sciences*. Big Island, Hawaii.

Donabedian, A. (1988). *Quality assessment and assurance: unity of purpose, diversity of means, Inquiry, 25*, 173-192.

Donaldson, W.G. (1995). Manufacturers need to show greater commitment to customer-service. *Industrial Marketing Management, 24*, 421–430.

Dromey, R. G. (1995). A model for software product quality. *IEEE Transactions on Software Engineering, 21*(2), 146-162.

Ferris, J. M. (1994). Using standards as a security policy tool. *StandardView, 2*(2), 72-77.

Grigoroudis, E. & Siskos, Y. (2002). Preference disaggregation for measuring and analysing customer satisfaction: The MUSA method, *European Journal of Operational Research, 143*, 148-170.

Harvey, J., (1998). Service Quality: A tutorial. *Journal of Operations Management, 16*, 583-597.

Hasin, M. A. A., Seeluangsawat, R., & Shareef, M.A. (2001). Statistical measures of customer satisfaction for hospital health-care quality assurance: a case study. *International Journal of Health Care Quality Assurance, 14*(1), 6-14.

Hebert, M. (2001). Telehealth success: Evaluation framework development. *Presented at Medinfo*. 10 (Pt 2), pp. 1145-9.

Hwang, Li-Jen J., Eves, A., Desombre, T. (2003). Gap analysis of patient meal service perceptions. *International Journal of Health Care Quality Assurance, 16*(3), 143-153.

Hysell, D. (1999). ISO 9001: Traditions before and after. ACM Special Interest Group for Design of Communication. *Presented at the proceedings of the 17th annual international conference on Computer Documentation*. New Orleans, Louisiana, United States, (pp. 99-104), ISBN: 1-58113-072-4.

Juran, J.M. (1988). Juran's Quality Control Handbook. In J.M. Juran, (Ed.) *Fourth edition*, New York: McGraw-Hill Book Company.

Kam, L.E. and Chismar, W.G. (2003), A self-disclosure model for personal health information.

HICSS. In *Proceedings of the 36th Annual Hawaii International Conference on System Sciences (HICSS'03) - Track 6 - Volume 6*, (pp.161.2), ISBN: 0-7695-1874-5.

Kandampully, J. (1997). Firms should give loyalty before they can expect it from customers. *Managing Service Quality, 7(2)*, 92-94.

Kastania, A.N. (2004). Telemedicine models for primary care. In R. Latifi (Ed), *Establishing telemedicine in developing Countries: from inception to implementation.*. Amsterdam: IOS Press.

Kastania, A.N. (2004). Data mining challenges in the design of Telemedicine platforms. In R. Latifi, (Ed.), *Establishing telemedicine in developing countries: from inception to implementation.* Amsterdam: IOS Press.

Knatterud, G.L., Rockhold, F.W., George, S.L., Barton, F.B., Davis, C.E., Fairweather, W.R., Honohan, T., Mowery, R. and O'Neill, R. (1998). Guideliness for quality assurance in multicenter trials: A position paper. *Controlled Clinical Trials 19*, 477-493.

Keogh W., Atkins M.H., Dalrymple J.F. (2000). Data collection and the economics of quality: Identifying problems. In *Proceedings of the 4th International and 7th National Research Conference on Quality Management*. Sydney. Retrieved 24 December 2007 from http://mams.rmit.edu.au/kh85606qs2qn.pdf

Lewis, B.R and Mitchell, V.W. (1990). Defining and measuring the quality of customer service. *Marketing Intelligence and Planning, 8*, 11–17.

Liljander, V. and Strandvik, T. (1994). Estimating zones of tolerance in perceived service quality and perceived service value. *Int. Journal of Service Industry Management, 2*, 6–28.

Liljander, V. and Strandvik, T. (1997). Emotions in service satisfaction. *International Journal of Service Industry Management, 8*(2), 148 – 169.

Lin, B. and Kelly, E. (1995). Methodological issues in patient satisfaction surveys. *International Journal of Health Care Quality Assurance, 8*(6), 32-37.

Mardia, K.V., Kent, J.I., Bibby, M. (1979). *Multivariate analysis, 1st ed.* Academic Press.

Marchetti, C., Pernici, B., and Plebani, P.A. (2004). Quality model for multichannel adaptive information systems. In *Proceedings of the 13th international World Wide Web conference on Alternate track papers & posters.* New York, Quality of service, (pp.48 – 54). ISBN: 1-58113-912-8.

Malhotra N.K. and Birks H. (2003). *Marketing research, an applied approach.* Harlow: Prentice Hall.

McCall, J., Richards, P. and Walters, G. (1977), *Factors in software quality.* RADC-TR-77-369, US Department of Commerce.

Merkouris, A., Yfantopoulos, J., Lanara, V., Lemonidou, C. (1999). Developing an instrument to measure patient satisfaction with nursing care in Greece. *Journal of Nursing Management, 7*, 91-100.

Moumtzoglou, A., Dafogianni, C., Karra, V., Michailidou, D., Lazarou, P. and Bartsocas, C. (2000). Development and application of a questionnaire for assessing parent satisfaction with care. *Int J Qual Health Care, 12*(4), 331-337.

Nejmeh, B. A. (1995). Process cost and value analysis. *Communications of the ACM, 38*(6), 19-24.

Oliver, R. L. (1996). *Satisfaction: A behavioral perspective on the consumer.* McGraw-Hill Education,.

Ovretveit, J. (2000). The economics of quality. *International Journal of Health Care Quality Assurance, 13*(5), 200-207.

Parasuraman, A., Zeithaml, V., Berry, L.L. (1985). A conceptual model of service quality and its implications for future research. *Journal of Marketing, 49*, 41-50.

Parasuraman, A., Berry, L. L., Zeithaml, V. A., (1988). SERVQUAL: A multiple-item scale for measuring customer perceptions of service quality. *Journal of Retailing, 64*, 12–40.

Parasuraman, A., Berry, L.L. and Zeithaml, V. A. (1991). Understanding customer expectations of service. *Sloan Management Review*, 39-48.

Perkins, W.St. (1993). Measuring customer satisfaction. *Industrial Marketing Management, 22*, 247–254.

Plsek P. E. (1999). Quality improvement methods in clinical medicine. *Pediatrics, 103*(1), 203-214.

Rada, R., (1996). ISO 9000 reflects the best in standards. *Communications of the ACM, 39* (3), 17-20.

Robinson, St. (1999). Measuring service quality: current thinking and future requirements. *Marketing Intelligence & Planning, 17*(1), 21-32.

Robledo, M. A. (2001). Measuring and managing service quality: Integrating customer expectations. *Managing Service Quality, 11*(1), 22-31.

Roine, R., Ohinmaa, A., Hailey, D. (2001). Assessing telemedicine: A systematic review of the literature. *Canadian Medical Association Journal, 165*(6), 765-771.

Rose, R., Uli, J., Abdul, M. and Ng, K. (2004). Hospital service quality: a managerial challenge. *International Journal of Health Care Quality Assurance, 17*, 146–59.

Saiedian, H. and McClanahan, L. (1995). A study of two frameworks for quality software process, presented at the Symposium on Applied Computing. In *Proceedings of the 1995 ACM symposium on Applied computing, Nashville*. Tennessee, United States, (pp.434-439). ISBN:0-89791-658-1.

Saturno P. J., (1999). Quality in Health Care: models, labels and terminology. *International Journal for Quality in Health Care, 11*(5), 373-374.

Schuler, K. (1996). Preparing for ISO 9000 registration: the role of the technical communicator, ACM Special Interest Group for Design of Communication. In *Proceedings of the 13th annual international conference on Systems documentation: emerging from chaos: Solutions for the growing complexity of our jobs***.** Savannah, Georgia, United States, (pp.148-154). ISBN:0-89791-713-8.

Seddon, P. B., Staples, S., Patnayakuni, R. and Bowtell, M., (1999). Dimensions of information systems success. *Communications of the Association of Information Systems, 2*(20) .

Shortell, S.M., Bennett, C. L., and Buck, G. R. (1998). Assessing the impact of continuous quality improvement on clinical practice: What it will take to accelerate progress. *The Milbank Quarterly, 76*(4), 593-624.

Sohail, M. S. (2003). Service quality in hospitals: More favourable than you might think. *Managing Service Quality, 13*(9), 197- 206.

Taylor, K. L., O'Keefe, C. M., Colton, J., Baxter, R., Sparks, R., Srinivasan, U., Cameron, M. A., and Lefort, L. A. (2004). Service oriented architecture for a health research data network. In *Proceedings of the 16th International Conference on Scientific and Statistical Database Management*, (pp.443- 444).

Teas, R. K. (1993). Expectations, performance evaluation and consumers' perceptions of quality. *Journal of Marketing, 57*, 18-34.

Thomas, W. and Cerino, D. A. (1995). Predicting software quality for reuse certification, presented at the Annual International Conference on Ada. In *Proceedings of the conference on TRI-Ada '95: Ada's role in global markets: solutions for a changing complex world*. Anaheim, California, United States, (pp.367-377). ISBN: 0-89791-705-7.

Ungureanu, V. (2001), A regulated approach to certificate management, ACSAC. In *Proceedings of the 17th Annual Computer Security Applications Conference*, (pp 377). ISBN: 0-7695-1405-7.

Ward, W.A. and Venkataraman, B. (1999). Some observations on Software Quality. In *Proceedings of the 37th annual Southeast regional conference.* (CD-ROM), Article No. 2. ISBN:1-58113-128-3.

Whitney, C. W., Lind, B. K. and Wahl, P. W. (1998). Quality Assurance and Quality Control in Longitudinal Studies. *Epidemiologic Reviews, 20*(1), 71-80.

Zimeras S., Lambrinoudakis C., Fournaridis G., Fournaridis I. (2005). An IT-based questionnaire system for the evaluation of healthcare services using electronic sampling techniques. *The Journal on Information Technology in Healthcare, 3*, 239–47.

Zimeras, S., Kostagiolas P. and Lambrinoudakis C. (2007). Quality evaluation in healthcare based on the assessment of services expectation using a web-based questionnaire system and adaptive sampling techniques. *The Journal on Information Technology in Healthcare, 5*(1), 50-58.

KEY TERMS

Telehealth Quality: The quality measurement of telehealth services should be based on product characteristics that contribute to user satisfaction and on product attributes that can be present or absent. In order to measure quality, the user view, the developer view, the product view and the value-based view should be considered.

Telehealth Reliability: Reliability is the probability that software will not cause the failure of the system for a specified time under specified conditions. For the reliability assessment, models exist that present graphically the number of failures of system operation in the time. When users think for software quality they usually mean the reliability on the basis of the existing reliability model: IEEE/ANSI standard 982.2. The code should be reliable according to the deviating views of individuals that develop software, check software or are users of software. A developer-based view focuses on software faults; if the developer has grounds for believing that the system is relatively fault-free then the system is assumed to be reliable. On the other hand a user-based view emphasizes the functions of the system and how often they fail.

Section IX
Data Evaluation, Validation, and Quality Aspects

Chapter XXXI
Quality of Health Information on the Internet

Kleopatra Alamantariotou
City University London, UK

ABSTRACT

Recent statistics show that the World Wide Web has now grown to over 100 million sites: a phenomenal expansion in only 15 years (Mulligan 2007). It has been estimated that there are 100,000 sites offering health related information (Wilson 2002). As the amount of health information increases, the public find it increasingly difficult to decide what to accept and what to reject (Burgess 2007). Searching for information on the internet is both deceptively easy and the same time frustratingly difficult (Kiley 2002). The challenge for consumers is to find high quality, relevant information as quickly as possible. There has been ongoing debate about the quality of information aimed at patients and the general public and opinions differ on how it can be improved (Stepperd 1999). The purpose of this chapter is to provide a brief overview of the different perspectives on information quality and to review the main criteria for assessing the quality of health information on the internet. Pointers are provided to enable both clinicians and patients find high quality information sources. An understanding of these issues should help health professionals and patients to make effective use of the internet..

INTRODUCTION

Health information includes information for staying healthy, preventing and managing disease, and making other decisions related to health and health care. It includes information for making decisions about health products and health services. It may be in the form of data, text, audio, and/or video. (Dzenowagis 2001)

The Internet provides a powerful tool for patients seeking medical information. It offers consumers access to a wealth of health and medical information that can enable them to take responsibility for their own health (Linkous 1999). Information is the communication or reception of knowledge. Such communication occurs in great part through the recording of knowledge(Taylor 2004). Some commentators predict that in the near future the Internet will be an important vehicle for delivering information and medical care. Tom Ferguson coined the term "e Patients" to define those people who were empowered to find medical answers for themselves, rather than rely on any single individual's opinion or interpretation. Virtual children's Hospital based the Internet's first medical Web site since 1993(Risk 2003).

The number of health related Web sites is rising with more 70,000 sites available to patients in 2000. A 2006 survey of 5,007 U.S. adults found that 84% of consumers claimed to have researched a health-related topic online in the past 12 months. (Fox 2006). Another survey reported that eighty percent of American Internet users (some 113 million adults) have searched for information on at least one of seventeen health topics. (Fox 2006). 75% of all adults on line (47% of all adults) use the Internet to look for health information. This amounts to 98 million adults nationwide. (David 2003). On average those who look for health information online do so on average 3.3 times every month(Fox 2006).

Faced with this explosion of online information the main challenge facing today's information consumer is how to find high quality information that meets their personal needs, within an acceptable time frame. But whilst everyone agrees that information quality is an important consideration, the concept of quality is problematic since in medicine there are often gray areas where the evidence-base is poor, making it difficult to determine a gold standard (Lewis 2005) Quality is an inherently subjective assessment, which depends on the type of the information needed, the type of the information searched for, and the particular qualities of the consumer (Wilson 2002). Experts believe that formal methods are needed to describe and assess information quality. Naumann maintains that "quality is the main discriminator of data and data sources on the Web" (Naumann 2001).

The paradox of quality as Robert Pirsing notes is the fact that "even though quality cannot be defined, you know what quality is" (Pirsing 1974). Although the typical consumer may be able to produce and define what quality means to them, each individual's perception of the quality of health information will vary depending upon their current circumstances and quality requirements (Burgess 2007).

A recurrent concern about online health information is that anyone is free to publish. Websites are set up by individuals, patient, charities, activist groups, commercial bodies either selling a product, as well as by health care professionals. The overwhelming majority of these resources are informal, quite often with no clinical input (Potts 2006).

RISKS POSED BY POOR QUALITY INFORMATION

It has never been easier for members of the public to access health information. In the twenty-first century it is taken for granted that patients may browse the Internet for the information about their condition, contact other patients by e-mail, send e-mails to their doctor or use touch screen kiosks in order to get health information (Jones et al 2005). But many believe there is a downside to this development. They fear that while the quantity of information has expanded exponentially, the same is not true for its quality. There is a concern in many professional groups about the potential harm associated with the use of poor quality health information. The quality of health information is of a particular concern because misinformation could be a matter of life and death (McClung 1998, Crocco 2002).

Harm in this context may be defined as adverse events or bad outcomes, either physical or emotional or financial, that occur from acting on materials or information and medication obtained from a Web site. On the other hand Crocco and collegues found only a few cases in the literature of harm associated with poor quality of health information on the Internet . In particular the authors report on a systematic review of peer-reviewed literature, to evaluate the number and characteristics, of reported cases of harm associated with the use of health information obtain on the Internet.(Crocco 2002).

In addition one way to demonstrate the amount of dubious health information online is to carry out a free text search using the phrase 'cancer cure'. The Web sites retrieved from this search contain cure-all remedies, based on scant or no medical evidence. At http://www.1cure4cancer.com for example, visitors are informed that Vitamin B17 kills cancer cells. The site fails to disclose the results of clinical trials into the effectiveness of this treatment. Ekman (2005) has investigated the prevalence and quality of interactive risk sites on the Internet. He found that the number of cancer risk sites increased by 50% between 2001-2002. Ekman's research study found that that the overall quality of the documentation on the cancer risk sites was poor. The majority of the cancer risk sites do not give reliable risks estimates. Similarly Lee et al (2003) found that thirty two percent of bladder cancer information sites contained inaccurate information. One critical problem was outdated data, rather than incurrent information.

Many of those searching for health information are looking for advice not about illness but ways of staying healthy or improving health. Furthermore disease information, material about weight control, and facts about prescription drugs top the lists of interests for health seekers. Many Website dealing with lifestyle choices and health are scams, particularly sites which shortcuts to weight loss and improvements in personal performance. Such sites frequently are devoid of scientific evidence, relying instead on anecdotes where personal experiences are presented as facts without references. Quite often sites with biased information only present one side of the argument. (Kiley 2003).

A longitudinal study (Pandolfini 2002). concluded that the quality of health information on the Internet had improved over the last 5 years. Nonetheless, the author concluded that people should continue to be alert as online information is not always accurate. In the absence of editorial controls, information may be of low quality and potentially harmful (Bower 1996). Poor interpretation of written information on medicines has been

Table 1. Wesite monitoring health frauds and quackery

Quackwatch — http://www.quackwatch.com • A member of Consumer Federation of America • A nonprofit corporation whose purpose is to combat health-related frauds, myths, fads, fallacies, and misconduct.
National Council Against Health Fraud — http://www.ncahf.org • A private, non-profit, voluntary health agency that focuses upon health misinformation, fraud and quackery as public health problems (NCAHF 2007).
Health Care Reality Checked and alternative medicine — http://www.hcrc.org (Kiley 2003).
American Council on Science and Health (ACSH) — http://www.acsh.org • A consumer education consortium concerned with issues related to food, nutrition, chemicals, pharmaceuticals, lifestyle, the environment and health • An independent, nonprofit organization (ACSH 2003).

shown to lead to anxiety and poor compliancy to therapy. Therefore there is a need for promoting and educating consumer search and appraisal skills when using this information. For instance as Peterson(2003) indicated educating customer to find information on medicines may help them use their medicines in safer and more effective way(Peterson 2003).

There are various Internet sites which monitor health frauds and quackery. These are summarised in Table 1.

REVIEW OF INITIATIVES TO IMPROVE QUALITY OF HEALTH INFORMATION

The quality of health information on the Internet became a subject of interest to healthcare professionals and consumers groups in the mid-1990s (Gagliardi 2002). This concern is prompted by a desire to prevent of physical, mental, and emotional harm caused by wrong, misleading, inappropriate, false, information to member of the public who use the Internet to seek or receive health information, products, and services (Dzenowagis 2001).

There have been a host of initiatives aimed at establishing criteria for judging the quality of online health information. These have produced policy document, tools to assist the development, implementation and evaluation process and various methods to determine how well Web-sites comply with the standards(in which case they can display a kitemark). The hope is that if developers adhere to the quality criteria, end users will be able to readily identify reputable sites (Ekman 2005). The European Union has also drafted guidelines on quality criteria for health Websites. However, there is no international consensus for how to deal with the quality issue problem (Jadad 1998, Eysenbach 1998).

The organizations who have created guidelines for evaluating health related Websites include

- Health On the Net (HON)
- American Medical Association
- Internet Health Care
- Coalition Hi-Ethics
- MedCertain

None of these guidelines have been systematically applied to a broad set of Web pages and conditions. Furthermore little research has been conducted to empirical assess what a consumer might find while searching on Internet (Berland et al 2002).

In conclusion the emphasis of the responsibility for the future access and quality of health information is placed on the medical informatics leaders who must understand: medicine and information disciplines. Health professionals need to be able to direct patients of good quality health information included health related Websites (Shepperd 1999).

The Judge Health guidelines were developed in partnership between Contact a Family (a UK charity) and the Information Society Research and Consultancy Group at Northumbria University (www.northumbria.ac.uk/isrc).

In addition the Judge project, supported by the Health Foundation developed guidelines in order to judge the quality of health information Web sites. Two sets of guidelines were produced: (i) to help health consumers make informed choice about Web sites.(ii) to assist some support groups to produce good quality Web sites. These were made available via www.judgehealth.org.uk.

The guidelines comprise four sections:

i. How to produce good quality information;
ii. How to design good quality Web sites;
iii. How to market Web sites;
v. How to help consumers use health information (Barnett 2006).

One of the more successful quality initiatives schemes has been developed by the Geneva based Health On Net Foundation (HON). The initiative is an expression of a self-regulatory mechanism. Self-regulation of the health Internet remains a powerful driver of the pursuit of quality standards for health information on the Internet (Dzenowagis 2001).

The HON code originally consisted of eight broad principles for medical Webmasters. Central to this code is the principle that any medical information must only be given by medically trained and qualified professionals. Where this condition cannot be met there must be clear confirmed that a piece of advice was given from a non-medically qualified individual or organization (HON 2007). To some extend other principles of the code are concerned with how clearly the source of both data and funding for a site can be determined. HON has stepwise taken a more active approach in actually "reviewing" and verifying applications. It is certain that sites displaying a HONcode are not necessary better than those do not comply with these criteria (Lewis 2005).

In 2002 the European commission published a communication called "quality Criteria for Health related Web site" based on a workshop in Brussels . The Quality criteria include Transparency and Honesty, Authority, Privacy and Data protection, Accountability, Responsible Up dating information, Editorial policy and accessibility (E-europe 2002).

According to (e-Europe 2002) quality criteria should address issues of both supplier and user education. In particular one document that simultaneously tell suppliers how to comply with key quality criteria and in order to educate users what to expect from a good health Web site. Needless to say that the quality criteria should address both passive information-giving sites as well as sites that allow for transactions between service or users and information providers.

Moreover the Health Summit Working Group selected defined and evaluated seven major criteria for assessing the health quality information : Credibility, content, disclosure, links, design, interactivity, and Caveats.

Criteria for Evaluating Internet Health Information (Health Summit Working Group H.S.W.G):

- **Credibility:** Includes the source, currency, relevance/utility, and editorial review process for the information. A site should display the name and logo of the institution or organization responsible for the information. Furthermore the date of the original information is based and the date that post on the Web.
- **Content:** Must be accurate and complete, and disclaimer provided. In particular clinical or scientific evidence that supports a position should be clear and understandable. Also a disclaimer describing the purpose and scope authority and currency of the information should be provided.
- **Disclosure:** Web sites is important to provide disclosure including the purpose of the Web site and the profile as result user can understand the intent of the organization or individual. In particular includes informing the user of the purpose of the site, as well as any profiling or collection of information associated with using the site.
- **Links:** Evaluated according to selection, architecture, content, and back linkages. Especially critical to the quality of an Internet Web site are its external resources and links connections to other Web sites that confirm the information that provided .
- **Design:** Encompasses accessibility, logical organization (navigability), and internal search capability. In particular the Web sites must be easy to use. The design including graphics, text and links is important in order to delivery and use of any Web information.
- **Interactivity:** Web sites should include a feedback mechanism for users in order to offer their comment, corrections, and criticisms, and as result raise questions about

the information provide. This make the Web site accountable to its user and allowing information exchanged to many individuals.

- **Caveats:** Clarification of whether site function is to market products and services or is a primary information content provider (HSWG 1999).

In addition The eHealth Code of Ethics is developed as a set of guiding principles aimed at health Internet stakeholders worldwide. In January 2000, about 50 experts in providing health information on line attended the "e-health" summit on the ethics providing information on the Internet in Washington. The code of ethics addresses issues of quality, privacy security and confidentiality and commercial behaviour (Eysenbach 2004). The goal of the E-health code of ethics is to ensure that people can confidently and with full understanding of know risks realize the potential of the Internet in managing their own health (Dzenowagis 2001). In conclusion the e-health code of ethics places a border on other organization developing quality standards for Internet health information.

HI-Ethics Code of Conduct consisted of 14 principles, and was developed by a group of leading for-profit consumer health information Web sites (Lewis 2005). Established on May 2000 current members is 15 companies and current membership fee are 6000 dollars. The rules developed are intended to assure that Internet health services reflect high quality criteria and ethical standards. Also health information is trustworthy and protected. Needless to say that consumers are able to distinguish on line health services that follow the Hi-Ethics principles from those that do no t(Hi-Ethics 2007, Dzenowagis 2001). Sustainability of the Hi-Ethics Code of Conduct is Vulnerable to the burdens placed on member companies, citizens and the ability of Hi-Ethics to maintain the currency of the principles. (Dzenowagis 2001). Furthermore AMA code of America Medical Association (Winker 2000). The mission of AMA is to promote the art and science of medicine and the betterment of public health. Guidelines for Medical and health information site on the Internet and Principles Govern AMA Web sites has been established since 2000 by AMA. Providers are Web site of the American Medical Association Medem (www.medem.com) The development of guidelines begin in 1999 where health information on the Web are based on those that govern medical journals , including peer-review process, authorship, sponsorship and the principles of privacy and confidentiality (Dzenowagis 2001, AMA 2007). These are governance tools indended for use by the developers of AMA . Also other organizations have adopted these guidelines for use.

It is certain that all the sets of criteria derive from similar roots. These roots are the principles of privacy, honesty, confidentiality, currency, accuracy, prevalence, consent , disclose and accountability. Quality criteria for patients decision and health information are relevant to patients and health care professionals, health care services and policy makers, all of whom is necessary to be confident about the developing and testing quality tools that undergone before their release (Elwyn 2006). For instance factors affecting the quality of an information source, the issues associated with the accessibility of a resource, the overall design and layout of the information and the ease of using of materials are secondary to the content issues (Intute 2006). At that point that we may be able to understand and examine in more depth the goal of helping patients to have the best quality information in order to take the best health decisions.

Promoting quality criteria for health information means better health. The benefits and outcomes of using health information are many. According to David et al (2003) on line questionnaire produced by the British Life and Internet Project, a total of 93 per cent said that the information had helped in understanding more about an illness or injury and a relatively high 57 per cent of responders said that that the information found was sufficient for them to act upon to improve their health. Moreover a total 26 per cent said that the information found had affected their decision about whether to see a doctor. In conclusion what have we learned from quality of health information on Internet is that consensus is important, collaboration and dissemination are crucial. Furthermore the cost of implementation is too high, also user and provider indifference is real. Moreover citizens education is a difficult and important task. In addition quality criteria are not enough and technology and understanding need to be promoted. As result more research needs to be done on : poor quality and health outcomes, on consumers behaviour, and better international collaboration and dissemination(Risk 2003).

EXAMPLES OF TOOLS FOR ASSESSING THE QUALITY OF CONSUMER HEALTH INFORMATION

Several groups have developed interactive Internet tools to educate consumers. These tools help users to assess the quality themselves(Eysenbach 2004).A further application of the code of good conduct takes the form of a user guidance tool. In particular with a code is demonstrated not by a label, but by a link to a guidance tool which invites the user to check if a site comply the quality criteria. Such tools may be specific to a particular type of information, such as DISCERN **(http://www.discern.org.uk/)** where developed to assess the quality of health information on treatment choices(Charnock 1998, Charnock 1999) Areas covered are: bias in the material, a clear statement of aims, references and additional sources of support and information, uncertainty, risks and benefits (including those of opting for no treatment), and treatment options. Moreover DISCERN(http://discern.org.uk) provides a brief questionnaire through which users gain a valid and reliable way of assessing the quality of written information on treatment choices. Similarly NETSCORING which uses a questionnaire of 49 criteria falling into eight categories: credibility, content, links, design, interactivity, quantitative aspects, ethics, and accessibility (e-Europe 2002). In conclusion another user guidance system is QUICK (www.quick.org) where provides children with a step by step guide to assessing health related information on Internet (Eysenbach 2002).

The Health Information Quality Assessment Tool **(hitiWeb.mitretek.org/iq)** — the Health Summit Working Group in North America (hitiWeb.mitretek.org/hswg) is currently developing a reliable and valid appraisal tool for users of health information on the Internet (Mitretek 1999). The main areas currently covered are credibility, content, disclosure, links, design, interactivity, and caveats (information on the function of the site). When looking for health information most Internet users start with a generic search engine. Very few check the source and date of the information they find (Fox 2006).

HEALTH WEBSITES AND SEARCH ENGINES

Health information can be extremely useful, empowering us to make important health decisions. Given the wealthy of information available through the Internet and other sources it is important to be able to assess its quality. This can be difficult because health information is constantly changing.

Web sites should provide clear and conspicuous notice of their information practices. It was thought that the greater the number of sites visited, the greater the like hood of a healthy behavior outcome. This based on an information model that argues that not all sites will present the information in the same way and design. Users benefit from collecting information from a number of sites. In particular they find it easier to collect the information and because jumping from site to site means that users can compare the information and become more knowledgeable (David 2003).

Below we provided some searchable catalogues to good quality health Web sites .

EXAMPLES OF HIGH QUALITY HEALTH WEB SITES

NHS Direct on line (http://www.nhsdirect.nhs.uk): The forefront of 24 hour health care delivery telephone and e-health information services during day and night. Provide information and advice about health and based in United Kingdom.

Healthfinder (http://www.healthfinder.gov/): Is a gateway consumer health information Web site whose goal is to improve consumer access to selected health information from a government agencies. The developer and sponsor of this site is the office of Disease Prevention and Health Promotion.

In particular is a US government site that provides access to health information from a range of sources, including government agencies and professionals organizations.

HON Health on Net Foundation (http://www.hon.ch/): An international not profit organization. It provides a databases of evaluation health materials and also provides the use of the HON Code and help unify the quality of medical and health information available.

MEDLINE PLUS (http://www.nlm.nih.gov/medlineplus): Is the National Library of Medicine, and part of National institute of Health. Provides access to a wide range of databases and health related organizations.

Patient UK (http://www.patient.co.uk): Designed to direct non-medical people in the United Kingdom to information about health related issue.

Organising Medical Networked Information (OMNI) (http://www.omni.ac.uk): OMNI provides access to good quality biomedical and health information Websites worldwide. It has been developed for medical professionals first and it based at the university of Nottingham in United Kingdom.

Provide good quality biomedical and health information by the Internet worldwide.

HealthWeb(http://healthWeb.org): Is a site established by librarians and information professionals from major academic medical institution in the Midwest. The site also provides "user Guides" developed to help consumers use Internet resources more effectively.

National Electronic Library for Health (NeLH) (http://www.nelh.nhs.uk): Extend Nhs library service to patient and the public. Provide easy access to health information and to the best current knowledge.

HebsWeb Health education Board of Scotland (http://www.hebs.scot.nhs.uk): The Web site for the Health Education Board of Scotland. In particular the site provide access to a wide range of consumer health information resources.

NOAH: New York Online Access to Health (http//:www.noah-health.org/): Is a unique collection of state local, and federal health resources for consumers. NOAH'S mission is to provide hifh quality, full term information for consumers, timely and relevant.

National Institutes of Health (http://www.nih.gov/health/consumer): Provides access to database of consumer health information published by the US National Institute of Health.

NHS in England (http://www.nhs.uk/): Health Web site is based in England, in particular is giving straightforward information presented in words, pictures video and audio about health living.

Best Treatments (http://www.besttreatments.co.uk/): In association with BMJ(British Medical Journal clinical evidence is a Web site for patients and doctors. In particular is providing the best research evidence about the treatments for many medical conditions.

Medem (http://medem.com): A new site launched in the fall of 2000, is a project of the leading medical societies in the United States. The site was developed to provide a trust online source for credible, comprehensive, and clinical healthcare information secure and confidential.

National Women's Health Information center(http://www.4women.gov/): Is gateway to selected women's health information resources. Its purpose to provide information about prevention, diagnosis and treatment of the illnesses and health conditions that affect them. Is sponsored by the U.S public Health Services office on women's Health.

IPEX (http://www.dipex.org): Is a Web site based in Oxford in England. Has a wide variety of personal experience of health and illness. People talking about their experience of illness and health issues.

Diabetes123(http://www.Diabetes123.com/): Is an organization whose mission is give information in online diabetes care, improving quality and reducing the cost of care by increasing the understanding of providing traditional products and services for the treatment of diabetes.

Contact a family (http://www.cafamily.org.uk): Is the only United Kingdom wide charity providing advice, information and support to the parents of all disabled children. Also parents can get in contact with other families both on a local and national basis.

StartHere (http://www.starthere.org/bigpage1.htm): Offer a variable service to citizens, providing useful information across a broad range of health topics.

EQUIP (Electronic Quality Information for Patients) (http://www.equip.nhs.uk/index.html#top): The Web site is based in west Midlands region NHS England and offer a variable links health Web sites. It was created in response to government requirements for improvements in information available to patients.

Health Education Board Scotland (http://www.healthscotland.com/): Is a National agency for health improvement from gathering evidence, to planning delivery and evaluation of a range of health topics and life stages.

Clinical Evidence (http://www.clinicalevidence.com): Is a new kind of decision support resource. BMJ clinical evidence systematic reviews summarise the current state of knowledge and uncertainty about the prevention and treatment of clinical conditions, based on searches and appraisal of the literature.

PathCAL (http://www.pathcal.ac.uk/): Is a set of 129 Web-based tutorials in order to help students understand the basic pathological principles of disease exploiting techniques in learning psychology

National Patient Safety Foundation (NPSF) (http://www.npsf.org/)/(www.centreforhig.demon.co.uk): Is a central resource in order to facilitated the production and dissemination of high quality patient information for health services users. The trust provides information as part of the health information services and NHS direct include large library information and databases.

Center of Disease Control and prevention(http://www.cdc.gov/): An agency of the department of Health and Human services is dedicated to promoting health quality of life by preventing and controlling disease, there are also sections on health topics in the news and health hoaxes (Williamson 2006, Killey 2003, Childs 2003, Shepperd 1999, Fox 2002).

SEARCH ENGINES

According to Fox(2002) A typical health seeker goes on line to see what can find without getting advice about where or how to search from anyone including medical professionals or friends.

You can use some search engines if you can not find what you need from the gateways. Here are some examples of search engines.

- **Google** (http://www.google.co.uk)
- **AlltheWeb** (http://www.alltheWeb.com)
- **Yahoo** (http://www.yahoo.com)

- **MedHunt** (http://www.hon.ch/MedHunt)
- **Mirago** (http://www.mirago.co.uk)
- **Excite** (http://www.Excite.com)
- **Allsearchengines.com** (http://www.All-searchengines.com)
- **Medstory** (http://www.medstory.com)

LEARNING HOW TO SEARCH

There are free on line tutorials by organizations or libraries. Here are some sites that provide free on line tutorial in order to develop Internet skills:

- The online Netskills Interactive Course (TONIC) Since 1995 Netskills has delivered high quality professional training services to the education public in the UK and beyond (http://www.netskills.ac.uk/onlinecourses/tonic/).
- Resource Discovery Network (RDN) Virtual Training Suite (http://www.rts.rdn.ac.uk) or http://www.intute.ac.uk is a free on line service providing you with access to the very best Web resources for education and research. In particular the service is created by a networked of UK universities and partners. The databases characterized of high quality information.
- Quality information checklist: www.quick.org.uk/menu.htm provides children with a step by step guide to assessing health related information on the Internet.
- DISCERN www.discern.org.uk is a brief questionnaire for users to validate information or treatment choice. (Childs 2003).

CONCLUSION

Health information has been variously described as the foundation for better health. The complexity of the issues surrounding quality of health information in the context of the health Internet has been shown (Dzenowagis 2001).

On demand side, there are different users of information. The usual position searching for information based on quality is to find the best available item that meet patient needs (Burgess 2007). The existence of the pseudo-health segment of information producers and users complicates efforts to introduce quality standards for health information on the Internet. Trustworthy health information from well known source on the Internet needed for the growing user population (Ekman 2005). Qualitative data are needed to design educational and technological innovations to guide consumers to high quality information (Eysenbach 2002).

Since no international consensus for quality criteria exists has as impact the responsibility falls on the medical organizations institutions and societies. It is important that organizations such as medical universities and governmental agencies to provide trustworthy high quality health information on Internet (e-Europe 2002) Experts from around the world will be invited to share their knowledge and experience. The international partnership for health informatics education(IPHIE) dares from 1999 and seeks to maintain, improve and promote medical and health informatics training and education through international collaboration(Murphy 2007).

It is now to be expected that national and regional health authorities, and private medical Web sites owners will implement the quality criteria and to develop information campaigns to educate site developer and citizens about minimum quality standards for health related Web sites.

REFERENCES

ACSH (2003). American Council on Science and Health. Retrieved 25 June 2007 from, http://www.acsh.org

AMA (2007). American Medical Association. Retrieved 28, June 2007 from, http://www.ams.assn.org

Barnett D., Grey J., Langrick C (2006). Developing a support group Web site use of the judge health guidelines. *Health information on Internet journal, 53*, p3.

BBC (2003b). Student died after buying Web drugs. *BBC News*. Retrieved 28, June 2007 from http://news.bbc.co.uk/1/hi/england/3130187.stm

BBC (2004). Millions illiterate about health. *BBC News*. Retrieved 28, June 2007 from http://news.bbc.co.uk/1/hi/health/3530874.stm

Beland, G. K., Ellott .M. N, Moralles, L. S., Algazy JZ, Kravite RL, Broder MS., Kanouse D.E, Munoz J. A., Yang K.,M. C. Glynn E. A. (2002). Health information on Internet. *Accessibility, Quality and Readability In English and Spanish, 285*(20), 2612-2621.

Bower H. (1996). Internet sees growth of unverified health claims. *BMJ 318*(381).

Burgess, M.S.E, Gray, W.A, Fiddian N.J(2007). Using quality criteria to assist in information searching. International Journal of information quality. Vol 1, No1, pp83-99.

Charnock, D.(1998). *The DISCERN handbook: Quality criteria for consumer health information*. Abingdon: Radcliffe Medical Press.

Charnock, D., Shepperd S., Gann B., Needham G. (1999). DISCERN — an instrument for judging the quality of consumer health information on treatment choices. *J Epidemiol Community Health 53*, 105-111.

Childs, S. (2003). *Summary how to search the Internet for health information*. Retrieved 10, June 2007 from www.judgehealth.org.uk/print.htm

Crocco A. G, Keever M. V, Jadad A. R(2002). Analysis of cases of Harm Associated with use of health information on the Internet. *JAMA , 287*(21), 2869-2871.

David, N., Huntington, P., Gunter B., Russell C., Withey, R. (2003). *The British and their use of the Web for Health information and advice: A survey*. Retrieved 28, June 2007 from, http://www.emeraldinsight.com/0001-253X.htm

E-Europe (2002). Commision of the European communities. Quality criteria for Health related Websites. *J. Med Internet res. 4*(3), e15.

Ekman, A., Hall, P., Litton, J. E. (2005). Can we trust cancer information on the Internet? A comparison of interactive cancer risk sites. *Cancer causes and control Journal, 16*, 65-772.

Eysenbach, G. (2004). Recent advances Consumer health informatics. Clinical review. *BMJ, 320*.

Elwyn, G., O'Conor, A., Stacey, D., Volk, R., Edwards., A, Coulter, A., Thomson, R., et al (2006). Developing a quality criteria frame work for patients decisions aids: online international Delphi, consensus process. *BMJ 333*, 417.

Eysenbach G., Diepgen T. C., Gray J. A. M., et al (1998). Towards quality management of medical information on the Internet. Evaluation labelling and filtering of information. *BMJ 317*, 1496-1502.

Eysenbach, G., Kohler, C. (2002). How do consumers search for and appraise health information on the World Wide Web. *BMJ 324*, 573-577.

Fox, S. (2006). *Online health search*. Retrieved 15 of June 2007 from, http://www.pewInternet.org/pdfs/PIP_Online_Health_2006.pdf

Gagliardi, A., Jadad, A. R. (2002). Examinations of instruments used to rate quality of health information on the Internet. Chronicle of a voyage with an unclear destination. *BMJ 324*, 569-573.

General Accounting Office (1996). *Consumer health informatics-emerging issues*. Washington, DC,

Grandinetti, D. A. (1994). Doctors and the Web help your patients surf the Net safety. *Medical Economics, 77*(5), 186-8.

Hi-Ethics, Inc. (2007). Retrieved 29 June 2007 from http://www.hiethics.com

HON (Health on Net Foundation) (2007). Retrieved 22, June 2007 from http://www.hon.ch/HONcode/Conduct.html

Intute (2006). Intute: Health and life sciences evaluation guidelines. Retrieved 28 June 2007 from http://www.intute.ac.uk/healthandlifesciences/

Jones, R., Gann, B., Duman M., Murphy, J.(2005). *Consumer health informatics.* DH V2

Jadad A. R., Gagliardi, A. (1998). Rating health information on the Internet: navigating to knowledge or to label. *JAMA, 279*, 611-614.

Kiley, R. & Graham, E. (2002). The patient's Internet handbook. *Royal Society of Medicine.*

Kiley, R.(2003). *Medical information on the Internet. A guide for health Professionals.* Churchill Livinstone.

Lewis, D., Eysenbach, G., Kukafka R., Stavri, P.Z., Jimison H. B. (2005). *Consumer health informatics. informing consumers and improving health care.* Springer Publications

Linkous, J.(1999). American telemedicine Association Issues Advisory on the use of the medical Web sites. Retrieved from http://www.atmeda.org/news/072899.html

McClung, H. J., Murray, R. D., Heitlinger, L. A. (1998). The Internet as a source for current patient information. *Padiatrics 101*, E2.

Mitretek Systems Innovative Technology in the Public Interest (2007). Retrieved 2, June 2007 from hitiWeb.mitretek.org/hswg

Mulligan, Z.(2007) GP specialist e-library. *Health information on Internet. 55*, 5.

Murphy, J. (2007). International perspectives and initiatives. *Health information and Libraries Journal. 24*(1), 62-68.

Murphy, J. (2007). *Workshop—Consumer Health Information.* City Univercity London

Naumann, F. (2001). From databases to information systems information quality makes the difference. In *Proceedings of Int. Cont on information Quality(ICIQ).* Boston, MA, USA, (pp 244-260).

NCAHF (2007) National Council Against Health Fraud. Retrieved 25, June 2007 from http:// www.ncahf.org/

Pandolfini, C., Bonati, M. (2002). Follow up of quality of public oriented health information on the World Wide Web: Systematic re-evaluation. *BMJ 32497337*, 82-583.

Peterson, G., Aslani, P., Williams, K. (2003). How do consumers search for and appraise information on Medicines on the Internet? A qualitative study Using focus groups. *J. Med Internet Res 5*(4), e 33.

Pirsig, R. M.(1974). *Zen and the art of motorcycle maintence.* New York: Bantam Books.

Potts, H. M. M. (2006). Is e-health progressing faster than e-health researchers? *J.Med Internet Res 8*(3), e24.

Quackwatch (2007) Retrieved 25, June 2007 from http://www.quackwatch.org/00AboutQuackwatch/mission.html

Risk, A (2003). Quality of health information on Internet, achievements lessons and the future. *Conference Puebla Mexico Crics VI Birem.* Retrieved 5, July 2007 from http//:www.paho.org/English/PD/IRM/risk.pdf

Risk, A., Dzenowags, J (2001). Review of Internet Health information Quality Initiatives. *J.Med Internet Res. 3*(4), e28.

Shepperd S., Charnock D., Gann, B.(1999). Education and debate. Helping patient access high quality health information. *BMJ 319*, 764-766.

Silberg, W. et al (1997). Assessing, controlling and assuring the quality of medical information on the Internet. *JAMA, 277*(15), 1244-1245.

Taylor, A. G. (2003). *The organization of information.* 2nd edition Libraries Unlimited publications.

Talley, C. R. (1997). Editorial: Trouble on the Internet. *American Journal of Health-System Pharmacy, 54.*

Williamson, L. (2006). What's new. *Health information on the Internet, 50,* 12.

Wilson, P. (2002). How to find the good and avoid the bad or ugly: A short guide to tools for rating quality of health information on the Internet. *BMJ 324*, 598-602.

Winker, M. A., Flanagin A.,Chi-Lum B, et al (2000). Guidelines for medical and health information sites on the Internet. *JAMA 283*, 1600-1666.

Wyatt, J. C. (1997). Commentary: Measuring quality and impact of the World Wide Web. *BMJ, 314*, 1879-1881.

Ziebland, S., Chapple, A., Dumelow, C., Evans, J., Prinjha, S., Rozmovits, L. (2004). How the Internet affects patient's experience of cancer a qualitative study. *BMJ 328*, 364.

KEY TERMS

Consumer Health Informatics: Consumer health informatics is the branch of medical informatics that analyses consumers' needs for information; studies and implements methods of making information accessible to consumers; and models and integrates consumers' preferences into medical information systems. Consumer informatics stands at the crossroads of other disciplines, such as nursing informatics, public health, health promotion, health education, library science, and communication science, and is perhaps the most challenging and rapidly expanding field in medical informatics; it is paving the way for health care in the information age.

Health Information: Health information is required for a wide variety of purposes, including building knowledge and understanding of health conditions; helping people to decide when they need to seek specialist help; supporting choices in relation to treatment, management or social care options; identifying, choosing and accessing appropriate healthcare providers; and educating patients and the public about public health risks and about primary and secondary prevention.

Internet: The Internet is a world wide, publicly accessible series of interconnected computer networks that transmit data by packet switching using the standard Internet protocol (IP). It is a "network of networks" that consists of millions of smaller domestic, academic, business, and government networks, which together carry various information and services, such as electronic mail, online chat, file transfer, and the interlinked Web pages and other resources of the World Wide Web (WWW).

Quality: Quality is an inherently subjective assessment, which depends on the type of the information needed, the type of the information searched for, and the particular qualities of the consumer. Experts believe that formal methods are needed to describe and assess information quality.

Chapter XXXII
A Practical Approach to Computerized System Validation

Kashif Hussain
University of Valenciennes et Hainaut de Cambrésis, France

Shazia Yasin Mughal
University of Valenciennes et Hainaut de Cambrésis, France

Sylvie Leleu-Merviel
University of Valenciennes et Hainaut de Cambrésis, France

ABSTRACT

This chapter provides a practical approach to computerized system validation (CSV) for the pharmaceutical organizations for the users dealing with the validation. Validation package including plan, responsibilities, and documentation needed and created during the validation are also discussed. Any computer system can be validated utilizing the techniques described here. These activities address the organization commitment to implement the underlying system in order to improve, ensure and maintain the quality standards. The CSV is described as a reference and an orientation guide to understand the related quality processes. The activities presented here should be useful for initiating and conducting the principal tasks of validation. This chapter reflects a quick guide and addresses one of the "non-technical" aspects of CSV methodology. A clear approach is presented that defines the CSV activities and provides an efficient means of validation to new and existing systems, applications, and environments within the organization.

INTRODUCTION

CSV, short for computerized system validation, represents a major step forward for companies seeking to acquire regulatory requirements and to establish documentation proof of every activity to acquire validation. But to take full advantage of its potential cost and timesavings, many pharmaceutical organizations need to do more than simply use a traditional validation method. In recent years the introduction of computer systems for data handling in the pharmaceutical industry has increased (Friedli et al. 1998). Over the last three decades, the pharmaceutical industry has increasingly used computerized system to support the product development, less time in registration of patent, product development, manufacturing, and production, etc. The failure to validate a computerized system can have a significant financial and business implications from regulatory authorities including cancellation, delay in the issue of a license, delay in submission to regulatory authorities, negative publicity, removal of distribution of a product or recall of a product, shutdown of the manufacturing plant, etc (McDowall, 1995; Wingate, 2003).

Validation is vital and in fact, if pharmaceutical organizations aren't careful, they may run into several roadblocks that could derail the implementation and ultimately cost them more money over the validation of computerized system. Official inspections concentrate more and more on validation of computerized systems due to Good Manufacturing Practices (GMP) (Hoffmann et al., 1998).

World wide regulatory authorities (Food and Drug Administration - FDA, EC - European Council, AFSSAPS - French Agency of Health Safety of Health Products, Health Canada, and others) assure that all products are safe and effective and that's why impose certain conditions on the pharmaceutical organizations to ensure and maintain the critical quality processes. These authorities make it sure that all critical processes are validated and meet the required compliance before approving the license to the manufacturer. These requirements are provided in various forms like GxPs: Good (Clinical, Laboratory, Manufacturing) practices, BPF (Bonnes Pratiques de Fabrication), etc. All regulatory authorities consider the public health safety as the first priority and focus on pharmaceutical organizations to achieve all necessary measures to meet this challenging responsibility.

Companies have long relied on investments in validation activities (people, processes and technology) to provide more effective service. Invariably, such initiatives are often focused on the service variables within a company's control. Recent demands, however, have compelled organizations to look for the ways to enhance their validation process with capabilities similar to extreme requirements in performance and scalability.

A number of papers are available on the topics of validation, computerized system and system life cycle approach. However, few have combined and blended these topics into a practical set of principles for CSV. This is the ambitious task of our chapter. It provides a logical approach and comprehensive treatment of validation and also explains how the roles and responsibilities involved can improve the validation. For the validation specialist, the objective is to improve the utility and conformance of the system in validation. Such validation must always be designed from the point of view of the manager, user and compliance requirements. In order to achieve this, it is necessary that the validation activities are understood in the aforementioned context. This chapter investigates the role of validation activities to accelerate the development of business-specific validation.

COMPUTERIZED SYSTEM

Several definitions are available to define computerized system including European Parliament in the Annex-11 (computerised system) relating to the respect of medicinal products for human use and investigational medicinal products for human use (EC, 2003); the FDA's definition of computerized system (FDA, 1987a).

Computerized system may include operating environment (Unix, DOS, NT, etc) programming language (Basic, C++, Java, etc), data base (Oracle, Access, DB2, etc), any software, hard disk, processor, network materiel, data input, electronic processing and the output of the information to be used either for reporting or automatic control. It may include automated manufacturing equipment, process control systems, automated laboratory equipment, laboratory data capture system, clinical or manufacturing database systems, etc (Hussain et al. 2006).

The elements of a computerized system are shown in Figure 1.

We consider the definitions of validation used by the regulatory authorities. We put together all steps of validation that can help pharmaceutical organizations validate their computerized system through controlled specialization. We describe the steps and documentation required to better focus on validation and how to avoid barriers to achieving successful validation. We provide a road map for efficiently deploying validation methodology.

Figure 1. Elements of a computerized system

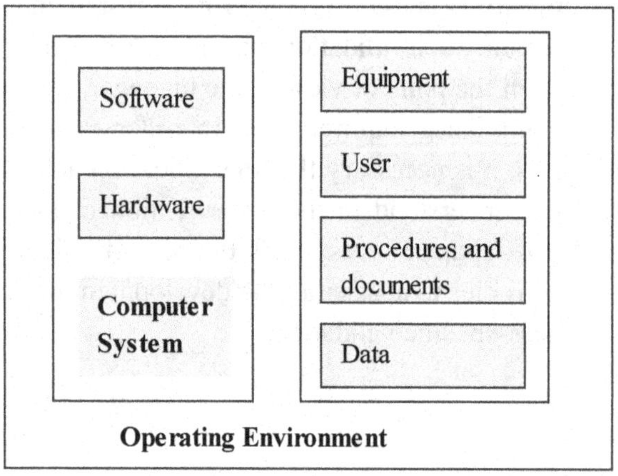

VALIDATION APPROACH

The FDA defines computerized system as "Computerized System means, for the purpose of this guidance, computer hardware, software, and associated documents (e.g., user manual) that create, modify, maintain, archive, retrieve, or transmit in digital form information related to the conduct of a clinical trial" (FDA, 1987a, 1987b).

The compliance with regulations, from the regulatory authorities (FDA, 1987a, 1987b; EC, 2003; Ministry of Health & Social Protection, France, 2004) expect all concerned computerized systems to ensure consistent product quality. A mature validation process can ease regulatory inspections, audits and reduce the risk of noncompliance (McDowall, 1995).

Validation of computerized system is a regulatory requirement for FDA, therefore, validation can be treated as a proof of its suitability which is linked with the whole system lifecycle to ensure that the system meets the user requirements, ensures compliance expectations and will be properly maintained to guarantee a secure environment with accurate, reliable, and traceable information throughout its lifecycle (Hussain et al. 2006).

The need of the computerized system being validated must be clearly understood along with the magnitude of validation efforts commensurate with the risk associated with the system (FDA, 2002). CSV is based on provision of documented evidence which provides a higher degree of assurance that a control system will consistently operate according to predefined specifications. The control system may refer to any part of computerized system (software, hardware, interface, communication medium to process other equipments or computers, etc) (Glennon, 1998).

VALIDATION APPROACH OF THE COMPUTERIZED SYSTEM

The clear understanding on quality validation is meant to enhance the overall validation process and provide assistance in completing validation in a cost effective manner. The principles of good practices for the use of computerized system via validation are now well established as they means by which quality is built into development of these systems. Major phases of the validation of a computerized system producing documented evidence are the following (Hussain et al. 2006).

- Network and infrastructure
- Validation master plan
- User requirements specification (URS)
- Risk analysis
- Supplier audit and vendor selection
- Legal requirements
- Functional specification
- Validation strategy planning
- Design specification
- Code review
- Implementation phase
- Testing phase
    - User acceptance testing (UAT)
- Qualification Phase
    - Installation qualification (IQ)
    - Operational qualification (OQ)
    - Performance qualification (PQ)
- Standard operating Procedures (SOPs)
- Trainings
- Verification and release phase
- Final validation report
- Maintenance and regular review
- Change management (CM)
- Decommissioning

Here we present a quick guide for all phases of validation including key activities.

ROLES AND RESPONSIBILITIES RELATED TO VALIDATION

It is the top management responsibility to ensure that all relevant computerized systems are validated according to the organization policy and regulatory requirements. The organization must have the clear policy and means to make the system validated and maintained through formal organization procedures. Along with planning and monitoring validation activities, all validation activities should be reviewed. The completion of validation activities should be documented to provide all necessary information. We describe in the following paragraph the responsibilities that can be related to the validation of computerized system. Roles and responsibilities will vary between organizations and there is no fix role to lead the validation process.

Figure 2. Different phases of validation

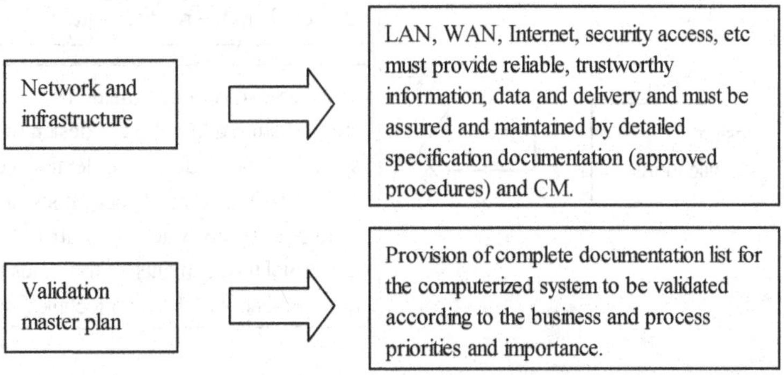
Network and infrastructure
LAN, WAN, Internet, security access, etc must provide reliable, trustworthy information, data and delivery and must be assured and maintained by detailed specification documentation (approved procedures) and CM.
Validation master plan
Provision of complete documentation list for the computerized system to be validated according to the business and process priorities and importance.

continued on following page

Figure 2. continued

USR	Defining the user's requirements and constraints is URS. It should answer what user wants to do or what the system is required to do for its users.
Risk Analysis	It includes strategy and methodology, risk associated with different parts, and action plan to minimize these risks. It should answer the solution against all risks identified.
Supplier Audit and Vendor Selection	A supplier audit is required to ensure the supplier is able to provide the services required with all necessary documentation. The audit includes verification of QMS, standards, tools used, programming standards, working conditions, market repute, development methodology, customer support, and CM, etc.
Legal requirements	Whenever external service providers are involved, legal contracts, service level agreements (SLA) must be incorporated and assured that regulatory requirements of the company are confirmed.
Functional Specifications	The purpose is to define how the computerized system to be delivered will satisfy the user requirements. It includes identification of any constraints on or potential deviations from the established requirements. It should answer what the system should do and how it should do that.
Validation Strategy planning	The purpose is to formalize the validation process, the validation strategy, the responsibilities and the release strategy applicable to the related system.
Design Specifications	The purpose is to document the infrastructure and software design of the system including adequate details to enable it to be built and maintained. It should answer how the system will satisfy the functional requirements. It translates the requirements of URS into technical solution.

continued on following page

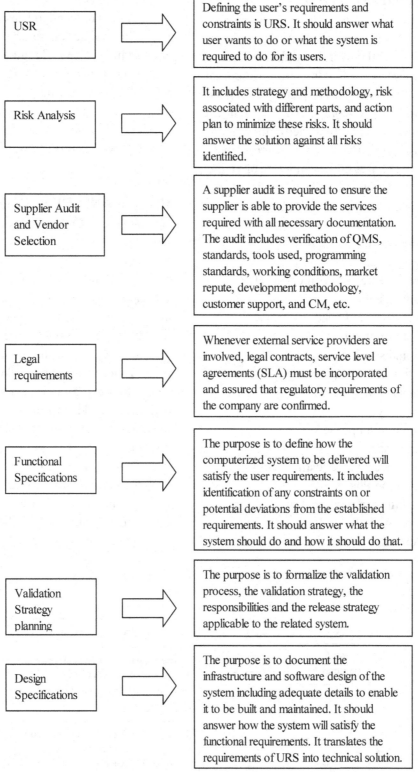

Figure 2. continued

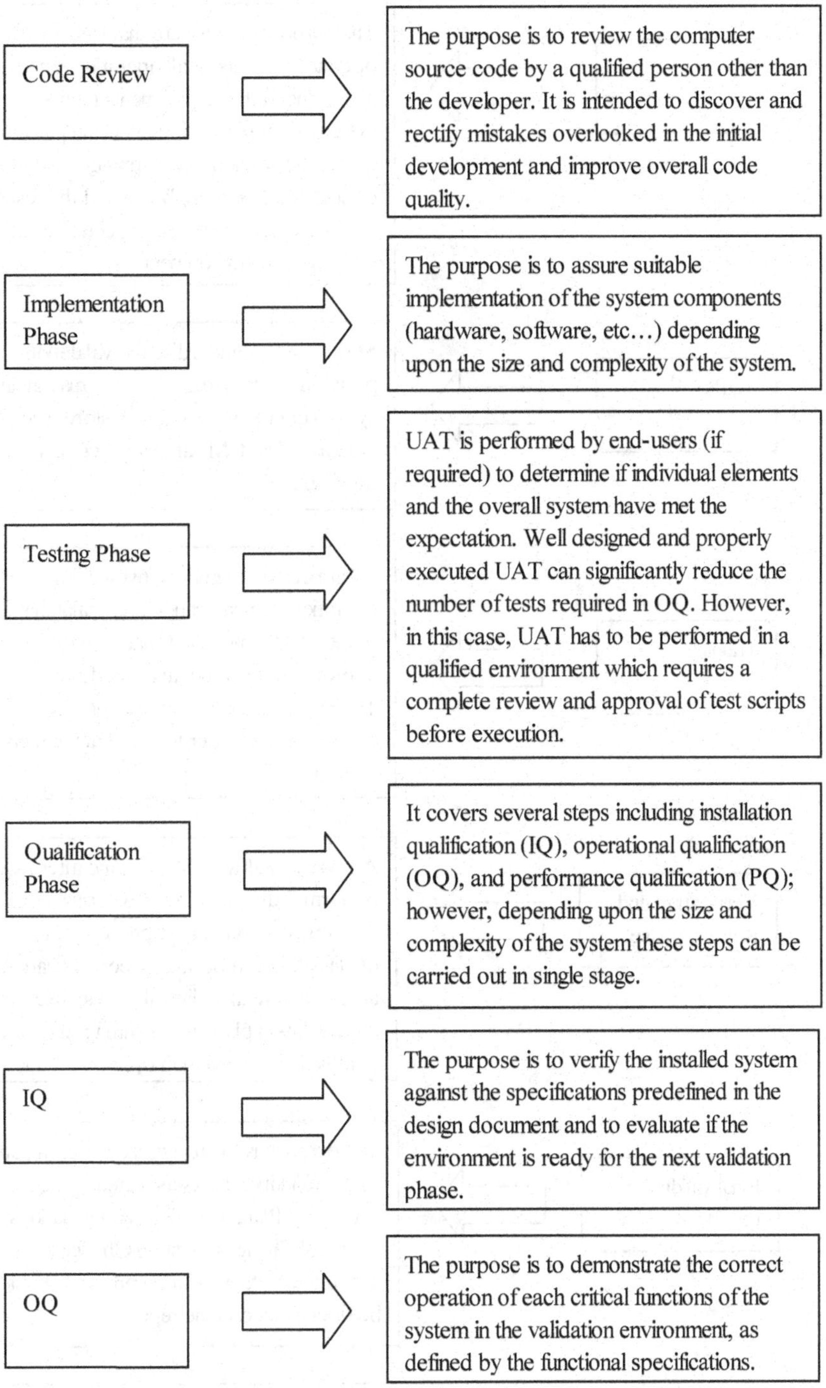

Code Review
The purpose is to review the computer source code by a qualified person other than the developer. It is intended to discover and rectify mistakes overlooked in the initial development and improve overall code quality.
Implementation Phase
The purpose is to assure suitable implementation of the system components (hardware, software, etc…) depending upon the size and complexity of the system.
Testing Phase
UAT is performed by end-users (if required) to determine if individual elements and the overall system have met the expectation. Well designed and properly executed UAT can significantly reduce the number of tests required in OQ. However, in this case, UAT has to be performed in a qualified environment which requires a complete review and approval of test scripts before execution.
Qualification Phase
It covers several steps including installation qualification (IQ), operational qualification (OQ), and performance qualification (PQ); however, depending upon the size and complexity of the system these steps can be carried out in single stage.
IQ
The purpose is to verify the installed system against the specifications predefined in the design document and to evaluate if the environment is ready for the next validation phase.
OQ
The purpose is to demonstrate the correct operation of each critical functions of the system in the validation environment, as defined by the functional specifications.

continued on following page

Figure 2. continued

PQ	The purpose is to assure that system operates throughout all operating ranges according to the requirements (stable system, operational documents in place, trained personnel) over a pre-defined period of time and is in compliance and the results are in accordance to the expectations and in its actual use environment.
SOPs	SOPs are to standardize the validation procedure performance. SOPs may include system operation, backup, restore, security, data handling, CM, disaster recovery, training, etc.
Training	All concerned members involved in operation, administration and maintenance of the system must be trained on the appropriate operational procedures. Training should be performed in a test environment in order to avoid any effects on system.
Verification and Release phase	A review of all activities is done after PQ to perform final system release verification, data transfer plan if any, process qualification and performance verification if any, to assure all deliverables identified in the validation plan and to sum up the completion of validation cycle.
Final validation report	The purpose is to summarize the completion of the validation tasks as stated in the Validation Plan. Test Results, Deviations, Protocol Changes, System Changes generated in the validation process should be documented in the report.
Maintenance and regular review	The purpose is to ensure the validated status of a system that is maintained after go-live. This phase should continue until the system is decommissioned.

continued on following page

Figure 2. continued

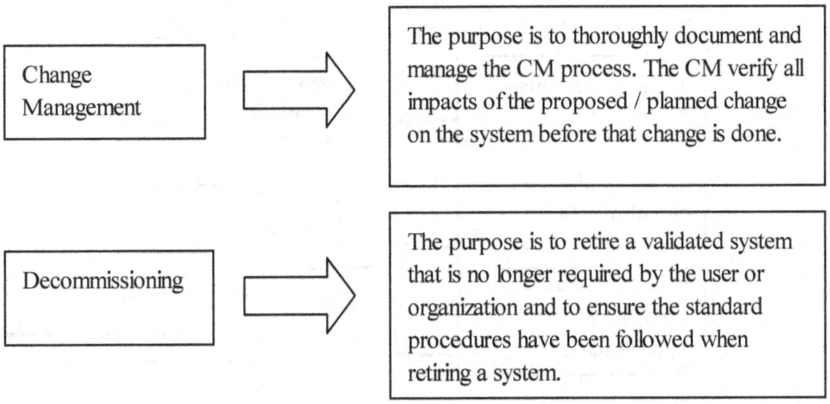

Throughout the validation process a package of documentation should be maintained that contains the required working documentation of the process. The validation plan and validation reports are often some of the first documents to be examined by GxP regulatory authorities inspecting a pharmaceutical or healthcare facility (Trill, 1996). Key validation documents must include change control records (Wingate, 2003) as CM is the required key operation for information system of pharmaceutical organizations. It ensures that CM process does not severely alter

Table 1. Function and responsibilities for key validation activities

Function	Responsibility
The validation team is responsible for	• All validation activities performed within a project, including the validation strategy and documentation; • Leading the validation; • Obtaining, preparing, and/or review the validation deliverables (protocols, reports, etc.); • Coordinating and performing all system qualification tests.
The supplier/vendor of the system is responsible for	• Specifying, designing, creating, and testing the computer system in accordance with a quality assurance system; • Preparing functional specifications (if applicable) and the entire technical documentation (including the user manual) of the system; • Defining and performing the unit tests or integration tests or the FAT (Factory Acceptance Test).
Quality assurance team is responsible for	• Defining the validation methodology in accordance with applicable regulations; • Providing guidance and assistance for the implementation of the validation methodology and preparing the validation deliverables; • Performing suppliers' audits; • Reviewing and approving all validation deliverables in order to make sure that the documents are in compliance with applicable regulatory requirements and with the organization procedures; • Performing internal audits.
System owner is responsible for	• For the compliance of the computerized system and integrity of related data; • For assuring that a validation team is in place and that the required documentation is created and maintained and that the changes to the system are managed and controlled; • Ultimately, the system owner is responsible for the validation of the system and for maintaining its validated status. The system owner must be able to present the validation file and the change control file to the health authorities at any time.
The user as members of the validation group is responsible for	• Preparing the user requirements specification; • Performing qualification tests of the computerized system; • Preparing and issuing SOPs and instructions for the use of the system (if applicable).

Figure 3. Key validation deliverables (procedures and documents)

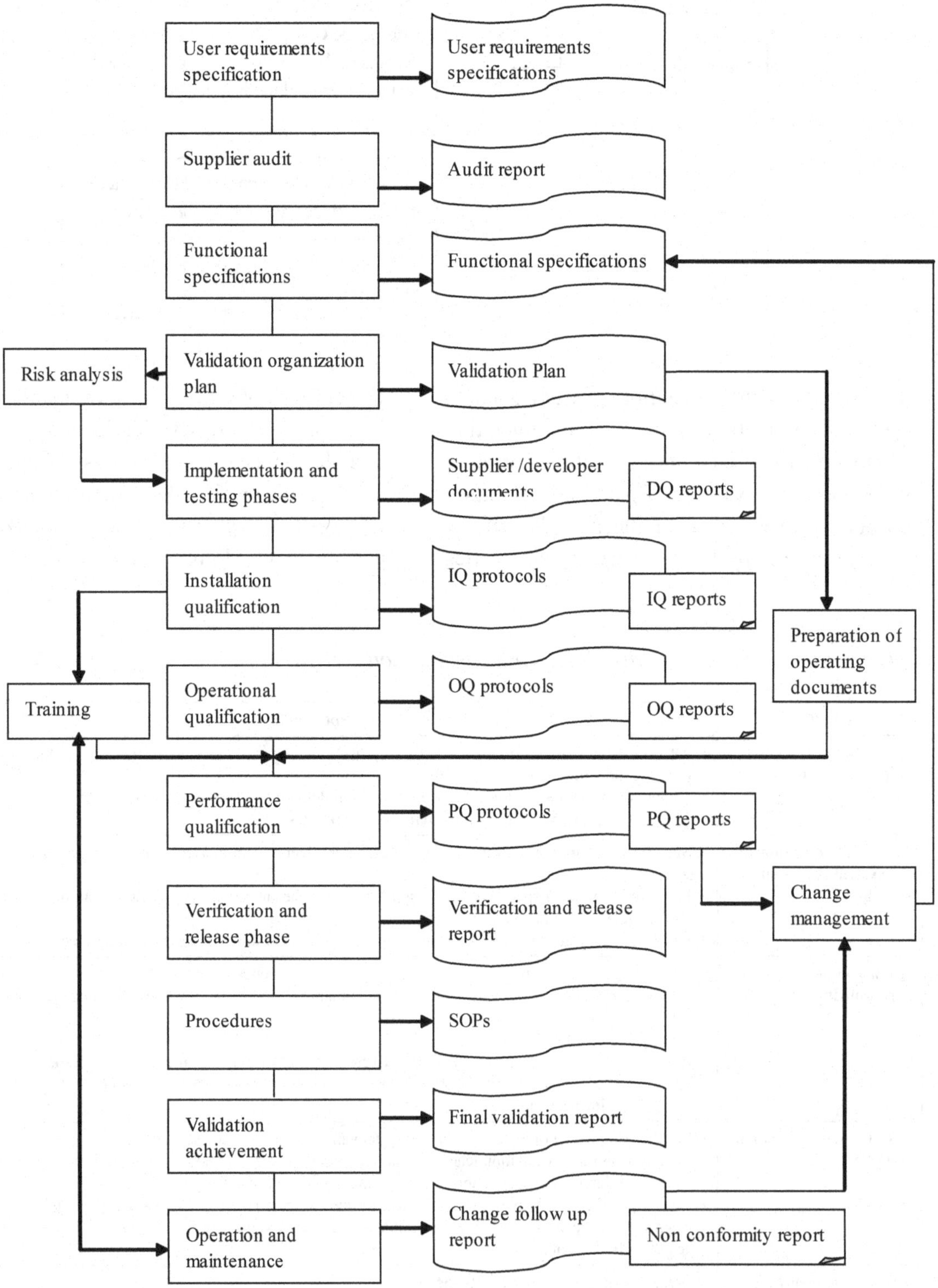

the system functionality, integrity, availability, stability or security, etc, by involving an excellent documentation to track all approved and planned changes (Hussain and Mughal, 2006). Attempts to aster the formidable problems of validation have led to standardizing and formalizing documents and validation techniques and to incorporating the documentation function into the validation life cycle. The key elements and documents of the validation are indicated in Figure 2.

DISCUSSION

Once the final validation report is issued, the system should be maintained and a regular review is required. The system owner is responsible for the operation and monitoring of the system. Various activities can be helpful for smooth operation including:

- All the non-conformities of the software or equipment should be are tracked to remove these non-conformities.
- All system changes follow change request addressed through a CM procedure.
- The functional specifications document must be regularly updated to integrate the changes made to the computerized system.
- All the changes in the software and equipment must be reported in the computerized system logbook in accordance with SOPs.
- Qualification tests must be planned either following any change to the system or routinely.
- Audits may be performed at any time by quality teams to make sure that organization rules are followed, and to check that the system is still under control.

A clear approach to validation can help minimize the communication gap between the validation specialist and the system user. The validation process should include the general scope of the system including high level design features, the teams responsible for the validation, a clear time-frame, and a brief summary of other supporting documentation that need to be addressed in order to use the system (Carter, 2005). As can be seen, there are many stages to go through before the system is fully operational; thus the acquisition of CSV must not be undertaken lightly. Validation at the end of the life cycle must be complimented by verification at each stage, as it is a more cost effective approach (McDowall, 1995). CSV goes through a number of stages from the time they are conceived until decommissioning that is a life cycle. The validation life cycle concept is useful because it provides a disciplined approach for the development and operation of CSV. The tasks identified as belonging to a specific stage of the cycle are important as they contain coherent framework for organization of the validation process.

CONCLUSION

CSV theory and practices have undergone radical changes in the past three decades; these changes are certain to accelerate. The validation experts of the future must be able to cope with the environment that is system oriented and in compliance. The implications of validation are great when applied to the information system. The purpose of the validation of a computerized system is to make sure that the system and its use are in compliance with applicable regulatory requirements. It provides guidelines to assure that the system is in compliance with all functional, reliability, integrity and security requirements and its operation is under control, and any changes of such systems are well managed through change management. Validation should be regarded as part of an integrated concept to ensure the quality, safety, and efficacy of pharmaceuticals (Ermer, 2001). The validation life cycle sets forth a logical order for the events; that take place in the validation of a system and it encompasses problems and risks that occur during the validation of a system.

We define the approach required and the responsibilities involved in the validation of computerized systems used by pharmaceutical organizations in a regulated context (GxP, BPx). In order to obtain the maximum benefit from CSV, the respect of procedures, organisation and company's commitment to support and maintain the system is essential. The system owner, quality assurance and validation teams and users mutually play an important role to make a validation successful.

ACKNOWLEDGMENT

We have had the benefit of discussion, careful reading, critique and guidance on validation concepts and application from several pharmaceutical industry experts of CSV and CM all of whom prefer to remain anonymous. These discussions have added considerably to its contents and organization. We are particularly thankful to the associate editor and two anonymous reviewers of this handbook for invaluable feedback that greatly improved this chapter.

REFERENCES

Carter, E.R. (2005). Systems validation: Application to statistical programs. *BMC Medical Research Methodology, 5*, 3.

EC (2003). *Directive of 2003/94/EC, of 8 October 2003, laying down the principles and guidelines of good manufacturing practice in respect of medicinal products for human use and investigational medicinal products for human use*. Volume 4, Medicinal Products for Human and Veterinary Use: Good Manufacturing Practice. In Annex 11: Computerised system, (pp 11). Retrieved April 13, 2005 from http://pharmacos.eudra.org/F2/eudralex/vol-4/home.htm.

Ermer, J. (2001). Validation in pharmaceutical analysis, Part 1, an integrated approach. *Journal of Pharmaceutical and Biomedical Analysis, 24*, 755-767.

FDA (2002). General principles for software validation medical devices. *Guidance for Industry, Final Guidance*, January.

FDA (1987a). Guidelines on general principles of process validation. *US Food and Drug Administration*. Retrieved March 12, 2007 from, http://www.fda.gov/cder/guidance/pv.htm

FDA (1987b). General principles of validation. *Food and Drug Administration, Center for Drug Evaluation and Research*. Rockville, MD.

Friedli, D., Kappeler, W., Zimmermann, S. (1998). Validation of computer systems: Practical testing of a standard LIMS. *Pharmaceutica Acta Helvetiae, 72*, 343-348.

Glennon, B. (1997). Control system validation in multipurpose biopharmaceutical facilities, *Journal of Biotechnology, 59*, 53–61.

Hoffmann, A., Kähny-Simonius, J., Plattner, M., Schmidi-Vckovski, V., Kronseder, C. (1998). Computer system validation: An overview of official requirements and standards. *Pharmaceutica Acta Helvetiae, 72*, 317-325.

Hussain, K., S. Y. Mughal., S. Leleu-Merviel. (2006). Computerized systems validation: a quality approach in the pharmaceutical industry. In Athina Lazakidou (Eds.), *Handbook of research on informatics in healthcare and biomedicine*. Hershey, PA, USA: Idea Group Reference.

Hussain, K., S.Y. Mughal. (May 7-10, 2006). Change Management, key factor in pharmaceutical organizations (existing information systems approach). *IEEE Canadian Conference on Electrical and Computer Engineering – IEEE-CCECE*. Ottawa, Canada.

Ministry of Health and Social Protection, France. (2004). Décrets, arrêtés, circulaires. *Journal Officiel de la République française, Text 23 sur 95, 21st August*. Retrieved July 10, 2006 from, http://agmed.sante.gouv.fr/htm/3/pta/ptaa1_190804.pdf

McDowall, R. D. (1995). Practical computer validation for pharmaceutical laboratories. Journal of Pharmaceutical and Biomedical Analysis, 14, pp 13-22.

Trill, A. J. (March 26-27, 1996). Regulatory requirements for computer validation, computer systems validation: A practical approach. *Management Seminar*. London.

Wingate, G. (2003). *Computer Systems validation - quality assurance, risk management, and regulatory compliance for pharmaceutical and healthcare companies*. CRC Press, 1st edition.

KEY TERMS

21 CFR Part 11: FDA code of US Federal Regulations, Title 21, Part 11 (21 CFR Part 11) Electronic Records; Electronic Signatures applicable since 1997 that defines parameters by which pharmaceutical companies can author, approve, store, and distribute records electronically.

Acceptance Testing: Functional acceptance tests of the system performed with the supplier/developer.

AFSSAPS: Stands for French Health Products Safety Agency is the French authority for all safety decisions taken concerning health products from their manufacturing to their marketing, i.e.: medicinal products, raw materials for pharmaceutical use, organs, tissues and cells and products of human and animal origins, etc.

BPF: Stands for "Bonnes Pratiques de Fabrication" in french. It is the equivalent of GMP.

cGMP: Stands for current good manufacturing practice is an international set of quality regulations and guidelines applicable to the manufacture, testing and distribution of drugs, medical devices, diagnostic products, biological for human or veterinary use, etc. FDA ensures quality product applicable to GMP via 21 CFR Part 210 and 211 regulations.

Change Management (CM): The complete set of processes employed for tracking all changes from existing and new systems, applications, and environments defined by a respective pharmaceutical regulatory conformance and to mange systematically the effects of change.

Code Review: A process to detect possible coding errors, implement path analyses and determine adherence to design specifications and standards by reviewing the source code.

Computerized System: A system that includes software, hardware, application software, operating system software, supporting documentation, e.g. automated laboratory systems, control systems, manufacturing, clinical, or compliance monitoring database systems, etc…

Design Qualification (DQ): Documented evidence that the specifications, design, and implementation of the computerized system (hardware and software) are appropriate for their intended use.

DRP: Stands for disaster recovery plan is the plan for business continuity in the event of a disaster that destroys business resources. The goal of DRP is to recover the technical infrastructure that supports business continuity, in the event of a serious incident in the least possible time.

FDA: Stands for Food and Drug Administration, the branch of US federal government which approves new drugs for sale and is responsible for ensuring the safety and effectiveness of all drugs, biologics, vaccines, and medical devices, including those used in the diagnosis, treatment, regulation, etc.. for USA.

Functional Specification: It defines what the system should do, and what functions and facilities are to be provided. It provides a list of design objectives for the system (GAMP 4).

GCP: Stands for good clinical practice is an international set of quality regulations and guidelines for design, conduct, monitoring, recording, auditing, analysis, and reporting of studies applicable to the clinical or human studies in the evaluation of drugs, medical devices, biological product, etc... FDA ensures quality product applicable to GCP via 21 CFR Part 50, 54 & 56.

GAMP: Stands for good automated manufacturing practice is a technical sub-committee of the International Society of Pharmaceutical Engineering (ISPE). Its goal is to encourage and promote a better understanding of the regulation and role of automated systems in the pharmaceutical industry.

GLP: Stands for good laboratory practice embodies an international set of quality regulations and guidelines applicable to the non-clinical studies in the evaluation of drugs, medical devices, biological product, etc... GLP provides a framework within which FDA ensures laboratory studies are planned, performed, monitored, recorded, reported and archived under 21 CFR Part 58.

GxP / BPx: GxP / BPx is generalization of any quality guidelines used in the pharmaceutical industry that groups together the following compliance practices, cGMP: Current Good Manufacturing Practice, GLP: Good Laboratory Practice, GCP: Good Clinical Practice.

Installation Qualification (IQ): Documented evidence that the computerized system (hardware and software) is installed in accordance with the requirements of the manufacturer and of the user and that the supplier documentation is in place.

Operation Qualification (OQ): Documented evidence that, under anticipated conditions, the system or a part of the system operates in accordance with the pre-established functional specifications.

Performance Qualification (PQ): Verification that, under actual operating conditions, the computerized system operates as expected and that the results (actual data) are as expected.

Quality Management: Quality management is a continuous process that aims at quality improvement and overall performance in all processes and activities in the organization.

SLA: Stands for Service Level Agreement and provides the predefined and standard level of services available in the organization and ease the process to establish a solution-specific SLA.

SOP: Stands for Standard Operating Procedure is a written document that describes in details how a particular procedure or method is executed for repetitive use. It is generally intended to standardize the procedure performance.

Supplier: Entity (external company or internal department) that designs and produces the computerized system.

Validation: Documented evidence providing a high degree of assurance that a specific process under consideration does what it purposes to do. Validation deals with the entire system lifecycle to ensure a system satisfies user requirements, meets compliance expectations and adequately maintained to provide a secure environment with accurate, reliable, and traceable information from conception to retirement. The term is also used to describe the overall validation approach including qualification. Validation includes but is not limited to manufacturing processes, equipments, computerized system, etc.

Validation Plan: A plan created by the customer to define validation activities, responsibilities and procedures.

Vendor Audit: A systematic and independent examination to determine whether quality activities and related results comply with a documented quality system and whether this documented quality system is implemented effectively and is suitable to achieve the contractual requirements placed by the customer.

Chapter XXXIII
Organization and Evaluation of Experimental Measurements of Ergophysiological Data with the Method of SF12V2

Bill Ag Drougas
HATRLab, Greece & Higher Technological Institute of Epirus, Greece

Maria Sevdali
Higher Technological Institute of Kalamata, Greece

ABSTRACT

Ergophysiology as a division of the Physiology and helps us today to understand what happens in the human body and movement and how we are able to create models and methodologies to understand these mechanisms especially when we recognize something different and or any disability. Focuses on the human Biokinetics and the ability of the human body to create movement with various mechanisms and methods. These mechanisms are Biological, Chemical and Physical mechanisms and is the most important part of the human body and life. There are many problems today existed from various internal or external conditions and parameters for the human movement. If we'll recognize these problems we will be able to create methodologies to work in to serious scientific directions to help these people. These problems sometimes are very big and very important for the daily person's life especially with the existence of various other pathological problems in to the modern environment. Many of these problems give us informations about the personal kinetic ability status of any person. With the application of this statistical method of SF12V2 we are able organize and select a lot of personal information from different persons and to recognize different problems in to their own daily life. There are a numerous of recognized similar problems today about the daily kinetics ability level in to different ages. We can recognize the personal health level and the kinetics ability of different persons with some statistical tools and methods.

One of these tools is the SF12V2 statistical method. This is a very important tool to organize the selected data from various individuals and to take informations about their health and kinetics ability level using simply ergophysiological research methodologies. This one helps us to recognize every parameter in to the personal daily life activities and work inside or outside their family life or in to their job.Asking people we can take much information about their kinetic ability and their health level. The importance of this method is that the SF12V2 tool helps us to organize the answers for any similar existed problem and also to organize the experimental measurements of other Ergophysilogical data. SF12V2 helps us to recognize problems in to any level age or to search for individuals with any personal disability or any kinetic problem. In this chapter we analyze the special and newest methods used from the SF12V2 tools as we worked in the last year in Greece to recognize different problems in to many individuals. This Statistical methodology is very simple but still with a lot of different applications such as the Ergophysiology and the different levels of health.

INTRODUCTION

Today the Mathematics Science created many different tools to organize different but similar selected data from any research and to search informations about different subjects. This method called statistics. Firstly in United States presented the SF36 as a statistical instrument to recognize the level of the public health.

The SF36 is a multipurpose, short-form health survey with only 36 questions. It yields an 8 scale profile of functional health and well-being scores as well as psychometrically – based physical and mental health summary measures and a preference-based health unity index. It is a generic measure, as opposed to one that targets a specific age, disease, or treatment group (Sevdali M. and Petropoulou M. 2004).

The SF12V2 is a reflected version 2.0 of the SF-36 is so a newest recognized statistical method which uses the questions to select data especially in to the field of the personal health. The SF12V2 is a part of the SF12 statistical method of searching informations with the method of organizing the answers of different questions.

In this chapter we present the applications of this statistical tool especially in to the field of the Ergophysiology and in to the division of the Experimental Ergophysiology measurements such as kinetics ability, flexibility etc (Drougas Ag. Bill 2001).

We are able to organize the questions of the SF12V2 using some of them to search data from Ergophysiological parameters such as Physical Functioning-PF, Role Physical –RP, Bodily Pain-BP, General Health-GH, Vitality-VT, Social Functioning-SF, Role Emotional-RE, Mental Health-MH, Physical Component Summary-PCS, Mental component summary –MCS and the ability of kinetics and physical activity.

In the Ergophysiology this is very important and represents the personal kinetics ability and adaptability of the human body (Drougas B. 2002)

BACKGROUND

The Sort Form - SF36 questions method is a statistical methodology to select scientific informations directly from the persons who are participated in to the research and firstly used in the United States of America between 1970's and 1980's for the adults health research. This method of analyzing different selected data is very useful in to many applications in the division of the public health.

Today is a very important research and statistical tool officially in to more than 50 countries worldwide and have the official trade mark of quality of the IQOLA (Health Related Quality of Life). Past research methodologies were the official tools that created from Stewart and Ware in the 1992 with 40 different health meanings representing 149 different questions. This number of questions was very big not only for the researcher but also for any individual participating in the research. So just a little later in 1998 established another more simple tool with 36 questions in to only 8 health meanings.

Two years later resented the SF36V2 which is a newest tool after the simply SF36 cutting the 25% from the first questions (Sevdali M. and Petropoulou M. 2004). The philosophy of research by the SF is to recognize the answers between 0 and 100. When the score from the answers is less than 50 the individual's health level is very low (www.sf36.com)and if the score is over 50 the individual's personal health level is good. There are today many publications about the SF (Hurst N.P., Lambert C.M., Forbes J., Lochhead A.,Majior k., Lock P 2000) One of the most complete indepented accounts of the development of the SF36 along with a critical commentary offered from Mc Dowell and Newell (Mc Dowell and Newell 1996)

ISSUES

The aim of this chapter is to present the effects and the applications of the newest SF12V2 statistical methods in to the research and organization of various experimental measurements of Ergophysiological data especially in to the human kinetics and movement ability. The SF12V2 modern statistical methodology of selecting data is a very good tool today especially in the field of personal or national health.

Using simply questions we are able to make a diagram of their health level and then to organize a scientific statistical methodology for the future and level of their health and of course to

Figure 1.

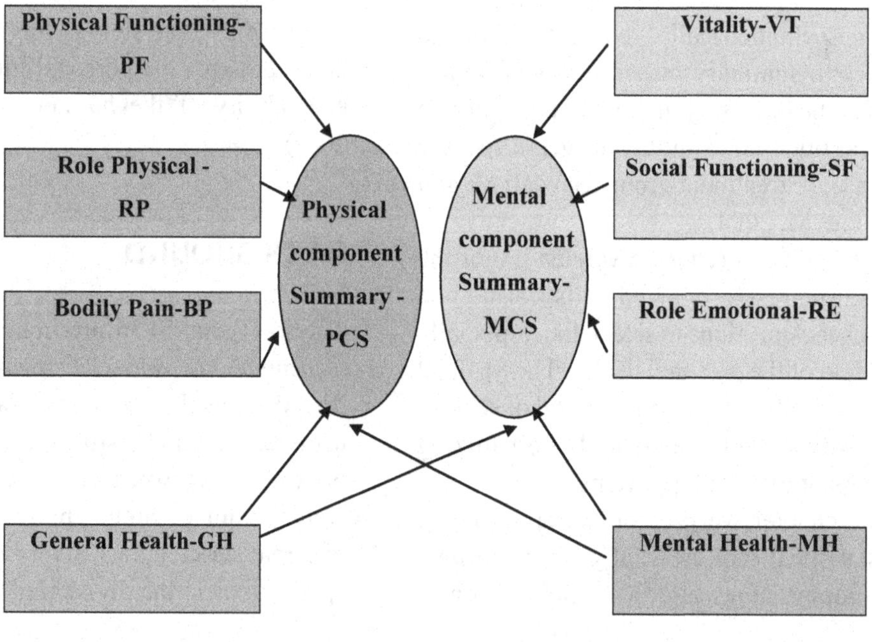

give directions and applications of rehabilitation if it is possible.

This chapter presents the applications of the latest statistical method of SF12V2 as a tool to take information about various experimental Ergophysiological data (Drougas Ag. Bill 2004G).

In the area of the Ergophysiology research with the SF12V2 we are able to search and recognize the following parameters which is summarized in Figure 1.

All the applications and methodologies presented in to various tables and statistical diagrams in to different categories for personal and popular health applications.

Also will present the methodology of the use of this modern statistical toll SF12V2 to take and to organize informations directly and personally from the citizens. This will help any researcher to use the SF12V2 tool in to many more research directions and applications not only in to the field of the Ergophysiological applications

So we are able to see how the modern environment and the daily personal kinetic ability may help researchers and individuals not only to recognize any Ergophysiological problem but also to establish programs and directions to help his/her self or to work with the health professionals for better and scientific popular health programs.

With this application we are able also to organize a project data base of Ergophysiological and high quality informations of human behavior which will help researchers and individuals in to searching methodologies and directions (Drougas Ag. B. 2006). This will give them the opportunity to establish or to recognize personal or national health and rehabilitation programs for the public health.

Table 1 summarizes some of the 1st level of questions of the SF12V2 tool which helped us in to the Ergophysiological parameters.

The following question help us to receive informations about the physical health or the emotional problems and this is as follows

Table 1.

A general question about your health, answering with one of the following (Excellent, very good, good, fair, poor)

Vigorous Activities such as running, lifting heavy objects, participating in strenuous sports

Moderate Activities such as moving a table, pushing a vacuum cleaner, bowing, or playing golf

- Lifting a carrying groceries
- Climbing several flights of stairs
- Climbing one flight of stairs
- Bending, kneeling, or stooping
- Walking more than a mile
- Walking several hundred yards
- Walking one hundred yards
- Bathing or dressing your self

The answers of the aforementioned questions must be between a lot, a little, none at all and give us information about a physical and typical day of the person.

In the following Table 2 summarized the 2ed level of questions. These questions give us informations for the past 4 weeks of how much of the time had the person any of the following problems with his/her work or other regular daily activities as a result of his/her physical health. This helps us to understand the last 4 weeks ability.

Table 2.

• Cut down on the amount of time you spent on work or other activities
• Accomplished less than you would like
• Were limited in the kind of work or other activities
• Had difficulty performing the work or other activities (example, it took extra effort)
• All the answers must be between: All of the time, Most of the time, Some of the time, a little of the time and None of the time.

During the past 4 weeks, to what extent has your physical health or emotional problems interfered with your normal social activities with family, friends, neighbors, or groups.

- **The typical answers are between:** Not at all, Slightly, Moderately, Quite a bit, Extremely.

The next question may help us to have informations about the disability and the pain something very important in to our research and is the following:

How much bodily pain have you had during the past 4 weeks?

- **Answers are between:** None, Very Mild, Mild, Moderate, Severe, Very Severe

The next question helps us to see the importance of the pain during a daily life and in to various activities of the person and this is as follows.

During the past 4 weeks, how much did pain interfere with your normal work (including both work outside the home and housework)?

- **The answers of this question must be between :** Not at all, a little bit, Moderately, Quite a bit, Extremely

Table 3 summarizes the next level of questions which gives us information about other daily problems and how much of the time he/she had any of the following problems with the work or other regular daily activities as a result of any emotional problems (such as feeling depressed or anxious).

All the answers must be between: All of the time, Most of the time, Some of the time, a little of the time and None of the time.

The next question also give us informations about of the past 4 weeks how much of the time he/she has his/her physical health or emotional problems interfered with any social activities (like visiting friends, relatives, hobbies etc)

The answer must be between : All of the time, Most of the time, Some of the time, a little of the time and None of the time.

There are some more questions about the person's psychological level but these questions are not possible to give us Ergophysiological answers and information.

All the above questions give us a lot of different informations about the ability and the activity

Table 3.

• Cut down on the amount of time you spent on work or other activities
• Accomplished less than you would like
• Did work or activities less carefully than usual

of the person. With the answers we are able to organize the level of similar answers and to find the problems by the SF with the answers between 0 and 100. When the score from the answers is less than 50 the individual's health level is very low (www.sf36.com)and if the score is over 50 the individual's personal health level is good. In to the application of the Ergophysiological measurements we are able to know the kinetics adaptability and the ability of the person to participate in to various daily activities during his/her life. This will help us to search for any other similar pathological problems or any disabilities.

FUTURE TRENDS

The SF12V2 is a serious and simply statistical tool in the modern statistics. Especially in the field of the experimental measurements of the Ergophysiology the SF12V2 tool give us many informations about any activities in the daily life or the work and for the social life of one person. This helps us to create directions, politics and methodologies about the personal health to help these people in to his/her home with simple exercises and methodologies and always with the affiliation of the special scientists.

We are able to use the SF12V2 questions as a recognized tool to organize different selected data in the field of the Ergophysiology and to have answers from different applications in to a group of persons during their own daily life. We are also able to organize more similar questions in to similar fields of the public health to take statistical informations in to various experimental measurements and applications.

This statistical tool helps us also to select informations directly from individuals just in to a few minutes having answers and their thoughts about their health level.

It would be great to work with the SF12V2 in to many more applications and to induct more questions with Ergophysiological applications in to different ages.

REFERENCES

Drougas, B. (2003). Applications of teleinformatics in medicine. *TEI of Epirus*, 2001, pp 24-29

Drougas, Ag. B (April – June 2001). Kinetics & Flexibility for the Human Body. *Karate Voice Newspaper,* page 9

Drougas, Ag. B (2002). Study of the ability of the kinetic adaptability by combinable movements. *Exercise and Society Journal 31,* 371,372 .

Drougas, Ag. B. Telemedicine (2004a). *Applications in a contemporary environment, Edition,* pp 47-55.

Drougas, Ag. B. (2003). Theory and laboratory applications for the lesson teleinformatics and applications in Medicine Department of Teleinformatics. *ATEI of Epirus*, pp 25-47

Drougas, Ag. B. (2004B). *Care and the Modern technologies*, pp 45-67

Drougas, Ag. B.(2004G). Rehabilitation by new technologies.*Research and Theory Journal Issue. 1/04*, 12-15.

Drougas, Ag. B. (2004c). Virtual reality and health manual of the laboratory of the teleinformatics and applications in Medicine, Department of Teleinformatics. *ATEI of Epirus*, pp 10-22

Drougas Ag. B. (2006). Virtual reality simulation in human applied kinetics and ergo-physiology. *Encyclopedia of Informatics in Health Care and Biomedicine*. University of Piraeus Greece: IGI Publications

Hurst N.P., Lambert C. M., Forbes J., Lochhead A.,Majior k., Lock, P. (2000). Does waiting matter? A randomized controlled trial of new non-urgent rheumatology out-patient referrals. *Rheumatology 2000*, 369-376

Mc Dowell I, Newell C.(1996). *Measuring health: A guide to rating scales and questionnaires (second edition).* New York: Oxford University Press

Muller, Nordhorn J. Roll, S. Willich, S. N. (2004). Comparison of the short form(SF)-12 health status instrument with the SF36 in patients with coronary heart disease. *Heart 2004*, 523-527. BMJ Publishing Group & British Cardiac Society.

Sevdali M.,Petropoulou M.,(2004). *Measuremed of health levels using the evaluation method sf36: Comparative study of 2 hospital units.* H.O.U. of Patra, Greece, pp 7-16

KEY TERMS

Biokinetics: Is an integral part of the multidisciplinary sports medicine approach. This profession utilises physical activity as the primary therapeutic modality in preventative health care and improvement of physical condition, as well as final phase rehabilitation for cardiac, orthopaedic, and chronic disease population groups. Biokineticists perform a comprehensive, functional assessment on each patient and then prescribe scientifically based exercise programmes based on their evaluation findings. These findings determine whether the patient has poor cardiovascular and respiratory function, muscle weakness or imbalances, inflexibility or instability or poor neuromuscular co-ordination. The word Biokinetics is taken from the Greek word "BIOS" which means "life" and "KINESIS" which means "movement". In other words the maintenance of quality of life through use of physical activity.

Ergophysiology: Is a scientific part of the Physiology science which focuses on the human Biokinetics and the ability of the human body to create movement with various mechanisms and methods. These mechanisms are Biological , Chemical and Physical mechanisms and is the most important part of the human body and life.

Ergophysiology Mechanism: Energy metabolism and muscular work. Energy sources, reserves and replenishment. Special features of the different types of muscle fibbers. Anaerobic, aerobic exercise, lactate threshold. Exercise and disuse induced adaptations to the cardiovascular, the hormonal and neuromuscular systems. Thermoregulation. Basics of nutrition.

IQOLA: Means Health Related Quality of Life. This is to recognize the level of quality of personal life of different persons and ages.

SF12V2: Is an important statistical tool which focuses in to some vital groups of questions with different level of answers which are able to give us infromations about the health level of any individual. Especially in the field of the experimental measurements of the Ergophysiology the SF12V2 tool give us many infromations about any activities in the daily or the work and social life of one person. This helps us to create directions, politics and methodologies to help these people in to his/her home with simple exercises and methodologies with the affiliation of the special scientists. This is the newest tool of the SF36 Statistical tools.

The Sort Form - SF36: The SF36 as a statistical instrument to recognize the level of the public health. Is a number of different questions method and statistical methodology to select scientific informations directly from the persons who are participated in to the research and firstly used in the United States of America between 1970's and 1980's for the adults health research. This method of analyzing different selected data is very useful in to many applications in the division of the public health. The SF36 is a multipurpose, short-form health survey with only 36 questions. It yields an 8 scale profile of functional health and well-being scores as well as psychometrically – based physical and mental health summary measures and a preference-based health unity index. It is a generic measure, as opposed to one that targets a specific age, disease, or treatment group.

Chapter XXXIV
Ubiquitous Risk Analysis of Physiological Data

Daniele Apiletti
Politecnico di Torino, Italy

Elena Baralis
Politecnico di Torino, Italy

Giulia Bruno
Politecnico di Torino, Italy

Tania Cerquitelli
Politecnico di Torino, Italy

ABSTRACT

Current advances in sensing devices and wireless technologies are providing a high opportunity for improving care quality and reducing the medical costs. This chapter presents the architecture of a mobile healthcare system and provides an overview of mobile health applications. Furthermore, it proposes a framework for patient monitoring that performs real-time stream analysis of data collected by means of non-invasive body sensors. It evaluates a patient's health conditions by analyzing different physiological signals to identify anomalies and activate alarms in risk situations. A risk function for identifying the instantaneous risk of each physiological parameter has been defined. The performance of the proposed system has been evaluated on public physiological data and promising experimental results are presented. By understanding the challenges and the current solutions of informatics appliances described in this chapter, new research areas can be further investigated to improve mobile healthcare services and design innovative medical applications.

INTRODUCTION

Technological advances in sensing devices, miniaturization of low-power microelectronics, and wireless networks enable the design and exploitation of wireless devices capable of autonomously monitoring human health conditions to improve mobile healthcare services for patients and health professionals. Mobile health applications may play a key role in saving lives by allowing timely assistance, in collecting data for medical research, and in significantly cutting the cost of medical services. Hence, advances in health information systems and healthcare technologies offer a tremendous opportunity for improving care quality while reducing cost [Lee, 2006]. Non-invasive medical sensors measuring vital signs (e.g., temperature, heart rate, blood pressure, oxygen saturation, serum glucose), integrated into tiny intelligent wearable accessories (e.g., watches [http://www.skyaid.org/LifeWatch/life_watch.htm]), are currently under development [Jovanov, 2005]. Wearable devices allow an individual to closely monitor changes in her or his vital signs for extended periods of time and provide a comprehensive view of a patient's condition. These devices can be integrated into a general health system architecture to continuously monitor patient health status and timely recognize life-threatening changes. Hence, an important issue in this context is the real-time analysis of physiological signals to characterize the patient condition and immediately identify dangerous situations.

This chapter describes the architecture of a mobile healthcare system and provides an overview of health applications. Furthermore, it proposes a flexible framework called IGUANA (Individuation of Global Unsafe Anomalies and Alarm activation) to perform stream analysis of physiological data to monitor a patient's health condition, by analyzing physiological measures collected by means of a set of wearable sensors. The real-time analysis exploits data mining techniques for assessing the instantaneous risk of monitored people. To allow ubiquitous analysis, real-time processing is performed on mobile devices (e.g., Pocket PCs and smart phones). When a dangerous situation is detected, an immediate intervention may be requested by raising an alarm (e.g., phone call, SMS) to the closest medical centre.

MOBILE HEALTH SYSTEM ARCHITECTURE

The overall architecture of a mobile health system (see, e.g., [Jones, 2006], [Apiletti, 2006]) is shown in Figure 1. It may be composed by some or all of the following subsystems:

- A body sensor network
- A wireless local area network
- A GSM network

Each individual (patient) wears a set of sensors that monitor physiological signals. These sensors, which are integrated into non-invasive objects, are connected to the user's device (also called personal server, e.g., a smart phone or a PDA) through a short range communication link (e.g., Bluetooth), in charge of transmitting recorded signals. The device may locally elaborate the incoming signals to immediately detect life-threatening situations. The set of wearable sensors and the mobile device form the body sensor network.

The second subsystem allows the communication between the user's mobile device and the elaboration centre, possibly by means of an infrastructure node (e.g., an access point). Communication with the elaboration centre may occur when recorded data is transferred to the system for off-line analysis or to backup/gather historical data. Finally, through the GSM network an alert message may be sent to the closest medical centre to request prompt medical intervention when a risk situation is detected.

Figure 1. General architecture of a mobile health system

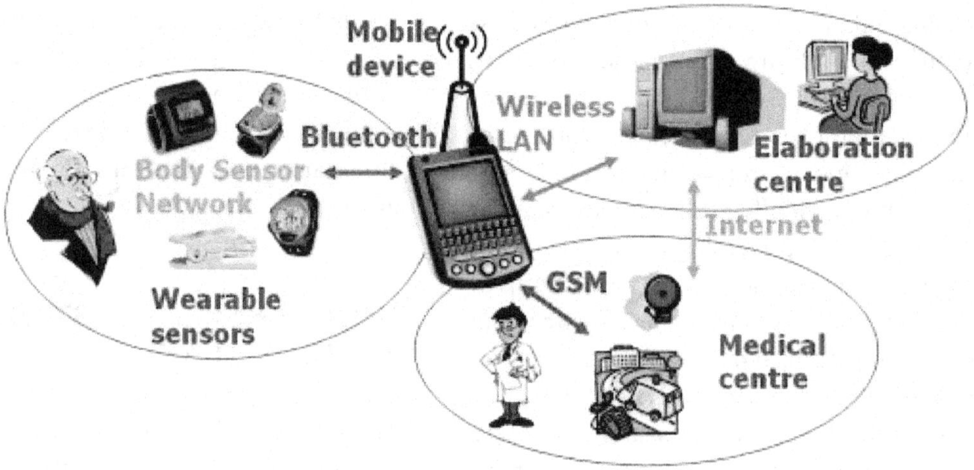

A more detailed description of each subsystem is presented in the following.

Body Sensor Network. A body sensor network consists of multiple sensing devices capable of sampling and processing one or more vital signs (e.g., heart rate, blood pressure, oxygen saturation, patient activity, body temperature) or environmental parameters (e.g., patient location, environment temperature and light). Furthermore, these devices are able to transfer relevant gathered measurements to a personal server (i.e., a mobile device like a personal digital assistant or a smart phone) through a wireless personal network implemented using ZigBee (based on the IEEE 802.15.4 standard) or Bluetooth (defined in the IEEE 802.15.1 specifications).

According to the type and nature of a healthcare application the frequency of relevant events (e.g., sampling, processing, and communicating) is set. Sensors periodically transmit their status and gathered measurements. Power consumption reducing strategies are exploited to extend battery life. Furthermore, since sensing devices are placed strategically on the human body, as tiny wearable accessories they must satisfy requirements for minimal weight, miniature form-factor, and low-power consumption to allow extended health monitoring time.

Several efforts have been devoted to the design of wearable medical systems ([Axisa, 2003], [Varady, 2002]) and the reduction of power consumption of medical body sensors ([Anliker, 2004], [Cheng, 2004], [Branche, 2005]). For example in [Axisa, 2003] the authors describe a system for the measurement of the nervous system activity by means of a smart shirt and a smart glove, which use textiles with sensors and wires for communication. Instead, in [Anliker, 2004], the authors describe several ways to reduce power consumption by choosing passive sensors, activating the display back-light only when the user presses a button, putting special care in the analog processing unit design, reducing clock frequency, and replacing a discrete analog board with an ASIC. In [Branche, 2005] a method to minimize LED driving currents, lowering the overall power requirement of a reflectance mode pulse oximeter, is described.

Wireless LAN (WLAN). Once the physiological data have been collected by means of the body sensor network and transferred to the personal server, this device may send them to an elaboration centre through the WLAN. By means of the WLAN the personal server can reach an Internet access point to communicate with medical centre services (e.g., off-line physicians' analysis). The elaboration centre is generally a computer which locally stores historical physiological signals collected during everyday monitoring and provides a powerful graphical user interface to show time series of physiological data. The elaboration centre is particularly convenient for in-home monitoring of elderly patients.

Many efforts have been devoted to integrate mobile devices (e.g., PDAs) and WLAN technology [Lin, 2004]. Through the WLAN an Internet access point is reached to transfer in real time the patient's signals to a remote central management unit, where medical staff can access and analyze the physiological data. Also the framework proposed in [Wu, 1999] is focused on a medical mobile system which performs real-time telediagnosis and teleconsultation. Patient measures are collected by a DSP-based hardware, compressed in real time, and sent to the physicians in hospital.

GSM Network. If the mobile device is equipped with appropriate intelligence, it can process the physiological data locally and automatically generate alarms when life-threatening events are detected [Manders, 1996]. When the device identifies a dangerous situation, it can send an alarm to the medical centre. In this way, data are transmitted only when needed and data compression can be avoided. In [Varshney, 2006] the authors concentrate on improving transmission of emergency messages, which must be reliably delivered to healthcare professionals with minimal delays and no message corruption. They propose a network solution for emergency signal transmission using ad hoc wireless networks, which can be formed among patient-worn devices.

The core of the overall architecture is the mobile device which records physiological values from wearable sensors, transmits vital signs to the elaboration centre, locally elaborates them to detect dangerous situations, and sends alert messages to request prompt medical intervention. Connectivity with other architectural components employs different technologies. While the mobile device interfaces to the body sensor network through a network coordinator that implements ZigBee or Bluetooth protocols, it exploits mobile telephone networks (e.g., GSM) or WLANs to reach an Internet access point for communicating with the medical server. Furthermore, the mobile device is also a critical point of the architecture. Since portable appliances work with different constraints (e.g., power consumption, memory, battery), the analysis of physiological signals performed on mobile devices requires optimized power consumption and short processing response times which are important research topics in different computer science areas.

HEALTH CARE APPLICATIONS

Since health care applications of intelligent systems are becoming pervasive, sensor technologies have been exploited for patient monitoring. Furthermore, medical staff and patients can benefit from the monitoring process by applying automatic real-time knowledge extraction algorithms. Hence, an important issue in this context is the analysis of physiological signals performed on mobile devices, which requires optimized resource-aware algorithms.

In [Lin, 2004] the authors propose a monitoring system, which integrates PDAs and WLANs. Through the WLAN, the patient's measures are sent to a remote management unit, where the medical staff can analyze the data. In [Wu, 1999] the architecture of a medical mobile system is proposed. It performs real-time telediagnosis and teleconsultation. Patient data are gathered by a DSP-based device, compressed in real time, and sent to physicians. The main advantage of these approaches is the simplicity of the architecture, which does not require any intelligence to the devices, since the analysis is performed in the elaboration centre. However, since this architecture introduces a delay for data transmission, it may cause a delay in detecting a critical condition. Furthermore, it requires the presence of physicians to monitor patients also in normal conditions.

If the mobile device is a smart appliance, it can elaborate the measures locally and trigger alarming actions [Manders, 1996]. When dangerous conditions are detected, the medical centre can be automatically warned. Thus, only when unsafe situations occur, data are actually transmitted.

One step further towards the elaboration on mobile devices is proposed in [Gupta, 2004] where a PDA is exploited to receive data from medical sensors and to transmit them over bandwidth-limited wireless networks. The authors specifically address the problems of managing different medical data (e.g., vital bio-signals and images), developing an easy interface (user-oriented for physicians) to view or acquire medical data, and supporting simultaneous data transfers over low bandwidth wireless links.

Many efforts have been dedicated to improving hardware and connectivity among devices ([Lorincz, 2004], [Jones, 2006]), but less attention has been devoted to investigating analysis techniques to assess the current risk level of a patient. However, the definition of efficient algorithms that automatically detect unsafe situations in real time is a difficult task. In [Varady, 2002] an algorithm to discover physiological problems (e.g., cardiac arrhythmias) based on a-priori medical knowledge is proposed. Physiological time series recorded through sensors may be exploited for learning usual behavioral patterns on a long time scale. Any deviation is considered an unexpected and possibly dangerous situation. More recently, in [Sharshar, 2005] the extraction of temporal patterns from single or multiple physiological signals by means of statistical techniques (e.g., regression) is proposed. Single signal analysis provides trend descriptions such as increasing, decreasing, constant and transient. Instead, multiple signal analysis introduces a signal hierarchy and provides a global view of the clinical situation. Furthermore, a machine learning process discovers pattern templates from sequences of trends related to specific clinical events. The above mentioned solutions either are limited to specific physiological signals, or require some kind of a-priori information, such as fixed thresholds, or address related but different problems, such as detecting long term trends.

THE IGUANA FRAMEWORK

The IGUANA (Individuation of Global Unsafe Anomalies and Alarm activation) framework is based on the overall architecture shown in Figure 1. It performs real-time stream analysis of data collected by a body sensor network on a mobile device and evaluates a patient's health conditions by analyzing different clinical signals to identify anomalies and activate alarms in risk conditions.

The building blocks of the framework are shown in Figure 2. Since risk conditions depend on the specific disease or patient profile, we first perform a training phase in which the framework automatically learns the common and uncommon behaviors. Given historical physiological data, IGUANA creates different risk models tailored to specific conditions (e.g., a specific disease) or patient profiles. The training phase is performed off-line in the elaboration centre and different models of patients and diseases can be created. The most suitable model for the current monitored patient is exploited in the risk evaluation phase.

Since patient conditions depend on the contribution of several physiological signals (i.e., heart rate, blood pressure, oxygen saturation), we devise a global risk function to evaluate the risk indicator for the patient at each instant. The proposed risk function combines different components. Each component models a different type

Figure 2. Building blocks of the IGUANA framework

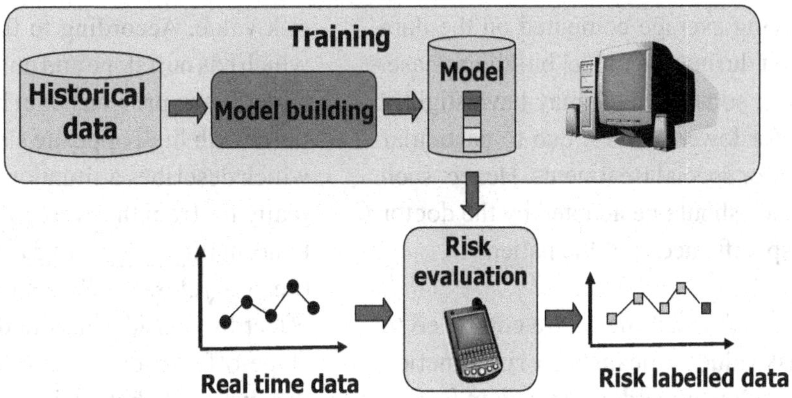

of deviation from the standard behavior, such as the difference from the moving average value to evaluate a long term trend, or the difference from the previous measure to detect quick changes. Furthermore, standard conditions for patients may be represented by a normality band, whose upper and lower bounds are denoted as normality thresholds. Outside these thresholds, the risk of a patient additionally increases. Higher danger levels are denoted by a higher risk value of the risk function.

During the on-line classification phase, IGUANA processes real-time streams of measures collected by sensors. For each measure, the risk value is computed by means of the proposed risk function to evaluate the current patient condition. If a dangerous situation is detected, an alarm (e.g., phone call, SMS) can be sent to the closest medical centre to request prompt medical intervention.

Risk Function

The idea of quantifying the health status of a patient by means of his/her physiological signals is based on the comparison between current conditions and the common behavior derived by the analysis of previously collected data. We define as dangerous a situation in which the patient exhibits a deviation from a standard conduct described by the model. The model can be tailored to the different clinical conditions of a patient. We base our risk evaluation on a function that combines different components. Each component assesses a kind of deviation from the normal clinical behavior. The same risk function is applied to all physiological signals. However, different weights may be assigned for each signal, according to its importance in the global clinical condition evaluation and its specific physiological characteristics. The risk of each measure depends on the following components, which are depicted in Figure 3.

1. **Offset:** It is the difference between the current measure and the moving average value. Since the moving average is the mean value of the measures in a given time window, the offset shows long term trends related to the current situation of a given patient.
2. **Slope:** It is the difference between the current and previous measures. Its purpose is to detect quick changes. Hence, it shows short term trends.
3. **Dist:** It is the difference between the current value and the closest of two thresholds, named "normality thresholds". Normality thresholds define a range outside which the

patient risk increases because of excessively high (or low) values. They are estimated as the maximum and minimum values of the moving average computed on the data analyzed during the model building phase. However, some patients may have slightly higher (or lower) values, due to particular diseases or special treatments. Hence, such thresholds should be adapted by the doctor to the specific needs of the patient.

The above risk components are combined to compute a risk value by means of the risk function in Box 1, where w_o, w_s, and w_d are weight factors for the different risk components.

A higher risk is associated with a point with high offset and slope, because it is far from the moving average of the signal and it is on a trend which increases the distance. Points with low offset and slope correspond to a lower risk value, because the signal, even if far from its moving average, shows a stabilizing trend, because its distance is decreasing. This concept is expressed in the first term of the function (i.e., $|w_o \cdot Offset + w_s \cdot Slope|$), but it is not sufficient to properly estimate the risk value. According to this term only, a point which has null slope and null offset (i.e. a measure equal to the previous one) has the same risk as a point with high opposite slope and offset values, which describes a situation where the measure is really far from the average but quickly returning to normality. The second term in the risk formula (i.e.,$w_r \cdot \sqrt{Offset^2 + Slope^2}$) takes into account this effect by considering the distance of a point in slope-offset coordinates from the origin. Finally, the dist contribution is added as third term. It increases the risk associated with measures outside the normality thresholds range. The weights w_s, w_o, and w_d are parametric functions of slope, offset, and dist respectively. The coefficient w_r is a function of w_o and w_s. Each weight is in the range [0,1] and can be different for positive and negative component values. This approach allows a wide degree of flexibility in the risk evaluation, thus

Figure 3. Risk components used in the risk function

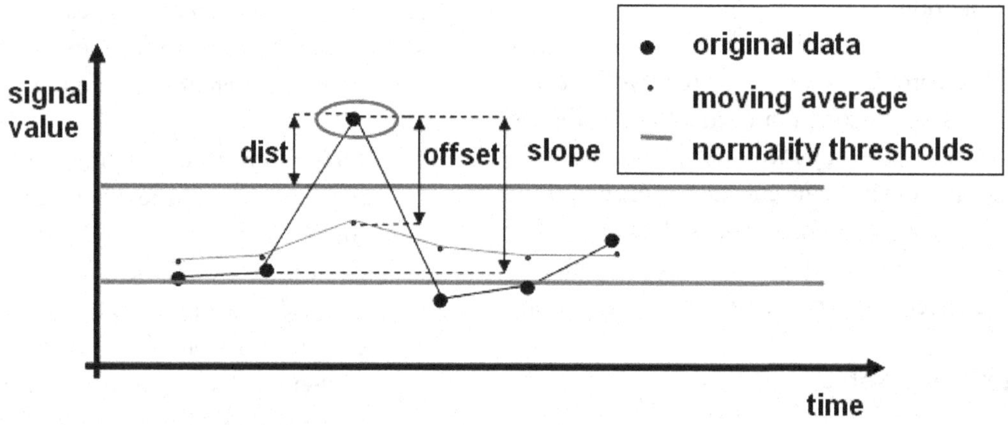

Box 1.

$$F_{risk} = |w_o \cdot Offset + w_s \cdot Slope| + w_r \cdot \sqrt{Offset^2 + Slope^2} + w_d \cdot Dist$$

suiting different characteristics of physiological signals. For example, while increases in peripheral blood oxygen saturation are beneficial, decreases are relevant to risk evaluation. By considering only negative component values the correct interpretation of the physiological behavior is provided (e.g., positive and negative offset values can be easily associated with different weights).

Training Phase

In the training phase we analyzed historical clinical data to automatically model normal and unsafe situations. The most infrequent situations are considered as representative of risky situations and are exploited to model dangerous states, while common behaviors yield a model of standard (normal) states. Since situations depend on the specific disease or patient profile, different models can be built. After computing for every measure its corresponding risk components (offset, slope and dist), the model building step is performed in three parts:

- **Measure clustering:** Clustering is separately applied to the offset, slope and dist measures, to partition them in (monodimensional) clusters, characterized by homogeneous values. IGUANA is currently based on a hierarchical clustering technique, but the generality of our framework allows us to exploit any suitable clustering algorithm. Different selection issues are discussed in the Experimental Results section. At the end of this phase, for each considered sensor stream, a collection of classes for offset, slope and dist values is available, each characterized by upper and lower bounds.
- **Measure risk computation:** The risk associated with each physiological signal (or measure) is computed by applying the risk function to the offset, slope and dist risk levels. Measure risk is divided into a finite number of values by means of a discretization step.
- **Global risk computation:** The clinical situation of a patient depends on every physiological signal at the same instant. Since different physiological signals give different contribution to the global risk according to the specific disease or clinical conditions, we allow different weights for each signal in the global risk computation. For example, considering heart rate and body temperature of a heart patient, the weight of the heart rate signal should be higher than the weight of the body temperature signal in the global risk computation. Since we focused our analysis on identifying unsafe anomalies which can lead to vital threat, we consider only vital signals and even a single high risk measure is enough to show an unsafe trend. For this reason, the global risk associated with the clinical situation of the patient at a given instant is defined as the highest risk level among those assigned to every physiological signal at the same instant.

Real-Time Risk Evaluation Phase

Real time streams of measures incoming from different sensors are initially processed separately, but the same operations are applied to all of them and at the end the results are combined into a unique value indicating the risk factor of the current clinical situation. Before starting the analysis, the value of each incoming measure is compared with user-defined absolute thresholds to determine whether it is outside a given range. If so, it is directly assigned the highest risk level.

Examples of user defined thresholds for some vital signals are:

- Heart rate: 40-150 beats per minute;
- Arterial blood pressure (systolic): 80-220 mmHg;
- Arterial blood pressure (diastolic): 40-120 mmHg;

- Peripheral blood oxygen saturation: 90-100%.

Next, the offset, slope and dist components are computed for the incoming measure. The needed information is: (i) the previous measure, (ii) the previous moving average value, and (iii) the normality threshold values. A risk level is assigned to each component, by comparing the current values with the predefined classes stored in the model itself. The risk associated with each physiological signal (or measure) is computed by applying the risk function to the offset, slope and dist risk levels. In this step, the user-defined weight parameters (see Section "Risk function") are exploited. Next, the maximum risk among all synchronous measures is assigned as global risk level. If the obtained global risk level is above a user-defined threshold, an alarm may be triggered.

EXPERIMENTAL RESULTS

We validated our approach by means of several experiments addressing both the effect of varying several parameters of the framework (i.e., clustering algorithm selection, sliding window width, sampling frequency, and risk function weights), the performance of its current implementation, the required resources and the battery average lifetime. While experiments for the model building phase have been performed off-line using a typical desktop PC, the classification phase has been extensively tested on mobile platforms.

Datasets

We validated the IGUANA framework with sensor measures publicly available on the Internet and collected by PhysioBank, the PhysioNet archive of physiological signals (www.physionet.org/physiobank), maintained by the Harvard-MIT Division of Health Sciences and Technology.

We analyzed 64 patient records from the MIMIC-numerics database (Multiparameter Intelligent Monitoring for Intensive Care) [http://www.physionet.org/physiobank/ database/mimicdb], for whom the medical information we needed had been recorded and who were more than 60 years old. MIMIC-numerics is a section of the larger MIMIC database whose data is represented in the numeric format displayed in the digital instrumentation used for patient monitoring in hospitals. Since the MIMIC database collects data from bed-side ICU (Intensive Care Unit) instrumentation, the clinical situations of the patients we analyzed were extremely serious, allowing us to the test our approach in such utmost conditions. For our purpose, in the MIMIC-numerics database we chose 4 physiological signals considered significant of a patient's health conditions: (i) heart rate (HR) [beats per minute], (ii) systolic arterial blood pressure (ABP-sys) [mmHg], (iii) diastolic arterial blood pressure (ABP-dias) [mmHg], and (iv) peripheral blood oxygen saturation (SpO_2) [percentage]. Original measures from the MIMIC-numerics database are provided every second. NA-threshold values (see Section "Real-time Risk Evaluation Phase") were determined according to medical literature. PhysioNet also provides PhysioToolkit, a library of software for physiological signal processing and analysis. We used some PhysioToolkit tools (e.g., the rdsamp utility/command) for extracting the desired data from the databases and during the preprocessing phase.

Clustering Algorithm Selection

We considered many clustering techniques (e.g., partitioning, hierarchical, and density-based). We focused on partitioning and hierarchical techniques [Han, 2000], which were available in the statistical open-source environment R [http://www.r-project.org/]. Partitioning algorithms, such as k-means, performed worse than hierarchical algorithms, because they clustered also normality situations in different risk levels. Figure 4(a) shows this wrong behaviour. Hierarchical clustering algorithms may use different methods to compute the inter-cluster distance. In our context, the average linkage method yields better results than single linkage (which forms chains of points), or complete linkage, or ward. Figure 4(b) shows clusters obtained by applying the average linkage method. We finally observe that the clustering algorithm is a single, modular component of our framework. Any suitable algorithm may be easily integrated in place of the current one.

Sliding Window Size

The size of the sliding window models the effect of the recent past on the current situation. The longer the sliding window, the less the moving average follows any sharp trend of a measure. Decreasing the sliding window size increases the rapid adaptation of risk evaluation to abrupt changes in a measure. The offset is the risk component affected by variations of the sliding window. It is based on the moving average value, which is strongly affected by the sliding window length. The variation of the sliding window size allows the IGUANA framework to adapt to different patient conditions. When a small sliding window size is considered, sudden changes in physiological values are quickly detected as potential risk conditions. However, due to therapy side effects or a very active life style, some patients may be allowed to have quick changes in physiological values without being in danger. In this case, a longer sliding window may smooth the effect of a short, abrupt change in the context of a normal, steady situation.

Sampling Frequency

The sampling frequency value directly affects the alarm activation delay. Every measure is assigned a risk level, which can potentially trigger an alarm. Hence, a dangerous situation can be identified within the next measure, which is in a sampling period time. For example, to identify a heart failure soon enough to have good chances of life-saving intervention by an emergency staff, the longest alarm activation delay should be 15 seconds. Longer delay values may be suitable for different purposes. The IGUANA framework is able to easily adapt to diverse sampling frequencies. Since sensor measures may be provided with different frequencies, in this context the adaptability of the IGUANA framework becomes essential. When the sampling frequency is high, even subtle, short anomalies are detected, while a longer sampling period hides some of the sharpest spikes, but correctly identifies the remaining unsafe situations.

Risk Function Weights

Risk function weights are among the most important parameters of the framework, because they directly determine the effect of each risk component (slope, offset, and dist) on the computed risk value. Hence, a physician is allowed to customize this setting to the clinical conditions of the patient and to the kind of anomalies to be detected. We report the results of some experiments performed to show the separate effect of the different risk components. All experiments are performed on the same sample dataset. They have no direct medical value, but demonstrate the adaptability of the framework to a wide range of situations. In Figure 4(c) and Figure 4(d) risk evaluation is only based on the offset component (slope and dist weights are set to zero). Risk rises with the distance between the measured value and the moving average. Such setting allows a physician to reveal deviations from a stationary behaviour dynamically evaluated. In this case, positive or negative spikes in the signal time series are identified as dangerous situations. To separately analyze positive and negative contributions of the offset component, the offset weight w_o is set to 1 only for positive offset values in Figure 4(c), and only

Figure 4. Experimental results for different parameters of the framework

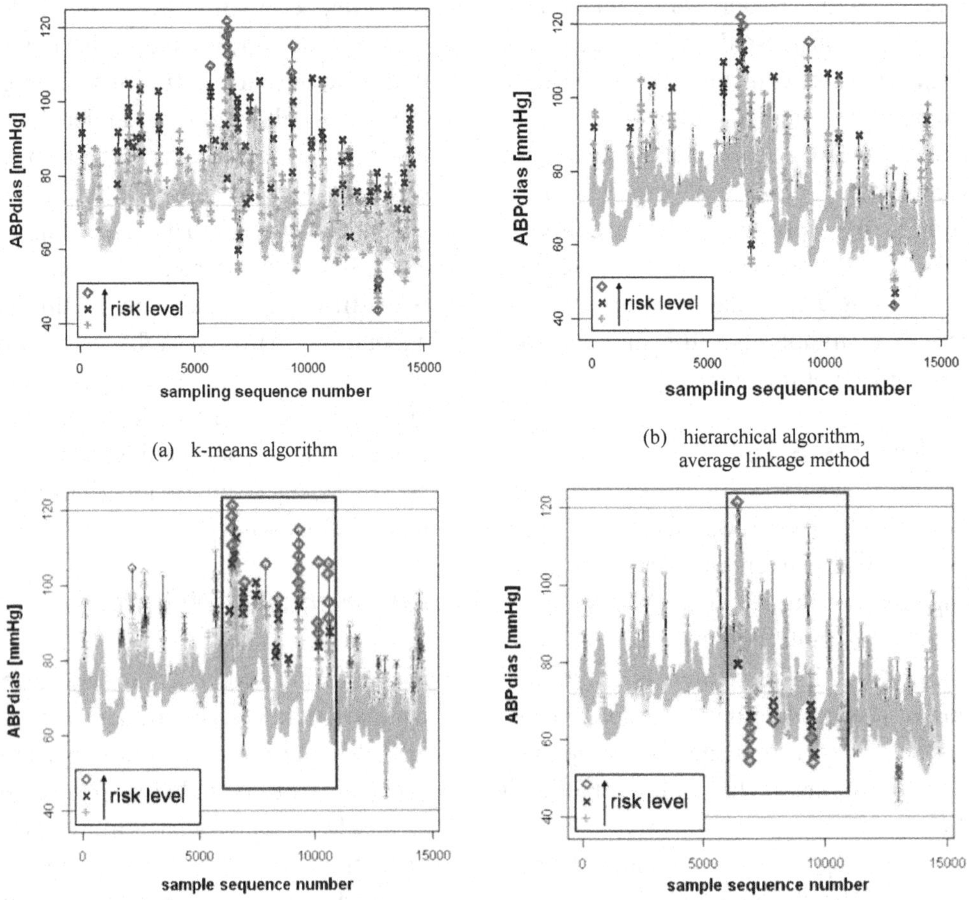

(a) k-means algorithm

(b) hierarchical algorithm, average linkage method

(c) positive offset only (

d) negative offset only

for negative offset values in Figure 4(d). When it is necessary to identify abrupt increases in a given measure, the slope risk component should be considered. This kind of analysis allows a physician to focus on rapid changes in the physiological behaviour of the patient.

Performance

In our experiments, we evaluated the performance of the IGUANA framework both for the off-line model building phase and for the on-line classification phase. Model building experiments have been performed on an AMD Athlon64 3200+ PC with 512 Mb main memory, Windows XP Professional operating system and R version 2.1.1. As expected, the k-means algorithm is about 60 times faster than the hierarchical algorithm and shows a better scalability with increasing data cardinality. However, since model creation is performed off-line, the selection of the clustering algorithm has been based on the quality of generated clusters, rather than performance. With hierarchical clustering algorithms, different methods for computing inter-cluster distance may be adopted. Different distance computation methods show a negligible effect on performance. Hence, again, the selection of the average linkage distance method was driven by cluster quality issues. Models with thousands of measures, generated by means of hierarchical clustering, are created in tens of minutes.

Performance of the classification phase is more critical, since this task is performed on-line. Furthermore, to be able to deliver real-time classification of incoming sensor data, the time requested by the classification of a single measure has to be less than the sampling period of the sensors.

Since mobile health applications have specific requirements in terms of power consumption and resources, they need to be evaluated directly on the scene. We performed experiments with a mobile version of IGUANA developed for both the Pocket PC and the Smartphone architectures. In Figure 5 a sample screenshot of the mobile application is presented. The instantaneous risk of each monitored vital sign is denoted as a number ranging from 1 to 5 (ABPsys, systolic blood pressure; ABPdias, diastolic blood pressure; HR, heart beat rate; SpO2, peripheral blood oxygen saturation). To the right, the global risk is shown, together with the remaining battery power.

Results are promising, since the Smartphone battery proved to last many hours. Memory resources are estimated to be in the order of the hundreds of bytes for the data structures, while the complete application can be run on a 2 Mbyte equipped Smartphone without restrictions. Since each measure requires around 0.5 ms to be processed by the mobile application, real-time measure classification can be performed even at high sampling frequency. These experiments highlight both the adaptability and the efficiency of the proposed approach.

Figure 5. Screenshot of the mobile application

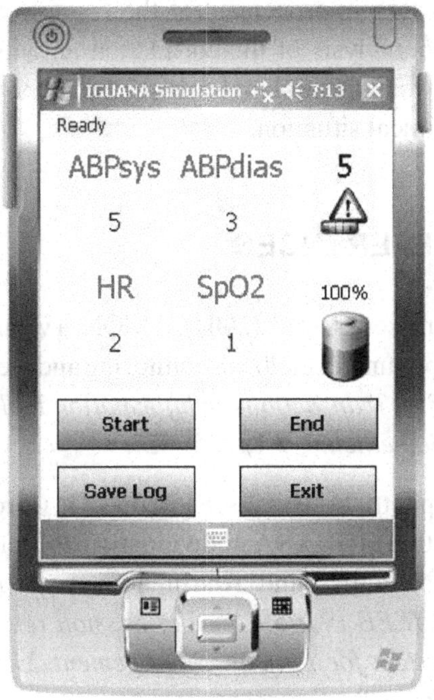

CONCLUSION

In this chapter we have introduced the architecture of a mobile healthcare system to collect and analyse physiological signals for ubiquitous patient monitoring. We reviewed some of the relevant recent literature on health care applications and we proposed a flexible framework to perform the real-time analysis of clinical data collected by means of a body sensor network.

We illustrated the effectiveness of our framework by analysing publicly available clinical data, by investigating different physiological signals, and by estimating its performance. An off-line analysis is performed to build a model tailored to a specific patient or disease. On-line analysis classifies each measured value with a risk level according to the previous model. Experiments, performed on both personal PCs and mobile devices (smart phones and Pocket PCs), show the adaptability of the proposed approach and its computational efficiency.

There are a number of directions in which the proposed framework can be extended. Since our aim was to detect dangerous situations, we have analyzed vital signs, by considering each signal independently. However, physiological signals can be correlated and contribute in different ways to the global risk computation. Hence, a further improvement of the framework will be the analysis of the correlation among different physiological signals which contribute to a global clinical situation.

REFERENCES

Anliker U., et al. (2004). AMON: a wearable multiparameter medical monitoring and alert system. *IEEE Transactions on Information Technology in Biomedicine, 9*(1), 415–427.

Apiletti, D., Baralis, E., Bruno, G., Cerquitelli, T. (2006). IGUANA: Individuation of Global Unsafe ANomalies and Alarm activation. *Presented at IEEE IS '06 - Special Session on Intelligent System for Patient Management.* London, (pp 267-272).

Axisa, F., Dittimar, A., Delhomme, G. (2003). Smart clothes for the monitoring in real time and conditions of physiological, emotional and sensorial reaction of human. In *Proceedings of the 2 Annual International Conference of the IEEE EMBS*, (pp. 3744-3747).

Branche, P., Mendelson, Y., (2005). Signal Quality and Power Consumption of a New Prototype Reflectance Pulse Oximeter Sensor. *Presented at IEEE Northeast Bioengineering Conference,.* Hoboken, NJ, (pp 42- 43).

Cheng, P.-T., Tsai, L.-M., Lu, L.-W., Yang, D.-L., (2004). The design of PDA-based biomedical data processing and analysis for intelligent wearable health monitoring systems. *Presented at IEEE International Conference on Computer and Information Technology*, (pp 879 - 884).

Gupta, S., Ganz, A. (2004). Design considerations and implementation of a cost-effective, portable remote monitoring unit using 3G wireless data networks, presented at IEEE EMBS, San Francisco, CA, USA, pp. 3286-3289.

Han, J., Kamber, M., (2000). Data Mining: Concepts and Techniques, Series Editor Morgan Kaufmann Publishers. The Morgan Kaufmann Series in Data Management Systems, Jim Gray.

Jones V., et al. (2006). Mobihealth: mobile health services based on body area networks. In *Technical Report TR-CTIT-06-37 Centre for Telematics and Information Technology.* University of Twente, Enschede.

Jovanov, E., Milenkovic A., Otto C., de Groen P. C. (2005). A wireless body area network of intelligent motion sensors for computer assisted physical rehabilitation. *Journal of NeuroEngineering and Rehabilitation, 2*,(6).

Lee I., et al. (2006). High-Confidence Medical Device Software and Systems. *Computer 39*(4), 33-38.

Lin, Y.-H., et al. (2004), A Wireless PDA-Based Physiological Monitoring System for Patient Transport. *IEEE Transactions on Information Technology in Biomedicine, 8*(4), 439-447.

Lorincz, K., et al. (2004). Sensor networks for emergency response: Challenges and opportunities. *IEEE Pervasive Computing, 3*(4), 16-23.

Manders, E., Dawant, B. (1996). Data acquisition for an intelligent bedside monitoring system. *Presented at IEEE Engineering in Medicine and Biology Society*, Amsterdam, pp 1987-1988.

Sharshar, S., Allart, L., Chambrin, M. C., (2005). A new approach to the abstraction of monitoring data in intensive care. *Lecture Notes in Computer Science, 3581*, 13–22.

Varady P., Benyo Z., Benyo B. (2002), An open architecture patient monitoring system using standard technologies. *IEEE Transactions on Information Technology in Biomedicine, 6*(1), .95–98.

Varshney, U., (2006). Transmission of emergency messages in wireless patient monitoring: routing and performance evaluation. *Presented at IEEE*

Hawaii International Conference on System Sciences, vol. 5, (pp 91- 100).

Wu, H.-C., et al., (1999). A mobile system for real-time patient-monitoring with integrated physiological signal processing. *Presented at IEEE BMES/EMBS Joint Conference*, vol.2, (pp.712).

KEY TERMS

ABPdias: Diastolic Arterial Blood Pressure. Diastole is the period of time when the heart relaxes after contraction. The diastolic pressure is the lowest pressure in the cardiac cycle (i.e., in the relaxing). A typical value for a healthy adult human is approximately 80 mmHg.

ABPsys: Systolic Arterial Blood Pressure. Systole is the contraction of the chambers of the heart, driving blood out of the chambers. The systolic arterial blood pressure is defined as the peak pressure in the arteries, which occurs near the beginning of the cardiac cycle (i.e., in the contraction). A typical value for a healthy adult human is approximately 120 mmHg.

Bluetooth: Radio standard and communications protocol (i.e., IEEE 802.15.1 standard) for wireless personal area networks characterized by short transmission ranges (1-100 m). It has been designed for low power consumption and it is based on low-cost transceiver microchips in each device.

Global System for Mobile Communications Gsm (Originally from Groupe Spécial Mobile):. It is the most popular standard for mobile phones in the world. GSM is a cellular network, which means that mobile phones connect to it by searching for cells in the immediate vicinity. GSM networks operate in four different frequency ranges and use a variety of voice codecs.

Heart Rate (HR): The heart rate describes the frequency of the cardiac cycle. It is a vital sign and usually it is calculated as the number of contractions (heart beats) of the heart in one minute and expressed as "beats per minute" (bpm). When resting, the adult human heart beats at about 70 bpm (males) and 75 bpm (females), but this rate varies among people.

Personal Digital Assistant (PDA): It is a handheld computer, also known as pocket or palmtop computer. A typical PDA has a touch screen for data entry, a memory card slot for data storage, IrDA and USB ports for connectivity. Wi-Fi and Bluetooth are often integrated in newer PDAs.

Smartphone: It is a full-featured mobile phone with personal computer like functionalities. Applications for enhanced data processing and connectivity can be installed on the device, and may be developed by the user. Smart functionalities may include miniature keyboard, touch screen, operating system, and modem capabilities.

Saturation of Peripheral Oxygen (SpO_2):. It measures the percentage of haemoglobin binding sites in the bloodstream occupied by oxygen. It is usually evaluated by a non-invasive pulse oximeter, which relies on the light absorption characteristics of saturated haemoglobin to give an indication of oxygen saturation.

Wireless Local Area Network (WLAN): It is a network which uses a modulation technology based on radio waves to enable communication among devices in a limited area, without using wires. Among benefits of WLAN there are: convenience, cost efficiency, mobility, expandability, and ease of integration with other networks and network components.

ZigBee: Name of a specification for a suite of high level communication protocols using small, low-power digital radios based on the IEEE 802.15.4 standard for wireless personal area networks. The ZigBee 1.0 specification was ratified on December 14, 2004 and is available to members of the ZigBee Alliance.

Section X
Ethical, Legal, and Other Issues in E-Health

Chapter XXXV
Chaotization of Human Systems by Technical Electromagnetic Fields

Manfred Doepp
Holistic DiagCenter, Germany

ABSTRACT

In our energy diagnostic department we noticed more and more cases with irrational stimulus-reaction-patterns and with a chaotic regulation state of the autonomous systems. We found an explanation by the 'Switching phenomenon'. However, in addition to earlier results a new cause came up, it is the electrosmog exposure. We used three criteria to clarify the findings: A) a negative reaction on a pulsating magnetic field, B) a positive reaction on a brain synchronization procedure, and C) the frequency distribution analysis of skin resistance values approximated by a lognormal (order) or by a bell curve (chaos). A retrospective evaluation over 4 years (435 patients) was performed. Results: 1) a positive correlation between the criterium A) and a chaotic tendency in C), and 2) a significant difference between reactions before and after the synchronization procedure B). The hypothesis of an electrosmog-induced chaotization of autonomous systems becomes likely.

INTRODUCTION

Around 1976 Goodheart, the founder of the Applied Kinesiology (AK), described a phenomenon which he named '**Switching**".

His definition said "not foreseeable neurological dys-organisation" (Goodheart, 1985). It means a changeover of the regulation systems of the organism. As predominating causes he found alcohol dependence and food allergies with high histamine. In 1985 Leaf added a discovery which was referred as „disturbance of laterality" (Leaf, 1987). Callahan broadened the spectrum when he described a „psychological reversal" (Callahan, 1998). At that not the hemispheres are separate, however, the conscious and the subconscious parts of the brain

In 2002 (Doepp & Edelmann, 2002/1) we published the frequent presence of Switching states through electro-magnetic waves exposure (**electrosmog**). The regulations are chaotified in the subcortical brain and the vegetative nervous system. This means, that the intellect (the cerebrum rind) may function as usually further, one hardly notices this state, however, the **autonomous systems** and brain parts are fragmented and desynchronized (Frick, 2002; Frick, 2005; Hillert, 1998; Landgrebe, 2006; Levallois, 2002; Lyskov, 2001; Sandstrom et al. 2003).

Our entrance to this problem field worked about the **meridian diagnostics** whose discoveries go ahead of the clinical symptoms around months or years. What could that mean for normal citizens? We then may be temporarily and partly no more ourselves, one becomes ‚cool' instead of authentic. However, if someone is in the Switching state, the brain can be defragmentated and resynchronized. We compiled for this purpose four practices that can be carried out over 30 seconds each:

1. Eyebrow massage above cross, with the thumb under that and the four fingers above that.
2. Rubbing gently over the hairy head, with four fingers from the forehead to the neck, with both hands after each other.
3. Dot massage over and under the lips, done with the small fingertips, with both hands after each other.
4. Ear conch massage with the fingers above cross.

Another testing procedure is the **frequency distribution analysis** performed by means of Chi-square and Kolmogorov-Smirnov analysis of the approximation to the lognormal and the normal curve (Doepp & Edelmann 2002/1; Doepp et al. 2002/2; Doepp & Edelmann 2006; Popp

Figure 1. Chaos in the state of switching

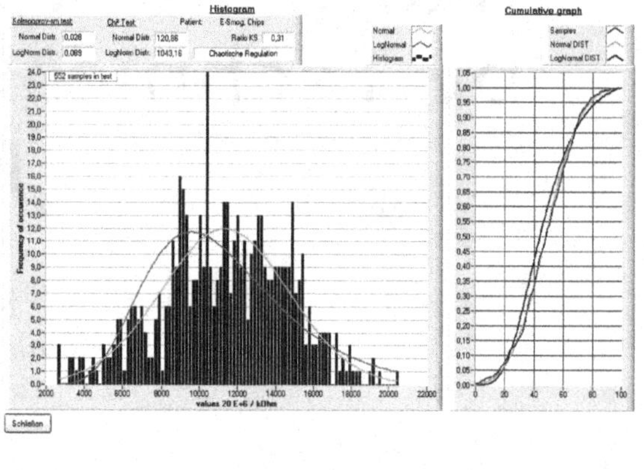

Figure 2. Fragmentation in the state of Switching

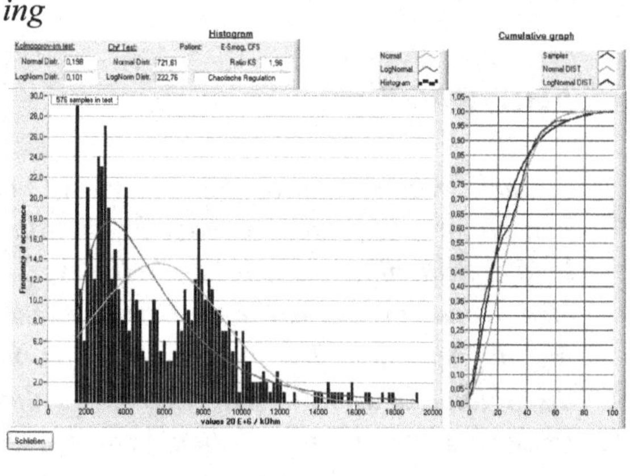

Figure 3. Order after the synchronization practices

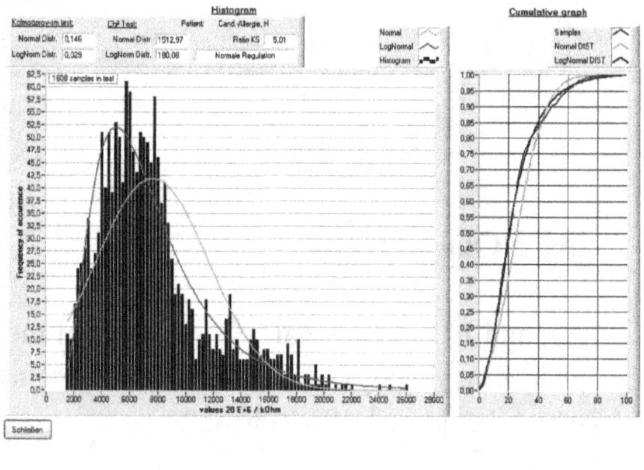

1987; Sachs 1969; Zhang & Popp 1996). A patient in the Switching state shows a chaotic (Figure 1) or a fragmented distribution (Figure 2) and after performing the synchronization practices a lognormal pattern (Figure 3) meaning a regulatory state of order. If the data are collected via a body system (e.g. the net of meridians) it is a system analysis.

PROBLEM FORMULATION

Up to now the question of Switching of the systems of the organism is known in the Applied Kinesiology, however, has not yet been examined by digital methods. Especially the cause of an electrosmog exposure for this phenomenon has not been evaluated. This should be performed.

Material and Methods

Four hundred and thirty five randomized patients from the routine energy medicine diagnostics from 2002 until 2006 received an evaluation of their dates and of their **frequency distributions** retrospectively. As an electrosmog exposure we used a pulsating magnetic field (9 Hz, 50 μT, 5 minutes in the back), and as a resynchronization procedure the four practices previously described. The following parameters were taken into consideration: A) a negative reaction on the pulsating magnetic field, B) a positive reaction on a brain synchronization procedure, and C) the frequency distribution analysis of skin resistance values histograms approximated by a lognormal (LN, order) or by a normal curve (N, chaos).

PROBLEM SOLUTION

Results

In Table 1 the changes (%) of the three parameters A), B), and C) produced by a pulsating magnetic field before and after the synchronization practices of 435 patients are listed.

- **Parameter A:** Change of the skin resistance values of 24 meridian end points,
- **Parameter B:** Change of the resistance values after the four procedures,
- **Parameter C:** Change of the sum of N/LN ratios of the statistical analysis of the frequency distributions (Doepp & Edelmann 2006).

All parameters are significantly different before and after the synchronization practices. The magnetic field application as a representative for technical electrosmog produces an increase of the skin resistance values and a chaotic regulation pattern of the systems of the organism, all this before a synchronization procedure which means in a presumable state of Switching. After the synchronization procedure the negative effects

Table 1. The results of the 3 parameters

	Before synchronization		
Parameter	A	B	C
Mean	- 22,4	+ 15,6	1,34
SD	14,1	6,7	0,96
	After synchronization		
Mean	+ 4,1	+ 2,7	3,12
SD	6,8	1,95	1,85
Significance	p < .01	p < .01	p < .05

Table 2. Correlation coefficients, r =

	Before synchronization		
	A	B	C
A	/	.45	.69
B	/	/	.34
	After synchronization		
A	/	.32	.40
B	/	/	.27

are reduced and the chaotic regulatory situation is normalized.

A regression analysis between the three parameters was performed. The correlation coefficients are listed in Table 2. The highest and significant correlation was found between the parameters A and C before synchronization. This means that in a presumable state of Switching the effect of an electrosmog exposure on the skin resistance and a chaotic regulation tendency are connected to each other. After the synchronization treatment of the Switching there is a low correlation only.

Discussion

In this chapter two subjects are combined which have not been investigated yet: the effects of electrosmog on the regulation systems of the organism and the state of a Switching of the autonomous centres in the central nervous system (CNS). It is usually detected by means of paradoxical results within testing procedures of the energy medicine. We tested the effects of a representative technical electrosmog – a pulsating magnetic field application – on three biological and biometric parameters. In order to distinguish the states of Switching and of normal regulations, a procedure was developed consisting of four synchronization practices.

The hypotheses were: 1) many people nowadays have an exposure to electrosmog and so are living at times in the state of Switching which means a desynchronization of the CNS regulation abilities, 2) in a state of Switching a magnetic field exposure has different effects in comparison to normal regulations, and 3) the state of Switching may be normalized by several special practices which are able to resynchronize the CNS. According to our results the hypotheses are more reliable than before, however, a proof will need prospective studies. A further assumption is that the rise of allergies in the populations of the civilized countries may be connected with the regulatory chaos which – among other reasons - may be a result of the increasing technical electrosmog.

The **chaos theory** supplies the reason that the best adaptation is guaranteed - as conditions are changing continuously in the environment - through the inherent order in a chaos (Feigenbaum 1978; Gebelein & Heite 1950; Gerz 1996; Prigogine & Stengers 1981), or through the deterministic chaos of non-linear and/or dissipative systems, respectively. A Gaussian distribution is too confused and a lognormal distribution is too inflexible and does not allow creativity, so naturally a combination of both developed in the evolution of man. It is represented by the Golden Section relationship (Doepp & Edelmann 2006). According to our results technical electrosmog is able to shift the regulatory centres from the equilibrium towards a lability up to a chaos. Several authors found similar results ('electrical hypersensitivity') by other methods like Holter ECG (Sandstrom et al. 2003)). It has to be concluded that a certain, however, increasing percentage of the population becomes hypersensitive to electrosmog, usually with negative effects on the CNS.

CONCLUSION

We evaluated retrospectively the results of 435 patients who received a meridian diagnostics (skin resistance measurements) and a frequency distribution analysis (Chi square and Kolmogorov-Smirnov tests, normal and lognormal distributions), both, before and after a synchronization procedure in order to remove the state of Switching of the CNS. As a representative for technical electrosmog we used the pulsating magnetic field emissions of a flat coil with a low radiation intensity.

In summary: the phenomenon of a regulatory chaos seems to be a reality in our civilization. This negative development may be particularly a result of the ubiquitous technical electrosmog. The regulatory centres of the central nervous system can become desynchronized, fragmented and chaotizised. The phenomena can be detected by energy medicine, biometric techniques, and special ECG methods. This should be taken into consideration in Medical Informatics and E-health, too.

REFERENCES

Callahan, K.L. (1998). *Twelve keys for living: Possibilities for a whole*, Healthy Life, Jossey-Bass, 1998.

Doepp, M., & Edelmann, G. (2002). The switching of the brain as an addiction-like condition: Interference of the meridians by electrosmog? *AKU 30*(3), 133-139.

Doepp, M., Edelmann, G., Cohen, S., Popp, F.-A., Yu, Y. (2002). A new procedure for the judgement of the health state with the aid of the frequency distribution of the conductivity values of the skin. *Erfahrungsheilkunde, 51*, 3–11.

Doepp, M., & Edelmann, G. (2003). Clinical evaluation of the frequency distribution analysis of biological data. *Erfahrungsheilkunde,* 12, 818-824.

Doepp, M., & Edelmann, G. (2006). System patterns of the human organism and their heredity, 375-382, In Lazakidou, A. A. (ed.), *Handbook of Research on Informatics in Healthcare and Biomedicine*. Hershey PA: Idea Group Inc.

Feigenbaum, M. J. (1978). Quantitative universality for a class of nonlinear transformations. *Journal Statistical Physics, 19*, 25.

Frick, U. et al. (2002). Risk perception, somatization, and self report of complaints related to electromagnetic fields – a randomized survey study. *Int. J. Hyg. Environ. Health, 205*, 353-360.

Frick, U. et al. (2005). Comparison perception of singular transcranial magnetic stimuli by subjectively electrosensitive subjects and general population controls. *Bioelectromagnetics 26*, 287-298.

Gebelein, H., & Heite, H.-J. (1950). About the imbalance of biological frequency distributions. *Klin. Wochenschrift, 28*(41).

Gerz, W. (1996). *Textbook of the Applied Kinesiology (AK) in the natural medicine practice.* Munich: AKSE-publisher, 1996. ISDN: 3-00-000616-8.

Goodheart, G.J. jr. (1985). *You'll be better – the story of applied kinesiology.* Geneva, Ohio: AK Printing.

Hillert, L. et al. (1998). Cognitive behavioural therapy for patients with electric sensitivity – a multidisciplinary approach in a controlled study. *Psychother. Psychosom, 67*, 302-310.

Landgrebe, M., Hauser, S., Langguth, B., Hajak, G., Eichhammer, P. (2006). Transcranielle Magnetstimulation zur neurobiologischen Charakterisierung somatoformer Störungen. *Nervenheilkunde, 25*, 653-656.

Leaf, D.W. (1987). *Applied Kinesiology Flowchart Manual* (private ed.). Plymouth, Massachusetts.

Levallois, P. (2002). Hypersensitivity of human subjects to environmental electric and magnetic field exposure: A review of the literature. *Environ. Health Perspect. 110*, Suppl. 4, 613-618.

Lyskov, E. et al. (2001). Neurophysiological study of patients with perceived 'electrical hypersensitivity. *Int. J. Psychophysiol., 42*, 233-241.

Popp, F.-A. (1987). *New horizons in medicine (2nd ed.).* Heidelberg, Germany: Haug.

Prigogine, I., & Stengers, I. (1981). *Dialog with the nature: New ways of scientific thinking.* Munich, Germany: Piper.

Sachs, L. (1969). *Statistical evaluation methods.* Berlin, Germany: Springer.

Sandstrom, M. et al. (2003). Holter ECG monitoring in patients with perceived electrical hypersensitivity. *Int. J. Psychophysiol., 49*, 227-235.

Zhang, Ch., & Popp, F.-A. (1996). Log-normal distribution measure of physiological parameters and the coherence of biological systems. In Ch. Zhang, F.-A. Popp, & M. Bischof (Eds.), *Current developments of biophysics,* (pp. 102-111). Hangzhou University Press.

KEY TERMS

Autonomous Systems: Inside the human organism several systems are existing which are all regulated by feedback mechanisms in order to maintain a parameter concerned around its mean value. Some of those controlled systems are: heart rate frequency, blood pressure, perfusion rate, immune system, lymphatic system, hormonal system, breath rate, oxigen supply, meridian system, skin temperature, ... All those systems may be used in order to generate accumulations of biological data.

Chaos Theory: The bipolar organized universe is represented in the organism by the extreme abnormal states of chaos and rigidity. The chaos theory supplies the fact that the best adaptation is guaranteed through the inherent order in a chaos or through the deterministic chaos of non-linear and/or dissipative systems. Without chaos there is no creativity and no evolution. A stable equilibrium would contradict the will of the Creator of the universe and of each person and soul. So, in spite of their disadvantages the chaotic aspects of life are necessary.

Electrosmog: Electromagnetic fields with the whole existing range of frequencies and wave lengths are forming an ubiquitous chaotic situation. The human organism uses waves like those, too. A lot of electricity conducting structures belong to the human body. So, biological antennas go into resonance with the technical electrosmog. Desinformation and manipulations are a possible result. Human feedback systems may become labile up to a chaotic situation. Sensible persons are producing a hypersensitivity.

Frequency Distributions: Biological data are collected which are generated by a randomized procedure of a measuring principle concerning any system of the organism. There should be more than 500 data. They are plotted in a graph, with the measured values on the x- and the frequencies on the y-axis, so producing a distribution pattern.

Frequency Distribution Analysis: The distribution pattern is compared with a normal curve (N, Gaussian) and a lognormal curve (LN). Two mathematical methods are used for that purpose: the Chi square- and the Kolmogorov Smirnov-analysis. Both are able to analyse the adaption of the person's values distribution by the two curves.

Meridian Diagnostics: The net of meridians is one of the body regulation systems. According to the Traditional Chinese Medicine (TCM) 12 paired meridians are existing in man. In order to determine their functional states the electrical resistance in the beginning or the end points ('Ting points') of those meridians is measured, left and right means in 24 points. The important conductance showing the energetic state is reciprocal to the resistance. The test runs are performed 20 up to 100 times per patient under different and randomized circumstances.

Switching: A brain working normally is synchronized with active association paths between all parts. Several negative influences (long-lasting disstress, allergy, addiction, dependance, electrosmog) produce a desynchronization= fragmentation = dissoziation inside the brain which is called "Switching". The cerebrum rind/intellect is not disturbed, however, the contact to the emotions, the subconscious centres, and the autonomous centres does not work any more. This results in paradoxical and irrational stimulus-reaction-patterns. The person is no longer a whole entity.

System Analysis: The human organism allows the detection of huge amounts of data describing the function of the systems. For each of those data collections mathematical and statistical evaluations may be applicated in order to find out the normal ranges and to control the agreement of a person's results with those of a normal population (sex and age dependant). Significances are calculated. Chaos and rigidity are typical abnormal situations.

Chapter XXXVI
Demographic Differences in Telehealth Policy Outcomes

Mary Schmeida
The Cleveland Clinic, USA

Ramona McNeal
University of Northern Iowa, USA

ABSTRACT

This chapter is an analysis of demographic variables influencing policy outcomes with online health information searches in the general U.S. public. This study is based on The Internet and American Life Daily Tracking Survey, August 2006 from the Pew Research Center for the People and the Press. Multivariate regression statistical technique is used to explore changes in individual level behavior following the search for online medical information. The data show individuals in most need of healthcare services (poor, less educated, and minority groups) and those with a recent demand for services, are more likely to make changes to improve their health after accessing online medical information.

INTRODUCTION

The public sector in the U.S. is increasingly using the Internet to provide information, deliver services, and interact with citizens, businesses, and other government agencies (West, 2003, 2004). There are numerous reasons for the government adoption of electronic government (e-government) practices that "refer to the delivery of information and services via the Internet or other digital means" (West, 2004, pp 2). E-government is expected to deliver services and information around the clock, making government more efficient and transparent to the public (Tolbert and Mossberger, 2006; West, 2003). The adoption of these practices may make government more responsive through its ability to provide communication options that are quicker and more convenient for users (Thomas and Streib, 2003).

Telehealth is an important example of e-government that takes on many forms. Although there is no consensus on its definition, the United States Congress defines telehealth as the use of electronic information and telecommunication technology to support long-distance clinical healthcare; patient and professional health-related education; public healthcare and administration (U.S. House of Representatives 2157, 2001). In practice, telehealth is understood as the inclusion of telemedicine plus other on-line social services.

Regardless of how telehealth is defined, this new medium for delivering medical services has been adopted with the goal to improve the accessibility of public and private healthcare, service quality and clinical outcomes. It is often implemented as a way to provide cost-effective healthcare. However, if we examine all the different aspects of telehealth in the U.S.—technology-enabled delivery, regulation and enabling legislation (state policies), and healthcare information available online, we find a unifying theme of broadening healthcare access. Telehealth practices may act to expand healthcare services through improving the dissemination of health information by Internet to the public, facilitating Internet based second opinions on disease management, improving consultative services to rural facilities and has the potential to reduce medical errors (Schmeida, 2005).

Despite the hopes for telehealth (as well as other forms of e-government), there is also a literature suggesting that these service delivery advancements will not live up to expectation. One barrier to the Internet for expanding healthcare access is the Internet cleavages that exist among United States citizens---people who do and do not use the Internet. These differences in Internet usage are based on a number of socioeconomic factors including age, income, education and race. The variation in Internet practices attributed to these socioeconomic factors has been linked to underlying inequalities in Internet access and technological skills, along with psychological barriers (Mossberger, Tolbert and Stansbury, 2003; Stanley, 2003). This suggests that e-government will only act to widen the gap between those that do and do not benefit from telehealth services.

Supporting this literature on Internet inequalities is research examining the differences in online health information searches among the various socioeconomic groups in the U.S. (Schmeida and McNeal, 2007). In exploring differences among socioeconomic groups in searching for Medicare and Medicaid information online, Schmeida and McNeal (2007; 2006) find some disparities are narrowing as the elderly and poor in need of these publicly subsidized health insurance programs are online searching for information at the U.S. Centers for Medicare & Medicaid Services Web site. Services and information obtainable at this Web site include eligibility criteria, enrollment procedures, Medicare plan options, local physicians and medical suppliers, pharmacy directory and healthcare chat rooms. In addition, beneficiaries can obtain personal information on their benefits and services. However, people without Internet access and experience, remain disadvantaged in accessing this critical information that can link them to needed healthcare services, suggesting that e-government service delivery advancements may not be living up to expectation.

This current research on Internet healthcare information and government services only represents an initial step in exploring the impact of online health searches and does not discuss the policy implication of these findings. To minimally understand the healthcare consequences of disparities in Internet usage in the U.S., one needs to examine if telehealth is changing how citizens take care of themselves and others. This chapter discusses these behavioral outcomes and the policy implications. In exploring this issue, this chapter will first examine the literature on barriers to the promises of e-government with a focus on the digital divide. Next, it will outline government policy toward eliminating barriers to Internet use. Finally, multivariate regression analysis will be used to empirically test the impact of one example of telehealth (seeking medical information online) and behavior directed toward improving and maintaining health.

THE REALITIES OF INTERNET USAGE IN THE UNITED STATES

Despite the promises of e-government, there is a literature suggesting there are barriers to realizing its possibilities in the United States. One reason is cleavages that exist between those who have and do not have access to this technology. These differences in access are referred to as the "digital divide." There is an extensive body of literature finding that Internet access is not distributed equally in the U.S. based on socioeconomic factors (Pew Internet & American Life Project, 2003; Mossberger, Tolbert and Stansbury, 2003).

Mossberger, Tolbert and Stansbury's (2003) research found gaps based on income, education, age and race/ ethnicity that continue to exist even after strides toward digital inclusion. The study indicated that Asian Americans had the highest predicted probability of access followed by whites with Latinos and African Americans significantly trailing behind. Furthermore, Internet access has not been adopted equally based on region and geography. West and Miller (2006) find U.S. regional disparities in Internet accessibility, privacy and security with southern states having lower levels of Internet connectivity.

Another barrier to widespread e-government is lack of technological skill. The use of e-government requires skills, such as being able to use a computer mouse and knowing how to find Internet information. Younger individuals are more likely to carry these skills because of Internet exposure in school. Respondents to the Pew Internet and American Life Project 2003 survey, *Ever-Shifting Internet Population*, were asked why they do not go online. Forty-six percent of respondents indicated they lack the technological ability to navigate the Web because of its complexity.

Mossberger, Tolbert and Stansbury (2003) find that computer technology skills can be summarized into two broad categories. The first category (technical competencies) includes the necessary skills to use hardware and software such as typing and using a mouse. The second (information or basic literacy) concerns the ability to determine what information is obtained from the Internet for specific tasks (Mossberger, Tolbert, and Stansbury, 2003: pp. 38). Their study shows the individuals lacking the technology skills necessary for Internet use includes those older, less educated, less affluent, Latino, and African American. Since these factors are the same as those associated with the "digital divide," they may work to exacerbate the gaps in usage based on access.

While the findings from the Mossberger, Tolbert and Stansbury (2003) study point to socioeconomic factors as predictors of the skill divide, other research adds psychosocial variables to the list of barriers to developing technological skills. Stanley's (2003) research found motivation as a significant element of digital skill development. Her research examined "new computer users," or individuals with limited experience and "non-computer users," those with minimal or no computer ability to determine what factors acted as a barrier in developing computer skills. The individuals in her study were primarily low income and had resisted obtaining computer skills until economic motives (finding a job, gaining a promotion, or getting a better job) led them to seek training. The findings revealed that psychological barriers (such as computer fear and poor self-concept) were more important than education in preventing computer skill development (Stanley, 2003: pp. 410-13). All of these study findings suggest there are potential barriers to the development of e-government use in the U.S., despite its promises.

U.S. GOVERNMENT POLICY ADDRESSING UNEVEN INTERNET USAGE

Although the federal government has pushed for adoption of e-government practices, its policies for eliminating Internet use disparities has been fragmented and piecemeal. Policy with the Clinton administration stressed public access strategies, emphasizing connectivity in libraries and schools with funding authorized by the Telecommunications Act of 1996. Two of these programs which provided more flexible funding were largely eliminated under the Bush administration.. The Technology Opportunities Program (TOP), offered grants for public Internet access and technology projects to solve social problems (Edutopia News, 2004). The Community Technology Centers Program provides matching grants for state-local, and nonprofit sectors providing public access in the community. Program funding fell from $32 billion to only $5 million in the 2005 budget (Edutopia News, 2004).

The government is addressing regional disparities to Internet use by mandating private-sector telephone companies to improve access and affordability of Internet to rural America. The Telecommunications Act of 1996, for example, keeps rural policy on the same trajectory as urban policy by requiring that companies provide affordable telehealth utilities in rural America as they do to urban counterparts in the same state (Schmeida, 2005). Recent Congressional hearings also target reform in the Federal Communications Commission universal service fund subsidizing rural Internet services for elementary and secondary schools public libraries and not-for-profit rural healthcare providers (U.S. House of Representatives, 2006).

Under the Clinton administration, libraries provided public access for computers and the Internet and a source for Internet training. Studies conducted by the University of Washington revealed that 30% of library patrons have no other Internet access. Job search is especially important for low-income library users, and medical information searches are prevalent in rural areas (Gates Foundation, 2004).

Under the Bush administration, policy for eliminating Internet use disparities switched from providing public access to improving Internet skills through the requirements of "The No Child Left Behind Act." Since implementing this policy, there has been progress in providing more technology in the schools (Kleiner and Lewis, 2003). Yet, schools face shortages in funding for computer maintenance and support staff and in some districts partly rely on students for technical support.

The review of the current U.S. policies regarding e-government and unequal Internet usage reveals contradictory policies. On the one hand, the federal government has strongly encouraged government units to adopt e-government practices for providing information and services. Yet, there are gaps in Internet usage based on a number of demographic factors limiting individual citizens who can benefit from the practices. This is coupled with policies addressing the disparities in Internet use that can at best be described as fragmented and piecemeal. What are the consequences of such conflicting policies with regard to telehealth? Is telehealth practice aiding those in greatest need of healthcare services, or resulting in greater inequality of service delivery?

DATA AND MEASUREMENT

In an attempt to address these questions, this chapter utilizes *The Internet and American Life*

Daily Tracking Survey, August 2006; conducted for the Pew Research Center for the People and the Press, by the Princeton Survey Research Associates. The Pew survey is a random digit dial national telephone survey conducted in August 2006 and has a sample size of 2,928. In this study, we limit our exploration to the 1,594 respondents who reported searching for healthcare information online. Our dependent variable is represented by a count of the number of 6 healthcare activities an individual performed following a health information search online, see Table 1.

Since the current literature (Schmeida and McNeal, 2007; 2006; Mossberger et al, 2003) suggests that demographic and region factors are important in determining searches for online health information, variables are included for age, gender, education, income, full-time employment, part-time employment, African American, Asian American, Latino, Northeast , Midwest and the West regions. Age is in years and gender is measured using a binary variable coded 1 for male and 0 for females. Education is measured using a 7-point scale, ranging from less than a grade-eight education to a Ph.D. education.

Table 1. Dependent variable- searching for health information online (Pew Internet and American Life Project, 2006)

Did the information you found online affect a decision about how to treat an illness or condition?
Did the information you found online change your overall approach to maintaining your health or the health of someone you help take care of?
Did the information you found online change the way you cope with a chronic condition or manage pain?
Did the information you found online affect a decision about whether to see a doctor?
Did the information you found online lead you to ask a doctor new questions, or to get a second opinion from another doctor?
Did the information you found online change the way you think about diet, exercise, or stress management?

The income measure is based on an 8-point scale where 1 indicates that family income ranges from $0 to $10,000 and 8 signifies a family income of $100,000 or more.[1] A binary variable is used for full-time employment coded 1 for full-time and 0 other wise, a similar variable is used for part-time employment. To control for race and ethnicity, dummy variables are included for African Americans, Asian Americans, and Latinos with non-Hispanic whites as the reference group. Three variables are used to measure region---Northeast, Midwest and West with South as the reference group. Measures for need/ demand were also added including recent medical care experience, recent medical diagnosis and recent medical emergency. Each is binary coded 1 for yes and 0 for otherwise.[2]

FINDINGS

Since the dependent variable represents a count of different behavioral health outcomes/ action to online health information searches, a Poisson regression model in Table 2 is reported. A number of demographic factors were found to statistically predict policy outcomes. Contrary to expectation, many demographic groups who are least likely to have Internet access at home are most likely to have taken health-related action to the health information they searched on the Internet. Our model shows the less-educated, poor, African Americans, Latinos and those living in the south were more likely to have taken action after reading online healthcare information. Additionally, people with a recent new medical diagnosis and recent medical emergency experience were also more likely to have taken action. Table 2 shows the coefficient for education is statistically significant and negative. As education decreases, the probability of behavioral outcomes increases even after controlling for age, gender, income, employment, race, ethnicity, geography, and demand. The less educated are not only less likely to have

Table 2. Poisson regression models- health behavior outcomes to online health searches

VARIABLES	β (se)	p>|z|
Age	.001(.002)	.727
Male	-.039(.049)	.428
Education	**-.053(.017)**	**.002**
Income	**-.028(.013)**	**.032**
Full-time Employment	-.025(.058)	.664
Part-time Employment	-.129(.085)	.127
African American	**.288(.075)**	**.000**
Asian American	.162(.176)	.359
Latino	**.212(.105)**	**.044**
Northeast Region	-.038(.070)	.588
Midwest Region	**-.104(.061)**	**.086**
West Region	.019(.065)	.773
Recent Medical Care Experience	.094(.070)	.181
Recent Medical Diagnosis	**.141(.053)**	**.008**
Recent Medical Emergency	**.110(.050)**	**.027**
Constant	1.274 (.133)	.000
Pseudo R^2	.0301	
LR chi^2 (15)	80.52	
N	657	

Poisson regression estimates with standard errors in parentheses. Unstandardized coefficients reported. Reported probabilities are based on two-tailed tests. Statistically significant coefficients at .10 or less in bold (Pew Internet and American Life Project, 2006).

Internet use at home (Mossberger et al., 2003) but those who do have access and searched for health information online are more likely to take some health-related action after their searches.

The coefficient for income is also significant and negative. The poor are more likely to take health-related steps after an online health information search than the wealthy. Our model also indicates that minority groups (African American and Latino) were statistically more likely than Caucasians to take action after online searches. Region is also a significant predictor in our model. The coefficient for *Midwest Region* was significant and negative. This suggests that residents of the South searching for health information online have a greater chance of taking action following their search than those living in the Midwest.

Two demand variables were important predictors in our model. We find the online health searchers who have had some type of recent interface with the health system are more likely to take some type of health-related action after their online information searches. The variable for *Recent Medical Diagnosis* was significant and positive. Individuals who either personally or had someone close recently diagnosed with a chronic medical condition (such as asthma, diabetes, heart disease, or high blood pressure) and then searched for health information online had a greater chance for taking some type of action after the search. The factor *Recent Medical Emergency* was also significant and positive. Individuals (or someone close) who had faced a serious medical emergency or crisis and then searched for information online had a greater chance for taking a health-related action.

DISCUSSION

Our chapter attempts to explore the differences in policy outcomes with online health information searches in the general U.S. public. It goes beyond the current research exploring differences based on demographic factors in the use of telehealth without exploring the consequences of these inequalities. The outcomes under study are the health behaviors that occur as an effect to online health information searches at home---seeking a second opinion from another doctor, changing self-care practices, changing one's way of pain management, among other.

We find that certain demographic variables are statistically associated with behavioral outcomes of online health information searches. The demographic groups found in this study (less educated, poor, African American, Latino) to act on online healthcare information are surprisingly the same groups found least likely to have Internet access and Internet literacy skills for the U.S. In other words, those least likely to use the Internet are most likely to take steps toward improving their health if they do access healthcare information online. We also find that severity of need/ demand to online searches (individual facing medical crisis and new medical diagnosis) is important in influencing the health-related behaviors that occur after online health information searches are made.

How do we settle the contradiction in our findings? Why are those individuals who are least likely to have Internet access and the necessary skills to use it, most likely to benefit from healthcare searches online? To answer this question, we turn to previous work by Mossberger, Tolbert and Stansbury (2003). They found that even though African Americans and Latinos were less likely than similarly-situated whites to have home computers or home Internet access, to use the Internet as frequently, to report sufficient skills, or to use the Internet at all, they were more likely than whites to express positive attitudes about technology. Additionally, they found that African Americans were statistically more likely than whites to use the Internet for activities, such as job search and online classes. Mossberger and Tolbert (2005) resolved the contradiction in their earlier findings through using hierarchical linear modeling to illustrate that factors, such as concentrated poverty and racial segregation are responsible for what seem like racial differences in Internet usage. Their research indicated that factors, such as community educational attainment and median income, explained more of the variation in frequency of Internet use than individual characteristics.

The findings of this chapter and the research by Mossberger and Tolbert (2005) are somewhat reassuring. Despite fears that those individuals most likely to benefit from e-government would be left out, they appear to be using the Internet to access services, such as healthcare, education and job searches. Furthermore, this chapter shows those most in need of healthcare services are more likely to take measures to improve their health after reading health/ medical information online. However, there is also indication that the policies enacted in the U.S. to alleviate gaps in Internet use are insufficient and under stress. Libraries have become the temporary solution for inequalities in Internet access and skill. Nevertheless, they are showing the strain of this responsibility as funding of public libraries is insufficient to keep up with Internet access demand (Bertot, McClure, Jaeger, and Ryan, 2006; Gates Foundation, 2005). Given the potential for telehealth and other forms of e-government to help deliver services and information to citizens, there is a significant need for a holistic policy for closing the gap between those who do and do not access the Internet.

REFERENCES

Bertot, J., McClure, C., Jaeger, P., Ryan, J. (2006). *Public libraries and the Internet 2006: study results and findings*. Retrieved from http://www.ala.org/ala/washoff/contactwo/oitp/papersa/papers.cfm

Edutopia News. (2004). *Ed-tech funding reduced for 2005*. Retrieved 1, December 2004 from, http://www.edutopia.org/products/changeformat.php

Gates Foundation. (2004). U.S. library program: summary of research reports. Retrieved from http://www.gatesfoundation.org/Libraries/USLibraryProgram/Evaluation/default.htm

Gates Foundation. (2005). U.S. public libraries providing unprecedented access to computers, the Internet, and technology training. Retrieved from http://www.gatesfoundation.org/Libraries/USLibraryProgram/Announcements/Announce-050623.htm

Jacobus, C., Lichtenstein, E., Cybernet Medical. (June 2006). Telehealth outcomes. Available Online: www.cybernetmedical.com

Kleiner, A., Lewis, L. (2003). Internet access in U.S. public schools and classrooms: 1994-2002 (NCES 2004-011). *U.S. Department of Education. Washington, D.C.: National Center for Education Statistics.*

Mossberger, K., Tolbert, C., Stansbury, C. (2003). *Virtual inequality beyond the digital divide.* Washington, DC: Georgetown University Press.

Mossberger, K., Tolbert, C. (2005). Race, place and information technology. *Report prepared for the U.S. Department of Housing and Urban Development.* Grant H-21439RG.

Pew Internet and American Life Project. (April 16, 2003). *The ever-shifting Internet population: A new look at Internet access and the digital divide.* Retrieved from http://www.pewinternet.org/reports/.

Pew Internet and American Life Project. (August 2006). *Daily tracking survey.* Retrieved from http://www.pewinternet.org/

Schmeida, M. (December 2005). *Telehealth Innovation in the American States.* Dissertation. Ann Arbor, MI: ProQuest.

Schmeida, M., McNeal, R. (2007). The telehealth divide: disparities to searching public health information online. *Journal of Health Care for the Poor and Underserved, 18*(3), 549-563.

Stanley, L. (2003). Beyond access: psychosocial barrier to computer literacy. *The Information Society, 19,* 407-416.

Tolbert, C., Mossberger, K. (2006). The effects of e-government on trust and confidence in government. Public Administration Review, vol 66, 3, pp. 354-369.

Thomas, J., Streib, G. 2003. The new face of government: citizen-initiated contacts in the era of e-government. *Journal of Public Administration Research and Theory, 13*(1), 83-102.

U.S. House of Representatives, Committee on Small Business Hearing. (May 3, 2006). *Future of rural telecommunications: is universal service reform needed?,* CIS-NO: 2006-H721-24. (pp. 1-78).

West, D. (September 2003), State and federal e-government in the United States (2003). Center for Public Policy, Brown University, Retrieved from www.insidepolitics.org/egovt03us.pdf

West, D. (2004). E-government and the transformation of service delivery and citizen attitudes. *Public Administration Review, 64*(1), 15-27.

West, D., Miller, E. (2006). The digital divide in public e-health: barriers to accessibility and privacy in state health department Web sites. *Journal of Health Care for the Poor and Underserved, 17,* 652-666.

KEY TERMS

Demographics: Population statistics about socioeconomic factors such as gender, age, education, income, marital status, ethnicity, etc.

Electronic Government (E-Government): The delivery of information and services online through the Internet or other digital means (West, D.M., 2000; p. 2)

Internet: A worldwide computer network that is capable of linking all network users.

Poisson Regression: A linear model, Poisson regression analysis is used when the response variable represents counts.

Telehealth: The term is often interchanged with telemedicine. There is no consensus on its definition. However, the United States Congress defines it as the use of electronic information and telecommunications technologies to support public health and health administration,long-distance clinical healthcare, patient and professional health-related education (H.R. 2157, 2001). An example of e-government.

Telehealth Policy: An electronic government policy that uses the Internet to improve accessibility of public and private and non-profit healthcare services in rural and urban areas, while improving the quality of services at lower service costs.

Technological Skill: Skills, such as being able to use a computer mouse and knowing how to find Internet information. Younger individuals are more likely to have developed these skills because of Internet exposure in school. A barrier to widespread e-government is lack of technological skill.

U.S. Internet Cleavages: Internet cleavages that exist among United States citizens---people who do and do not use the Internet, and can be based on a number of socioeconomic and psychological factors.

ENDNOTES

1. This variable is further defined as the total 2005 family income from all sources, before taxes (Pew Internet and American Life Project, 2006).
2. The variable *Recent Medical Care Experience* asks: "In the last 12 months have you visited a doctor or medical clinic for any reason, including check-ups or visits to the emergency room or hospital outpatient department?" The variable *Recent Medical Diagnosis* asks: "In the last 12 months have you or has someone close to you been diagnosed with a chronic medical condition, such as asthma, diabetes, heart disease, or high blood pressure?" *Recent Medical Emergency* asks: "In the last 12 months have you or has someone close to you faced a serious medical emergency or crisis?" (Pew Internet and American Life Project, 2006).

Compilation of References

A&D. (2007). *Blood pressure monitor.* Retrieved from http://www.lifesourceonline.com

Aamodt, A., & Plaza, E. (1994). Case based reasoning: Foundational issues, methodological variations and system approaches. *AI Communications* 7(1), 39-59.

Abbott, S & Dambergs, Y. (2003). *Raymond Lull's ars magna*. Retrieved December 28, 2006 from http://lullianarts.net/cont.htm

Abston, C. K., Pryor, A.T., Haug, P.J., Anderson J.L. (1997). Introducing practice guidelines from a hospital database. Presented at the *Proc/AMIA Annu Fall Symp (1997)*, (pp. 168–172).

Accreditation Council for Continuing Medical Education (2003). *ACCME annual report data.*Retrieved from: http://www.accme.org

ACSH (2003). American Council on Science and Health. Retrieved 25 June 2007 from, http://www.acsh.org

Advani, A., Shahar, Y., Musen, M. A., Medical Quality Assessment by Scoring Adherence to Guideline Intentions (2002). *Journal of the American Medical Informatics Association, 9*(6), S92-S97.

Afga. (2007). Retrieved February 2007 from http://www.agfa.com/en/he/index.jsp

Afrin J. A., Whittemore KR (1997). A telemedicine success story. *Carolina Health Services Review, 4,* 225-231.

Agarwal, R. and Prasad, J. (1999). Are individual differences germane to the acceptance of new information technologies? *Decision Sciences, 30*(2), 361-375.

Aiken L. H., Clarke S. P., Sloane D. M., Sochalski J. and Silber J. H. (2002). Hospital nurse staffing and patient mortality, nurse burnout, and job dissatisfaction. *JAMA.* Retrieved from http://www.webmm.ahrq.gov/perspective.aspx?perspectiveID=7

AIM. (2001). *Shrouds of time: History of RFID.* Retrieved January 20, 2006, from http://www.aimglobal.org/technologies/rfid/resources/shrouds_of_time.pdf

Ajzen, I. and Fishbein, M. (1980). *Understanding attitudes and predicting social behavior,* Englewood Cliffs: Prentice Hall, New Jersey.

Akdemir, O., & Koszalka, T. (in-press). Investigating the relationships among instructional strategies and learning styles in online environments. *Computers and Education.*

Akdemir, O., & Koszalka, T. (Oct 2005). Expository and discovery learning compared: Their effects on learning outcomes of online students. Presented at *Association of Educational Communication and Technology 2005 annual conference*. Orlando, FL.

Akerkar SM & Bichile LS (2004). Health information on the internet: patient empowerment or patient deceit? *Indian Journal of Medical Sciences, 58,* 326.

Akrich M. (1994). Comment sortir de la dichotomie technique/société : Presentation des diverses sociologies de la technique. De la préhistoire aux missiles balistiques : De lintelligence sociale des techniques. *La Découverte Latour & Lemonnier*, 105-131.

Alavi, M., & Leidner, D. (1999). Knowledge Management Systems: Emerging Views and Practices from the Field. *Proceedings of the Thirty-second Annual Hawaii International Conference on System Sciences-Volume 7 - Volume 7*, 7009.

Alessi, N. (2002).Telepsychiatric care for a depressed adolescent. *Journal of the American Academy of Child & Adolescent Psychiatry, 41*(8), 894-895.

Alexandria, V. (2006). *Number of independent pharmacies on the rise, impact of medicare part D looms on the horizon.* Retrieved from http://www.ncpanet.org/media/releases/2006/~number_of_independent_pharmacies_on_the_04-28-2006.php.

Alonso G., Casati, F., Kuno H. and Machiraju V. (2003). *Web services, concepts, architectures and applications.* Springer.

Al-Shahrour, F., Dopazo J. (2005). Ontologies and functional genomics. In *Data Analysis and Visualization in Genomics and Proteomics.* Azuaje, F., Dopazo J. (Eds.). New York, NY: John Wiley & Sons, pp. 99-112.

AMA (2007). American Medical Association. Retrieved 28, June 2007 from, http://www.ams.assn.org

American College of Physicians Research Center (2004). *Member survey: Report of findings.* October 2004.

Amouh, T., Gemo, M., Macq, B., Vanderdonckt, J., Wahed, A., Reynaert, M.S., Stamatakis, L., Thys, F. (2005). Versatile clinical information system design for emergency departments. *IEEE Transactions on Information Technology in Biomedicine, 9*(2), 174-183.

Andersen, R., Rice, T.H. & Kominski, G.F. (2001). *Changing the U.S. health care system: Key Issues in health services, policy and management.* Josswey-Bass.

Anderson, R.J. (1996). *Security in clinical information systems.* British Medical Association.

Angeles, R. (2005). RFID technologies: Supply-chain applications and implementation issues. *Information Systems Management, 22*(1), 51-65.

Angelopoulou, P., Kangis, P., Babis, G. (1998). Private and public medicine: A comparison of quality perceptions. *Int. Journal of Health Care Quality Assurance, 11*(1), 14-20.

Anliker U., et al. (2004). AMON: a wearable multiparameter medical monitoring and alert system. *IEEE Transactions on Information Technology in Biomedicine, 9*(1), 415–427.

Anliker, U., Ward, J.A., Lukowiez, P., Tröster, G., Dolveck, F., Baer, M., Keita, F., Schnecker, E., Catarsi, F., et.al. (2004, December). A wearable multiparameter medical monitoring and alert syste. *IEEE Transactions on Information Technology in Biomedicine, 8*(1), 415-425.

ANSI/IEEE Std. 1471-2000 (2000). *Recommended practice for architectural description of software intensive systems.*

Aoki N, Dunn K, Johnson-Throop K. A., Turley J. P. (2003). Outcomes and methods in telemedicine evaluation. *Telemed J E Health, 9*(4),393-401.

Apache. (2007). *Axis2, Axiom, Tomcat.* Retrieved from http://ws.apache.org/

Apiletti, D., Baralis, E., Bruno, G., Cerquitelli, T. (2006). IGUANA: Individuation of Global Unsafe ANomalies and Alarm activation. *Presented at IEEE IS '06 - Special Session on Intelligent System for Patient Management.* London, (pp 267-272).

Arellano, M. G.,Weber, G. I.. (1998). Issues in identification and linkage of patient records across an integrated delivery system. *J Healthc Inf Manag, (12)*, 43-52.

Argyris, C., & Schoen, D. (1978). *Organization learning: A theory of action research.* Reading, MA: Addision-Wesley.

Argyris, C., & Schön, D. A. (1995). Organizational Learning II: Theory. *Method and Practice (Reading, MA: Addison-Wesley).*

Arts, D. G. T., de Keizer, N. and Scheffer, G. J. (2002). Defining and improving data quality in medical registries: A literature review, case study, and generic framework. *J Am Med Inform Assoc, 9*(6), 600-611.

Ash, G. (2006). *Traffic engineering and QoS optimization of integrated voice & data networks.* Morgan Kaufmann Series in Networking.

Ashburner, M., Ball, C.A., Blake, J.A., Botstein, D., Butler, H., Cherry, J.M., Davis, A.P., Dolinski, K., Dwight, S.S., Eppig, J.T., Harris, M.A., Hill, D.P., Issel-Tarver, L., Kasarskis, A., Lewis, S., Matese, J.C., Richardson, J.E., Ringwald, M., Rubin, G.M., Sherlock, G. (2000). Gene ontology: tool for the unification of biology. *The Gene Ontology Consortium. Nature genetics, 25* (1):25-9

Ashburner, M., Ball, C.A., Blake, J.A., Botstein, D., Butler, H., Cherry, J.M., Davis, A.P., Dolinski, K., Dwight, S.S., Eppig, J.T., Harris, M.A., Hill, D.P., Issel-Tarver, L., Kasarskis, A., Lewis, S., Matese, J.C., Richardson, J.E., Ringwald, M., Rubin, G.M., Sherlock, G. (2000) Gene ontology: tool for the unification of biology. The Gene Ontology Consortium. *Nature Genetics*, *25*(1), 25-29.

Asif, Z., & Mandviwalla, M. (2005). Integrating the supply chain with RFID: A technical and business analysis. *Communications of the Association for Information Systems, 15*, 393-427.

AT&T. (2007). Natural Voices speech synthesis software. Retrieved from http://www.research.att.com/~ttsweb/tts/

Athanasopoulos, A., Gounaris, Sp., Stathakopoulos, V. (2001). Behavioural responses to customer satisfaction: An empirical Study. *European Journal of Marketing,35*,(5/6), 687-707.

Averill, E. (1994). Reference models and standards. *StandardView*, 2(2), 96-109.

Axisa, F., Dittimar, A., Delhomme, G. (2003). Smart clothes for the monitoring in real time and conditions of physiological, emotional and sensorial reaction of human. In *Proceedings of the 2 Annual International Conference of the IEEE EMBS*, (pp. 3744-3747).

Badenoch D., Tomlin A. (2004). How electronic communication is changing health care: Usability is main barrier to effective electronic communication systems. *BMJ 2004, 328*, 1564-1566.

Bakker A. (2004). Access to EHR and access control at a moment in the past: a discussion of the need and an exploration of the consequences. *Int J Med Inform, (73)*, 267-70.

Balas, E.A., Jaffrey, F., Kuperman, G.J., Boren, S.A., Brown, G.D., Pinciroli, F. and Mitchell, J.A. (1997). Electronic communication with patients: evaluation of distance medicine technology. *JAMA*, *278*(2), 152-159.

Baldwin G (1999). AMA warns doctors on dangers of Web pill pushing. amednews.com *The Newspaper for America's Physicians*. Retrieved from www.ama-assn.org/amednews/1999/pick_99/biza0719.htm

Bandura, A. (2002). Social cognitive theory of mass communication. In J. Bryant & D. Zillman (Eds.), *Media effects: Advances in theory and research* (pp. 121-154). Mahwah, NJ: Erlbaum.

Bankman, I. N. (2000). *Handbook of medical imaging: Processing and analysis*. Academic Press.

Barnes, K. (2006). *RFID exploding into pharma industry*. Retrieved September 3, 2006, from http://www.in-pharmatechnologist.com/news/ng.asp?n=64786-gartner-frost-and-sullivan-rfid

Barnett D., Grey J., Langrick C (2006). Developing a support group Web site use of the judge health guidelines. *Health information on Internet journal, 53*, p3.

Barnett, O. (1990). Computers in medicine. *JAMA, (263)*, 2631-2633.

Barua, A and A.B. Whinston (1999). *Measuring the Internet Economy*. Center for E-Commerce Research, University of Texas at Austin, October 1999, pp 3.

Basdogan, C., De, S., Kim., J., Munivandi, M., & Srinivasan, M.A. (2004). Haptics in minimally invasive surgical simulation and training. *IEEE Computer Graphics and Applications (special issue on Haptic Rendering–Beyond Visual Computing), 24*(2), 56-64.

Bashshur R. L., Sanders J. H., Shannon G. W., (1997). *Telemedicine: Theory and practice. springfield*. ILL. C.C. Thomas Publisher, Ltd.

Bashur R. (1997). *Telemedicine and the health care system in telemedicine, theory and practice*. Thomas, Charles C. (Ed.). Springfield, pp. 5-35.

Bass L., Clements P. and Kazman R. (2003). software architecture in practice, 2nd edition. *SEI series in software engineering*.Addison-Wesley.

Bassett, M. T., & Krieger, N. (1986). Social class and black-white differences in breast cancer survival. *American Journal of Public Health, 76*, 1400-1403.

BBC (2003b). Student died after buying Web drugs. *BBC News*. Retrieved 28, June 2007 from http://news.bbc.co.uk/1/hi/england/3130187.stm

BBC (2004). Millions illiterate about health. *BBC News*. Retrieved 28, June 2007 from http://news.bbc.co.uk/1/hi/health/3530874.stm

Beale, T. (2002). Archetypes: constraint-based domain models for future-proof information systems. In *OOPSLA 2002 Workshop on Behavioural Semantics*. Retrieved from http://www.deepthought.com.au/it/archetypes/archetypes new.pdf

Beale, T. (2005). The openEHR Integration Information Model. openEHR Reference Model. *The openEHR foundation.*

Beale, T. and Heard, S. (2003). Archetype definitions and principles. *The openEHR foundation.*

BearingPoint. (2005). *Large healthcare organizations are embracing RFID.* Retrieved September 4, 2006, from http://www.nahit.org/cms/index.php?option=com_content&task=view&id=157&Itemid=148

Becker, M. Y.,Sewell, P. (2004). Cassandra: flexible trust management, applied to electronic health records.

Becker, Moritz, Y., Sewell, Peter (2005). Cassandra: Flexible trust management applied to electronic health records. Published as *Technical Report UCAM-CL-TR 648.* University of Cambridge, Computer Laboratory, (pp 214).

Beland, G. K., Ellott .M. N, Moralles, L. S., Algazy JZ, Kravite RL, Broder MS., Kanouse D.E, Munoz J. A., Yang K.,M. C. Glynn E. A. (2002). Health information on Internet. *Accessibility, Quality and Readability In English and Spanish, 285*(20), 2612-2621.

Bell,S.G.L Lohse and E.J.Johnson (1999). *Predictors of Online Buying Behaviors,Communications of the ACM, 42*(12) December 1999, 32-38.

Bemmel, J.V. and Musen, M.A. (eds.). *Handbook of medical informatics*, Springer.

Benini, L. and DeMicheli, G. (2002). Networks on Chips: A New Paradigm for Component-Based MPSoC Design. *IEEE Computer.*

Benini, L. and DeMicheli, G. (2002). Networks on chips: a new paradigm for component-based MPSoC Design. *IEEE Computer.*

Benneyan J.C., Lloyd R. C., Plsek P. E. (2003). Statistical process control as a tool for research and healthcare improvement, *Qual Saf Health Care, 12*, 458-464.

Beolchi, L.(Ed). (2003). *Medical informatics in :Telemedicine glossary 5th edition, working document*, p. 748.

Bergmo T. S. (1997). An economic analysis of teleconsultation in otorhinolaryngology. *J Telemed Telecare, 3*, 194–199.

Berner, E.,Moss, J. (2005). Informatics Challenges for the Impending Patient Information Explosion. *J Am Med Inform Assoc,* 12, 614-7.

Berners-Lee T, Hendler J, Lassila O. The semantic web. *Scientific American.* April 2002.

Bertot, J., McClure, C., Jaeger, P., Ryan, J. (2006). *Public libraries and the Internet 2006: study results and findings.* Retrieved from http://www.ala.org/ala/washoff/contactwo/oitp/papersa/papers.cfm

Beyer, M., Kuhn, K.A., Meiler, C., Jablonski, S. and Lenz, R. (2004). Towards a flexible, process-oriented IT architecture for an integrated healthcare network. *Proceedings of the 2004 ACM Symposium on Applied Computing.* Nicosia, Cyprus (pp. 264-271).

Bez, A., (2005). *Emergency medicine.* Retrieved from http://telehealth.hrsa.gov/pubs/tech/ems.htm

Birkland, A., Yona, G. (2006). BIOZON: a hub of heterogeneous biological data. *Nucleic Acids Research, 34*(Database issue), D235-D242.

Bishop J. E., O'Reilly R. L., Maddox K., et al.(2002). Client satisfaction in a feasibility study comparing face-to-face interviews with telepsychiatry. *J Telemed Telecare 8*, 217–221.

Blezek, D.J., Robb, R.A., & Martin, D.P. (2000). Virtual reality simulation of regional anesthesia for training of residentes. *Presented at the 33rd Hawaii International Conference on System Sciences*, (pp. 1-8). IEEE CS Press.

Blobel, B. (2002). Evaluation and harmonisation of electronic healthcare record architecture approaches. *Business Briefing: Global Healthcare,* 1-5.

Blobel, B. (2004). Authorisation and access control for electronic health record systems. *Int J Med Inform,* 73, 251-7.

Blois, M.S. and Shortliffe, E.H. (1990). The computer meets medicine: Emergence of a discipline in Medical Informatics. *Computer Applications in Health Care, 20.*

Bloomfield, B.P. (1991). The role of information systems in the UK National Health Service: Action at a distance and the fetish of calculation. *Social Studies of Science 21*, 701-734.

Bodenreider, O. (2004). The Unified Medical Language System (UMLS): integrating biomedical terminology. *Nucleic Acids Research*, *32*(Database issue), D267-D270.

Bodenreider, O., Mitchell, J.A., McCray, A.T. (2005). Biomedical Ontologies. In: Altman, R.B., Dunker, A.K., Hunter, L., Jung, T.A., Klein, T.E. (Eds.). *Proceedings Pacific Symposium on Biocomputing 2005.* Hackensack, NJ: World Scientific Publishing Co., Inc., pp. 76-78.

Bodenreider, O., Nelson, S.J., Hole, W.T. & Chang, H.F. (1998). Beyond synonymy: exploiting the UMLS semantics in mapping vocabularies (pp. 815-819). *Proceedings AMIA Fall Symposium* American Medical Informatics Association

Bodenreider, O., Stevens, R. (2006). Bio-ontologies: current trends and future directions. *Briefings in Bioinformatics*, *7*(3), 256-274.

Bodie, G. D., Dutta, M. J., Basu, A., & Anderson, J. G. (2007, November). *Explaining demographic differences in online health information seeking: An initial test of the integrative model of e-health Use.* Paper presented at the annual convention of the National Communication Association, Chicago, IL.

Boland JR, R., & Teknasi, R. (1999). Perspective making and perspective taking in communities of knowing. *Shaping Organization Form: Communication, Connection, and Community.*

Bonifacio, M., Bouquet, P., & Traverso, P. (2002). Enabling distributed knowledge management. managerial and technological implications. *Novatica and Informatik/Informatique*, *3*, 23-29.

Booho Yang, Harry H. Asada, S. Rhee, (1999, October). Design of an Artifact-Resistive, Finger-Ring Plethysmographic Sensor. *MIT Home Automation and Healthcare Consortium*, Progress Report No.2-4.

Booth, N., Jain, N.L., and Sugden B. (1999). *The TextBase project — implementation of a base level message supporting electronic patient record transfer in English general practice.* Proceedings of the AMIA Annual Symposium, 691-5.

Boquete,L., Bravo, I., Barea, R., Ascariz, J.M.R., and Martin, J.L.(2005, May). Practacal laboratory project in telemedicine: Supervision of electrocardiograms by mobile telephony. *IEEE Transactions on Education, 48*,(2).

Bose U., McLaren P., Riley A., et al.(2001). The use of telepsychiatry in the brief counseling of non-psychotic patients from an inner-London general practice. *J Telemed Telecare 7*(suppl. 1), 8–10.

Bott, O. J. (2004). Electronic health record: Standardization and implementation, 2nd. *OpenECG Workshop.* Berlin, Germany, pp. 57-60.

Bountis C, Kay J. An integrated knowledge management system for the clinical laboratories: an initial application of an architectural model. Health data in the Information Society. In *Proceedings of MIE 2002. IOS Press.* Amsterdam 2002; 562-567

Bourke, M.K. (1994). *Strategy and architecture of health care information systems.* Springer.

Bower H. (1996). Internet sees growth of unverified health claims. *BMJ 318*(381).

Brady, M.K., Cronin, J.J., Brand, R.R. (2002). Performance-only measurement of service quality: A replication and extension. *Journal of Business Research, 55*, 17– 31.

Branche, P., Mendelson, Y., (2005). Signal Quality and Power Consumption of a New Prototype Reflectance Pulse Oximeter Sensor. *Presented at IEEE Northeast Bioengineering Conference,*.Hoboken, NJ, (pp 42- 43).

Bray, T. (2005). *RSS 2.0 and Atom 1.0 compared.* Retrieved http://www.tbray.org/atom/RSS-and-Atom.

Bredegaard, K. (2000). National standardisation of electronic health care records in Denmark. *Toward an Electronic Health Record Europe 2000*, 98-102.

Breeden, L., Cisler, S., Guilfoy, V., Roberts, M., & Stone, A. (1998). *Computer and communications use in low-income communities: Models for the neighborhood transformation and family development initiative.* Baltimore, MD: Annie E. Casey Foundation.

Brickell, E., Denning, D., Kent, S., Mahler, D. and Tuchman, W. (1993). SKIPJACK Review. *Interim Report.*

British Standards Institution, BSI (2005). Information technology. Security techniques. Information security management systems. Requirements. British Standard / ISO/IEC / 18-Oct-2005/ ISBN: 0580467813.

Brodey B. B., Claypoole K. H., Brodey I. S., et al.(2000): Satisfaction of forensic psychiatric patients with remote telepsychiatric evaluations. *Psychiatric Services 51,* 1305–1307.

Brody, D. S., Miller, S. M., Lerman, C. E., Smith, D. G., & Caputo, G. C. (1989). Patient perception of involvement in medical care: Relationship to illness attitudes and outcomes. *Journal of General Internal Medicine, 4,* 506-511.

Brostoff, S., Sasse, M. A., Chadwick, D., Cunningham, J., Mbanaso, U.,Otenko, S. (2005). "R-What?" Development of a role-based access control (RBAC) policy-writing tool for e-scientists. *Software - Practice and Experience, (38)***,** 835-856.

Brown F. W. (1998). Rural telepsychiatry. *Psychiatr Serv; 49,* 963-964.

Brown, J. S., & Duguid, P. (1991). Organizational learning and communities of practice. *Organization Science, 2,* 40-57.

Brown, N. and Reynolds, M. (2000). Strategy for production and maintenance of standards for interoperability within and between service departments and other healthcare domains. *Short Strategic Study CEN/TC 251/N00-047, CEN/TC 251 Health Informatics.* Brussels: Belgium.

Brown, N., (1995). *History of telemedicine, TIE.* Retrieved from http://tie.telemed.org/telemed101/topics/telemedicine_history.asp

Budgen, D., Rigby, M., Brereton, P. and Turner, M. (2007). *A data integration broker for healthcare systems. IEEE Computer 40*(4), 34-41.

Burdea, G. (1999). Haptic feedback for virtual reality. *Presented at the Virtual Reality and Prototyping Workshop,* (pp. 87-96).

Burgess, M.S.E, Gray, W.A, Fiddian N.J(2007). Using quality criteria to assist in information searching. International Journal of information quality. Vol 1, No1, pp83-99.

Burl M.C., Fowlkes C., Roden J., Stecher A., Mukhtar S. (1999). Diamond Eye: A distributed architecture for image data mining. Presented in *SPIE Thirteenth International Symposium On Aerospace/Defense Sensing, Simulation and Controls.*

Business Week (2000). *The E.biz., 25,* May 15 2000, pp 44.

Butler, T., Kendra, J., Grimley, R., Taylor, B. (1996). Can we measure the effectiveness of our organizations. *International Journal of Health Care Quality Assurance, 9*(5), 37-38.

Callahan, K.L. (1998). *Twelve keys for living: Possibilities for a whole,* Healthy Life, Jossey-Bass, 1998.

Cameron, K.S. and Whetten, D.A. (1983). Some Conclusions about Organisational Effectiveness. In K.S. Cameron and D.A. Whetten, (Eds.). *Organisational Effectiveness: A Comparison of Multiple Models.* New York: Academic Press, (pp. 261-277).

Canadian Institute for Health Information (2006). Understanding family physician usage of electronic health records in Canada. *Results From the 2004 National Physician Survey,* (pp. 1-11).

Capner M. (2000). Videoconferencing in the provision of psychological services at a distance. *J Telemed Telecare 6,* 311–319.

Cappiello, C., Francalanci, C., Pernici, B. (2004). Data quality assessment from the user's perspective, Information Quality in Informational Systems. In *Proceedings of the 2004 international workshop on Information quality in information systems.* Paris, France, (pp.68 – 73), ISBN:1-58113-902-0.

Care2x. (2007). *Hospital information system.* Retrieved from http://www.care2x.org

Carter, E.R. (2005). Systems validation: Application to statistical programs. *BMC Medical Research Methodology, 5*, 3.

Catizone, C. (2002). Colorado state board of pharmacy news. Retrieved fromhttp://www.nabp.net

CENENV 12265. (1997). *Medical informatics {electronic healthcare record architecture*. European Prestandard ENV 12265. European Committee for Standardization. Brussels: Belgium.

CEN/TC 251. *European committee for standardization - technical committee on health informatics*. Retrieved from http://www.centc251.org/.

CEN/TC251 (1999). ENV 12251: Health Informatics - Secure user identification for health care management and security of authentication by passwords. *European Standards in Health Informatics.* CEN.

Center for Disease Control and Prevention (CDC). (2004). Fact sheet: Racial/Ethnic health disparities. Retrieved April 24, 2006, from http://www.cdc.gov/od/oc/media/pressrel/fs040402.htm

Chan F. H. Y., Lam F. K. and Hui Z. (1998), Adaptive thresholding by variational method. *IEEE Transaction on Image Processing. 7*(6), 468-473.

Chan F. Y., Soong B., Lessing K., et al (2000). Clinical value of real-time tertiary fetal ultrasound consultation by telemedicine: preliminary evaluation. *Telemed J, 6*, 237–242.

Charnock, D.(1998). *The DISCERN handbook: Quality criteria for consumer health information.* Abingdon: Radcliffe Medical Press.

Charnock, D., Shepperd S., Gann B., Needham G. (1999). DISCERN — an instrument for judging the quality of consumer health information on treatment choices. *J Epidemiol Community Health 53*, 105-111.

Chau, P.Y.K. (2001). Influence of computer attitude and self-efficacy on IT usage behaviour. *Journal of End User Computing, 13*(1), 26-33.

Cheng, P.-T., Tsai, L.-M., Lu, L.-W., Yang, D.-L., (2004). The design of PDA-based biomedical data processing and analysis for intelligent wearable health monitoring systems. *Presented at IEEE International Conference on Computer and Information Technology*, (pp 879 - 884).

Childs, S. (2003). *Summary how to search the Internet for health information.* Retrieved 10, June 2007 from www.judgehealth.org.uk/print.htm

Choi, J., Yoo, S., Park, H., Chun, J. (2006). MobileMed: A PDA-based mobile clinical information system. *IEEE Transactions on Information Technology in Biomedicine*, 10(3), 627-635.

Chow C.K. and Kaneko R. (1972). Automatic boundary detection of the left ventricle from cineangiograms. *Comp. Biomed. Res. 5*, 443-452.

Christensen, G.E. (1998). MIMD vs SIMD parallel Processing: a case study in 3D medical image registration. *Parallel Computing, 24*, 1369-1383.

Christov, I. and Bortolan, G. (2004). Ranking of pattern recognition parameters for premature ventricular contractions classification by Neural Networks. *Physiological Measurement, 25*(5), 1281-1290.

Chryssanthou, Anargiros (2006). Gathering of digital evidence in a computer network : Problems & possible solutions. School of officers in research and informatics. *Informational leaflet in informatics & technology, issue 28*, May 2006.

Chryssanthou, Anargiros & Apostolakis, Ioannis (2006). Network forensics: Problems and solutions. In *Proceedings of the 2nd National Conference with International Participation, Electronic Democracy.* Athens, ACCI.

Chryssanthou, Anargiros & Kastania, Anastasia (2006). Quality & Security in medical information systems. *Health Review, Tome 17, Issue 100*, pages 42-45.

Chryssanthou, Anargiros (2006). Security of information systems in health environments. *6th National Conference on Public Health & Medical Services.* Athens.

Chu, Y. & Gantz, A. (2004, December). A mobile teletrauma system using 3G networks. *IEEE Transactions on Information Technology in Biomedicine, 8*,(4), 457-461.

Chute, C. (2000). Clinical Classification and Terminology -Some History and Current Observations *Journal of the American Medical Informatics Association, 7*(3), 298–303.

Chuva MT, Fernandes MT, Correia C, Barbosa L, Silva MJ, Gomes MJ, Moreira MM, Gomes MM, Vinhas MS, Dias M, Moreira M,Ferreira A. (2006). Attitudes and opinions of patients and healthcare professionals about the use of coomputers in primary care – systematic review. *IX Jornadas Científicas dos Estudantes de Medicina. Faculdade de Medicina da Universidade do Porto.*

Classic episodes in telemedicine. Treatment by telegraph (1917). *Excerpt from the obituary of John Joseph Holland (1876-1959).* JTT.1997;3:223.

Clements P., Bachmann F., Bass L., Garlan D., Ivers J., Little R., Nord R. and Stafford J. (2002). Documenting software architectures. *SEI series in software engineering.* Addison-Wesley.

Cline, R., & Haynes, K. (2001). Consumer health information seeking on the Internet: The state of the art. *Health Education Research, 16*, 671-679.

Clunie, D. A. (2005). PixelMed Java DICOM toolkit. Retrieved October 2005 from http://www.pixelmed.com/, Accessed in

Coiera, E. (1998). Guide to medical informatics, the internet and telemedicine. *Chapman and Hall Medical 2nd Edition*, ISBN 0 412 75710 9 (book review. BMJ. 316, 158).

Coiera, E. (2003). *Guide to health informatics*, Arnold.

Coldwell, J., Wells, J. (2003). Students' perspective of online learning', In G. Davies & E. Stacey (Eds.), *Quality education@a distance.* Norwell, MA: Kluwer Academic Publishers Group, (pp. 101-108).

Collen, M.F. (1986). Origins of medical informatics. *West J Med. (145)6*, 778–785.

Collen, M.F. (1994), The origins of informatics. *Journal of the American Medical Informatics Association, (1)2* 91-107.

Commission, A. (1995). For your information: a study of information management and systems in the acute hospital.

COMPACCS Study (2000). *JAMA*, pp 284:2762.

Conway, T., Willcocks, S. (1997). The role of expectations in the perception of health care quality: developing a conceptual model. *International Journal of Health Care Quality Assurance, , 10*(3), 131–140.

Cook, D.A., Dupras, D.M.. (2004). A practical guide to developing effective Web-based learning. *Journal of General Internal Medicine, 19*, 698-707. Retrieved from: http://www.blackwell-synergy.com

Coonan, G. M. (2002). Making the most of mobility. *Health Management Technology, 23*(10), 32-36.

Costlow, D., (2004), Telehealth companies poised for market growth. *Design News*. Retrieved from http://www.designnews.com/article/CA404920.html?text=telemedicine

Cotten, S. R., & Gupta, S. S. (2004). Characteristics of online and offline health information seekers and factors that discriminate between them. *Soc Sci Med*, 1795-1806.

Cowie, M. R., & Mosterd, A., & Wood, D. A., & Deckers, J.W., & Poole-Wilson, P. A., & Sutton, G. C. (1997). The epidemiology of heart failure. *European Heart Journal, 18*, 208-255.

Crichard M (2003). Privacy and electronic communications. *Computer Law and Security Report, 19*, 299-303.

Crocco A. G, Keever M. V, Jadad A. R(2002). Analysis of cases of Harm Associated with use of health information on the Internet. *JAMA , 287*(21), 2869-2871.

Crowson, R. (1970). *Classification and biology* London: Heinemann Educational Books Ltd.

Cruz-Correia R, Vieira-Marques P, Costa P, Ferreira A, Oliveira-Palhares E, Araújo F,Costa-Pereira A. (2005). Integration of Hospital data using Agent Technologies – a case study. *AICommunications special issue of ECAI, (18)*, 191-200.

Cruz-Correia R, Vieira-Marques P, Ferreira A, Oliveira-Palhares E, Costa P,Costa-Pereira A. (2006). Monitoring the integration of hospital information systems: how it may ensure and improve the quality of data. *Stud Health Technol Inform (121)*, 176-182.

Cruz-Correia, R., Vieira-Marques, P., Costa, P., Ferreira, A., Oliveira-Palhares, E., Araujo, F.,Costa-Pereira, A. (2005). Integration of hospital data using agent technologies - a case study. *AI Communications, (18)*, 191-200.

Cruz-Correia, R., Vieira-Marques, P., Ferreira, A., Oliveira-Palhares, E., Costa, P.,Costa-Pereira, A., 2006. Monitoring the integration of hospital information systems: how it may ensure and improve the quality of data. *Stud Health Technol Inform, (121)*, 176-182.

Cuevas C. et al. (2003).Telepsychiatry in Canary Islands: user acceptance and satisfaction. *J Telemed Telecare, 9*, 221-224.

Currell, R., Urquhart, C., Wainwright, P., & Lewis, R. (2000). Telemedicine versus face to face patient care: Effects on professional practice and health care outcomes. Retrieved June 4, 2007, from http://www.cochrane.org/reviews/en/ab002098.html

Czerwinski, S. J., & Abramowitz, A. D. (2001). *Telecommunications: Characteristics and choices of internet users*. Retrieved April 8, 2006. from http://www.gao.gov/new.items/d01345.pdf.

Dadoun, G. (1992). ISO 9000 a requirement for doing business. IBM Centre for Advanced Studies Conference. In *Proceedings of the 1992 conference of the Centre for Advanced Studies on Collaborative research*. Toronto, Ontario, Canada, SESSION: Software engineering environment, vol.1, (pp. 433-437).

Dambergs, Y. translator. (2003). *Raymond Lull: ars magna* Retrieved December 28, 2006 from http://lullianarts.net/agu/contents.htm

Daveport, T. *H, and Prusak, L Working Knowledge: How Organizations Manage What They Know*. Boston. MA: Harvard Business School Press.

David, N., Huntington, P., Gunter B., Russell C., Withey, R. (2003). *The British and their use of the Web for Health information and advice: A survey.* Retrieved 28, June 2007 from, http://www.emeraldinsight.com/0001-253X.htm

Davis, F.D. (1989). Perceived usefulness, perceived ease of use, and user acceptance of information technology. *MIS Quarterly, 13*(1), 319-340.

Davis, F.D. (1993). User acceptance of information technology: system characteristics, user perceptions and behavioral impacts, *Int J Man-Machine Studies, 38*, 475-487.

Davis, F.D., Bagozzi, R.P. and Warshaw, P.R. (1989). User acceptance of computer technology: a comparison of two theoretical models. *Management Science, 35*(8), 982-1003.

Davis, F.D., Bagozzi, R.P. and Warshaw, P.R. (1992). Extrinsic and intrinsic motivation to use computers in the workplace. *Journal of Applied Social Psychology, 22*(14), 1111-1132.

Dawson, S. L., Kaufman, J. A. (1998). The Imperative for Medical Simulation. In *Proceedings of the IEEE,* 86/3, pp. 479-483.

DB Kendall, SR Levine. Perspective: Pursuing The Promise Of An Information-Age Health Care System. Health Affairs, USA 1998

DCMTK. (2005). The DICOM Offis toolkit. Retrieved December 2005 from http://dicom.offis.de/

De Chazal, P., O'Dwyer, M. and Reilly, R. (2004). Automatic classification of heartbeats using ECG morphology and heartbeat interval features. *IEEE Trans. Biomedical Eng., 51*(7), 1196-1206.

De Chazal, P., O'Dwyer, M. and Reilly, R. (2004). Automatic classification of heartbeats using ECG morphology and heartbeat interval features. *IEEE Trans. Biomedical Eng., 51*(7), 1196-1206.

Deftereos, S., Lambrinoudakis, C., Andriopoulos, P., Farmakis, D., and Aessopos, A. (2001). A java-based electronic healthcare record software for beta-thalassaemia. *Journal of Medical Internet Research, 3*(4), e33.

Deitsch S. E., Frueh B. C., Santos A. B. (2000). Telepsychiatry for post-traumatic stress disorder. *J Telemed Telecare 6*, 184-186.

Delacy, M. (1999). Nosology, mortality and disease theory in the eighteenth century *Journal of the History of Medicine, 54*, 261-284.

DeLone, W. H. and McLean E. R. (2002). Information success revisited. *Presented at Hawaii International Conference on System Sciences.* Big Island, Hawaii.

DeMeis, R., (2002), Hospitals to go. *Design News.* Retrieved from http://www.designnews.com/article/CA217944.html?text=telemedicine

Department of Health - Estates and Facilities Division

(2007). *Using mobile phones in NHS hospitals*, (pp.5-10). Retrieved from http://www.dh.gov.uk/en/Publicationsandstatistics/Publications/PublicationsPolicyAndGuidance/DH_074396

Detmer, D.E. (2003). Building the national health information infrastructure for personal health, health care services, public health and research. *BMC Medical Informatics and Decision Making 3*, 1-40.

Dev, P., Montgomery, K., Senger, S., Heinrichs, W.L., Srivastana, S., & Waldron, K. (2002). Simulated medical learning environment on the Internet. *Journal of the American Medical Informatics Association, 9*(5).

DeVaul, R., Sung, M., Gips, J, and Pentland, A. (2003). Mithril 2003: Applications and architecture. *Seventh IEEE Symposium on IEEE Wearable Computers*, pp 4-11.

Dick, R.,Steen, E., 1997. *The Computer-based patient record: An essential technology for healthCare.*

Dick, W., Carey, L., & Carey, J. (2005). *The systematic design of instruction- sixth edition.* Boston, MA: Allyn and Bacon.

DICOM Supplement 85 (2004). Web Access to DICOM Persistent Objects (WADO). *Joint DICOM standards committee / ISO TC215 Ad Hoc WG on WADO, final text.* Retrieved from ftp://medical.nema.org/medical/dicom/_nal/sup85 ft.pdf.

DICOM. (2004). Digital imaging and communications in medicine. *NEMA Standards Publication PS 3, National Electrical Manufacturers Association*. Rosslyn: VA, USA.

DiMaio, S.P., & Salcudean, S.E. (2005). Interactive simulation of needle insertion models. *IEEE Transactions on Biomedical Engineering,52*(7), 1167–1179. IEEE CS Press.

Dixon R, Grubb PA, Lloyd D, Kalra D. (2001). Consolidated list of requirements. *EHCR Support Action Deliverable 1.4. European Commission DGXIII.* Retrieved from http://www.chime.ucl.ac.uk/HealthI/EHCR-SupA/del1-4v1_3.PDF.

Doepp, M., & Edelmann, G. (2002). The switching of the brain as an addiction-like condition: Interference of the meridians by electrosmog? *AKU 30*(3), 133-139.

Doepp, M., & Edelmann, G. (2003). Clinical evaluation of the frequency distribution analysis of biological data. *Erfahrungsheilkunde,* 12, 818-824.

Doepp, M., & Edelmann, G. (2006). System patterns of the human organism and their heredity, 375-382, In Lazakidou, A. A. (ed.), *Handbook of Research on Informatics in Healthcare and Biomedicine*. Hershey PA: Idea Group Inc.

Doepp, M., Edelmann, G., Cohen, S., Popp, F.-A., Yu, Y. (2002). A new procedure for the judgement of the health state with the aid of the frequency distribution of the conductivity values of the skin. *Erfahrungsheilkunde, 51*, 3–11.

Dolin R. H., Alschuler L., Boyer S. et. al. (2006). HL7 clinical document architecture, release 2. *Journal of American Medical Informatics Association, 13*, 30-39.

Dolin RH, Alschuler L, Beebe C., et al. (2001). The HL7 clinical document architecture. *J Am Med Inform Assoc., 8*(6), 552–69.

Donabedian, A. (1988). *Quality assessment and assurance: unity of purpose, diversity of means, Inquiry, 25*, 173-192.

Donaldson, W.G. (1995). Manufacturers need to show greater commitment to customer-service. *Industrial Marketing Management, 24*, 421–430.

Doyle DJ (1995). Surfing the Internet for patient information: the personal clinical Web page. *Journal of the American Medical Association, 274,* 1586.

Doyle DJ (1996). Informational clinical consulting via the Internet. *Canadian Medical Association Journal, 154,* 1180.

Doyle DJ (2007). Medical Conditions with Airway Implications. Available: http://anestit.unipa.it/anestit/gta/medical-airway.html

Dromey, R. G. (1995). A model for software product quality. *IEEE Transactions on Software Engineering, 21*(2), 146-162.

Drougas Ag. B. (2006). Virtual reality simulation in human applied kinetics and ergo-physiology. *Encyclopedia of Informatics in Health Care and Biomedicine.* University of Piraeus Greece: IGI Publications

Drougas B. (2003). *Applications of Teleinformatics in Medicine.* ATEI of Epirus 2001.

Drougas, Ag. B (2002). Study of the ability of the kinetic adaptability by combinable movements. *Exercise and Society Journal 31,* 371,372 .

Drougas, Ag. B (April – June 2001). Kinetics & Flexibility for the Human Body. *Karate Voice Newspaper,* page 9

Drougas, Ag. B. (2003). Theory and laboratory applications for the lesson teleinformatics and applications in Medicine Department of Teleinformatics. *ATEI of Epirus*, pp 25-47

Drougas, Ag. B. (2004B). *Care and the Modern technologies*, pp 45-67

Drougas, Ag. B. (2004c). Virtual reality and health manual of the laboratory of the teleinformatics and applications in Medicine, Department of Teleinformatics. *ATEI of Epirus*, pp 10-22

Drougas, Ag. B. Telemedicine (2004a). *Applications in a contemporary environment, Edition*, pp 47-55.

Drougas, Ag. B.(2004G). Rehabilitation by new technologies.*Research and Theory Journal Issue. 1/04*, 12-15.

Drougas, B. (2003). Applications of teleinformatics in medicine. *TEI of Epirus*, 2001, pp 24-29

Drucker, P. (1994) The age of social transformation. *The Atlantic Monthly*, (Nov), pp. 53–80.

Dutta, M. J., & Bodie, G. D. (2008). Web searching for health: Theoretical foundations and connections to health related outcomes. In A. Spink & M. Zimmer (Eds.), *Web searching: Interdisciplinary perspectives.* New York: Peter Lang Publishing.

Dutta, M. J., Bodie, G. D., & Basu, A. (2008). Health disparity and the racial divide among the nation's youth: Internet as an equalizer? In A. Everett (Ed.), *The MacArthur Foundation Series on Digital Media and Learning: Race and Ethnicity*: MIT Press.

Dutta-Bergman, M. J. (2004a). A descriptive narrative of healthy eating: A social marketing approach using psychographics in conjunction with interpersonal, community, mass media and new media activities. *Health Marketing Quarterly, 20*, 81-101.

Dutta-Bergman, M. J. (2004b). Developing a profile of consumer intention to seek out additional health information beyond the doctor: Demographic, communicative, and psychographic factors. *Health Communication, 17*, 1-16.

Dutta-Bergman, M. J. (2004c). Health attitudes, health cognitions, and health behaviors among Internet health information seekers: Population-based survey [Electronic Version]. *Journal of Medical Internet Research*, 6, e15. Retrieved August 22, 2005 from http://www.jmir.org/2004/2/e15.

Dutta-Bergman, M. J. (2006). Media use theory and internet use for health care. In M. Murero & R. Rice (Eds.), *The internet and health care: Theory, research, and practice* (pp. 83-103). Mahwah, NJ: Erlbaum.

Eadie, L. H., Seifalian, A.M., Davidson, B.R., (2003). Telemedicine in surgery. *British Journal of Surgery Society Ltd, 90*(6), 647-658.

EC (2003). *Directive of 2003/94/EC, of 8 October 2003, laying down the principles and guidelines of good manufacturing practice in respect of medicinal products for human use and investigational medicinal products for human use.* Volume 4, Medicinal Products for Human and Veterinary Use: Good Manufacturing Practice. In Annex 11: Computerised system, (pp 11). Retrieved April 13, 2005 from http://pharmacos.eudra.org/F2/eudralex/vol-4/home.htm.

Eckstein, R., Brown, D. C., Kelly, P. (1999). *Using Samba, 1st Edition.* O'Reilly & Associates, Inc. .

Eco, U. (1993). *La ricerca della lingua perfetta nella cultura europea* Rome-Bari: Gius Laterza & Figli

Edutopia News. (2004). *Ed-tech funding reduced for 2005.* Retrieved 1, December 2004 from, http://www.edutopia.org/products/changeformat.php

E-Europe (2002). Commision of the European communities. Quality criteria for Health related Websites. *J. Med Internet res. 4*(3), e15.

Efferth, T. (2002). E-learning in medicine at the virtual campus rhineland-palatinate. In *Proceedings of the 7th International Conference on the Medical Aspects of Telemedicine.* Regensburg, Germany.

Eichelberg, M., Aden T., Riesmeier J., Dogac A., Laleci G. (2006). Electronic health record standards – a brief overview. In *Proceedings of the 4th International Conference on Information and Communications Technology (ICICT 2006).* Cairo, Egypt.

Eichelberg, M., Aden, T., Riesmeier, J., Dogac, A., and Laleci, G. B. (2005). A survey and analysis of Electronic Healthcare Record standards. *ACM Computing. Surveys, 37*(4), 277-315.

Ekman, A., Hall, P., Litton, J. E. (2005). Can we trust cancer information on the Internet? A comparison of interactive cancer risk sites. *Cancer causes and control Journal, 16*, 65-772.

Elwyn, G., O'Conor, A., Stacey, D., Volk, R., Edwards., A, Coulter, A., Thomson, R., et al (2006). Developing a quality criteria frame work for patients decisions aids: online international Delphi, consensus process. *BMJ 333*, 417.

emmel, J.H.V. (1984). *The structure of medical informatics - Medical Informatics. (9)*, p. 175.

Engelmann, U., Schröter, A., Baur, U., Werner, O., Schwab, M., Müller, H. and Meinzer, H.-P. (1998). A three-generation model for teleradiology. *IEEE Transactions on Information Technology in Biomedicine, 2*(1), 20–25.

Epocrates. (2007). *Prescription software.* Retrieved from http://www.epocrates.com

Ericson, C. (2005). *Real time collision detection.* Morgan Kaufmann. Elsevier.

Ermer, J. (2001). Validation in pharmaceutical analysis, Part 1, an integrated approach. *Journal of Pharmaceutical and Biomedical Analysis, 24,* 755-767.

Eysenbach G, Sa ER, Diepgen TL. (1999) *Cyber medicine.* Interview by Clare.

Eysenbach G., Diepgen T. C., Gray J. A. M., et al (1998). Towards quality management of medical information on the Internet. Evaluation labelling and filtering of information. *BMJ 317,* 1496-1502.

Eysenbach, G. (2000). *Consumer health informatics. BMJ, (320)*, 1713-16.

Eysenbach, G. (2004). Recent advances Consumer health informatics. Clinical review. *BMJ, 320.*

Eysenbach, G., & Diepgen, T. L. (1999). Labeling and filtering of medical information on the Internet. *Methods of Information in Medicine, 38*, 80-88.

Eysenbach, G., Kohler, C. (2002). How do consumers search for and appraise health information on the World Wide Web. *BMJ 324*, 573-577.

Ezquerra N., Capell S., Klein L. and Duijves P. (1998). Model-guided labelling of coronary structure. *IEEE Transactions on Medical Imaging, 17*(3), 429-441

Fadlee, M., Rasid, A., and Woodward, B. (March, 2005). Bluetooth Telemedicine Processor for Multichannel Biomedical Signal Transmission via Mobile Cellular Networks. *IEEE Transactions on Information Technology in Biomedicine, 9*(1), 35-43.

Fan, R. Ceded, L., Toser, O. (2005). Java plus XML: a powerful new combination for SCADA systems. *Computing & Control Engineering Journal, 16*(5), 27-30.

Fanberg, H. (2004). The RFID revolution. *Marketing Health Services, 24*(3), 43-44.

Farr, W. (1839). *First Annual report of the Registrar General* London: W. Clowes and Sons

FDA (1987a). Guidelines on general principles of process validation. *US Food and Drug Administration.* Retrieved March 12, 2007 from, http://www.fda.gov/cder/guidance/pv.htm

FDA (1987b). General principles of validation. *Food and Drug Administration, Center for Drug Evaluation and Research.* Rockville, MD.

FDA (2002). General principles for software validation medical devices. *Guidance for Industry, Final Guidance*, January.

Feigenbaum, M. J. (1978). Quantitative universality for a class of nonlinear transformations. *Journal Statistical Physics, 19*, 25.

Feldman, R. H. L., & Fulwood, R. (1999). The three leading causes of death in African Americans: Barriers to reducing excess disparity and to improving health behaviors. *Journal of Health Care for the Poor and Undeserved, 10*, 45-71.

Ferguson, Tom (2002). "From patients to end-users". *British Medical Journal, 324*, 555-556.

Ferreira A, Correia A, Silva A, Corte A, Pinto A, Saavedra A, Pereira A, Pereira AF, Cruz-Correia R,Antunes L. (2007a). Why facilitate patient access to medical records. *Studies in Health Technology and Informatics, (127)*, 77-90.

Ferreira A, Cruz-Correia R, Antunes L, Farinha P, Oliveira-Palhares E, Chadwick D. W,Costa-Pereira A. (2006). How to Break Access Control in a Controlled Manner. *CBMS2006.* Salt Lake City, USA.

Ferreira A, Cruz-Correia R, Antunes L, Oliveira-Palhares E, Farinha P,Costa-Pereira A. (2005). How to start modelling access control in a healthcare organization. *10th International Symposium for Health Information Management Research.* Greece.

Ferreira A, Cruz-Correia R, Antunes L,Chadwick D W. (2007b). Access Control: how can it improve patients' healthcare? *Studies in Health Technology and Informatics, (127)*, 65-76.

Ferreira, A., Correia, R., Antunes, L., Palhares, E., Marques, P., Costa, P., da Costa Pereira, A. (2004). Integrity for electronic patient record reports. *Proceedings of the 17th IEEE Symposium on Computer-Based Medical Systems (CBMS'04)*, (pp. 4-9).

Ferris, J. M. (1994). Using standards as a security policy tool. *StandardView, 2*(2), 72-77.

Finch, C. (1999). Mobile computing in healthcare. *Health Management Technology, 20*(3), 64-65.

Fischer-Homberger, E. (1970). Eighteenth-century nosology and its survivors *Medical History, 14*(4), 397-403.

Fogel, J., Albert, S. M., Schnabel, F., Ditkoff, B. A., & Neugut, A. I. (2003). Racial/Ethnic differences and potential psychological benefits in use of the internet by women with breast cancer. *Psycho-Oncology, 12*, 107-117.

Fogel, K. (2005). *Producing open source software.* O'Reilly Media, Inc. ISBN: 0-596-00759-0

Fogg, B.J. & Tseng, Hsiang (1999). The elements of computer credibility. In *Proceedings of CHI'99.* Pittsburgh, PA.

Forester Research (1998). *US Online Business Trade According to Forester Research*, Press release. December 17, 1998.

Forester Research, power ranking for top Consumer Sites (1999). Retrieved November 19, 1999 from http://www.forester.com

Forrest, C.B. and Starfield, B. (1998). Entry into primary care and continuity: the effects of access. *Am J Public Health, 88*(9), 1330-1336.

Foster I. and Kesselman C. (1999). *The grid blueprint for a new computing infrastructure*. Morgan Kaufmann Publishers.

Fox, S. (2005a). *Digital divisions.* Washington, DC: Pew Internet & American Life Project.

Fox, S. (2005b). *Health information online: Eight in ten internet users have lookedfor health information online, with increased interest in diet, fitness, drugs, health insurance, experimental treatments, and particular doctors and hospitals* Washington, DC: Pew Internet & American Life Project.

Fox, S. (2006). *Online health search.* Retrieved 15 of June 2007 from, http://www.pewInternet.org/pdfs/PIP_Online_Health_2006.pdf

Freimuth, V. S., Stein, J. A., & Kean, T. J. (1989). *Searching for health information: The Cancer Information Service Model.* Philadelphia: University of Pennsylvania Press.

Frick, U. et al. (2002). Risk perception, somatization, and self report of complaints related to electromagnetic fields – a randomized survey study. *Int. J. Hyg. Environ. Health, 205*, 353-360.

Frick, U. et al. (2005). Comparison perception of singular transcranial magnetic stimuli by subjectively electrosensitive subjects and general population controls. *Bioelectromagnetics 26*, 287-298.

Friedli, D., Kappeler, W., Zimmermann, S. (1998). Validation of computer systems: Practical testing of a standard LIMS. *Pharmaceutica Acta Helvetiae, 72*, 343-348.

Friedman C,Wyatt J. (2006). *Evaluation methods in biomedical informatics*, Springer.

Fuchs, B., & Lieber, J., & Mille, A., & Napoli, A. (1999). Towards a unified theory of adaptation in case based reasoning. In Althoff, K.-D. et. al. (Eds.). *Case Based Reasoning Research and Development* (pp.104-117). Berlin: Springer.

Fukuyama, Francis (1995). *Trust—the social virtues and the creation of prosperity*. New York: The Free Press.

Gagliano, D., (1998). Wireless Ambulance Telemedicine May Lessen Stroke Morbidity. *Telemedicine Today,* 1998, *6*(1), 21.

Gagliardi, A., Jadad, A. R. (2002). Examinations of instruments used to rate quality of health information on the Internet. Chronicle of a voyage with an unclear destination. *BMJ 324*, 569-573.

Gammon D., Sorlie T., Bergvik S., Hoifodt T. S. (1998). Psychotherapy supervision conducted by videoconferencing: a qualitative study of users experiences. *J Telemed Telecare, 4*(suppl. 1),33 5.

Ganesan, P., Venugopalan, R., Peddabachagari, P., Dean, A., Mueller, F., and Sichitiu, M. (2003). Analyzing and modeling encryption overhead for sensor network nodes. *Wireless Sensor Networks and Applications (WSNA 2004).* San Diego, CA.

Ganesan, P., Venugopalan, R., Peddabachagari, P., Dean, A., Mueller, F., and Sichitiu, M. (2003). Analyzing and Modeling Encryption Overhead for Sensor Network Nodes. *Wireless Sensor Networks and Applications (WSNA 2004).* San Diego, CA.

Gans, D., Kralewski, J., Hammons, T., Dowd B. (2006). Medical groups' adoption of electronic health records and information systems. *Health affairs (Project Hope), 24*(5), 1323-1333.

Garg, A.X., Adhikari, N.K.J., McDonald, H., Rosas-Arellano, M.P., Devereaux, P.J., Beyene, J., Sam, J., and Haynes, R.B. (2005). Effects of computerized clinical decision support systems in practitioner performance and patient outcomes: A systematic review. *Journal of the American Medical Association, 293*, 1223–1238.

Gates Foundation. (2004). U.S. library program: summary of research reports. Retrieved from http://www.gatesfoundation.org/Libraries/USLibraryProgram/Evaluation/default.htm

Gates Foundation. (2005). U.S. public libraries providing unprecedented access to computers, the Internet, and technology training. Retrieved from http://www.gatesfoundation.org/Libraries/USLibraryProgram/Announcements/Announce-050623.htm

Gay, E. G. (1998). A State's use of the electronic medical record: a means to address Arkansas' health care responsibilities to her children-promoting access to cost-effective care. *International Journal of Technology Management, 15*, 458-469.

Gazette. (2005). *RFID in the pharma supply chain.* Retrieved September 2, 2006, from http://www.rfidgazette.org/2005/11/rfid_in_the_pha.html

Gebelein, H., & Heite, H.-J. (1950). About the imbalance of biological frequency distributions. *Klin. Wochenschrift, 28*(41).

General Accounting Office (1996). *Consumer health informatics-emerging issues*. Washington, DC,

General Electric. (2007). *General Electric Healthcare Company*. Retrieved February 2007 from http://www.gehealthcare.com/worldwide.html

Gerasimov B., Oxijuk A., Gulak N., (2006). Estimation of efficiency of the systems for support of decision-making. In *System of Support of Decision Making Theory and Practice*.Kiev, 25-7. (rus.)

Gerz, W. (1996). *Textbook of the Applied Kinesiology (AK) in the natural medicine practice.* Munich: AKSE-publisher, 1996. ISDN: 3-00-000616-8.

Giardina, M. (1992). Interactivity and intelligent advisory strategies in a multimedia learning environment: Human factors, design issues and technical considerations. In M. Giardina (Ed.), *Interactive multimedia learning environments,* New York: Springer -Verlag, (pp. 48-66).

Gilbert, L., & Moore, D. (1998). Buidling interactivity in Web courses: Tools for social and instructional interaction. *Educational Technology, 38*, 29-35.

Gillette, B. (2001). Promoting wellness programs results in a healthier bottom line. *Managed Health care Executive, 11*(2), 45-46.

Glencross, M. & Chalmers, A. (2005). High fidelity collaborative virtual environments. *Presented at the 4th*

International Conference on Virtual Reality, Computer Graphics, Visualization and Interaction in Africa (tutorial notes). AFRIGRAPH.

Glennon, B. (1997). Control system validation in multipurpose biopharmaceutical facilities, *Journal of Biotechnology, 59*, 53–61.

Glowniak, J. V. (1995). Medical resources on the Internet. *Ann Intern Med., 123*, 123-31.

Goodheart, G.J. jr. (1985). *You'll be better – the story of applied kinesiology.* Geneva, Ohio: AK Printing.

Goos, K. (1996). *Fallbasiertes klassifizieren: Methoden, integration und evaluation.* Sankt Augustin: Infix Verlag.

Grabowski, B., & Small, R. (1997). Information, instruction, and learning: A hypermedia perspective. *Performance and Improvement Quarterly, 10*(1). 156-166.

Grandinetti, D. A. (1994). Doctors and the Web help your patients surf the Net safety. *Medical Economics, 77*(5), 186-8.

Greek Data Protection authority. (1997). *Individuals protection against the processing of personal sensitive data.* (Law 2472/1997).

Greenberg, SJ. (1997). The "Dreadful Visitation": public health and public awareness in seventeenth-century London. *Bulletin of the Medical Library Association 85(4)*, 391-401.

Greenes, R., Shortliffe, E. (1990). Medical Informatics: an emerging academic discipline and institutional priority. *JAMIA, (263)*, 1114-20.

Greenes, R.A. and Shortliffe, E.H. (1990). Medical Informatics, In: An emerging academic discipline and institutional priority. *Journal of the American Medical Association, (263) 8*, 1114-1120.

Greenes, R.A. and Siegel, E.R. (1987). Characterization of an emerging field, In: approaches to defining the literature and disciplinary boundaries of medical informatics. *Symp Comp Appl Med Care*, 411–415.

Griffith S., Kalra D., Lloyd D., and Ingram D. (1995). A portable and communicable architecture for electronic healthcare records: The good European Healthcare Record Project (AIM project 2014). Greenes, R. A. and others, eds. *Medinfo 8*(1995), 223-226.

Grigoroudis, E. & Siskos, Y. (2002). Preference disaggregation for measuring and analysing customer satisfaction: The MUSA method, *European Journal of Operational Research, 143*, 148-170.

Grimson, J., Grimson, W. & Hasselbring, W. (2000). The SI challenge in health care. *Communications of the ACM, 43*(6), 48-55.

Grimson, J., Grimson, W., Berry, D., Stephens, G., Felton, E., Kalra, D., Toussaint, P., and Weier, O.W. (1998). A CORBA-based integration of distributed electronic healthcare records using the synapses approach. *IEEE Trans Inf Technol Biomed, 2*(3), 124-38.

Gritzalis S (2004). Enhancing privacy and data protection in electronic medical environments. *Journal of Medical Systems, 28*, 535-547.

Grover, V. and Ramanlan (1999). Six Myths of Information and Markets: Information Technology Networks, Electronic Commerce and the Battle for Consumer Surplus. *MIS Quarterly 23*(4) December 1999.

Grunwald, T., & Crosbie-Massay, C. (2006). Guidelines for cognitively efficient multimedia learning tools: Educational strategies, cognitive load and interface design. *Academic Medicine, 81*, 213-223.

Guan, L.; Kung, S.Y.; Larsen, J. (2001). *Multimedia image and video processing.* New York: CRC Press.

Gunkel, D. J. (2003). Second thoughts: Toward a critique of the digital divide. *New Media & Society, 5*, 499-522.

Gunn PP, Fremont AM, Bottrell M, Shugarman LR, Galegher J, & Bikson T (2004). The Health Insurance Portability and Accountability Act Privacy Rule: a practical guide for researchers. *Medical Care, 42*, 321-327.

Gunn, C., Hutchins, M., & Adcock, M. (2005b). Combating latency in haptic collaborative virtual environments. *Presence: Teleoperators and Virtual Environments, 14*(3), 313-328.

Gunn, C., Hutchins, M., Stevenson, D., Adcock, M., & Youngblood, P. (2005a). Using collaborative haptics in remote surgical training. *Presented at the Eurohaptics Conference and Symposium on Haptic Interfaces for*

Virtual Environment and Teleoperator Systems, (pp. 481-482).

Gupta, S., Ganz, A. (2004). Design considerations and implementation of a cost-effective, portable remote monitoring unit using 3G wireless data networks, presented at IEEE EMBS, San Francisco, CA, USA, pp. 3286-3289.

Gura, N., Patel, A., Wander, A., Eberle, H., and Shantz, S. (2004). Comparing elliptic curve cryptography and RSA on 8-bit CPUs. *Workshop on Cryptographic Hardware and Embedded Systems (CHES 2004)*. Cambridge, MA.

Gura, N., Patel, A., Wander, A., Eberle, H., and Shantz, S. (2004). Comparing elliptic curve cryptography and RSA on 8-bit CPUs. *Workshop on Cryptographic Hardware and Embedded Systems (CHES 2004)*. Cambridge, MA.

Gurjit Kaur , Neena Gupta (2006). *Journal of Evolution and Technology, 15*(1), 23-35

Hackos JoAnn,Redish Janice. (1998). *User and task analysis for interface design* Wiley.

Hailiang Mei, Ing Widya, Aart van Halteren, Bayu Erfianto, (2006, December). A flexibile vital sign representation framework for mobile healthcare. *International Conference on Pervasive Computing Technologies for Healthcare*. Innsbruck, Austria.

Haluck, R. et al., (2002). Reliability and validity of endotower, a virtual reality trainer for angled endoscope navigation. In J.D. Westwood et al. (Eds.), *Medicine meets virtual reality*. IOS Press

Hammond, K., Helbig, S., Benson, C.,BM, B.-S. (2003). Are electronic medical records trustworthy? Observations on copying, pasting and duplication. *AMIA Annual Symposium*.

Han, C., Rengaswamy, R., Shea, R., Kohler, E., and Srivastava, M. (2005). SOS: A dynamic operating system for sensor networks. *Third International Conference on Mobile Systems, Applications, and Services (Mobisys 2005)*. Seattle, WA.

Han, J., Kamber, M., (2000). Data Mining: Concepts and Techniques, Series Editor Morgan Kaufmann Publishers. The Morgan Kaufmann Series in Data Management Systems, Jim Gray.

Haris K., Efstratiadis S., Maglaveras N., Pappas C., Goruassas H. and Loruidas G. (1999). Model-based morphological segmentation and labelling of coronary angiograms. *IEEE Transactions on Medical Imaging, 18*(10), 1003-1015

Harrington, J. J. (1993). *IEEE P1157 MEDIX: A standard for open systems medical data interchange*. Institute of Electrical and Electronic Engineers, New York City, NY

Harris S, 2003. *CISSP All-in-one exam guide*. McGraw-Hill Osborne Media.

Harrop, P., & Das, R. (2006). *RFID in healthcare 2006-2016*. Cambridge, UK: IDTechEx.

Harvey, J., (1998). Service Quality: A tutorial. *Journal of Operations Management, 16*, 583-597.

Hasin, M. A. A., Seeluangsawat, R., & Shareef, M.A. (2001). Statistical measures of customer satisfaction for hospital health-care quality assurance: a case study. *International Journal of Health Care Quality Assurance, 14*(1), 6-14.

Hasman, A., Haux, R. and Albert, A. (1996). *A systematic view on medical informatics, (51)* 3,131-139.

Hassmann U., Merk L., Nicklous, M.S., Stober, T., Korhonen P., Khan P. and Shelness N. (2003). *Pervasive computing: The mobile world*. Springer

Hassol A, Walker JM, Kidder D, Rokita K, Young D, Pierdon S et al. (2004). Patient experiences and attitudes about access to a patient electronic health care record and linked web messaging. *Journal of the American Medical Informatics Association, 11*, 505-513.

Hastings, S., Kurc, T., Langella, S., Catalyurek, U., Pan, T., & Saltz, J. (2003). Image processing for the grid: a toolkit for building grid-enabled image processing applications. In *Proceedings of the 3rd IEEE/ACM International Symposium on Cluster Computing and the Grid*. 36-43.

Haux, R. (1996). Medical informatics. In, once more towards systematization. *Methods Inf Med., (35)*3, 189-92 (abstract).

Hawkridge, D. (1999) Distance learning: International Comparisons. *Performance Improvement Quarterly, 12*(2) 9-20.

He X., Wu Q., Liu D. and Zheng L.H. (2003). A Distributed and Parallel Edge Detection Scheme within Spiral Architecture. In *Proceedings of Visualization, Imaging and Image Processing 393* (pp 303-311).

Health and Medicine (1998). *The wall Street journal reports.* October 19, 1998.

Health Insurance Portability and Accountability Act of 1996 (HIPAA) (1996). P.L. 104-191 Enacted H.R. 3103, August 21, 1996 110 Stat. 1936, codified 42 U.S.C. 1320.

Health Insurance Portability and Accountability Act of 1996 (HIPAA) (1996). P.L. 104-191 Enacted H.R. 3103, August 21, 1996 110 Stat. 1936, codified 42 U.S.C. 1320.

Healthgrid Association & Cisco Systems. (2004). *Healthgrid whitepaper.* Retrieved from http:// whitepaper. healthgrid.org.

Healy, J.C. (2004). Applications relating to health. fifth research and development framework programme 1998-2002. *Office for Official Publications of the European Communities.* Luxembourg, ISBN: 92-894-7432-7. Retrieved from http://ec.europa.eu/information_society/activities/health/docs/publications/fp5-ehealth-applications-relating-to-health.pdf

Hebert, M. (2001). Telehealth success: Evaluation framework development. *Presented at Medinfo.* 10 (Pt 2), pp. 1145-9.

Heinemann, T.D.B. (1996). Medicine and books.In: *Medical Informatics. BMJ* (313), 1270.

Heinisch, R. H., & Weber, R., & Martins, A., & Barcia, R. M. (1998). Representing medical decision making strategies in a CBR system. In *Proceedings of the 6th German Workshop on Case based Reasoning - Foundations, Systems, and Applications.* Berlin.

Héja, G., Surján, G., Lukácsy, G., Pallinger, P., Gergely, M. (2007). GALEN based formal representation of ICD10. *International Journal of Medical Informatics, 76,* 118–123

Hettler, B. (1984). Wellness: encouraging a lifetime pursuit of excellence. *Health Values, 8*(4), 13-17.

Hi-Ethics, Inc. (2007). Retrieved 29 June 2007 from http://www.hiethics.com

Higgins, R., Cavendish, S., & Gregory, R. (2006). Class half-empty? Pre-registration house officer attendance at weekly teaching sessions: Implications for delivering the new Foundation Programme curriculum. *Medical Education, 40,* 877-883.

Hillert, L. et al. (1998). Cognitive behavioural therapy for patients with electric sensitivity – a multidisciplinary approach in a controlled study. *Psychother. Psychosom, 67,* 302-310.

Hilty D. M., Sison J. I., Nesbitt T. S., Hales R. E. (2000). Telepsychiatric consultation for ADHD in the primary care setting (letter). *J Am Acad Child Adolesc Psychiatry 39,* 15-16

Hindman, D. B. (2000). The rural-urban digital divide. *Journalism & Mass Communication Quarterly, 77,* 549-560.

HL7 2.5 (2000). HL7. Application protocol for electronic data exchange in healthcare environ- ments, version 2.5. *ANSI Standard.* Ann Arbor: MI, USA.

HL7 CDA Release 2.0 (2005). The HL7 version 3 standard: Clinical data architecture, release 2.0. *ANSI Standard.*

HL7 RIM. HL7. *Reference information model.* Retrieved from http://www.hl7.org/library/data-model/RIM/modelpage non.htm

HL7 V3. HL7. *Version 3 message development framework.* Retrieved http://www.hl7.org/library/mdf99/mdf99.pdf

Hludov, S., Meinel, C., Noelle, G. and Warda, F. (1999). Pacs for teleradiology. *12th IEEE Symposium on Computer-Based Medical Systems.*

Hoffman, J. J., Hoelscher, M. L., & Sherif, K. *Social capital, knowledge management, and sustained superior performance.*

Hoffmann, A., Kähny-Simonius, J., Plattner, M., Schmidi-Vckovski, V., Kronseder, C. (1998). Computer system validation: An overview of official requirements and standards. *Pharmaceutica Acta Helvetiae, 72,* 317-325.

Hoffmann, M., Loser, K., Walter, T., & Herrmann, T. (1999). A design process for embedding knowledge management in everyday work. *Proceedings of the international ACM SIGGROUP conference on Supporting group work*, 296-305.

Hogan, W.,Wagner, M. (1997). Accuracy of data in computer-based patient records. *J Am Med Inform Assoc, (4)*, 342-355.

Hohnloser, J., Fischer, M., Konig, A.,Emmerich, B. (1994). Data quality in computerized patient records. Analysis of a haematology biopsy report database. *Int J Clin Monit Comput, (11)*, 233-40.

Holle, R., Zahlmann, G. (1999). Evaluation of telemedical services. *IEEE Transactions on Information Technology in Biomedicine, 3*(2), 84-91.

HON (Health on Net Foundation) (2007). Retrieved 22, June 2007 from http://www.hon.ch/HONcode/Conduct.html

Hoppe, U. C., & Erdmann, E. (2004). *Herzinsuffizienz –fortschritte in diagnostik und therapie*. München: Urban & Vogel Medien und Medizin Verlag.

Horsch, A., Balbach, T. (1999). Telemedical Information Systems. *IEEE Transactions on Information Technology in Biomedicine, 3*(3), 166-175.

Hosseini, M., & Georganas, N.D. (2001). Collaborative virtual environments for training. *In the ACM Multimedia*. Ottawa, ON, Canada.

Hsia, D.C., Ahern, C.A., Ritchie, B.P., Moscoe, L.M. & Kurshat, W.M. (1992). Medicare Reimbursement accuracy Under the Prospective Payment System, 1985-1988 *Journal of the American Medical Association, 268*(7), 896-899.

Hsia, D.C., Kurshat, W.M., Fagan, N.B., Tebbut, J.A. & Kusserow, R.P. (1988). Accuracy of Diagnostic Coding for Medicare Patients under the Prospective Payment System *New England Journal of Medicine 318(6)*, 352-355.

Hsu, J., Huang, J., Kinsman, J., Fireman, B., Miller, R., Selby, J., et al. (2005). Use of e-Health services between 1999 and 2002: a growing digital divide. *Journal of the American Medical Informatics Association, 12*, 164-171.

Hu, P.J., Chau, P.Y.K., Sheng, O.R.L. and Tam, K.Y. (1999). Examining the technology acceptance model using physician acceptance of telemedicine technology. *Journal of Management Information Systems,* 16(2), 91-112.

Huang, D.W., Sherman, B.T., Tan, Q., Kir, J., Liu, D., Bryant, D., Guo, Y., Stephens, R., Baseler, M.W., Lane, H.C., Lempicki, R.A. (2007). DAVID Bioinformatics Resources: Expanded annotation database and novel algorithms to better extract biology from large gene lists. *Nucleic Acids Research, 35*(Web Server issue), pp. 1-7, Epub ahead of print.

Huang, M.P. and Alessi, N.E. (1998), An informatics curriculum for psychiatry. *Academic Psychiatry (22)*, 77-91.

Hull, D., Wolstencroft, K., Stevens, R., Goble, C., Pocock, M.R., Li, P., Oinn, T. (2006). Taverna: a tool for building and running workflows of services. *Nucleic Acids Research, 34*(Web Server issue), W729-W732.

Hung, K., Zhang, Y. (2003). Implementation of a WAP-based telemedicine system for patient monitoring. *IEEE Transactions on Information Technology in Biomedicine, 7*(2), 101-107.

Hurst N.P., Lambert C. M., Forbes J., Lochhead A.,Majior k., Lock, P. (2000). Does waiting matter? A randomized controlled trial of new non-urgent rheumatology outpatient referrals. *Rheumatology 2000*, 369-376

Hussain, K., S. Y. Mughal., S. Leleu-Merviel. (2006). Computerized systems validation: a quality approach in the pharmaceutical industry. In Athina Lazakidou (Eds.), *Handbook of research on informatics in healthcare and biomedicine*. Hershey, PA, USA: Idea Group Reference.

Hussain, K., S.Y. Mughal. (May 7-10, 2006). Change Management, key factor in pharmaceutical organizations (existing information systems approach). *IEEE Canadian Conference on Electrical and Computer Engineering – IEEE-CCECE*. Ottawa, Canada.

Hussein, R., Engelmann, U., Schroter, A., and Meinzer, H.P. (2004a). DICOM structured reporting: Part 1. Overview and characteristics. *Radiographics, 24*(3), 891-96.

Hussein, R., Engelmann, U., Schroter, A., and Meinzer, H.P. (2004b.). DICOM structured reporting: Part 2. Problems and challenges in implementation for PACS workstations. *Radio-graphics, 24*(3), 897-909.

Hwang, Li-Jen J., Eves, A., Desombre, T. (2003). Gap analysis of patient meal service perceptions. *International Journal of Health Care Quality Assurance, 16*(3), 143-153.

Hyler S. E., Gangure D. P. (2003). A review of the costs of telepsychiatry. *Psychiatr Serv, 54*, 976-980.

Hyler SE & Gangure DP (2004). Legal and ethical challenges in telepsychiatry. *Journal of Psychiatric Practice, 10*, 272-276.

Hysell, D. (1999). ISO 9001: Traditions before and after. ACM Special Interest Group for Design of Communication. *Presented at the proceedings of the 17th annual international conference on Computer Documentation.* New Orleans, Louisiana, United States, (pp. 99-104), ISBN: 1-58113-072-4.

Iakovidis, I. (1998). Towards personal health record: Current situation, obstacles and trends in implementation of electronic healthcare records in Europe. *International Journal of Medical Informatics, 52*(128), 105-117.

IBISWorld Australia Pathology Services Industry Market Research Report. Retrieved January 10, 2008, from http://www.ibisworld.com.au/industry/retail.aspx?indid=615&chid=1

ICT for Health (2006). Resource book of eHealth projects. *Office for official publications of the European Communities*. Luxembourg. Retrieved from http://ec.europa.eu/information_society/activities/health/highlights/2006/index_en.htm

IHE. (2005a). *IT infrastructure technical framework revision 2.0*. Retrieved from http://www.ihe.net/Technical Framework/index.cfm.

IHE. (2005b). *Cross-enterprise document sharing for maging (XDS-I)*. IHE Radiology TechnicalFramework, Supplement 2005-2006, Trial Implementation, Integrating the Healthcare Enterprise. Retrieved http://www.ihe.net/Technical Framework/upload/IHE RAD-TF Suppl XDSI TI 2005-08-15.pdf

Ilioudi, S., Lazakidou, A. (2007). Principles and effects of electronic communication systems between healthcare providers and managed care organizations. *International Journal of Electronic Healthcare*, ISSN (Online): 1741-8461, ISSN (Print): 1741-8453, Vol. 3, Nr. 4, pp. 468-478.

Image-I/O. (2006). Java advanced imaging image-I/O tools 1.1. Retrieved October 2006 from http://java.sun.com/javase/6/docs/technotes/guides/imageio/index.html

Ingram D., Griffith S., Maskens A.P., Kalra D., Lloyd D., and Southgate L. (1995). The Good European healthcare record project - the results of a three year project to design a common architecture for healthcare records across Europe AIM project A2014. *Future of Patient Records - Care for Records of Care. May 1995*, 415-419.

Institute, M. R., 2005. 7th annual survey of electronic health record trends and usage for 2005, Medical records institute. (2005). *Medical records institute, medical records institute.*

Intel Co., (2004). Understanding WiMAX and 3G for portable/mobile broadband wireless. *White Paper* (305150-001US).

International Electrotechnical Commission, IEC (2005). *Information technology - Security techniques - code of practice for information security management.* ISO/IEC/17799/ 01-Jun-2005.

International Electrotechnical Commission, IEC_2 (2005). *Information technology – security techniques – information security management systems – requirements.* ISO/IEC FDIS 27001:2005.

Intute (2006). Intute: Health and life sciences evaluation guidelines. Retrieved 28 June 2007 from http://www.intute.ac.uk/healthandlifesciences/

ISO 17432. (2004). *Health informatics - messages and communication - Web access to DICOM persistent objects.* International Standard IS 17432, International Organization for Standardization, Geneva, Switzerland.

ISO/TR 20514. (2005). *Health informatics - electronic health record - definition, scope and context.* Technical Report TR 20514. International Organization for Standardization. Geneva: Switzerland.

ISO/TS 18308. (2004). *Health informatics - requirements for an electronic health record architecture*. Technical Specification TS 18308. International Organization for Standardization, Geneva: Switzerland.

Istepanian R. S. H., Jovanov E. and Zhang Y. T. (2004). Guest editorial introduction to the special section on m-Health: Beyond seamless mobility and global wireless health-care connectivity, *IEEE Transactions on Information Technology in Biomedicine, 8*(4), 405- 414.

Istepanian, R.S.H., Jovanov, E., and Zhang, Y.T (2004, December). Guest editorial introduction to the special section on m-health: Beyond seamless mobility and global wireless health-care connectivity. *IEEE transactions on information technology in biomedicine, 8*(4), 405-413.

ITU. (2005). *Ubiquitous network societies: The case of radio frequency identification*. Retrieved January 20, 2006, from http://www.itu.int/osg/spu/ni/ubiquitous/Papers/RFID%20background%20paper.pdf

Jackson, L. A., Barbatsis, G., Biocca, F., Zhao, Y., von Eye, A., & Fitzgerald, H. E. (2004). Home Internet use in low-income families: Frequency, nature, and correlates of early Internet use in the HomeNetToo Project In E. P. Bucy & J. E. Newhagen (Eds.), *Media access: Social and psychological dimensions of new technology use*. Mahwah, New Jersey: Erlbaum.

Jacobus, C., Lichtenstein, E., Cybernet Medical. (June 2006). Telehealth outcomes. Available Online: www.cybernetmedical.com

Jadad A, Enkin M, Glouberman S, Stern A. (2006). Are virtual communities good for our health? *BMJ, 32*(7547).

Jadad A. R., Gagliardi, A. (1998). Rating health information on the Internet: navigating to knowledge or to label. *JAMA, 279*, 611-614.

Jadar, A. R., Delamothe, T. (2004). What next for electronic communication and health care? *BMJ 2004, 328*, 1143-1144.

Jafari, R., Dabiri, F., Brisk, P., and Sarrafzadeh, M. (2005a). Adaptive and fault tolerant medical vest for life critical medical monitoring. *20th ACM Symposium on Applied Computing (SAC 2005)*, March 2005. Santa Fe, NM.

Jafari, R., Dabiri, F., Sarrafzadeh, M. (2005b) .CustoMed: A power optimized customizable and mobile medical monitoring and analysis system. *ACM HCI Challenges in Health Assessment Workshop in conjunction with CHI 2005.* Portland, OR.

Jafari, R., Jindrich, D., Edgerton, V., Sarrafzadeh, M. (2006b). CMAS: Clinical movement assessment system for neuromotor disorders, *IEEE Biomedical Circuits and Systems Conference (BioCAS)*, London, UK.

Jafari, R., Noshadi, H., Ghiasi, S., Sarrafzadeh, M. (2006a). Adaptive electrocardiogram feature extraction on distributed embedded systems. *IEEE Transactions on Parallel and Distributed Systems special issue on High Performance Computational Biology (TPDS), 17*(8), 1-11.

JAI. (2006). Java advanced imaging 1.1.3. Retrieved September 2006 from http://java.sun.com/products/java-media/jai/

James, A., Wilcox, Y., Naguib, R.N.G. (2001). A telematic system for oncology based on electronic health and patient records. *IEEE Transactions on Information Technology in Biomedicine, 5*(1), 16-17.

Janz, B. D., Pitts, M. G., & Otondo, R. F. (2005). Information systems and health care II: Back to the future with RFID: Lessons learned - Some old, some new. *Communications of the Association for Information Systems, 15*.

Jarmulak, J., & Craw, S., & Rowe, R. (2001). Using case-based data to learn adaptation knowledge for design. In *Proceedings of the 17th IJCAI Conference*. Morgan Kaufmann, 1011-1016.

John L. Semmlow (2004). *Biosignals and biomedical image processing*. New York: Marcel Dekker.

John T. W. Yeow (2006). Biomedical sensors. *Wiley Encyclopedia of Biomedical Engineering*. University of Waterloo.

Johnson, J. D., & Meischke, H. (1991). Cancer information: Women's sources and content preferences. *Journal of Health Care Marketing, 11*, 37-44.

Johnson, J. D., & Meischke, H. (1993). A comprehensive model of cancer-related information seeking applied to magazines. *Human Communication Research, 19*, 343-367.

Jones V., et al. (2006). Mobihealth: mobile health services based on body area networks. In *Technical Report TR-CTIT-06-37 Centre for Telematics and Information Technology*. University of Twente, Enschede.

Jones, R., Gann, B., Duman M., Murphy, J.(2005). *Consumer health informatics*. DH V2

Jovanov, E., Milenkovic A., Otto C., de Groen P. C. (2005). A wireless body area network of intelligent motion sensors for computer assisted physical rehabilitation. *Journal of NeuroEngineering and Rehabilitation, 2*,(6).

Juran, J.M. (1988). Juran's Quality Control Handbook. In J.M. Juran, (Ed.) *Fourth edition*, New York: McGraw-Hill Book Company.

Kalra, D. (2006). Electronic health record standards. *IMIA Yearbook of Medical Informatics*, 136-144.

Kam, L.E. and Chismar, W.G. (2003), A self-disclosure model for personal health information. HICSS. In *Proceedings of the 36th Annual Hawaii International Conference on System Sciences (HICSS'03) - Track 6 - Volume 6*, (pp.161.2), ISBN: 0-7695-1874-5.

Kamaev I., Levanov V., Sergeev D., (2001). *Telemedicine: Clinical, organisational, law, technological, economical aspects*. N. Novgorod: NGMA,. (rus.)

Kaminski J. (2006). *Designing high quality health sites*. Retrieved from http://www.bellaonline.com

Kandampully, J. (1997). Firms should give loyalty before they can expect it from customers. *Managing Service Quality, 7(2)*, 92-94.

Kane B & Sands DZ (1998). Guidelines for the clinical use of electronic mail with patients. The AMIA Internet working group, task force on guidelines for the use of clinic-patient electronic mail. *Journal of the American Medical Informatics Association, 5,* 104-111.

Kanellos, M. (2005). *RFID tags used to track hurricane Katrina dead.* Retrieved September 2, 2006, from http://networks.silicon.com/lans/0,39024663,39152382,00.htm

Kareem, S.A., Baba, A. and Wahid, M.I.A. (2000). Research in medical informatics. *Health Informatics Journal, (6)*2, 110-115.

Karlinsky, H. (1999). Feature : *medical informatics, information technology, andpsychiatry, bulletin canadian psychiatric association.*

Karlof, C., Sastry, N., and Wagner, D. (2004). TinySec: A Link Layer Security Architecture for Wireless Sensor Networks. *Second ACM Conference on Embedded Networked Sensor Systems (SenSys 2004).* Baltimore, MD.

Kart, F., Moser, L.E. & Melliar-Smith, P.M. (2007). Reliable data distribution and consistent data replication using the atom syndication technology. *Proceedings of the International Conference on Internet Computing.* Las Vegas, NV, (pp. 124-132).

Kastania, A.N. (2004). Data mining challenges in the design of Telemedicine platforms. In R. Latifi, (Ed.), *Establishing telemedicine in developing countries: from inception to implementation.* Amsterdam: IOS Press.

Kastania, A.N. (2004). Telemedicine models for primary care. In R. Latifi (Ed), *Establishing telemedicine in developing Countries: from inception to implementation..* Amsterdam: IOS Press.

Kastner, R., Ogrenci, S., Bozorgzadeh, E., Sarrafzadeh, M. (2001) Instruction generation for hybrid reconfigurable systems. *IEEE/ACM Intl Conf Computer-Aided Design (ICCAD).*

Katz, S. and Moyer, C. (2004). The emerging role of online communication between patients and their providers. *Journal of General Internal Medicine, 19*(9), 978–983.

Kearsley, G. (1997). A guide to online education. Retrieved November 1, 2003, from http://gwis.circ.gwu.edu/~et1/online.html.

Keeling, P. et al., (2003). Safety and feasibility of prehospital thrombolysis carried out by paramedics. *BMJ Publishing Group Ltd., 327*(7405): 27–28.

Keogh W., Atkins M.H., Dalrymple J.F. (2000). Data collection and the economics of quality: Identifying problems. In *Proceedings of the 4th International and 7th National Research Conference on Quality Management.* Sydney. Retrieved 24 December 2007 from http://mams.rmit.edu.au/kh85606qs2qn.pdf

Kidney, G., & Puckett, E. (2003). Rediscovering the first principles through online learning. *Quarterly Review of Distance Education, 4*, 203-212.

Kiley, R. & Graham, E. (2002). The patient's Internet handbook. *Royal Society of Medicine.*

Kiley, R.(2003). *Medical information on the Internet. A guide for health Professionals.* Churchill Livinstone.

Kim, J., Park, J., Kim, K., Chee, Y., Lim,Y., and Park, K. (2007). Development of nonintrusive blood pressure estimation system for computer users. *Telemedicine and e-Health,* 13(1).

Kirbas C. and Queq F. (2003). *A review of vassel extraction techniques and algorithms*

Kleiner, A., Lewis, L. (2003). Internet access in U.S. public schools and classrooms: 1994-2002 (NCES 2004-011). *U.S. Department of Education. Washington, D.C.: National Center for Education Statistics.*

Kling R, 1991. Computerization and social transformations. Science, technology and human values. *Science, Technology and Human Values, (16)***,** 342-267.

Knatterud, G.L., Rockhold, F.W., George, S.L., Barton, F.B., Davis, C.E., Fairweather, W.R., Honohan, T., Mowery, R. and O'Neill, R. (1998). Guideliness for quality assurance in multicenter trials: A position paper. *Controlled Clinical Trials 19*, 477-493.

Kneebone, R. (2003). *Med Educ, 3*, 267-77.

Knitz M. (2005). *HIPPA compliance and electronic medical records: are both possible?* . Bowie State University: Maryland, Europe.

Knowles, M. (1984). *The adult learner: A neglected species.* Houston, TX: Gulf Publishing Company.

Koffler, D.,Galstad, E. (2002). *Nagios 1.x documentation.*

Koilias H, Kalafatoudis S, Mandila E. (2004). *Introduction in to informatics and the use of the computer. New technologies.* Kleidarithmos Publications Athens.

Koocher G. P., Morray E. (2000). Regulation of telepsychology: a survey of state attorneys general. *Professional Psychology, Research, and Practice 31*, 503–508.

Kopel H., Nunn K., Dossetor D.(2001). Evaluating satisfaction with a child and adolescent psychological telemedicine outreach service. *J Telemed Telecare, 7*(suppl 2), 35–40.

Korpman, R.,Lincoln, T. (1998). The computer-stored medical record: For whom ? *J Am Med Inform Assoc, (259)***,** 3454-3456.

Koszalka, T. & Bianco M. (2001). Reflecting on the instructional design of distance education for teachers: Learnings from the instructors. *Quarterly Review of Distance Education. 1*(2), 59-70.

Koszalka, T. & Ganesan, R. (2004). Designing Online Courses: A taxonomy to guide strategic use of features available in course management systems (CMS) in distance education. *Distance Education, 25*(2), 243-256.

Koszalka, T. (2001). Designing synchronous distance education: A demonstration project. *Quarterly Review of Distance Education. 2*(4), 333-346.

Koszalka, T. (May 2007). The nuts & bolts of creating an online curriculum: A primer in: principles for designing effective online instruction. Presented at the *2007 Pediatric Medicine Conference.* Toronto CA.

Kühn Pedersen, M., & Holm Larsen, M. (2000). Inter-Organizational Systems and Distributed Knowledge Management in Electronic Commerce. *Proceedings of IRIS, 23.*

Kyriacou, E. et al., (2003). Multi-purpose healthcare telemedicine systems with mobile communication link support, Biomed Eng Online. Retrieved from http://www.pubmedcentral.gov/articlerender.fcgi?tool=pmcentrez&artid=153497

Lai, F., Hutchinson, J., & Zhang, G. (2005). Radio frequency identification (RFID) in China: Opportunities and challenges. *International Journal of Retail & Distribution Management, 33*(11/12), 905-916.

Laird S.P., Wonng J.S.K., Schaller W.J. Ericksin B.J., de Groen P.C. (2003). Desing and implementation of an internet-based medical image viewing system. *The Journal of Systems and Software. Col. 66*, 167-181.

Lamb, A., & Smith, J. (2000). Ten facts of life for distance learning courses. *TechTrends, 44*(1), 12-15.

Lambrecht CJ. Telemedicine in trauma care: description of 100 trauma teleconsults. Telemed J 1997;3:265–268.

Lamming, M., Eldridge, M., Flynn, M., Jones, C., & Pendleburry, D. (2000). Satchel: providing access to any document, any time, anywhere. *ACM Transactions on Computer-Human Interaction, 7*(3), 322-352.

Landgrebe, M., Hauser, S., Langguth, B., Hajak, G., Eichhammer, P. (2006). Transcranielle Magnetstimulation zur neurobiologischen Charakterisierung somatoformer Störungen. *Nervenheil-kunde, 25*, 653-656.

Lave, J., & Wenger, E. (1991). Situated Learning: Legitimate Peripheral Participation (Learning in Doing: Social, Cognitive and Computational Perspectives). *Cambridge University.*

Lazakidou A. Hatzimitsis D. Evaggelou I. (2004). *Virtual World and New Technologies.* p.p 89-94. Kleidarithmos Publications, Athens.

Lazakidou A., Lazakidou G.(2004). *New Applications and futures in to the information community* p.p 77-88. Kleidarithmos Publications, Athens.

Lazakidou-Kafetzi, G., Lazakidou, A., Siassiakos, K. (2008). Computer supported collaborative work systems and communication services in health. *International Journal of Healthcare Technology and Management, Special Issue: Learning Environments in Health Sciences*, ISSN (Online): 1741-5144, ISSN (Print): 1368-2156, Vol. 9, Nr. 2, 2008.

Leaf, D.W. (1987). *Applied Kinesiology Flowchart Manual* (private ed.). Plymouth, Massachusetts.

Lee I., et al. (2006). High-Confidence Medical Device Software and Systems. *Computer 39*(4), 33-38.

Lee, I., Pappas, G.J., Cleaveland, R., Hatcliff, J., Krog. B.H., Lee, P., et al. (2006). High-confidence medical device software and systems. *Computer (special issue on Clinical Software Engineering), 39*(4), 33-38. IEEE CS Press.

Leff B., & Harper G. M. (2006). The reading habits of medicine clerks at one medical school: Frequency, usefulness and difficulties. *Academic Medicine, 81*, 489-494.

Legislation affecting telemedicine licensure (1995-1997) (2007). *Council on Licensure, Enforcement and Regulation.* Retrieved from www.clearhq.org/teletable2.htm

Lehner, F. and Nosekabel, H. (2002). The role of mobile devices in e-learning -first experience with a e-learning environment. In M. Milrad, H. U. Hoppe and Kinshuk (Eds.). *IEEE International Workshop on Wireless and Mobile Technologies in Education,* Los Alamitos, USA, (pp. 103-106).

Lehoux P, 2006. *The Problem of Health Technology: Policy Implications for Modern Health Care*, Routledge.

Lehoux P, Sicotte C,Denis J. (1999). Assessment of a computerized medical record system: disclosing its scripts of use. *Evaluation and Program Planning, (22)*, 439-453.

LeMoyne, R., Jafari, R., Jea, D., Srivastava, M., Sarrafzadeh, M. (2005) Fully quantified evaluation of myotatic stretch reflex. *Symp Neuroscience,* 2005.

LeMoyne, R., Jafari, R., Jea, D., Srivastava, M., Sarrafzadeh, M. (2005). Fully quantified evaluation of myotatic stretch reflex. *Symp Neuroscience,* 2005.

Lenz, R., Kuhn, K. (2002). *Integration of heterogeneous systems in hospitals.* Business briefing: data management and storage technology

Lepkowska-White, E. (2004). Online store perceptions: how to turn browsers into buyers? *Journal of Marketing Theory and Practice, 12*(3), 36-47.

Lesh, J. (1990). Systematics and the geometrical spirit. In Frangsmyr, T., Heilbron, J. L., & Rider, R.E. (eds). *The quantifying spirit in the 18th century.* Berkley: University of California Press. Retrieved June 29, 2007 from http://content.cdlib.org/ark:/13030/ft6d5nb455/?&query=quantifying%20spirit&brand=ucpress

Levallois, P. (2002). Hypersensitivity of human subjects to environmental electric and magnetic field exposure: A review of the literature. *Environ. Health Perspect. 110*, Suppl. 4, 613-618.

Levy, A.H. (1977). *Is informatics a basic medical science?* Proceedings of MEDINFO, 979.

Lewis, B.R and Mitchell, V.W. (1990). Defining and measuring the quality of customer service. *Marketing Intelligence and Planning, 8*, 11–17.

Lewis, D., Eysenbach, G., Kukafka R., Stavri, P.Z., Jimison H. B. (2005). *Consumer health informatics. in-*

forming consumers and improving health care. Springer Publications

Li S. L., Veeravalli B., Ko C. (2003), Distributed image processing on a network of workstations. *International Journal of Computers and Applications, 25*, 2.

Liederman EM & Morefield CS (2003). Web messaging: a new tool for patient-physician communication. *Journal of the American Medical Informatics Association, 10*, 260-270.

Liljander, V. and Strandvik, T. (1994). Estimating zones of tolerance in perceived service quality and perceived service value. *Int. Journal of Service Industry Management, 2*, 6–28.

Liljander, V. and Strandvik, T. (1997). Emotions in service satisfaction. *International Journal of Service Industry Management, 8*(2), 148 – 169.

Lin CT, Wittevrongel L, Moore L, Beaty BL, & Ross SE (2005). An Internet-based patient-provider communication system: randomized controlled trail. *Journal of Medical Internet Research, 7*, e47.

Lin, B. and Kelly, E. (1995). Methodological issues in patient satisfaction surveys. *International Journal of Health Care Quality Assurance, 8*(6), 32-37.

Lin, Y., Jan, I., Ko, P., Chen, Y., Wong, J., Jan, G. (2005, December). Wireless PDA based physiological monitoring system for patient transport. *IEEE Transactions on Information Technology in Biomedicine, 8*(4), 443-447.

Lin, Y.-H., et al. (2004), A Wireless PDA-Based Physiological Monitoring System for Patient Transport. *IEEE Transactions on Information Technology in Biomedicine, 8*(4), 439-447.

Lincoln, T.L. and Korpman, R.A. (1980). *Computers, health care, and medical information science. Science, (210)*4467, 257–63.

Lindberg, D.A., Humphreys. B.L. & McCray. A.T. (1993). The Unified Medical Language System. *Methods of Information in Medicine, 32*(4), 281-291.

Lindberg, D.A.B. (1987). *NLM long range plan*. Report of the Board of Regents, 1987, p.31.

Lindberg, D.A.B. and Schoolman, H.M. (1986). The National Library of Medicine and Medical Informatics. *West J Med., (145)*6, pp786–790.

Linkous, J.(1999). American telemedicine Association Issues Advisory on the use of the medical Web sites. Retrieved from http://www.atmeda.org/news/072899.html

Linneaus, C. (1776). *Genera Morborum* Retrieved June 13, 2006 from http://fermi.imss.fi.it/rd/bd#

Loeckx, D., Maes, F., Vandermeulen, D., & Suetens, P. (2004). *Non-rigid image registration using free-form deformations with a local rigidity constraint*. Lecture Notes in Computer Science. 3216, 639-646.

Lorincz, K., et al. (2004). Sensor networks for emergency response: Challenges and opportunities. *IEEE Pervasive Computing, 3*(4), 16-23.

Lowery, Julie C. (1998). 'Introduction to simulation in health care. In *Proceedings of the Winter Simulation Conference*, J. M. Charnes, D. M. Morrice, D.T. Brunner, and J. J. Swain, (Eds.). IEEE, Piscataway. New Jersey, (pp. 78-83).

Lussier, Y.A., Bodenreider, O. (2007). Clinical ontologies for discovery applications. In: Baker, C.J.O., Cheung, K.H. (Eds.). *Semantic Web: Revolutioning knowledge discovery in the life sciences*. New York, NY: Springer, pp. 101-119.

Lyskov, E. et al. (2001). Neurophysiological study of patients with perceived 'electrical hypersensitivity. *Int. J. Psychophysiol., 42*, 233-241.

Lyytinen, K., & Yoo, Y. (2002). Issues and challenges in ubiquitous computing. *Communications of the ACM, 45*(12), 63-65.

MacInnis, D. J., Moorman, C., & Jaworski, B. J. (1991). Enhancing and measuring consumers' motivation, opportunity, and ability to process brand information from ads. *Journal of Marketing, October*, 32-53.

Madden, M., & Rainie, L. (2003). *America's online pursuits: The changing picture of who's online and what they do*. Washington D.C.: Pew Internet and American Life Project. Accessed on April 24 from http://www.pewinternet.org/pdfs/PIP_Online_Pursuits_Final.PDF.

Madiope, M. (2004). Web-based instruction for critical care nursing science: Lessons learned. In *Proceedings of the World Conference on E-Learning in Corporate, Government, Healthcare, & Higher Education 2004, 1,* (pp. 814-818).

Maffezzoli, A., Masseroli, M. (2006). Chapter XLV: Genomic databanks for biomedical informatics. In: Lazakidou, A.A. (Ed.). *Handbook of Research on Informatics in Healthcare and Biomedicine*. Hershey, PA: Idea Group Inc., pp. 357-366.

Maheu, M., Allen, A., Whitten, P., (2001). *Ehealth, telemedicine, and telehealth : A guide to startup and success.* Jossey-Bass.

Maintz, J.B.A., & Viergever, A. (1998). A survey of medical image registration. *Medical Image Analysis, 2,* 1-36.

Malan, D.J., Welsh, M., and Smith, M. D., (2004) A public-key infrastructure for key distribution in tinyos based on elliptic curve cryptography. *First IEEE International Conference on Sensor and Ad Hoc Communications and Networks*, Santa Clara, California.

Malan, D.J., Welsh, M., and Smith, M.D. (2004) A public-key infrastructure for key distribution in tinyos based on elliptic curve cryptography. *First IEEE International Conference on Sensor and Ad Hoc Communications and Networks*, Santa Clara, California.

Malhotra N.K. and Birks H. (2003). *Marketing research, an applied approach.* Harlow: Prentice Hall.

Malhotra, Y. (2002). A Case for Knowledge Management: Rethinking management for the New world of Uncertainty and Risk. *BRINT Institute*.

Mamlin, J.,Baker, D., 1973. Combined time-motion and work sampling study in a general medicine clinic. *Medical Care, (11)*, 449-456.

Manders, E., Dawant, B. (1996). Data acquisition for an intelligent bedside monitoring system. *Presented at IEEE Engineering in Medicine and Biology Society*, Amsterdam, pp 1987-1988.

Maojo, V., Iakovidis, I., Martin-Sanchez, F., Crespo, J. and Kulikowski, C. (2001). Medical informatics and bioinformatics :European efforts to facilitate synergy. *Journal of Biomedical Informatics, (34)*, 423–427.

March, J. G. (1991). How Decisions Happen in Organizations. *Human-Computer Interaction, 6*, 95-117.

Marcheschi, P., Mazzarisi, A., Dalmiani, S., Benassi, A. (2004). HL7 clinical document architecture to share cardiological images and structured data in next generation. *Computers in Cardiology*, 617-620.

Marchetti, C., Pernici, B., and Plebani, P.A. (2004). Quality model for multichannel adaptive information systems. In *Proceedings of the 13th international World Wide Web conference on Alternate track papers & posters*. New York, Quality of service, (pp.48 – 54). ISBN: 1-58113-912-8.

Marculescu, D., Marculescu, R., Khosla, P. (2002). challenges and opportunities in electronic textiles modeling and optimization. *Design Automation Conference*, pp 175-180.

Marculescu, D., Marculescu, R., Khosla, P. (2002). Challenges and opportunities in electronic textiles modeling and optimization. *Design Automation Conference*, pp 175-180.

Mardia, K.V., Kent, J.I., Bibby, M. (1979). *Multivariate analysis, 1st ed.* Academic Press.

Marks, G. R., & Lutgendorf, S. K. (1999). Perceived health competence and personality factors differentially predict health behaviors in older adults. *Journal of Aging and Health, 11*, 221-239.

Martin, T., Jones, M., Edmison, J, and Shenoy, R. (2003). Towards a design framework for wearable electronic textiles. *Seventh IEEE International Symposium on Wearable Computers*, pp 190-199.

Masseroli, M., Bellistri, E., Franceschini, A., Pinciroli, F. (2007). Statistical analysis of genomic protein family and domain controlled annotations for functional investigation of classified gene lists. *BMC Bioinformatics, 8*(Suppl 1), S14, pp. 1-10.

Masseroli, M., Galati, O., Pinciroli, F. (2005). GFINDer: genetic disease and phenotype location statistical analysis and mining of dynamically annotated gene lists. *Nucleic Acids Research, 33(Web Server issue), W717-W723.*

Masseroli, M., Martucci, D., Pinciroli, F. (2004). GFINDer: Genome Function INtegrated Discoverer through dynamic annotation, statistical analysis, and mining. *Nucleic Acids Research, 32(Web Server issue), W293-W300.*

Masseroli, M., Pinciroli, F. *(2006).* Using Gene Ontology and genomic controlled vocabularies to analyze high-throughput gene lists: three tool comparison. *Computers in Biology and Medicine, 36*(7-8), 731-747.

Massey, T., Brisk, P., Dabiri, F., Sarrafzadeh, M. (2007). Delay aware, reconfigurable security for embedded systems. *Second International Conference on Body Area Networks (BodyNets 2007).* Florence, Italy.

Masys, D.R., Brennan, P.F., Ozbolt, J.G., Corn, M., and Shortliffe, E.H. (2000). Are medical informatics and nursing informatics distinct disciplines? The 1999 ACMI debate. *Journal of the American Medical Informatics Association, (7)*3, 304-312.

Mathieson, K., Peacock, E. and Chin, W.W. (2001). Extending the technology acceptance model: the influence of perceived user resources. *Information Systems, 32*(3), 86-112.

Mc Dowell I, Newell C.(1996). *Measuring health: A guide to rating scales and questionnaires (second edition).* New York: Oxford University Press

McCall, J., Richards, P. and Walters, G. (1977), *Factors in software quality.* RADC-TR-77-369, US Department of Commerce.

McCarty D., Clancy C (2002). Telehealth: implications for social work practice. *Social Work 47*,153–161.

McClung, H. J., Murray, R. D., Heitlinger, L. A. (1998). The Internet as a source for current patient information. *Padiatrics 101*, E2.

McClure, Stuart, Scambray, Joel & Kurtz, George (2003). *Hacking exposed, network security secrets and solutions.* McGraw Hill Osborn, (pp 408 -412).

McCray, A.T., Aronson, A.R., Browne, A.C., Rindflesch, T.C., Razi, A. & Srinivasan. S. (1993). UMLS knowledge for biomedical language processing. *Bulletin of the Medical Library Assocation, 81*(2), 184-194.

McDowall, R. D. (1995). Practical computer validation for pharmaceutical laboratories. Journal of Pharmaceutical and Biomedical Analysis, 14, pp 13-22.

McLaren P. et al. (2002). North Lewisham telepsychiatry project, *J Telemed Telecare, 8*,(2), 100.

MEDINFO, *Preliminary announcement for the Third World Conference on Medical Informatics*, MEDINFO 80, 1977. Retrieved from http://www.amia.org/history/what.html

MedSignals. (2007). *Electronic pillbox.* Retrieved from http://www.medsignals.com.

Menon, N. M., Lee, B., & Eldenburg, L. (2000). Productivity of information systems in the healthcare industry. *Information Systems Research, 11*(1), 83-92.

MERGE. (2007). Retrieved February 2007 from https://www.merge-emed.com/index.asp

Merkouris, A., Yfantopoulos, J., Lanara, V., Lemonidou, C. (1999). Developing an instrument to measure patient satisfaction with nursing care in Greece. *Journal of Nursing Management, 7*, 91-100.

Merrill, M. (1997). Instructional strategies that teach. *CBT Solutions,* 1-11.

Merrill, M.D. (2000). *First principles of instruction.* Retrieved December 5, 2007, from http://www.id2.usu.edu/Papers/5FirstPrinciples.PDF.

MeSH (medical subject headings) definition of medical informatics as defined in NLM's. Retrieved 10th January, 2007 from http://www.nlm.nih.gov/tsd/acquisitions/cdm/subjects58.html

Mezgar, Ivan (2005). Building trust in virtual communities. In Dasgupta, Subhasish (Ed.), *Encyclopedia of Virtual Communities and Technologies.* George Washington University, USA.

Miller R. H, Hillman J. M,Given R. S, 2004. Physician use of IT: results from the Deloitte Research Survey. *J Healthc Inf Manag, (18)*, 72-80.

Miller R. H,Sim I, 2004. Physicians' use of electronic medical records: barriers and solutions. *Health Aff (Millwood), (23)*, 116-26.

Ministers Committee (1997). Recommendation No. R (97) 5 of the Committee of Ministers to Member States on the Protection of Medical Data. IN Europe, C. o. (Ed.).

Ministers Committee (2004). Recommendation Rec(2004)17 of the Committee of Ministers to member states on the impact of information technologies on health care – the patient and Internet IN Europe, C. o. (Ed.).

Ministry of Health and Social Protection, France. (2004). Décrets, arrêtés, circulaires. *Journal Officiel de la République française, Text 23 sur 95, 21st August.* Retrieved July 10, 2006 from, http://agmed.sante.gouv.fr/htm/3/pta/ptaa1_190804.pdf

Mitretek Systems Innovative Technology in the Public Interest (2007). Retrieved 2, June 2007 from hitiWeb.mitretek.org/hswg

Mocanu, M.L., Dorobantu, M., Mocanu C., Burdescu, D. (2004). A distributed database system for glaucoma monitoring. *European Journal for Biomedical Informatics,* 50-58.

Moon, Jane (2005). Discussing health issues on the Internet. In Dasgupta, Subhasish (Ed.), *Encyclopedia of Virtual Communities and Technologies.* George Washington University, USA.

Moorman, C., & Matulich, E. (1993). A Model of consumers preventive health behaviors: The role of health motivation and health ability. *Journal of Consumer Research, 20*(2), 208-229.

Moreno A. (March 31 - April 1, 2003). Medical Applications of MultiAgent Systems. Workshop: Intelligent and Adaptive Systems in Medicine. Prague.

Morris, T.A. and McCain, K.W. (1998). *The Structure of Medical Informatics Journal Literature. J Am Med Inform Assoc, (5)*5, 448–466.

Mossberger, K., Tolbert, C. (2005). Race, place and information technology. *Report prepared for the U.S. Department of Housing and Urban Development.* Grant H-21439RG.

Mossberger, K., Tolbert, C., Stansbury, C. (2003). *Virtual inequality beyond the digital divide.* Washington, DC: Georgetown University Press.

Moumtzoglou, A., Dafogianni, C., Karra, V., Michailidou, D., Lazarou, P. and Bartsocas, C. (2000). Development and application of a questionnaire for assessing parent satisfaction with care. *Int J Qual Health Care, 12*(4), 331-337.

Mucic D. (2007). Telepsychiatry pilot-project in Denmark. WCPRR Jan : 3-9.

Muller, Nordhorn J. Roll, S. Willich, S. N. (2004). Comparison of the short form(SF)-12 health status instrument with the SF36 in patients with coronary heart disease. *Heart 2004,* 523-527. BMJ Publishing Group & British Cardiac Society.

Mulligan, Z.(2007) GP specialist e-library. *Health information on Internet. 55,* 5.

Murphy, J. (2007). International perspectives and initiatives. *Health information and Libraries Journal. 24*(1), 62-68.

Murphy, J. (2007). *Workshop — Consumer Health Information.* City Univercity London

Murray, C.J.L. and Lopez, A.D. (1997). Alternative projections of mortality and disability by cause 1990-2020: global burden of disease study. *The Lancet, 349*(9064), 1498-1504.

Musen, M.A. (2002). Medical informatics: searching for underlying components. *Methods Inf Med., (41)1,* 12-19.

Myers, J.D. (1986). Medical education in the information age, Proceedings of the Symposium on Medical Informatics. p. 3.

Mykkanen, J., Porrasmaa, J. Rannanheimo, J., and Korpela, M. (2003). A process for specifying integration for multi-tier applications in healthcare. *International Journal of Medical Informatics, 70,* 173-182.

MySQL. (2006). Retrieved August 2006 from http://www.mysql.com/

Nagendran, S., Moores, D., Spooner, R. and Triscott, J. (2000). Is telemedicine a subset of medical informatics? *Journal of Telemedicine and Telecare, (6)*2, pp51-52.

National Telecommunications and Information Administration (NTIA). (1999). *Falling through the net: Defining the digital divide.* Washington, DC: US Department of Commerce.

Naumann, F. (2001). From databases to information systems information quality makes the difference. In *Proceedings of Int. Cont on information Quality(ICIQ).* Boston, MA, USA, (pp 244-260).

Naval telemedicine (1998). Fleet lines up to provide live teleconsulting; telepsychiatry saves time and money on the high seas. *Telemedicine and Virtual Reality 3*(4), 40 - 47.

Navas-Delgado, I., Rojano-Munoz, M. del M., Ramirez, S., Perez, A.J., Andres Leon, E., Aldana-Montes, J.F., Trelles, O. *(2006).* Intelligent client for integrating bioinformatics services. *Bioinformatics, 22*(1), 106-111.

NCAHF (2007) National Council Against Health Fraud. Retrieved 25, June 2007 from http:// www.ncahf.org/

Nejmeh, B. A. (1995). Process cost and value analysis. *Communications of the ACM, 38*(6), 19-24.

Nelson SB (2006). Privacy and medial information on the Internet. *Respiratory Care, 51,* 183-187.

NEMA - National Electrical Manufacturers Association (2004). *Digital imaging and communications in medicine (DICOM) part 2: Conformance* PS3.2-2004, Rosslyn, VA .

NEMA - National Electrical Manufacturers Association (2007). *Digital imaging and communications in medicine (DICOM) part 5: Data Structures and Encoding Publication* PS 3.5-2007, Rosslyn, VA .

Neri, E., Thiran, J., Caramella, D., Petri, C., Bartolozzi, C., Piscaglia, B., Macq. B., Duprez, T., Cosnard, G., Maldague, B., De Pauw, J. (1998). Interactive DICOM image transmission and telediagnosis over theEuropean ATM network, *IEEE Transactions on Information Technology in Biomedicine, 2*(1), 35-38.

Nerlich M., Kretschmer R., (1998). The impact of telemedicine on health care management. In *Proceedings of the G 8 Global Health Care Applications Project (GHAP) Conference*. Regensburg, Germany, 21 November. Stud Health Technol Inform 1999; 64: 1-281

Nicolescu, C., & Jonker, P. (2000). Parallel low-level image processing on a distributed memory system. In *Proceedings of the 15th Workshop on Parallel and Distributed Processing,* 226-233.

Nilsson, M., & Sollenborn, M. (2004). Advancements and trends in medical case-based reasoning: An overview of systems and system development. In *Proceedings of the FLAIRS Conference*, AAAI Press, 178-183.

Nolle, L., Wong, K.C.P., & Hopgood, A.A. (2001). DARBS: a distributed blackboard system. *Research and Development in Intelligent Systems, 18*, 161-70.

Nonaka, I. (1998). The Knowledge-Creating Company. *The Economic Impact of Knowledge.*

Norris, A.C., (2002). *Essentials of telemedicine and Telecare*. Wiley.

Noumeir, R. (2003). DICOM structured report document type definition. *IEEE Transactions on Information Technology in Biomedicine, 7*(4), 318-328.

NTIA. (2000). *Falling through the net: Defining the digital divide*. Washington, DC: US Department of Commerce.

Nygren, E., Wyatt, J. C.,Wright, P. (1998). Helping clinicians to find data and avoid delays. *Lancet, (352)***,** 1462-6.

O'Brien J., Ezquerra N. (1994), Automated segmentation of coronary vessels in angiographic image sequences utilizing temporal, spatial and structural constraints. *Visualization in Biomedical Computing.*

O'Connell, B. (2004). Corporate wellness programs. *Biopharm International, 17*(10), 16-17.

O'Toole, R. V., Playter, R. R., Krummel, T. M., Blank, W. C., Cornelius, N. H., Roberts, W. R., Bell, W. J., Raibert, M. (1999). Measuring and developing suturing technique with a virtual reality surgical simulator. *Journal of the American College of Surgeons*, 189/1, 114-127.

Office of Health and the Information (2001). Toward electronic health records. *Highway Health.* Canada.

Ogle, W. (2001). transl. *Aristotle: De Partibus Animalium.* Retrieved June 24, 2007 from http://etext.lib.virginia.edu/toc/modeng/public/AriPaan.html

Ogrenci S, Bozorgzadeh E, Kastner R, Sarrafzadeh M. (2001a) A super-scheduler for embedded reconfigurable systems. *IEEE/ACM Intl Conf Computer-Aided Design (ICCAD).*

Ogrenci S, Bozorgzadeh E, Kastner R, Sarrafzadeh M. (2001a). A super-scheduler for embedded reconfigurable systems. *IEEE/ACM Intl Conf Computer-Aided Design (ICCAD).*

Ogrenci S, Bozorgzadeh E, Kastner R, Sarrafzadeh M. (2001b). SPS: A strategically programmable system. *Reconfigurable Architectures Workshop (RAW).*

Ogrenci S, Bozorgzadeh E., Kastner R., Sarrafzadeh M. (2001b). SPS: A strategically programmable system. *Reconfigurable Architectures Workshop (RAW).*

Oliver H (2002). Email and internet monitoring in the workplace: Information privacy and contracting-out. *Industrial Law Journal, 31,* 321-352.

Oliver N. and Flores-Mangas F. (2006). Healthgear: A real-time wearable system for monitoring and analyzing physiological signals. In *Proceedings of Int. Conf. on Body Sensor Networks (BSN'06).* MIT, Boston. USA.

Oliver, R. (1999). Exploring strategies for online teaching and learning. *Distance Education,* 20, 240-250.

Oliver, R. L. (1996). *Satisfaction: A behavioral perspective on the consumer.* McGraw-Hill Education,.

Olson, B., Koszalka, T., & Touhey, M., (May 2007). The nuts & bolts of creating an online curriculum. Presented at the *2007 Pediatric Medicine Conference*, Toronto CA.

Omar, A., Wahlqvist, M.L., Kouris-Blazos, A. and Vicziany, M. (2005). Wellness management through Web -based programmes. *Journal of Telemedicine and Telecare, 11*(S1), S8-11.

Omar, W.M. & Taleb-Bendiab, A. (2006). Service oriented architecture for e-health support services based on grid computing. *Proceedings of the IEEE International Conference on services oriented Computing,* Chicago, IL (pp. 135-142).

Otta, D. et al. (2005). *Virtual reality in surgical education, division of surgical oncology.* University of Missouri. Retrieved from http://www.vmasc.odu.edu

Ourselin, S., Stefanescu, R., & Pennec, X. (2002). Robust registration of multi-modal images: towards real-time clinical applications. In *Proceedings of the 5th International Conference on Medical Image Computing and Computer-Assisted Intervention*, 140-147.

Ovretveit, J. (2000). The economics of quality. *International Journal of Health Care Quality Assurance, 13*(5), 200-207.

PalaninathaRaja M., Wadhwa S., Deshmukh S. G. (2006). Cost-benefit analysis on eHealthcare services. *Ukr. z. telemed.med.telemat, 1*(4), 53-64.

Panchen, A.L. (1992). *Classification Evolution and the Nature of Biology* Cambridge: University Press

Pandolfini, C., Bonati, M. (2002). Follow up of quality of public oriented health information on the World Wide Web: Systematic re-evaluation. *BMJ 32497337,* 82-583.

Parasuraman, A., Berry, L. L., Zeithaml, V. A., (1988). SERVQUAL: A multiple-item scale for measuring customer perceptions of service quality. *Journal of Retailing, 64,* 12–40.

Parasuraman, A., Berry, L.L. and Zeithaml, V. A. (1991). Understanding customer expectations of service. *Sloan Management Review*, 39-48.

Parasuraman, A., Zeithaml, V., Berry, L.L. (1985). A conceptual model of service quality and its implications for future research. *Journal of Marketing, 49,* 41-50.

Park, C. W., & Mittal, B. (1985). A theory of involvement in consumer behavior: Problems and issues. In J. N. Seth (Ed.), *Research in Consumer Behavior* (Vol. 1, pp. 201-231). Greenwich, CT: JAI Press.

Pascoe, J., Ryan, N., & Morse, D. (2000). Using while moving: HCI issues in fieldwork environments. ACM Transactions on Computer-Human Interaction, vol. 7, 3, pp. 417-437.

Patel, V.L. and Kaufman, D.R. (1998). Medical informatics and the science of cognition. *Journal of the American Medical Informatics Association, 5(6)*, 489-492.

Pavlopoulos, S., Kyriacou, E., Berler, A., Dembeyiotis, S., and Koutsouris, D. (1999). A novel emergency telemedicine system based on wireless communication technology: AMBULANCE. *IEEE Transactions on Information Technology in Biomedicine, 2*(4), pp. 261-267.

Payandeh, et al. (2004). *On defining metrics for assessing laparoscopic surgical skills in a virtual training environment.* Simon Fraser University

Payton F.C, Lucas H. (2001). Health Care B2C Electronic Commerce. In *Proceedings of the 34th Hawaii International Conference on System Science,* 2001.

Payton F.C. and Brenman, P.F. (1999). *.How a community health information network is really used, communications of the ACM.* pp 85-89 December 1999

Penney, G.P., Weese, J., Little, J.A., Desmedt, P., Hill, D.L.G., & Hawkes, D.J. (1998). *A comparison of similarity measures for use in 2D-3D medical image registration. IEEE Transactions on Medical Imaging, 17*, 586-595.

Pereira J. (2003), Nuevo Enfoque en el desarrolo de un sistema de información de imágenes Médicas. *Una herramienta de apoyo a la toma de decisión clínica. Doctoral Thesis*. Universidade da Coruña.

Perez D., Crespo J., Anguita A., Pérez, J.L., Dorado J., Bueno G., Feliu V., Estruch A. and Heredia J. (2005). Biomedical Image Processing Integration Through INBIOMED: A Web Services-Based Platform. Lecture Notes in Bioinformatics. LNBI 3745 pp. 34-43.

Perkins, W.St. (1993). Measuring customer satisfaction. *Industrial Marketing Management, 22*, 247–254.

Perrig, A., Canetti, R. Tygar, J. D. and Song, D. (2002) The TESLA broadcast authentication protocol. *RSA Cryptobytes*.

Perry, M., O'Hara, K., Sellen, A., Brown, B., & Harper, R. (2001). Dealing with mobility: understanding access anytime, anywhere. *ACM Transactions TOCHI, 8*(4).

Pesch, D., Irvine, J. & Klepal, M. (2007). *Mobile communication systems and networks*. John Wiley & Sons.

Peterson, G., Aslani, P., Williams, K. (2003). How do consumers search for and appraise information on Medicines on the Internet? A qualitative study Using focus groups. *J. Med Internet Res 5*(4), e 33.

Petty, R. E., & Cacioppo, J. T. (1986a). *Communication and persuasion: Central and peripheral routes to attitude change*. New York: Springer-Verlag.

Petty, R. E., & Cacioppo, J. T. (1986b). The elaboration likelihood model of persuasion. *Advances in Experimental Psychology, 19*, 123-205.

Pew Internet and American Life Project. (April 16, 2003). *The ever-shifting Internet population: A new look at Internet access and the digital divide*. Retrieved from http://www.pewinternet.org/reports/.

Pew Internet and American Life Project. (August 2006). *Daily tracking survey*. Retrieved from http://www.pewinternet.org/

Picciano, A.G. (2001). *Distance learning: Making connections across virtual space and time*. Columbus, Ohio: Merrill Prentice Hall.

Pincus LB & Johns R (1997). Private Parts: A global analysis of privacy protection schemes and a proposed innovation for their comparative evaluation. *Journal of Business Ethics, 16*, 1237-1260.

Pinho C, Sá C, Mendes E, Santos E, Silva F, Sousa F, Gomes F, Abreu F, Mota F, Aguiar F, Faria F, Macedo F,Martins S. (2006). Electronic patient records - who should access what? Doctors' view. *Biostatistics and Medical Informatics Department - Faculty of Medicine of Porto*.

Pirsig, R. M.(1974). *Zen and the art of motorcycle maintence*. New York: Bantam Books.

Pitts V (2004). Illness and Internet empowerment: writing and reading breast cancer in cyberspace. *Health (London), 8*, 33-59.

Plsek P. E. (1999). Quality improvement methods in clinical medicine. *Pediatrics, 103*(1), 203-214.

Plsek P., Greenhalgh T. (2001). Complexity science. *BMJ 323*, 625-628, .

Pluim, J.P., Maintz, J.B.A., & Viergever, M.A. (2003). *Mutual information-based registration of medical images: a survey. IEEE Transactions on Medical Imaging, 22*, 986-1004.

Polley R. Liu, Max Q.-H. Meng, Peter X.Liu, Fanny F.L. Tong, M.Phil, and X.J. Chen, M.Phil, (2006). A telemedicine system for remote health and activity monitoring for the elderly. *Telemedicine and e-Health, 12(6).*

Pontes, M. C. F., & Pontes, N. M. H. (1996). Variables that influence consumers' inferences about physician ability and physician accountability for adverse health outcomes. *Health Care Management Review, 22*, 7–20.

Popp, F.-A. (1987). *New horizons in medicine (2nd ed.)*. Heidelberg, Germany: Haug.

PostgreSQL. (2007). Retrieved May 2007 from http://www.postgresql.org/

Potlapally, N. Ravi, S., Raghunathan, A., Jha, N. (2003). Analyzing the energy consumption of security protocols. *International Symposium on Low Power Electronics and Design (ISLPED 2003).* Seoul Korea.

Potlapally, N. Ravi, S., Raghunathan, A., Jha, N. (2003). Analyzing the energy consumption of security protocols. *International Symposium on Low Power Electronics and Design (ISLPED 2003).* Seoul Korea.

Potts, H. M. M. (2006). Is e-health progressing faster than e-health researchers? *J.Med Internet Res 8*(3), e24.

Prigogine, I., & Stengers, I. (1981). *Dialog with the nature: New ways of scientific thinking.* Munich, Germany: Piper.

Prince, M. (2002). Altering lifestyle through Internet fitness monitoring. *Business Insurance, 36*(14), T6 - T7.

Quackwatch (2007) Retrieved 25, June 2007 from http://www.quackwatch.org/00AboutQuackwatch/mission.html

Quantin, C., Binquet, C., Bourquard, K., Pattisina, R., Gouyon-Cornet, B., Ferdynus, C., Gouyon, J. B., Allaert, F. A., 2004. A peculiar aspect of patients' safety: the discriminating power of identifiers for record linkage. *Stud Health Technol Inform, (103)*, 400-6.

Rada, R., (1996). ISO 9000 reflects the best in standards. *Communications of the ACM, 39* (3), 17-20.

Rada, Roy (2005). Cancer patient-patient online discussion groups. In Dasgupta, Subhasish (Ed.), *Encyclopedia of Virtual Communities and Technologies.* George Washington University, USA.

Radin, Patricia (2006). To me, it's my life: Medical communication, trust, and activism in cyberspace. *Social science and Medicine, 62*, 591-601.

Raich, M. *Human Capital and Knowldge Management In the New Economy.* Retrieved from http://www.raich.net/

Rasband, W.S., (2006) ImageJ, U. S. National Institutes of Health, Bethesda. Maryland, USA, http://rsb.info.nih.gov/ij/, 1997-2006.

Ravi, S., Raghunathan, A., Kocher, P., and Hattangady, S. (2004). Security in embedded systems: design challenges. *ACM Transactions on Embedded Computing Systems. 3*,(3), 461-491.

Rector, A. (1999). Clinical terminology: why is it so hard? *Methods of Information in Medicine 38*(4–5), 239–252.

Rector, A., Nowlan, W. & Glowinski A. (1993). *Goals for concept representation in the GALEN project.* Proceedings of annual symposium of computer applications in medical care. (pp 414-418). American Medical Informatics Association

Reinartz, T., Iglezakis, I.; Roth-Berghofer, T. (2000). On quality measures for case base maintenance. In Blanzieri, E.; Portinale, L. (Eds.). *Advances in Case-Based Reasoning - Proceedings of the 5th European Workshop on Case-Based Reasoning.* Berlin: Springer Verlag, 247-259.

Rendina, M. C., Downs, S. M., Carasco, N., Loonsk, J., & Bose, C. L. (1998). Effect of telemedicine on health outcomes in 87 infants requiring neonatal intensive care. *Telemedicine Journal, 4*, 345-351.

Revolutionary Research on Virtual Surgery (2002). *Innovations Report, Forum for Science, Industry and Business.*

RFID. (2006). *The cost of RFID equipment.* Retrieved April 21, 2006, from http://www.rfidjournal.com/faq/20

Rhodes, R. S., Biesten, T. W., Ritchie Jr., W. P., Malangoni, M. A. (2003). Continuing medical education activity and american board of surgery examination performance. *Journal of the American College of Surgeons*, 196/4, pp. 604-609.

Rice, R. (2001). The Internet and health communication: A framework of experiences. In R. Rice & J. Katz (Eds.), *The Internet and health communication* (pp. 5-46). Thousand Oaks, CA: Sage.

Richart, R., 1970. Evaluation of a medical data system. *Computers and Biomedical Research, (3)*, 415-425.

Richter, M. M. (2003). Fallbasiertes Schließen. In Görz, G., & Rollinger, C.-R., & Schneeberger, J. (Eds.). *Handbuch der Künstlichen Intelligenz* (pp. 407-430), 4th ed. München: Oldenbourg Wissenschaftsverlag.

Rinkus S., Waljia M., Johnson-Throop K. A., Malin J., Turley J., Smith J., Zhang J. (2005). Human-centered design of a distributed knowledge management system. *Journal of Biomedical Informatics, 38*(1),4-17

Risk, A (2003). Quality ofhealth information on Internet, achievements lessons and the future. *Conference Puebla Mexico Crics VI Birem*. Retrieved 5, July 2007 from http//:www.paho.org/English/PD/IRM/risk.pdf

Risk, A., Dzenowags, J (2001). Review of Internet Health information Quality Initiatives. *J.Med Internet Res. 3*(4), e28.

Rivest, R. (1995). The RC5 encryption algorithm. *1994 Leuven Workshop on Fast Software Encryption.* pp. 86-96.

Rizzo, A.A., Klimchuk, D., Mitura, R., Bowerly, T., Buckwalter, Parsons, TD & Yeh, S.C. (2006). A virtual reality scenario for all seasons: the virtual classroom. *CNS Spectrums, 11*(1), 35-44.

Robinson, St. (1999). Measuring service quality: current thinking and future requirements. *Marketing Intelligence & Planning, 17*(1), 21-32.

Robledo, M. A. (2001). Measuring and managing service quality: Integrating customer expectations. *Managing Service Quality, 11*(1), 22-31.

Rodrigues, M.A.F., Silva, W.B., Barbosa-Neto, M.E., Gillies, D.F., Ribeiro, I.M.M.P. (2007). An interactive simulation system for training and treatment planning in orthodontics (article in press, doi: 10.1016/j.cag.2007.04.010). *Computers & Graphics*, Elsevier.

Rohlfing, T., & Maurer, C.R. (2003). Non-rigid image registration in shared-memory multi-processor environments with application to brains, breasts, and bees. *IEEE Transactions on Information Technology in Biomedicine, 7*, 16-25.

Roine, R., Ohinmaa, A., Hailey, D. (2001). Assessing telemedicine: A systematic review of the literature. *Canadian Medical Association Journal, 165*(6), 765-771.

Römer, K., Schoch, T., Mattern, F., & Dübendorfer, T. (2004). Smart identification frameworks for ubiquitous computing applications. *Wireless Networks, 10*(6), 689-700.

Rose, F.D., Brooks, B.M. & Rizzo, A.A. (2005). Virtual reality in brain damage rehabilitation: a review. *Cyber-Psychology & Behavior, 8*(3), 241-262.

Rose, R., Uli, J., Abdul, M. and Ng, K. (2004). Hospital service quality: a managerial challenge. *International Journal of Health Care Quality Assurance, 17*, 146–59.

Ross, D. (1977). *Aristotle.* London: Methuen & Co Ltd.

Ross, G (n.d.) Porphyry, Introduction to Aristotle's categories Retrieved June 9, 2007 from http://www.philosophy.leeds.ac.uk/GMR/hmp/texts/ancient/porphyry/isagoge.html

Rosse C, Mejino JL Jr. (2003) A reference ontology for biomedical informatics: the Foundational Model of Anatomy. *Journal of Biomedical Informatics 36,* (6):478-500.

Rosse, C., Mejino, J.L.V.Jr. (2003). A reference ontology for biomedical informatics: the Foundational Model of Anatomy. *Journal of Biomedical Informatics*, *36*(6), 478-500.

Rosser J. C., Jr., Prosst R. L., Rodas E. B., Rosser L. E., Murayama M., Brem H., (2000). Evaluation of the effectiveness of portable low-bandwidth telemedical applications for postoperative followup: initial results. *J Am Coll Surg, 191*, 196–203.

Rosset, A. ; Spadola L. and Ratib O. (2004) OsiriX: An open-source software for navigating in multidimensional DICOM images. *Journal of Digital Imaging, 17*(3), 205-216.

Roth-Berghofer, T. (2002). *Knowledge maintenance of case based reasoning systems - the SIAM methodology.* University of Kaiserslautern, Dissertation.

Rovner JA (2004). Making sense of HIPAA Privacy: solutions for complex compliance dilemmas. *Journal of Health Law, 37,* 399-427.

Ruskin P. E., Silver-Aylaian M., Kling M. A., et al.(2004). Treatment outcomes in depression: comparison of remote treatment through telepsychiatry to in-person treatment. *American Journal of Psychiatry, 161*(8), 1471-1476.

Sachpazidis, I. A., Ohl, R., Polanczyk, C. A., Torres, M. S., Messina, L. A., Sales, A. and Sakas, G. (2005). Applying telemedicine to remote and rural underserved regions in Brazil using eMedical consulting tool. *IEEE Engineering in Medicine and Biology -27th Annual Conference*, Shanghai, China.

Sachs, L. (1969). *Statistical evaluation methods.* Berlin, Germany: Springer.

Sadan B (2002). Patient empowerment and the asymmetry of knowledge. *Studies in Health Technology and Informatics, 90,* 514-518.

Safran C., Pompilio-Weitzner, Emery, G. K. D. and Hampers L., (2005). *Collaborative approaches to e-Health: Valuable for users and non-users, connecting medical informatics and bio-informatics.* R. Engelbrecht, et al. (Eds). (pp. 879-884).

Saiedian, H. and McClanahan, L. (1995). A study of two frameworks for quality software process, presented at the Symposium on Applied Computing. In *Proceedings of the 1995 ACM symposium on Applied computing, Nashville.* Tennessee, United States, (pp.434-439). ISBN:0-89791-658-1.

Salomon, M. Heitz, F. Perrin, G.R. & Armspach, J.P. (2005). A massively parallel approach to deformable matching of 3-D medical images via stochastic differential equations, *Parallel Computing 31*, 45-71.

Sam Burgiss, Rob Sprang, Joe Tracy, (2004). *Telehealth technology guidelines*. Retrieved from http://telehealth.hrsa.gov/pubs/tech/techhome.htm

Samuels A.(1999). International telepsychiatry: A link between New Zealand and Australia. *Aust N Z J Psychiatry, 33*(2), 284-6.

Sandstrom, M. et al. (2003). Holter ECG monitoring in patients with perceived electrical hypersensitivity. *Int. J. Psychophysiol., 49*, 227-235.

Saturno P. J., (1999). Quality in Health Care: models, labels and terminology. *International Journal for Quality in Health Care, 11*(5), 373-374.

Satyarthi, D., Raju, B.A.N, Dandapat, S. (2006). Detection of diabetic retinopathy in fundus images using vector quantization technique. In *Proceedings of the Annual India Conference*, (pp. 1-4).

Schaller, R. R. (1999). Moore's law: Past, present, and future. *IEEE Spectrum, 34*(6), 52-59.

Schaumont, P., Verbauwhede, I., Sarrafzadeh, M., and Keutzer, K. (2001). A quick safari through the reconfiguration jungle. *Design Automation Conference (DAC 2001).* Las Vegas, CA.

Schaumont, P., Verbauwhede, I., Sarrafzadeh, M., and Keutzer, K. (2001). A quick safari through the reconfiguration jungle. *Design Automation Conference (DAC 2001).* Las Vegas, CA.

Schicker, G., & Kaiser, C., & Bodendorf, F. (2007). Individualiserung von Prozessen und E-Services mithilfe von Case based Reasoning. In Oberweis, S., & Weinhardt, C., & Gimpel, H., & Koschminder, A., & Pankratius, V., & Schnizler, B., *eOrganisation: Service-, prozess-, market-engineering* (pp.713-730). Karlsruhe: universitätsverlag karlsruhe.

Schlais, D., & Davis, R. (2001). 'Distance learning through educational networks: The global view experience. In J. Stephenson (Ed.), *Teaching & learning online: Pedagogies for new technologies.* Sterling, VA: Stylus Publishing Inc., (pp. 112-126).

Schmeida, M. (December 2005). *Telehealth Innovation in the American States.* Dissertation. Ann Arbor, MI: ProQuest.

Schmeida, M., McNeal, R. (2007). The telehealth divide: disparities to searching public health information online. *Journal of Health Care for the Poor and Underserved, 18*(3), 549-563.

Schneier B, 2004. *Secrets and Lies: digital security in a networked world,* Wiley.

Schuler, K. (1996). Preparing for ISO 9000 registration: the role of the technical communicator, ACM Special Interest Group for Design of Communication. In *Proceedings of the 13th annual international conference on Systems documentation: emergingfrom chaos: Solutions for the growing complexity of our jobs.* Savannah, Georgia, United States, (pp.148-154). ISBN:0-89791-713-8.

Seddon, P. B., Staples, S., Patnayakuni, R. and Bowtell, M., (1999). Dimensions of information systems success. *Communications of the Association of Information Systems, 2*(20) .

Seelos, H.J. (1993). The empirical object of medical informatics. J Med Syst., vol.17, 2, 87-96.

Seely S. (2002), *Seguridad http y servicios web en ASP. NET.* Retrieved from http:// www.microsoft.com/spanish/msdn/articulos/archivo/111002/voices/httpsecurity.asp

Seinstra, F.J., Koelma, D., & Geusebroek, J.M. (2002). A software architecture for user transparent parallel image processing. *Parallel Computing. 28*, 967-993.

Senge, P. (1992). *The fifth discipline: The Art and practice of the learning organization.* London, Century Business.

Seo, J., Choi, J., Choi, B., Jeong, D., and Park,K.(2005). The development of a nonintrusive home-based physiologic signal measurment system. *Telemedicine and e-Health, 11(4)*, 487-495.

Sevdali M.,Petropoulou M.,(2004). *Measuremed of health levels using the evaluation method sf36:Comparative study of 2 hospital units.* H.O.U. of Patra, Greece, pp 7-16

Shaltis P., Wood L., Reisner A. & Asada H. (2005, September), Novel design for a wearable, rapidly deployable, wireless noninvasive triage sensor. *27th Annual International Conference of the IEEE/EMBS.* Shanghai, China.

Sharma, C., & Nakamura, Y. (2004). *Wireless data services: Technologies, business models and global markets.* Cambridge University Press.

Sharshar, S., Allart, L., Chambrin, M. C., (2005). A new approach to the abstraction of monitoring data in intensive care. *Lecture Notes in Computer Science, 3581*, 13–22.

Shepperd S., Charnock D., Gann, B.(1999). Education and debate. Helping patient access high quality health information. *BMJ 319*, 764-766.

Shim, J. P., Varshney, U., & Dekleva, S. (2006). Wireless evolution 2006: Cellular TV, wearable computing, and RFID. *Communications of the Association for Information Systems, 18*, 497-518.

Shortell, S.M., Bennett, C. L., and Buck, G. R. (1998). Assessing the impact of continuous quality improvement on clinical practice: What it will take to accelerate progress. *The Milbank Quarterly, 76*(4), 593-624.

Shortliffe, E.H. (1984). The science of biomedical computing, In: Pages JC, Levy AH, Gremy F, Anderson J (eds.), *Meeting the Challenge: Informatics and Medical Education.* Amsterdam, The Netherlands: North-Holland, 1-10.

Shortliffe, E.H. (1988). The state of the art in medical information sciences. In: Kuhn RL (Ed) *Frontiers of Medical Information Sciences.* New York: Praeger, pp 11–18.

Shortliffe, E.H. (1995). *Medical informatics meets medical education. JAMA (273)*, 1061-1065.

Shortliffe, E.H. and Garber, A.M. (2002). Training synergies between medical informatics and health services research, successes and challenges. *Journal of the American Medical Informatics Association, vol. 9*, 133-139.

Shortliffe, E.H., Perreault, L.E., Wiederhold, G. and Fagan, L.M. (1990). *Medical Informatics: computer applications in health care*, MA: Addison-Wesley.

Shortliffe, E.H., Perreault, L.E., Wiederhold, G. and Fagan, L.M. (eds.) (2001). *Medical Informatics: Computer Applications in Health Care and Bio*medicine, 2nd Edition, New York: Springer-Verlag.

Siassiakos, K., Ilioudi, S., Lazakidou, A. (2008). Simulation and learning environments in health care. *International Journal of Healthcare Technology and Management,* ISSN (Online): 1741-5144, ISSN (Print): 1368-2156, Vol. 9, Nr. 2, 2008.

Siden H. B., (1998). A qualitative approach to community and provider needs assessment in a telehealth project. *Telemed J, 4*, 225–235.

Silberg, W. et al (1997). Assessing, controlling and assuring the quality of medical information on the Internet. *JAMA, 277*(15), 1244-1245.

Simon, H. A. (1997). *Models of Bounded Rationality.* MIT Press.

Simonson, M., Smaldino, S., Albright, M., & Zvacek, S. (2003). *Teaching and learning at a distance.* Upper Saddle River, NJ: Merrill Prentice Hall.

Simpson J., Doze S., Urness D., Hailey D., Jacobs P.(2001).Telepsychiatry as a routine service -the perspective of the patient. J *Telemed Telecare; 7*, 155-60.

Skorin-Kapov, L., Vilendečić, D., Mikić, D. (2004). Experimental performance evaluation of networked virtual reality services. *Presented at the IEEE MELECON*, (pp. 661-664). IEEE CS Press.

Slee, V.N., Slee, D. & Schmidt, H.J. (2005). The tyranny of the diagnosis code. *North Carolina medical journal, 66*(5), 331-337.

Smith, A. D. (2005). Exploring radio frequency identification technology and its impact on business systems. *Information Management & Computer Security, 13*(1), 16-28.

Smith, D., Newell, L.M. (2002). A Physician's perspective: Deploying the EMR. *Journal of Healthcare Information Management, 16*(2), 71-79.

Smith, H., & Konsynski, B. (2003). Developments in practice X: Radio frequency identification (RFID) - An internet for physical objects. *Communications of the Association for Information Systems, 12*, 301-311.

Smith, J. P., & Kington, R. S. (1997). Race, socioeconomic status, and health in late life. In L. G. Martin & B. J. Soldo (Eds.), *Racial and Ethnic Differences in the Health of Older Americans*. Washington, DC: National Academy Press.

Smith, P., & Raga, T. (2005). *Instructional design-third edition.* Hoboken, NJ: John Wiley & Sons, Inc.

Smith, R. (1996). What clinical information do doctors need? *British Medical Journal, Oct. 313*, 1062-1068.

Sohail, M. S. (2003). Service quality in hospitals: More favourable than you might think. *Managing Service Quality, 13*(9), 197- 206.

Sokol, B. (2005). *RFID and emerging technologies market guide to healthcare*. Retrieved September 1, 2006, from http://www.rfidjournal.com/article/articleview/1534/1/1/

Song, X., Hwong, B., Matos, G., Rudorfer, A., Nelson, C., Han, M. & Girenkov, A. (2006). Understanding requirements for computer-aided healthcare workflows: Experiences and challenges. *Proceedings of the 28th International Conference on software engineering.* Shanghai, China, (pp. 930-934).

Sorvaniemi M., Ojanen E., Santamaki O. (2005). Telepsychiatry in emergency consultations: A follow-up study of sixty patients. *Telemed J E Health 11*(4),439-41.(ISSN: 1530-5627).

Southon G, Sauer C, Dampney K. (1999). Lessons from a failed information systems initiative: issues for complex organisations. *International Journal of Medical Informatics, 55*(1), Pages 33-46.

Sowa, J (1984). *Conceptual Structures: Information Processing in Mind and Machine.* Reading: Addison Wesley

Sowa, J. (2000). *Knowledge representation – Logical philosophical and computational foundations* Pacific Grove: Brooks/Cole cop.

Sprague L, 2004. Electronic health records: How close? How far to go? *NHPF Issue Brief*, 1-17.

Spring Framework. (2007). Retrieved from http://www.springframework.org/

Spyglass. (2006). *Providers not passive about RFID.* Retrieved September 5, 2006, from http://healthdatamanagement.com/HDMSearchResultsDetails.cfm?articleId=12499

SRI. (2007). *DynaSpeak speech recognition software.* Retrieved from http://www.sri.com/

Srinivasan, L. & Treadwell, J. (2005). *An overview of service oriented architecture, Web services and grid computing.* Retrieved from http://h71028.www7.hp.com/ERC/downloads/SOA-Grid-HP-WhitePaper.pdf

Stahl, A. (2003). *Learning of knowledge-intensive similarity-measures in case based reasoning.* University Kaiserslautern, Dissertation.

Stal, M.: OBJEKTspektrum (1999): Des Knaben Wunderhorn", Kommentare des Fachbeirats Komponenten-Forum. In *OBJEKTspektrum* 1/99, S. 18-20.

Stallings, W. (2005). *Cryptography and network security.* Prentice Hall.

Stanley, L. (2003). Beyond access: psychosocial barrier to computer literacy. *The Information Society, 19*, 407-416.

Stark, D.D., & Bradley, W.G. (1999). *Magnetic resonance imaging: third edition.* Mosby Publishing, USA.

Staves J., Davies A., Kay J., Pearson O., Johnson T, Murphy M. F. (2007). Electronic remote blood issue: a combination of remote blood issue with a system for end-to-end electronic control of transfusion to provide a "total solution" for a safe and timely hospital blood transfusion service. *Transfusion,* 2007 Dec

Stead, W.W. (1994). JAMIA – Why? *J Am Med Informatics Assoc., Vol. 1,* 75-76.

Steering Committee on the evaluation of medical information science in medical education. (1986). In *Proceedings of the symposium on medical informatics* (pp. 2-3). Washington, DC: Association of American Medical Colleges.

Stephan, E. (1996). *Observations on the bills of mortality.* Retrieved December 28, 2006 from http://www.ac.wwu.edu/~stephan/Graunt/graunt.html

Stevens, R., Baker, P., Bechhofer, S., Ng, G., Jacoby, A., Paton, N.W., Goble, C.A., Brass, A. (2000a). TAMBIS: Transparent Access to Multiple Bioinformatics Information Sources. *Bioinformatics, 16*(2), 184-185.

Stevens, R., Goble, C.A., Bechhofer, S. (2000b). Ontology-based knowledge representation for bioinformatics. *Briefings in Bioinformatics, 1*(4), 398-416.

Stewart, T. A. (1997). *Intellectual capital: the new wealth of organizations.* New York, NY, USA: Doubleday.

Stock-McIssac, M. (1999). Distance learning: The U.S. version. *Performance Improvement Quarterly, 12*(2), 21-35.

Strödter, D. (2000). *Therapie der Herzinsuffizienz.* Bremen: UNI-MED Verlag.

Subramanian, M., Ali, A.S., Rana, O., Hardisty, A. & Conley, E.C. (2006). Healthcare@Home: Research models for patient-centered healthcare services. *Proceedings of the 2006 International Symposium on Modern Computing* (pp.107-113).

Surján, G. & Balkányi, L. (1996). Theoretical considerations on medical concept representation. *Medical Informatics (London,) 21*(1), 61-68.

Surján, G. (1999) Questions on validity of International Classification of Diseases-coded diagnoses. *International Journal of Medical Informatics, 54(2),* 77-95.

Suzy, A., (1997). A survey of deformable modeling in computer graphics. *MERL Technical Report* TR-97-19, November 1997

Sveiby, K. E. (2004). *Methods for measuring intangible assets.* Retrieved from http://www. sveiby. com/articles/IntangibleMethods. htm

Tait, R.J., Schaefer, G., & Hopgood, A.A. (2006a). iDARBS – A distributed blackboard system for image processing. In *Proceedings of the 13th International Conference on Systems, Signals and Image Processing,* 431-434.

Tait, R.J., Schaefer, G., & Hopgood, A.A. (2006b). Towards high performance image registration using intelligent agents. In *Proceedings of the 13th International Conference on Systems, Signals and Image Processing,* 435-438.

Talley, C. R. (1997). Editorial: Trouble on the Internet. *American Journal of Health-System Pharmacy, 54.*

Talosig-Garcia, M., & Davis, S. W. (2005). Information-seeking behavior of minority breast cancer patients: an exploratory study. *Journal of Health Communication, 10*(Supplement 1), 53-64.

Tanenbaum A. S. (1988). *Computer networks, 2nd ed.* Englewood Cliffs, N.J: Prentice-Hall, .

Tang W. K., Chiu H., Woo J., et al.(2001). Telepsychiatry in psychogeriatric service: A pilot study. *International Journal of Geriatric Psychiatry 16,* 88–93.

Tang, P.C., McDonald, C.J. (2006). Electronic health record systems. In Cimino, J. J. and Shortliffe, E. H. (eds.) *Biomedical Informatics: Computer Applications in Health Care and Biomedicine (Health Informatics).* Springer-Verlag, New York, Inc.

Taylor, A. G. (2003). *The organization of information.* 2nd edition Libraries Unlimited publications.

Taylor, K. L., O'Keefe, C. M., Colton, J., Baxter, R., Sparks, R., Srinivasan, U., Cameron, M. A., and Lefort, L. A. (2004). Service oriented architecture for a health research data network. In *Proceedings of the 16th Interna-*

tional Conference on Scientific and Statistical Database Management, (pp.443- 444).

Taylor, K.L., Colton, C.M., Baxter, R., Sparks, R., Srinivasen, U., Cameron, M.A. & Lefort, L. (2004). A service oriented architecture for a health research data network. *Proceedings of the International Conference on Scientific and Statistical Database Management*, Santorini, Greece (pp. 443-444).

Teas, R. K. (1993). Expectations, performance evaluation and consumers' perceptions of quality. *Journal of Marketing, 57*, 18-34.

The American Board of Pediatrics (2007). Retrieved May 1, from https://www.abp.org/ABPWebSite/

The European parliament and the council of the European Union. (1995). *Directive 95/46/EC of the European Parliament and of the Council of 24 October 1995 on the protection of individuals with regard to the processing of personal data and on the free movement of such data.* Luxembourg. (Directive 95/46/EC).

Thomas, J., Streib, G. 2003. The new face of government: citizen-initiated contacts in the era of e-government. *Journal of Public Administration Research and Theory, 13*(1), 83-102.

Thomas, W. and Cerino, D. A. (1995). Predicting software quality for reuse certification, presented at the Annual International Conference on Ada. In *Proceedings of the conference on TRI-Ada '95: Ada's role in global markets: solutions for a changing complex world.* Anaheim, California, United States, (pp.367-377). ISBN: 0-89791-705-7.

Tight, M. (2002). *'Key concepts in adult education and training.* New York: RoutledgeFalmer.

Timmers P (1999) *Electronic commerce Strategies and Models for Business-To-Business.* New York NY: John Willey and Sons, Inc.

Timmons, S. (2001). Use of Internet by patients: Not a threat but an opportunity?', *Nurse Education Today, 21*(2), 104–109.

Titzer, B., Lee D., and Palsberg, J. (2005). Avrora: Scalable sensor network simulation with precise timing. *International Symposium on Information Processing in Sensor Networks (IPSN).* Los Angeles, California.

Tolbert, C., Mossberger, K. (2006). The effects of e-government on trust and confidence in government. Public Administration Review, vol 66, 3, pp. 354-369.

Tomas Ward (2001), *The Photoplethysmograph as an instrument for physiological measurement.* Department of Electronic Engineering, NUI Maynooth.

Treins, M., Curé, O., Salzano, G. (2006). On the interest of using HL7 CDA release 2 for the exchange of annotated medical documents. *Proceedings of the 19th IEEE Symposium on Computer-Based Medical Systems (CBMS'06)*, (pp. 524-532).

Trill, A. J. (March 26-27, 1996). Regulatory requirements for computer validation, computer systems validation: A practical approach. *Management Seminar.* London.

Tsiknakis, M., Chronaki, C.E., Kapidakis, S., Nikolaou, C. & Orphanoudakis, S.C. (1997). An integrated architecture for the provision of health telematic services based on digital library technologies. *International Journal of Digital Libraries 1*(3), 257-277.

Turner J. Kenneth, Gemma A., Campell and Feng Wang (2007, June). Policies for sensor networks and home care networks. In *Proceedings of 7th Int. Conf. on New Technologies for Distributed Systems*, pp. 237-284.

Twist, D. C. (2005). The impact of radio frequency identification on supply chain facilities. *Journal of Facilities Management, 3*(3), 226-239.

Tygar, Doug (1998 August 24-27). "Atomicity versus anonymity: Distributed transactions for electronic commerce. In *Proceedings of 24 International Conference on Very Large Databases (VLDB).* New York City

U.S. House of Representatives, Committee on Small Business Hearing. (May 3, 2006). *Future of rural telecommunications: is universal service reform needed?,* CIS-NO: 2006-H721-24. (pp. 1-78).

U.S. Institute of Medicine. Dick, R.S., Steen, E.B. & Detmer, D.E. (eds.) (1997). *The computer-based patient record - an essential technology for health care.* National Academy Press.

U.S. Institute of Medicine. Kohn, L.T., Corrigan, J.M. & Donaldson, M. (eds.). (2000). To *err is human: Building a safer health* system. National Academy Press.

Ungureanu, V. (2001), A regulated approach to certificate management, ACSAC. In *Proceedings of the 17th Annual Computer Security Applications Conference*, (pp 377). ISBN: 0-7695-1405-7.

Upham, R., (2004). The electronic health record: Will it become a reality?, Phoenix Health Systems, http://www.hipaadvisory.com/action/ehealth/EHR-reality.htm

USA Congress, 1996. HIPAA - Health Insurance Portability and Accountability Act IN Government, U. (Ed.), Public Law (pp. 104-191) 104th Congress.

Üstün, B., Jakob, R., Çelik, C., Lewalle, P., Kostanjsek, N., Renahan, M., Madden, R., Greenberg. M.., Chute, C., Virtanen, M. Hyman, S., Harrison, J., Ayme, S. & Sugano, K. (2007). *Production of ICD-11: The overall revision process* Geneva: World Health Organisation. Retrieved June 21 2007 from http://extranet.who.int/icdrevision/help/docs/ICDRevision.pdf

van Elst L, Dignum V, Abecker A. (2003). Towards agent-mediated knowledge management. *Agent-Mediated Knowledge Management: International Symposium AMKM 2003.* Stanford, CA, USA, March 24-26, revised and invited papers.

Varady P., Benyo Z., Benyo B. (2002), An open architecture patient monitoring system using standard technologies. *IEEE Transactions on Information Technology in Biomedicine, 6*(1), .95–98.

Varlamis, Iraklis & Apostolakis, Ioannis (2006). Use of virtual communities for the welfare of groups with particular needs. In *Proceedings of the 4th ICICTH International Conference on Information Communication Technologies in Health.*

Varlamis, Iraklis & Apostolakis, Ioannis (2007 February 18-20). Self supportive Web communities in the service of patients. In *Proceedings of IADIS International Conference on Web Based Communities* 2007. Salamanca, Spain.

Varshney, U. (2005). Pervasive healthcare: Applications, challenges and wireless solutions. *Communications of the Association for Information Systems, 16*, 52-72.

Varshney, U., (2006). Transmission of emergency messages in wireless patient monitoring: routing and performance evaluation. *Presented at IEEE Hawaii International Conference on System Sciences*, vol. 5, (pp 91- 100).

Venkatesh, V. and Davis, F.D. (2000). A theoretical extension of the technology acceptance model: four longitudinal field studies. *Management Science. 46*(2), 186-204.

Virtual medical worlds. (2006, April). Retrieved June 8, 2007, from http://www.hoise.com/vmw/06/articles/contentsvmw200604.html

Viswanath, K., & Finnegan, J. R. (1995). The knowledge gap hypothesis: Twenty-five years later. In B. R. Burleson (Ed.), *Communication Yearbook 19* (pp. 187-227). Thousand Oaks, CA.: Sage.

Vladzymyrskyy A. V. (2003). Klynycheskoe teleconsultirovanie. *Rukovodstvo dlya Vrachei [Clinical Teleconsultation. Manual for Physicians].* Sevastopol: OOO "Veber", 125 (rus.)

Vladzymyrskyy A. V. (2004). The Use of Teleconsultations in the Treatment of Patients with Multiple Trauma. *Europ J Trauma, 6*(30), 394-7.

Vladzymyrskyy A. V. (2005). Four years' experience of teleconsultations in daily clinical practice. *JTT, 6*(11), 294-97.

Vladzymyrskyy A., Chelnokov A., (2006). Relevance of telemedicine consultation. *Ukr.z.telemed.med.telemat, 1*(4), 99-100.

Vopel, O. Knowledge as resource and problem: the case of knowledge-intensive firms. In *Proceedings of I-KNOW'03.* Graz, Austria, July 2-4, 2003, 2003.

Vucetic, J. (2005). *Technological and business challenges and solutions for a successful emergency telemedicine venture*, IPSI-2005. MIT, Cambridge, MA

Vucetic, J., (2003). Telemedicine – the future of wireless internet applications. Invited Speaker, *Southeast US Wireless Symposium.* Winston-Salem, NC.

Wac K., Van Halteren A. Bults R. and Broens T. (2007). Context-aware QoS provisioning in an m-health service platform. *International Journal of Internet Protocol Technology, 2*(2), 102 – 108.

Wachter, G., (2001). Implications of HIPAA's Privacy Rule For Telemedicine, TIE, http://tie.telemed.org/legal/issues/hippa2001.asp

Waegemann C, 2003. EHR vs. CPR vs. EMR. *Healthcare Informatics online.*

Wainwright, C., & Wootton, R. (2003). A Review of Telemedicine and Asthma. *Disease Management & Health Outcomes, 11*, 557-563.

Ward, W.A. and Venkataraman, B. (1999). Some observations on Software Quality. In *Proceedings of the 37th annual Southeast regional conference.* (CD-ROM), Article No. 2. ISBN:1-58113-128-3.

Warfield, S.K., Jolesz, F., & Kikinis, R. (1998). A high performance approach to the registration of medical imaging data. Parallel Computing. 24(9), 1345-1368.

Warner, H.R. (1995). Medical informatics: A real discipline? *J Am Med Informatics Assoc., vol. 2, 4*, 207-214.

Watro, R., Kong, D., Cuti, S., Gardiner, C., Lynn, C., and Kruus, P. (2004). TinyPK : Securing sensor networks with public key technology. *2nd ACM Workshop on Security of Ad Hoc and Sensor Networks (SASN 2004).* Washington, D.C.

Watro, R., Kong, D., Cuti, S., Gardiner, C., Lynn, C., and Kruus, P. (2004). TinyPK : Securing sensor networks with public key technology. *2nd ACM Workshop on Security of Ad Hoc and Sensor Networks (SASN 2004).* Washington, D.C.

Webster, R. et al., (2005). Millersville University's research in haptic and surgical simulation. *A Joint Research Project in Surgical Simulation with the Penn State University College of Medicine.* Millersville University

Webster, R., Haluck, R., Mohler, B., Ravenscroft, B., Crouthamel, E., Frack, T., Terlecki, S., Sheaffer, J., (2002). Elastically deformable 3D organs for haptic surgical simulators. In *Proceedings of the Medicine Meets Virtual Reality Conference, MMVR '2002.* Newport Beach, CA, IOS Press, (pp 570-572).

Wee, C.C., McCarthy, E.P., Davis, R.B. and Phillips, R.S. (1999). Physician counseling about exercise. *JAMA. 282*(2), 1583-1588.

Weiser, M. (1993). Some computer science issue in ubiquitous computing. *Communications of the ACM, 36*(7), 74-84.

Weiss, R. (1999). Medical errors blamed for many deaths: As many as 98,000 a year in U.S. linked to mistakes. *The Washington Post.*

Wess, S. (1995): *Fallbasiertes problemlösen in wissensbasierten systemen zur entscheidungsunterstützung und diagnostik.* Sankt Augustin: Infix Verlag.

West, D. (2004). E-government and the transformation of service delivery and citizen attitudes. *Public Administration Review, 64*(1), 15-27.

West, D. (September 2003), State and federal e-government in the United States (2003). Center for Public Policy, Brown University, Retrieved from www.insidepolitics.org/egovt03us.pdf

West, D., Miller, E. (2006). The digital divide in public e-health: barriers to accessibility and privacy in state health department Web sites. *Journal of Health Care for the Poor and Underserved, 17*, 652-666.

Whitney, C. W., Lind, B. K. and Wahl, P. W. (1998). Quality Assurance and Quality Control in Longitudinal Studies. *Epidemiologic Reviews, 20*(1), 71-80.

Wiebusch, B., (2001), Telemedicine reduces mortality rate. *Design News.* Retrieved from http://www.designnews.com/article/CA83189.html?text=telemedicine.

Wilke, W., & Bergmann, R. (1998). Techniques and knowledge used for adaptation during case-based problem solving. In *Proceedings of the 12th International Conference On Industrial and Engineering Applications of Artificial Intelligence and Expert Systems, Lecture Notes in Computer Science* (pp. 497-506). Berlin: Springer Verlag.

Wilkins, John (1668). *An essay towards a real character, and philosophical. language* london: brouncker press. Retrieved from: http://reliant.teknowledge.com/Wilkins/

Wilkinson, M.D., Links, M. (2002). BioMOBY: an open source biological Web services proposal. *Briefings in bioinformatics, 3*(4), 331-341.

William Webb (2007). *Wireless communications: The future.* West Sussex, England: John Wiley & Sons Ltd. Key Words

Williamson, L. (2006). What's new. *Health information on the Internet, 50,* 12.

Wilson, D. C. (2001): *Case-base maintenance: the husbandry of experience.* Indiana University, Dissertation.

Wilson, P. (2002). How to find the good and avoid the bad or ugly: A short guide to tools for rating quality of health information on the Internet. *BMJ 324*, 598-602.

Wingate, G. (2003). *Computer Systems validation - quality assurance, risk management, and regulatory compliance for pharmaceutical and healthcare companies*. CRC Press, 1st edition.

Winker, M. A., Flanagin A.,Chi-Lum B, et al (2000). Guidelines for medical and health information sites on the Internet. *JAMA 283*, 1600-1666.

Winter A., Brigl B. and Wendt T. (2003). Modeling hospital information systems (Part 1), the revised three-layer graph-based meta-model 3LGM2. *Methods Inf. Med., 42*(5), 544—551.

Wiratunga, Ni., & Craw, S., & Rowe, R. (2002). Learning to adapt for case-based design. In *Proceedings of the 6th European Conference on Case Based Reasoning, Lecture Notes in Computer Science*, vol. 2416. Berlin: Springer Verlag, 421-435.

Wittrock, M. (1990). Generative processes of comprehension. *Educational Psychologist, 27*, 531-41

World Health Organisation (n.d.) *History of the development of the ICD* Retrieved June 27, 2006 from http://www.who.int/classifications/icd/en/HistoryOfICD.pdf

World Wide Web Consortium (W3C) (2004). *Web services architecture*. Retrieved from http:// www.w3.org/TR/ws-arch.

Wu, H.-C., et al., (1999). A mobile system for real-time patient-monitoring with integrated physiological signal processing. *Presented at IEEE BMES/EMBS Joint Conference*, vol.2, (pp.712).

Wyatt, J. C. (1997). Commentary: Measuring quality and impact of the World Wide Web. *BMJ, 314*, 1879-1881.

Wyatt, J.C. and Liu, J.L.Y. (2002). Basic concepts in medical informatics. *Journal of Epidemiology and Community Health, vol. 56*, 808-812.

Xu, Y., Sauquet, D., Zapletal, E., Lemaitre, D., and Degoulet, P. (2000). Integration of medical applications: the mediator service of the SynEx platform. *International Journal of Medical Informatics, 58-59*, 157-166

Yahoo! (2007). *LocalSearch APIs*. Retrieved from http:// developer.yahoo.com/search/local/.

Yoo, T.S. (2004). *Insight into images: Principles and practices for segmentation, registration, and image analysis*. A.K. Peters Ltd, USA.

Yoshino A., Shigemura J., Kobayashi Y., et al. (2001).Telepsychiatry: assessment of televideo psychiatric interview reliability with present- and next-generation internet infrastructures. *Acta Psychiatrica Scandinavica 104*, 223–226.

Youngblood, P., Parvati, D. (2005). A framework for evaluating new learning technologies in medicine. *AMIA Annu Symp Proc. 2005*, (pp. 1163).

Yu P., Wu M. X., Yu H. and Xiao G. C. (2006). The Challenges for the Adoption of M-Health. *IEEE International Conference on Service Operations and Logistics and Informatic*

Zaylor C., Whitten P., Kingsley C. (2000). Telemedicine services to a county jail. *J Telemed Telecare 6*(suppl 1), S93-S95.

Zeeberg, B.R., Feng, W., Wang, G., Wang, M.D., Fojo, A.T., Sunshine, M., Narasimhan, S., Kane, D.W., Reinhold, W.C., Lababidi, S., Bussey, K.J., Riss, J., Barrett, J.C., Weinstein, J.N. (2003). GoMiner: a resource for biological interpretation of genomic and proteomic data. *Genome Biology, 4*(4), R28, 1-8.

Zhang, Ch., & Popp, F.-A. (1996). Log-normal distribution measure of physiological parameters and the coherence of biological systems. In Ch. Zhang, F.-A. Popp, & M. Bischof (Eds.), *Current developments of biophysics,* (pp. 102-111). Hangzhou University Press.

Ziebland, S., Chapple, A., Dumelow, C., Evans, J., Prinjha, S., Rozmovits, L. (2004). How the Internet affects patient's experience of cancer a qualitative study. *BMJ 328*, 364.

Zimeras S., Lambrinoudakis C., Fournaridis G., Fournaridis I. (2005). An IT-based questionnaire system for the evaluation of healthcare services using electronic sampling techniques. *The Journal on Information Technology in Healthcare, 3*, 239–47.

Zimeras, S., Kostagiolas P. and Lambrinoudakis C. (2007). Quality evaluation in healthcare based on the assessment of services expectation using a web-based questionnaire system and adaptive sampling techniques. *The Journal on Information Technology in Healthcare, 5*(1), 50-58.

Zitova, B., & Flusser, J. (2003). Image registration methods: a survey. *Image and Vision Computing. 21*, 977-1000.

Zuckerman, A. M. (2000). Creating a version for the twenty-first century healthcare organization. *Journal of Healthcare Management, 45*(5), 294-305.

About the Contributors

Athina Lazakidou is lecturer in Health Informatics at the University of Peloponnese at the Department of Nursing in Sparta, Greece. From September 2002 she worked at the University of Piraeus, Greece as a teaching assistant, and at the Hellenic Army Academy & Hellenic Naval Academy, Greece as a visiting lecturer in informatics. Prior to that, she worked also as a visiting lecturer at the Department of Computer Science at the University of Cyprus (2000-2002). She did her undergraduate studies at the Athens University of Economics and Business (Greece) and received her BSc in computer science in 1996. In 2000, she received her PhD. in medical informatics from the Department of Medical Informatics, University Hospital Benjamin Franklin at the Free University of Berlin, Germany. She is also an internationally known expert in the field of computer applications in healthcare and biomedicine, with seven books and numerous papers to her credit. She was also editor of the "Handbook of Research on Informatics in Healthcare and Biomedicine", which is one of the best authoritative reference sources for information on the newest trends and breakthroughs in computer applications applied to healthcare and biomedicine. Her research interests include health informatics, e-Learning in medicine, software engineering, graphical user interfaces, (bio)medical databases, clinical decision support systems, hospital and clinical information systems, electronic medical record systems, distributed medical systems, telemedicine, and other applications in health care.

Konstantinos Siassiakos holds a diploma (1995) of electrical and computer engineer from the Department of Electrical and Computer Engineering Studies, University of Patras, Greece, and a PhD (2001) diploma from the Department of Electrical and Computer Engineering, National Technical University of Athens, Greece. Dr. K. Siassiakos currently works as visiting lecturer at the University of Piraeus at the Department of Informatics and at the Technological Educational Institute of Halkida in Greece. He has worked as an IT consultant at Ministry of Development (general secretariat of industry) on the Operational Programme 'Competitiveness' and as a researcher at the Department of Technology Education & Digital Systems, University of Piraeus. He has participated in various european research and development projects. His research interests include web-based learning systems in medicine and other areas, educational technologies, human computer interaction, quality assurance, management information systems in health organisations and other areas, business process reengineering, and e-government technologies.

* * *

Kleopatra Alamantariotou was born in Larisa, Greece on 8th of September 1980. From 2000 to 2004 she has studied Midwifery in Technological Education Institute in Athens, Greece. On April 2004 she has obtain her degree In Midwifery with the following dissertation thesis: "Ultrasonography and Biochemistry Indicators of Fetal Chromosomal Abnormalities at the First Trimester". From April 2005 until November 2007 she worked as a midwife in Chelsea Westminster hospital in London England in women's health department and in labor ward (2.5 years experience in maternity unit). During her work in London, she received also a Msc in midwifery in June 2007.

Luís Antunes is an Assistant Professor affiliated with the computer science faculty of the University of Porto, his main research interests are computational complexity and cryptography. He is the principal investigator of some projects financed by the Portuguese science foundation and the PhD advisor of some PhD students. Additionally he is in the coordinator of the first health informatics master course in Portugal

Daniele Apiletti is a PhD student of the Database and Data Mining Group at the Dipartimento di Automatica e Informatica of the Politecnico di Torino since January 2006. He holds a Master's degree in computer engineering from Politecnico di Torino (2005). His research interests are in the fields of bioinformatics and sensor data analysis. In the bioinformatics area, his research activities are focused on microarray data classification and feature selection techniques. In the area of sensor data analysis he is developing data mining techniques for physiological data processing on mobile devices.

Ioannis Apostolakis was born in Chania of Crete and studied Mathematics in University of Athens. He holds an MSc in informatics, operational research and in administration in Educational Units, and a PhD in health informatics. He has been for several years scientific researcher in the Department of the clinical therapeutics in University of Athens. He had been teaching in University of Athens and in Polytechnic University of Crete. Today he teaches to the post-graduate program of the National School of Public Health and to Panteion University.

Elena Baralis is full professor at the Dipartimento di Automatica e Informatica of the Politecnico di Torino since January 2005. She holds a Dr.Ing. degree in electrical engineering and a PhD in Computer Engineering, both from Politecnico di Torino. Her current research interests are in the field of databases, in particular data mining, sensor databases, and bioinformatics. She has published numerous papers on journal and conference proceedings. She has served on the program committees of several international conferences and workshops, among which IEEE ICDM, VLDB, ACM CIKM, DaWak, ACM SAC, PKDD. She has managed several Italian and EU research projects.

Ambar Basu is a doctoral candidate and graduate lecturer in the Department of Communication at Purdue University. He received his BA and MSc from Calcutta University in 1995 and has extensive experience working as a journalist. His research on health communication takes a culture-centered approach and explores the ways in which cultural meanings are co-constructed by participants in their interactions with the structures that surround their lives. This work has been published in journal such as *Health Communication* and *Qualitative Health Research*.

Graham D. Bodie (Ph.D., Purdue University 2008) is Assistant Professor in the Department of Communication Studies at Louisiana State University. His research explores the intersection between listening and information processing.

Christos Bountis (MSc, MD) studied medicine at the University of Genoa in Italy. His MD thesis explored the validity of applications of dedicated low-field magnetic resonance. Since January 2000 he has been working with Prof. Jonathan Kay at the Oxford Radcliffe Hospitals Trust on knowledge management and the clinical intranet. He is particularly interested in knowledge formation and delivery methods, health process automation, innovative medical testing technologies and point of care device prospects, particularly in relation to pathway integration, knowledge interaction and process sustainability, market effects and opportunities.

Philip Brisk received his BS, MS, and PhD degrees, all in computer science, from UCLA in 2002, 2003, and 2006 respectively. He is currently a postdoctoral researcher with the Processor Architecture Laboratory at Ecole Polytechnique Federale de Lausanne, in Switzerland.

Giulia Bruno is a PhD student of the Database and Data Mining Group at the Dipartimento di Automatica e Informatica of the Politecnico di Torino since January 2006. She obtained a Master's degree in computer engineering from Politecnico di Torino in September 2005. She is currently working in the field of data mining and bioinformatics. In particular, her activity is focused on the analysis of microarray gene expression data, gene network modelling, data cleaning and semantic information discovery. Her research activities are also devoted to classification of physiological signals in order to monitor patient conditions for clinical analysis.

Rafael Capilla is a graduate in computer science and holds a PhD by the Universidad Rey Juan Carlos of Madrid, Spain. He worked as a senior analyst for 2 years in a telecommunication company and more than eight years as a Unix system administrator. Currently, he is an assistant professor in the same university teaching on software architecture and Web programming. He is co-author of 1 book, 1 journal, and more than 25 referred conference papers. His research focuses on software architecture, product-line engineering, internet technologies, and mobile applications. Contact him at: rafael.capilla@urjc.es

Mario Ceresa received a Bachelor in Computer Science in 2004 from Politecnico di Milano, Italy and he is now attending a Master Degree program in Biomedical Engineering at Politecnico di Milano. His research interests are in neurosciences and bioinformatics and he has a solid background in computer programming and agents system for the Semantic Web.

Tania Cerquitelli is a post-doctoral researcher in computer engineering at the Politecnico di Torino since January 2007. She holds a PhD degree and a Master's degree in computer engineering, both from the Politecnico di Torino. She also obtained a Master's degree in computer science from Universidad De Las Américas Puebla. Her research activities are focused on the integration of data mining algorithms into database system kernels and on the exploitation of data mining techniques to analyze streaming data collected by sensor networks. She served in the program committee of DS2ME'08 and IADIS'06.

David Chadwick is a professor of information systems security at the University of Kent and the leader of the Information Systems Security Research Group. He specialises in public key infrastructures, privilege management infrastructures, trust management, privacy management and internet security research in general. Current research topics include: attribute aggregation, policy based authorisation, grid security, the management of trust, the delegation of authority and autonomic security. He actively participates in standardisation activities, is the UK BSI representative to X.509 standards meetings, the chair of the Open Grid Forum OGSA Authorisation Working Group, and the author of a number of Internet rafts, RFCs and OGF documents.His group are the creators of PERMIS (www.openpermis.org), an open source X.509 and SAML based authorisation infrastructure. PERMIS is part of the US NMI software suite, and is integrated with Globus Toolkit (version 3.3 onwards), Shibboleth and Apache.

Anargyros Chryssanthou studied applied informatics in Athens University of Economics and Business. He holds an MSc in information security and computer crime from the University of Glamorgan (Wales – UK). He has written and presented several articles in national conferences, concerning various aspects of computer security, from network forensics to cryptography, security management and ISO implementations of information security management systems (ISMS). He is currently employed by Coca Cola Hellenic Bottle and Company as a database reporting specialist.

Ricardo Cruz-Correia is an assistant lecturer and researcher at the Biostatistics and Medical Informatics Department at the Faculty of Medicine of the University of Porto, Portugal. His research interest is in the integration of heterogeneous healthcare information.He received his Master's Degree in computer science at the Faculty of Science of University of Porto. He is currently a PhD student at the Faculty of Medicine of the University of Porto.

Foad Dabiri received his BS degree in electrical engineering from Sharif University of Technology, Tehran, Iran in 2003. He joined University of California, Los Angeles in 2003 and currently he is working towards his PhD degree. His research area includes algorithm design and analysis for embedded systems with emphasis on power optimization and scheduling.

Isabel de la Torre Díez was born in Zamora, Spain, in 1979. She received the Engineer degree in telecommunications engineering from the University of Valladolid, Valladolid, Spain, in 2003. Currently, she is an assistant professor in the Department of Signal Theory and Communications at the University of Valladolid, where she is working towards the PhD degree. Her research has been mainly focused in development of telemedicine applications and EHR (Electronic Health Record) standards in ophthalmology.

Alfonso del Río is a graduate in computer science by the Universidad Rey Juan Carlos of Madrid (Spain). He worked as a senior analyst for 4 years for an aeronautical engineering company. From 2004 to 2005 he worked for a consulting firm developing software for hospitals and from 2005 he started in a new company leading the software integration team for medical solutions His research and interest focuses on internet technologies, telemedicine, mobile applications and system integration. Contact him at: alfonsodelrio@terra.es

Manfred Doepp currently works as research director at the Holistic DiagCenter which uses energy medicine methods in a holistic approach. He is member of the board of the German Society for Energy and Information Medicine (Stuttgart) and of the German Society for Vertebral und Systems Regulation (Rosenheim). He was active in the further development of meridian diagnostics (Prognos®) and segmentary diagnostics (Amsat-HC®) programs and devices. His special field is the clinical application of the frequency distribution analysis of biological data concerning medical decision making to receive an objective second opinion.

Julian Dorado de la Calle was born in 1970 in A Coruña, Spain. He finished his graduate in computer science in 1994; he became a PhD, with a special mention of European doctor. In 2004, he finished his graduate degree in biology. He has worked as a lecturer at the University of A Coruña more than eight years. Currently, he is working in the areas of bioinformatics, evolutionary computing, artificial neural networks, computer graphics and data mining.

D. John Doyle, MD, PhD is professor of anesthesiology, Cleveland Clinic Lerner College of Medicine of Case Western Reserve University and staff anesthesiologist, Department of General Anesthesiology, Cleveland Clinic. He has degrees in physics, electrical engineering, education and medicine, and is trained as an anesthesiologist. He has had a long-standing interest in computer technology in medical care, especially from the perspective of clinical, social and ethical issues.

Bill Ag. Drougas studied physics in the University of Ioannina Greece taking his university diploma BSc in Physics. He received his PhD in the University of Ioannina in the school of medicine in the Department of Physiology in the Unit of Ergophysiology and calculating physiology. Postgraduate research studies in Health Informatics and contemporary technologies in the Monash University of Australia in the Department of Medical Informatics. He studied and certified in the wireless communications from the Cleveland Institute of Electronics from Ohio USA. Also he studied educational technologies in the Indiana University USA. He teaches in the Highest Technological Educational Institute of Epirus in the department of Teleinformatics and telecommunications and is an associated researcher in various research groups world wide for modern technologies in medicine and ergophysiology. He is the author of 25 Books and published over 100 scientific research works worldwide for various scientific fields.

Mohan J. Dutta is associate professor of health communication, public relations and mass media and director of graduate studies in the Department of Communication at Purdue University. He received his B.Tech.(Honors) in agricultural and food engineering from the Indian Institute of Technology (IIT), Kharagpur, MA in mass communication from North Dakota State University and PhD in Mass Communication from the University of Minnesota. Professor Dutta is the 2006 Lewis Donohew Outstanding Scholar in Health Communication and conducts research on digital divide, healthcare inequities, and the culture-centered approach. His work has been funded by the MacArthur Foundation, National Science Foundation, and National Library of Medicine.

Ana Ferreira is an IT specialist at the Faculty of Medicine of the University of Porto and a PhD student with a joint supervision from the University of Porto in Portugal and the University of Kent in UK. Her current research is on access control for healthcare information systems. She has a BSc in computer science from the University of Porto and received her MSc in information security with distinction from the University of London, UK.

Raimir Holanda Filho is an Associate Professor at University of Fortaleza (UNIFOR), in the Center of Technological Sciences, where he advises graduate and undergraduate students. He received the PhD degree in computer science from Technical University of Catalonia (UPC), Barcelona, Spain, in 2005. He acts as a reviewer of *IEEE Transactions on Computer Networks*. Currently, he coordinates a project named "Tele-Health" that aims the development of a library with health contents. His main interest research areas are wireless communications, mobility, security, QoS, NGN, performance evaluation, and traffic modeling, characterization and classification.

Roberto Hornero was born in Plasencia, Spain, in 1972. He received the degree in telecommunication engineering and PhD degree from the University of Valladolid, Spain, in 1995 and 1998, respectively. He is currently "profesor titular" in the Department of Signal Theory and Communications at the University of Valladolid. His main research interest is nonlinear analysis of biomedical signals to help physicians in the clinical diagnosis. He founded the Biomedical Engineering Group in 2004. The research interests of this group are connected with the field of nonlinear dynamics, chaotic theory, and wavelet transform with applications in biomedical signal and image processing.

Kashif Hussain is a specialist in quality management and currently working as a quality maintenance analyst with *Volvo Powertrain* in the *Product Development Laboratory*, France. He worked for quality, validation and regulatory affairs for the pharmaceutical industry. He has lectured on quality management, cognitive designing, ergonomics and change management for the *WSEAS*, *IEEE*, *IFAC* and *IADIS*. Since 2005, he has been engaged in various activities related to validation and change management. *IEEE* and *Idea Group Publisher* have published his work on CSV and CM. He has extensive practical experience with wide range of quality management, production, maintenance, operation management for the automobile, pharmaceutical and cement industry. He has diversified experience with industry (*Toyota*, *Volvo*, *Sanofi Aventis*, *Askari Cement*) and the academic world. He can be reached by phone at +33 (0)624686485 and by email at seekashif@yahoo.com.

Christina Ilioudi graduated from the Department of Informatics, University of Piraeus, Greece. Her research interests include electronic communication systems, security in healthcare information systems, e-health systems, applications in health organisations and other areas.

Stamatia Ilioudi graduated from the Department of Informatics, University of Piraeus, Greece. She is currently a postgraduate student in Information Systems at the Athens University of Economics and Business. Her research interests include electronic communication systems, information systems, e-business, e-health systems, applications in health organisations and other areas.

Roozbeh Jafari received his BSc in electrical engineering in 2000 from Sharif University of Technology, Tehran, Iran. He received his MSc from SUNY at Buffalo, NY in electrical engineering in 2002. He received his MS and Ph.D in computer science from UCLA in 2004 and 2006 respectiveley. He spent one year visiting EECS departemnt at UC Berkeley as a post-doctotral researcher. He is currently an assistant professor in the Electrical Engineering department at the University of Texas at Dallas. His main research is primarily in the area of networked embedded system design and reconfigurable computing with emphasis in medical/biological applications and their algorithm design.

Carolin Kaiser is member of research staff and PhD student at the Department of Information Systems II of the University of Erlangen-Nuremberg in Germany. Her research focuses are business intelligence and knowledge based systems in e-business. During her recent research project she explores the development and deployment of decision support systems in e-health.

Firat Kart is a candidate for the PhD degree in electrical and computer engineering at the University of California, Santa Barbara, where he has served as a teaching assistant and a graduate student researcher. He received the BS degree in computer science from Bilkent University in Ankara, Turkey, and holds a MS degree in electrical and computer engineering from the University of California, Santa Barbara. His research interests include distributed systems, computer networks, service oriented architectures, Web services, Atom/RSS, databases, transactions and e-healthcare systems.

Anastasia Kastania was born in Athens, Greece. She received her BSc in mathematics and her doctor of philoshophy (PhD) degree from the National Capodistrian University of Athens. Research productivity is summarized in various articles (monographs or in cooperation with other researchers) in international journals, international conferences proceedings, international book series and international books chapters. She has participated in many research projects in Greece and in European Union. She is a member of ACM, AMIA, IEEE. She works in the Athens University of Economics and Business since 1987 and she collaborates with International and European organizations since 1991. Since July 2004 she is the Greek Chapter Chair of the IEEE Education Society.

Spyros Kitsiou is currently a PhD candidate with the Department of Applied Informatics at the University of Macedonia, Greece. Over the past five years, he has been involved as a Researcher in European-funded R&D programmes within the healthcare ICT domain. He has also worked as a Systems Analyst at the research centre of the Xerox Corporation in Rochester, USA. His current research interests include healthcare information systems, electronic healthcare records, clinical information systems, computer physician order entry systems, management of healthcare information systems, supply chain systems, systems analysis and design, e-business and e-commerce.

Olaf Kniemeyer was born in 1970. He studied biology and achieved his diploma in 1998 at the University of Bremen, Germany. He worked as a PhD student at the Max-Planck Institute for Marine Microbiology, Bremen and received his PhD in microbiology at the University of Bremen in 2001. Afterwards he started to work with fungi as a postdoc at the University of Sheffield, UK and at the University of Hannover, Germany. Since 2005 he has been working as the head of the Proteomics Group of the Department of Molecular and Applied Microbiology (A. Brakhage) at the HKI in Jena, Germany. His research interests are fungal proteomics and virulence of human-pathogenic fungi.

Tiffany A. Koszalka, PhD is an associate professor of instructional design, development & evaluation at Syracuse University. Her research focuses on the intersection among learning, instruction, and technologies. She explores uses of technologies and online instruction in university teaching for education, engineering, and medical domains and in pre-college instruction. She was awarded National Institute of Health (NIH), NASA, and National Science Foundation grants, and has been recognized as a Faculty Technology Associate for Syracuse University based on her practices of integrating technology into her own teaching. She collaborates with colleagues around the world and publishes widely on technology integration and distance education.

Dimitris Koutsouris was born in Serres, Greece in 1955. He received his Diploma in Electrical Engineering in 1978 (Greece), DEA in Biomechanics in 1979 (France), doctorat in genie biologie medicale (France), Doctorat d' Etat in Biomedical Engineering 1984 (France). Since 1986 he was research associated on the USC (Los Angeles), Rene Descartes (Paris) and associate professor at the Department. of Electrical & Computers Engineering of National Technical University of Athens. He is currently professor and chairman of the Department of Electrical & Computers Engineering of National Technical University of Athens and head of the Biomedical Engineering Laboratory. He has published over 100 research articles and book chapters and more than 150 conference communications. Recently ha has also been elected as president of the Greek Society of Biomedical Technology. Professor D. Koutsouris has been principal investigator in many European and national research programs, especially in the field of telematics applications in healthcare.

Cheon-Pyo Lee is a doctoral student in information systems at Mississippi State University. He received his MS/CIS degree from Georgia State University and MBA degree from Morehead State University. His research interests include SMEs IT adoption, mobile commerce, and business value of IT. **Azizah Omar** obtained her PhD in wellness management and marketing from Monash University, Australia. She is currently a lecturer of marketing at the School of Management, Universiti Sains Malaysia (USM). Her research interests including consumer behaviour, web-based marketing, service marketing and wellness management. She has presented and published her papers in several international conferences such as Nairobi, London, Mumbai, and Montreal. The author is also the Steering Committee member of Healthy Campus in USM.

Sylvie Leleu-Merviel is professor and working as the director of the *Laboratory of Communication Sciences*, France. Her research areas include new writing forms, production and informational intelligence. She did her PhD in automation and is leading the *DREAM* (development, research, teaching in audio visual and multimedia) which is to support the interaction among training, research and transfer. She is the Vice President of International Relations and Communications at the *University of Valenciennes* since October 2005 and is a member of *National Commission for French Universities*. She is the author of many books and has published numerous articles.

Maria Isabel López was born in Valladolid, Spain, in 1960. She received his degree in Medicine and PhD from the University of Valladolid in 1985 and 1991, respectively. She is currently "Associate Profesor" in ophthalmology in the Department of Surgery of the Medicine Faculty at the University of Valladolid and also works in the University Hospital of this town as a clinician. Her main research interest is teleophtalmology from a clinical point of view and ocular diabetes. She is the director of the ocular diabetes unit at the "Instituto de Oftalmobiología Aplicada" in the University of Valladolid. She is a member of the American Academy of ophthalmology and the Spanish Society of Retina and Vitreous.

Miguel López is a telecommunications professor in the University of Valladolid (Spain). He was born in Barcelona, Spain; in 1950. He has a PhD in telecommunications engineering from the Polytechnic University of Madrid, in 1982. Since 1991 he has been devoted to the promotion of information society in Castille and Leon region from several positions: Director of the Technical School of Telecommunications, R&D general manager of a telecommunications technological centre and also CEO of a cable telecommunications operator. Now, his research interests are biomedical signal, telemedicine, information society, and to contribute to the promotion of the entrepreneurial character of university.

Vicky Manthou works currently at the Department of Applied Informatics at the University of Macedonia in Thessaloniki, Greece. She received her BSc in management and administration, Louisiana State Univ., U.S.A., (1976) and Doctorate from Department of Applied Informatics, University of Macedonia, Thessaloniki, GR, (1991).

Marco Masseroli received the Laurea Degree in electronic engineering in 1990 from Politecnico di Milano, Italy, and a PhD in biomedical engineering in 1996 from Universidad de Granada, Spain. He is assistant professors at the Dipartimento di Elettronica e Informazione of Politecnico di Milano, where he teaches biomedical informatics and distributed systems. His research interests are in bioinformatics and medical informatics, focused on distributed Internet technologies, genomics databanks, and bio-ontologies to effectively manage, analyze, and semantically integrate genomics information with patient clinical and high-throughout genetic data. He is the author of many articles published in international journals and conference proceedings.

Tammara Massey (http://www.cs.ucla.edu/~tmassey) received her BS from the University of North Carolina, Wilmington and her MS degree in computer science in 2004 from Georgia Institute of Technology in Atlanta, Georgia. She is currently working towards her PhD in the Computer Science Department at the University of California, Los Angeles. Her research interests are in embedded medical systems, body sensor networks, and security and privacy. She is a student member of IEEE.

Victor W. A. Mbarika, PhD, has been in the forefront of academic research into ICT implementation in Africa. Dr. Mbarika is serving at Southern University and A&M Collete at Baton Rouge, Louisiana, USA and has received several NSF and State grants. Professor Mbarika has over 90 published works including three books, five book chapters, 31 journal papers in premier outlets such as *IEEE Transactions, CACM, JAIS, ISJ, The Information Society, Journal of the American Society for Information Sciences*, and over 45 papers at premier conferences such as IFIP, ICIS, DSI, AMCIS and HICSS. He has chaired several minitracks/workshops at DSI and AMCIS where he introduced the first minitrack on ICTs in developing countries. His publication outlets clearly reflects the impact he is having on the information systems, computer science, information science and engineering community.

Ramona McNeal is an assistant professor in political science at the University of Northern Iowa. She received her PhD from Kent State University in 2005. Her primary research and teaching areas are in public policy, American politics and quantitative research methods. Her chief research interests lie in technology and electoral politics including voting, elections, public opinion, interest groups and the media. She is equally interested in telecommunication policy such as e-government. She is under contract with MIT to write a new co-authored book "Digital Citizenship: The Internet, Society and Participation". She is published in several journals including *Social Science Quarterly, Political Research Quarterly* and *State Politics and Policy Quarterly*. Additionally, she maintains an active research agenda with forthcoming articles in *Government Information Quarterly, Public Administration Review* and *Telemedicine and e-Health.*

Louise E. Moser is a professor in the Department of Electrical and Computer Engineering at the University of California, Santa Barbara. Her research interests span the fields of computer networks, distributed systems and software engineering. Dr. Moser has authored or coauthored more than 230 conference and journal publications. She has served as an associate editor for the *IEEE Transactions on Computers* and an editor for *IEEE Computer* in the area of networks, and has also served on many conference program committees. She received a PhD in mathematics from the University of Wisconsin, Madison.

Gengxin Miao is a first year PhD student in electrical and computer engineering at the University of California, Santa Barbara, where she has served as a teaching assistant and a graduate student researcher. She received BS and MS degrees from the Department of Automation at Tsinghua University in Beijing, China. Her research currently focuses on Web Services, data mining and machine learning.

Davor Mucic was born in former Yugoslavia in 1962, educated psychiatrist in Denmark, with special interest in treatment of asylum seekers, refugees and migrants. Davor Mucic established Psychiatric Centre Little Prince, the only place for refugees and migrants from ex-Yugoslavia, Eastern Europe, the Middle East and Africa where the therapists speak the same languages as the clients. The centre has been frontier in developing of telepsychiatry in Denmark since 2003. Davor Mucic is the member of AEP (Association of European Psychiatry),WACP (World Association of Cultural Psychiatry), Danish Psychiatric Society and The Danish Society for Clinical Telemedicine. More information can be found on www.denlilleprins.org

Shazia Yasin Mughal has the Master's of science degree in computerization and human machine interaction from the *University of Valenciennes*. While earning this degree, she developed strong interest in ergonomics, computerized system and human machine interaction. She works in collaboration with *Laboratory of Communication Sciences*. Her participation in cognitive designing, and computerized system validation has given her fair experience in the above areas along with quality system management. She has contributed in many articles published and presented by *WSEAS* and *IEEE.*

Hyduke Noshadi received a BS degree in computer science from the University of California, Los Angeles (UCLA) in 2006. He is currently working toward the MS degree in computer science. His research interest is in embedded system design and analysis. He is a student member of the IEEE.

Francisco J. Nóvoa was born in Ourense, Spain, in 1974. He received the BS in Computer Science from the University of Deusto (Bilbao, Spain) in 1998. His research interests include telemedicine, medical information systems, information integration, DICOM, PACS and information systems security. Since 1998 he is a member of the Medical Computing and Radiological Diagnosis Center (IMEDIR Center) of the University of A Coruña. He is a research assistant at the Information and Communications Technologies at University of A Coruña. In addition that, he is a Cisco certified networking associate, Cisco certified design associate and Cisco certified networking professional.

Bradley Olson, MD, MEd is an assistant professor of pediatrics at SUNY Upstate Medical University where he is the associate program director for Resident Education and Curriculum Development. He earned his medical degree from Saint Louis University Medical School and completed his residency training in pediatrics at the National Naval Medical Center in Bethesda, Maryland. He recently obtained his Master's Degree of education in instructional design, development and evaluation from Syracuse University and has worked extensively with the School of Education faculty from Syracuse University on the development of online curriculum for pediatric resident education.

Juan Luis Pérez Ordóñez was born in Rianxo, Spain, on November 1976. He received the MS in Computer Science from the University of A Coruña, Spain, in 2004. His research interests include artificial neural network, evolutionary computation, telemedicine, medical information systems, DICOM and information systems security. He is a research assistant at the Department of Information and Communications Technologies at University of A Coruña and Department of Construction Technology at the same University. He is author of some book chapters, journal papers and conference papers. Since 2002 he is a member of the Medical Computing and Radiological Diagnosis Center (IMEDIR Center) of the University of A Coruña, and is a member of the Integrating the Healthcare Enterprise (IHE) society at Spain.

Konstantinos Perakis was born in Athens, Greece in 1979. He received his diploma in electrical & computer engineering from the National Technical University of Athens in October 2003. He received his MBA diploma in "techno-economical systems" from the National Technical University of Athens in 2006. Since November 2003 he has been a member of the Biomedical Engineering Laboratory as a PhD candidate. Mr. Perakis has been active in a number of European and national R&D programs, through which he has gained considerable experience in the field of Telematics Applications in Healthcare. He speaks both English and Spanish fluently and his current research interests include telemedical applications, medical signal processing, computer networks and more. He is a member of the Institute of Electrical and Electronics Engineers.

Jesús Poza was born in Soria, Spain, in 1978. He received the engineer degree in telecommunication engineering from the University of Valladolid, Valladolid, Spain, in 2003. He is currently a Lecturer in the Department of Signal Theory and Communications at the University of Valladolid. His main research interest is biomedical signal processing using time and frequency analysis.

Nupur Prakash, PhD, is professor and dean at University School of Information Technology, Guru Gobind Singh Indraprastha University (GGSIPU), Delhi India. She holds a PhD in engineering and technology and she has worked as a scientist at Central Scientific Instruments Organisation (CSIO), Chandigarh on microprocessor based cross correlation flow meter. She has also worked at Punjab Engineering College, Chandigarh and was the head of the department, computer science and engineering. She has been the principal of Indira Gandhi Institute of Technology at GGSIPU, Delhi. Her research interests include wireless communications, mobile computing, network security and cryptography. She has authored/presented 40 research papers in various national & international journals and conferences.

Maria Andréia F. Rodrigues is a professor at University of Fortaleza (UNIFOR). She holds a PhD degree in computer science from Imperial College, University of London, U.K. (1999). Professor Andréia has co-organized the *15th Brazilian Symposium on Computer Graphics and Image Processing (SIBGRAPI)* in 2002. She has co-chaired the *SIBGRAPI'05*, and served as a PC member of the *22nd ACM Symposium on Applied Computing (SAC'07), Special Tracks on Handheld Computing* and *Computer Applications* *in Health Care*. Currently, she is serving as a PC member of the *SIBGRAPI'07* and *ICCCN'07*, as well as a tutorial chair of the *SAC'08*, to be held 16-20 March 2008 in Fortaleza-CE, Brazil. Her research interests are in interactive computer graphics, virtual reality, and mobile technology.

Keeroo Sandhya (a Mauritian National) is presently working on her MBA at University of Mauritius. She is a graduate in information technology. Her path-breaking research on medical informatics – a multidisciplinary field of paramount necessity, presents unrivalled challenges to enhance ostensibly unyielding problems across the domain. She is honored to author a handy and an informative resource which would catalyze further research as well as contributing towards the win-win paradigm shift pertinent to wellness and treating illness. She is firm that this chapter shall help in identifying elusive broken links those still exist and eradicate problems of heterogeneity in clinical knowledge and will go a long way in improving quality of life of the populace at global level. She has authored a few more articles on healthcare information technology.

Jose A. Sánchez is graduated in physics by the Universidad Complutense of Madrid (Spain). He works as associated professor at the Universidad Politécnica of Madrid (UPM), Spain. He has worked in different research and development areas including videoconferencing systems and applications, network management and, more recently in wireless sensor networks, his main PhD research topic. Also, he has been involved in research and development projects funded by the European Union as well as in other management duties at the UPM. Contact him at: jsanchez@diatel.upm.es

Majid Sarrafzadeh (http://www.cs.ucla.edu/~majid) received his BS, MS and PhD in 1982, 1984, and 1987 respectively from the University of Illinois at Urbana-Champaign in Electrical and Computer Engineering. He joined Northwestern University as an assistant professor in 1987. In 2000, he joined the Computer Science Department at University of California at Los Angeles (UCLA). Dr. Sarrafzadeh is a fellow of IEEE and received an NSF Engineering Initiation award, two distinguished paper awards in ICCAD, and the best paper award in DAC.

Gerald Schaefer gained his PhD in Computer Vision from the University of East Anglia. He worked at the Colour & Imaging Institute, University of Derby as a Research Associate (1997-1999) and as Senior Research Fellow at the School of Information Systems, University of East Anglia (2000-2001). He joined the School of Computing and Informatics at Nottingham Trent University as a Senior Lecturer in 2001 and has recently joined Aston University in Birmingham. His research interests include colour image analysis, physics-based vision, image retrieval, and image coding.

Jacob Scharcanski has a PhD in systems design engineering (University of Waterloo, 1993), a MSc degree in computer science (1984) and a B.Eng. in electrical engineering (1981), both from the Federal University of Rio Grande do Sul (Brazil). His main areas of interest are image processing, computer vision, and medical imaging applications. Currently, he is an associate professor at the Instituto de Informática, Universidade Federal do Rio Grande do Sul, Porto Alegre, Brazil 91501-970. He authored and co-authored more than 80 publications in Books, Journals and Conferences, 2 patents, and has led to innovations in medical image storage and management. Dr. Scharcanski is a member of SBC, IEEE and PEO, and he has acted as associate editor and guest editor for 3 international journals. E-mail: [dwelfer,jacobs]@inf.ufrgs.br.

Mary Schmeida, PhD is adjunct faculty at Kent State University, Department of Political Science, and also Senior Researcher at the Cleveland Clinic. Her research focuses on e-government and health policy including the diffusion of communications innovation of telehealth policy across the states, Medicare reform, and the role of interest groups in health policy reform. She has authored many articles on telehealth innovation in health policy.

José A. Seoane was born in Ferrol, Spain, in 1980. He graduated in computing technical engineering at the University of A Coruña (A Coruña, Spain) in 2004.He is scientific/technical personnel of the same university since his graduation. His work lines are focused on the processing of digital images, artificial neural networks, information systems and distributed object systems.

Ankur Seth (an Indian National) is a healthcare technologist with experience of working in research labs and hospitals in Europe. He was instrumental in developing telesurveilance software for Inserm-France and implementing cross border videoconferencing solutions in HFZ-Germany/Switzerland. He also has rich and versatile experience in architecting big technology solutions for several IT organizations like TCS, ProQuest, and Adobe Systems. Ankur holds a Bachelor of technology in electronics engineering from Institute of Technology, Banaras Hindu University-Varanasi and is also a life member of Indian Association of Medical Informatics."

Maria Sevdali studied at the Management & Economic School of the Highest Technological Educational Institute of Kalamatas, in the management of health units & provision of medical services department. She has received her Master's degree (Master in Management of Health Units) in the Hellenic Open University, at the school of Social Science. Her post-graduated thesis is in the field "Measurement of Health Levels Using the Evaluation Method SF36 – Comparative study of 2 Hospital Units. She teaches at the Management of Hospitals department of the Highest Technological Educational Institute of kalamatas. She is the author of a book and published scientific research works, in the field of health, in Greece and in the USA.

J.P. Shim is professor of management information systems at the Mississippi State University. He has been on the faculty of University of Wisconsin and has been invited to Harvard Business School. Dr. Shim's research interests are in the areas of multimedia development and applications, strategic information systems, and decision support systems. He is the co-author of several books and has published 40 journal articles. He has presented over 60 papers at national and international conferences. He has received several awards, grants, and distinctions. He is a frequent invited speaker at numerous universities, research institutes, and companies in the United States, France, Korea, Taiwan, and Japan. He serves as an editorial board member for numerous journals.

P. Michael Melliar-Smith is a professor in the Department of Electrical and Computer Engineering at the University of California, Santa Barbara. Previously, he worked as a research scientist, and served as a project leader for a number of research projects, at SRI in Menlo Park, California. His research interests encompass the fields of distributed systems and applications, and network architectures and protocols. He has published more than 250 conference and journal papers in computer science and engineering. Dr. Melliar-Smith is a pioneer in the field of fault-tolerant distributed computing. He received a PhD in computer science from the University of Cambridge, England.

Sanjay Prakash Sood, M.Tech., is the director, C-DAC School of Advanced Computing in Mauritius and specializes in telemedicine & ehealth. Sood has pioneered telemedicine projects in India, Benin and Mauritius. He has been a telemedicine consultant to World Health Organisation; consultant biomedical engineer for a World Bank Project in Punjab, India. He is also associated with the United Nations (UN Office for Outer Space Affairs, Vienna) for telemedicine. He has been the principal resource person (medical informatics) for a premier Indian Govt. organization (C-DAC) and was the investigator/co-ordinator of National Telemedicine Project (development of telemedicine technology) in India. He has authored forty publications & articles including five chapters on cutting edge applications of IT in healthcare, Sood has been a member of the executive council of International Society for Telemedicine and eHealth. Sood is an international (professional) volunteer. He is a recipient of international scholarships and travel grants. Sood is currently researching (PhD) on diffusion & adoption of telemedicine technologies in the developing world. He may be contacted via www.spsood.com

György Surján is a physician in background. After more than 10 years clinical practice he is working in the field of medical informatics since about 15 years. He worked as chief information offices at several health care institutions. Recently he is the head of Department of Informatics at National Institute for Strategic Health Research. His main research interest lies in medical classifications, coding systems, knowledge representation and biomedical ontologies. He is a member of a number of professional organizations, standardization committees and participant of several EU and national projects.

Zhilbert Tafa was born in Ulcinj, Montenegro, on July 1974. In 1997 he received the BSc degree in electrical engineering and in 2006 the MSc in computer science, from the University of Montenegro. Mr Tafa is one of the founders of the APEG (Applied Electronics Group), founded in 2004. He worked as university lecturer and high school professor on computer networking, informatics and mathematics. He has been working as the collaborator on university electrical engineering projects as well as the technical manager in T-Com Montenegro. His current research interests include hardware/software design on Mobile Health and Home Telecare applications, wireless networking and software engineering. With his publications mostly on remote monitoring of biomedical signals, he has been present in many international conferences.

Roger Tait received an honours degree in computer science in 2003. Working as a software engineer designing and implementing algorithms for the modelling of human organs, he completed a placement year with the Forschungs-zentrum Karlsruhe - Institut für Angewandte Informatik (IAI). Currently he is a PhD student at Nottingham Trent University where he is carrying out research into image processing and artificial intelligence for use in non-destructive evaluation. His research interests include image registration for industrial and biomedical applications.

Miguel A. Valero, PhD, is graduated in telecommunications engineering in 1995 at Universidad Politécnica of Madrid (UPM), Spain. His doctoral thesis, defended in 2001, dealt with interactive telemedicine services and was awarded at national scope in 2002. He worked from 2001 to 2003 as a senior researcher at Group of Bioengineering and Telemedicine at UPM and, since 2003 works as associated professor at the same University. He is co-author of two books, 9 book chapters, 9 journals and 44 conference papers focused on health telematics services and systems, including multimedia, digital home, and broadband mobile communications. Contact him at: mavalero@diatel.upm.es

Iraklis Varlamis is a post-doctoral researcher in the Computer Science Department of Athens University of Economics and Business. His research interests vary from data-mining and knowledge management to virtual communities and their applications. He has written and presented several articles in international conferences, concerning the design and implementation aspects of virtual communities. For more information visit: http://wim.aueb.gr/iraklis

Noha Veiguela was born in Vegadeo, Spain, in 1981. She graduated in computing science at the University of A Coruña (A Coruña, Spain) in 2006. She has a research fellowship in the Department of information and communications technologies, University of A Coruña (Spain) and she is currently working on medical image and digital image processing for decision support.

Maro Vlachopoulou is a professor at the Department of Applied Informatics, University of Macedonia, Greece. Her professional expertise, research and teaching interests include marketing information systems, electronic commerce, e-business, e-marketing, internet marketing, ERP, CRM (Customer Relationship Management) systems, e-supply chain management, e-logistics and healthcare information systems. She participates in several European-funded R&D programmes in the above fields. She is also a member of the editorial board and a reviewer for several scientific journals, including the *International Journal of Production Economics, European Journal of Operation Research, International Journal of Physical Distribution and Logistics Management, Journal of Enterprise Information Management and International Journal of Business Information Systems.*

Anton V. Vladzymyrskyy was born in Donetsk (Ukraine) on 25.04.1977. Graduated Donetsk State Medical University in 2000 and began work in R&D Institute of Traumatology and Orthopedics as a physician. Since 2002 he holds MS degree, since 2003 – MD in 2001 in Institute was founded first in Ukraine Department of Informatics and Telemedicine headed by dr.Vladzymyrskyy (teleconsultations, systematic researches, educational process were provided). By his initiative in 2003 was founded "Ukrainian Journal of Telemedicine and Medical Telematics" which now cited by Index Copernicus. Since 2006 dr.Vladzymyrskyy – president of Association for Ukrainian Telemedicine and eHealth Development (national member of International Society for Telemedicine and eHealth – ISfTeH).

Jelena Vucetic is a founder and owner of Alpha Mission, Inc., a business and technology consulting firm in the Washington, D.C. area, whose focus is primarily in the telecommunications and high-tech industry. Dr. Vucetic is also a founder of a high-tech company that provides products for the wireless telecommunications market. She has more than 20 years of industrial experience in telecommunications and computer systems, including engineering, business development, marketing, sales, operations and manufacturing. In addition, Dr. Vucetic has served as an expert witness/consultant, and an adjunct professor and advisor in management and technology programs at several international universities. She holds a PhD degree in electrical engineering, Master's in business administration, Master's in computer science, and a BS degree in electrical engineering. Dr. Vucetic is a published author of numerous articles and four international patents in the area of wireless telecommunications.

Daniel Welfer is currently working towards his PhD degree in computer science at the Instituto de Informática, Universidade Federal do Rio Grande do Sul. He has a MSc degree in production engineering – information technology (2005) from the Federal University of Santa Maria (Brazil) and a

BSc degree in computer science (2003) from the University Regional do Noroeste do Estado do Rio Grande do Sul (Brazil). His areas of interest are medical imaging standards, PACS for teleradiology, radiological and hospital information systems. He currently is supported by CNPq (Brazilian National Research Council).

Stelios Zimeras works as lecturer at the Department of Statistics and Actuarial-Financial Mathematics at the University of the Aegean in Greece. His research interests include probability, statistics, and image processing.

Index

L

M

N

O

P

Q

R

S

T

U

V

W

Z